TARGET JIPMER

2018 – 2017

(May 2018, Nov. 2017 and May 2017)

(Model Questions with Solved Explanatory Answers)

"Get the inside edge! Authored by Jipmerites"

Volume 4

Dr. T. ARUN BABU
MD Pediatrics (JIPMER), DAA (CMC, Vellore), MBA (HM)
Fellow in Neonatal Perinatal Medicine (Canada)
Associate Professor and Head, Department of Pediatrics
All India Institute of Medical Sciences (AIIMS)
Mangalagiri, Andhra Pradesh
Puducherry – 605009
Website: www.drarunbabu.in

Peepee Publishers and Distributors (P) Ltd.®

TARGET JIPMER (Volume 4)

Published by
Pawaninder P. Vij and Anupam Vij

Peepee Publishers and Distributors (P) Ltd.
Head Office: 160, Shakti Vihar, Pitam Pura, Delhi-110 034 (India)

Correspondence Address:
7/31, First Floor, Ansari Road, Daryaganj
New Delhi-110 002 (India)
Ph: 41512412, 23246245, 9811156083
e-mail: peepee160@yahoo.co.in
e-mail: peepee160@gmail.com
www.peepeepub.com
join us on facebook.com/pp.publishers

First Edition: 2020

ISBN: 978-81-8445-277-8

Dedication

To my Parents, Teachers,
my wife Dr. Sharmila,
my kids Akshaya and Akash

Disclaimer:

This book fully complies with the non-disclosure agreement (NDA) levied by JIPMER. This book contains Model questions with solved explanatory answers. No questions included in this book have been obtained from any candidates registered for JIPMER exam. Any resemblance to the original JIPMER questions, if present, is purely coincidental. The author, contributors, publisher or sellers cannot be held responsible for any damage or loss caused to anyone, directly or indirectly.

PREFACE

We are very happy in bringing out yet another supplement of TARGET JIPMER book. Big thanks for making TARGET JIPMER series the best book for JIPMER PGMEE preparation. This book series was started with the sole purpose of making model JIPMER questions accessible to PG aspirants. The questions have been solved by a team of subject experts from reputed academic backgrounds. This book is tailor made for JIPMER PG entrance exam preparation. Most of our contributors are JIPMER alumni and have personally written JIPMER PG exams in the last few years and are well experienced and aware of the examination pattern. JIPMER questions are mostly taken from standard textbooks and articles. Though the pattern of JIPMER questions have changed in the last few years, the high yield area remains the same. You will understand this after going through all the volumes of 4th edition of TARGET JIPMER.

We have incorporated a systematic approach in solving each and every question which can be appreciated while reading this book. The schematic diagrams, tables, illustrations, bulleted key points and references are the highlights of this book and will make reading and understanding of the material easier and effective. Every solved question will have a valid reference citing a standard textbook or article in order to increase the credibility of the answers. The focused explanations should help you solve questions from same topics in the future easily.

I would like to thank all the contributors for their commitment and hard work that has led to the tremendous success of this book series. I wish to thank our publishers, Mr. Pawaninder Paul Vij and Mr. Anupam Vij, the Directors of Peepee Publishers and Distributors (P) Ltd., who have always been a pillar of support to our team. I would also like to thank our publishing team for their relentless efforts in releasing this book in a short notice. I am deeply indebted to students for their overwhelming support, feedback and critical appraisal. We are looking forward to hear your feedback and are fully committed in bringing out better editions in the future. For JIPMER students, a JIPMERITE tag is a matter of pride which they carry as a badge of honour throughout their professional life. For most others it is a dream. I believe and hope that this book will make your dream come true.

All the best!

T. Arun Babu

Website: *www.drarunbabu.in*

Email: *babuarun.t@gmail.com*

"Books are infinite in number and time is short. The secret of knowledge is to take what is essential."

–Swami Vivekananda

CONTRIBUTORS

Dr. T. Arun Babu, MD Pediatrics (JIPMER), DAA (CMC)
Fellow NPM (Canada)
Associate Professor and Head, Department of Pediatrics
All India Institute of Medical Sciences (AIIMS)
Mangalagiri, Andhra Pradesh
Puducherry – 605009
(Chief Editor)

Dr. Arul Varman, MD Psychiatry (JIPMER)
Assistant Professor, Department of Psychiatry
Indira Gandhi Medical College and Research Institute (IGMC&RI)
Puducherry – 605009
(Psychiatry)

Dr. Bharath Kumar V D, MD Pharmacology
Assistant Professor, Department of Pharmacology
BGS Global Institute of Medical Sciences
Bangalore, Karnataka
Dr. Bharath's Pharmacology MCQs and Discussion for PG Aspirants
(Pharmacology)

Dr. Dilip Kumar R, MD (JIPMER), MRCP (UK)
Consultant and Head, Department of Internal Medicine
Dr. Mehta's Hospitals, Chetpet, Chennai – 31
(Medicine)

Dr. Dinesh Kumar, MD Pediatrics
Assistant Professor, Department of Pediatrics
Indira Gandhi Medical College and Research Institute (IGMC&RI)
Puducherry – 605009
(Pediatrics)

Dr. Karthikeyan Pethusamy
Senior Resident and PhD Scholar, Department of Biochemistry
All India Institute of Medical Sciences (AIIMS)
New Delhi
(Biochemistry)

Dr. Krishna Kumar S, MD Physiology (AIIMS)
Assistant Professor, Department of Physiology
SRM Medical College Trichy Campus
Trichy – 621105
(Physiology)

Dr. Mohd Khaleel Ahmed, MD Radiology
NEET-PG Radiology National Faculty
(Radiology)

Dr. Mugunthan N, MS Anatomy, DNB, PhD, MBA
Professor of Anatomy
Sree Mookambika Institute of Medical Sciences
Kulasekaram, Kanyakumari District,Tamil Nadu – 629161
(Anatomy)

Dr. Mukul Mohindra, MS (Ortho), DNB, MNAMS,
Dip. SICOT (Belgium)
Fellow National Board (Arthroscopy and Sports Medicine)
Sports Injury Center, Safdarjung Hospital and VMM College
New Delhi
(Orthopaedics)

Dr. D. Pradeep, MS Gen Surg, MRCS (Edin)
Assistant Professor, Department of General Surgery
Shri Sathya Sai Medical College and Research Institute
Kancheepuram District, Tamil Nadu – 603108
(Surgery)

Dr. Prasanna S, MD Microbiology (AFMC, Pune)
Assistant Professor, Department of Microbiology
Shri Sathya Sai Medical College and Research Institute
Kancheepuram, Tamil Nadu – 603108
(Microbiology)

Dr. Rajamahendran, MS, MCh Gastro
Assistant Professor, Department of Surgical Gastroenterology
Government Villupuram Medical College
Villupuram – 605602
(Surgery)

Dr. Ranjith AR, MD Pathology (JIPMER)
Molecular Pathologist, Bangalore
(Pathology)

Dr. Sangeeta Dhanger, DA, DNB, MNAMS
Assistant Professor, Department of Anesthesiology
Indira Gandhi Medical College and Research Institute (IGMC&RI)
Puducherry – 605009
(Anesthesiology)

Dr. Satvinder Singh Bakshi, MS ENT (JIPMER), DNB
Associate Professor, Department of Otorhinolaryngology
Mahatma Gandhi Medical College and Research Institute (MGMC&RI), Pillaiyarkuppam,
Puducherry – 607 402
(ENT)

Dr. Sharmila Arun Babu, MS OBG (JIPMER)
Assistant Professor, Department of OBG
Indira Gandhi Medical College and Research Institute (IGMC&RI)
Puducherry – 605009
(OBG)

Dr. Sindhujha Sekar G (JIPMER), DGO, DNB OG
Department of Obstetrics and Gynecology
Rajiv Gandhi Government Women and Children's Hospital
Puducherry
(OBG)

Dr. Yogesh Bahurupi, MD PSM
Assistant Professor, Department of Preventive and Social Medicine
Indira Gandhi Medical College and Research Institute (IGMC&RI)
Puducherry – 605009
(PSM)

Dr. Suthanthira Kannan, MD Community Medicine
Senior Resident, Department of Community Medicine
Government Medical College, Manjeri, Kerala
(Community Medicine/PSM)

Dr. Udayashankar C, MD Dermatology (JIPMER), MBA (HM)
Professor and Head, Department of Dermatology
Indira Gandhi Medical College and Research Institute (IGMC&RI)
Puducherry – 605 009
(Dermatology)

Dr. Usha S Adiga, MBBS MD PhD
Professor, Department of Biochemistry
KS Hegde Medical Academy
Mangalore, Karnataka
(Biochemistry)

Dr. Venipriya, MS Ophthalmology
Senior Resident, Department of Ophthalmology
Indira Gandhi Medical College and Research Institute (IGMC&RI)
Puducherry – 605 009
(Ophthalmology)

Dr. Vinoth Kumar S, MD General Medicine
Assistant Professor, Department of General Medicine
Indira Gandhi Medical College and Research Institute (IGMC&RI)
Puducherry – 605 009
(General Medicine)

Dr. Yatiraj Singi, MD Forensic Medicine
Professor, Department of Forensic Medicine
Sree Mookambika Institute of Medical Sciences
Kulasekharam, District Kanya Kumari, Tamil Nadu
(Forensic Medicine)

ACKNOWLEDGEMENTS

Target JIPMER – Previous Edition Contributors

Dr. Balamurugan N, DCH, DNB, MRCPCH, Assistant Profesor, Department of Pediatrics, SLIMS, Puducherry.
Dr.Tejswita Rajpal Hande, MBBS, DGO, MUHS, Nashik.
Dr. Saranya K, MD Physio (JIPMER), Assistant Professor of Physiology, JIPMER, Puducherry.
Dr. Abarna Devi S, DDVL (JIPMER), MD Medicine, Assistant Professor of Medicine, ESIMC, Chennai.
Dr. Anshu Bahl, MD Anatomy (AIIMS), New Delhi.
Dr. Ankit Agarwal, MD RT (JIPMER), Senior Resident, GMCH, Chandigarh, Sector 32.
Dr. Dinesh Kumar, MD Pediatrics, Assistant Professor of Pediatrics, IGMC&RI, Puducherry.
Dr. Naga Dharshan Devendra, MD (JIPMER), Associate Professor and Course Director, Department of Biochemistry and Genetics, Trinity School of Medicine, Saint Vincent and Grenadines.
Dr. Saseendar S, MS (Ortho), DNB, Dip SICOT (Belgium), MNAMS, Care Sports Injury, Chennai.
Dr. Srirangaraj S, MD, Associate Professor, Department of Microbiology, MGMC&RI, Puducherry.
Dr. Sri Vengadesh Gopal, MS (JIPMER), Assistant Professor, Department of Surgery, IGMC&RI, Puducherry.
Dr. Sumanth MM, MD (JIPMER), DNB, Assistant Professor of Community Medicine, MMC&RI, Mysore, Karnataka.
Dr. Sentitoshi, (JIPMER) MD Forensic Medicine, Former Assistant Professor, MGMC&RI, Puducherry.
Dr. Asayas Bosco Chandrakumar, MS, Assistant Professor of Surgery, SLIMS, Puducherry.
Dr. Mahesh Nagappa, MD Anaes (JIPMER), DNB, MNAMS, Assistant Professor, SLIMS, Puducherry.
Dr. Sinhasan SP, MD, Associate Professor of Pathology, IGMC&RI, Puducherry.
Dr. Amiya Kumar Nath, MD (JIPMER), Assistant Professor of Dermatology, IGMC&RI, Puducherry.
Dr. Venkateswaran R, MD, Assistant Professor of Medicine, JIPMER, Puducherry.
Dr. Niranjan G, MD Biochem (JIPMER), Associate Professor of Biochemistry, AIIMS, Vijayawada.
Dr. VishnuKanth, MD (JIPMER), Assistant Professor, Department of Respiratory Medicine, JIPMER, Puducherry.
Dr. Dilli Kumar, MD (JIPMER), Associate Professor of Pediatrics, JIPMER, Puducherry.
Dr. Dilip Kumar R, MD (JIPMER), MRCP (UK), Dr. Mehta's Hospitals, Chetpet, Chennai 31.
Dr. Sachidananda Adiga, MD, Professor of Pharmacology, KS Hegde Medical Academy, Mangalore.
Dr. Usha Adiga, MD, Assistant Professor of Biochemistry, IGMC&RI, Puducherry.
Dr. Giriyanna Gowda, MD, Assistant Professor of Community Medicine, KIMS, Bangalore, Karnataka.
Dr. Gomathi Shankar V, MS (JIPMER), DNB, MNAMS, Assistant Professor of Surgery, JIPMER, Puducherry.
Dr. Karthik, MD Physiology (JIPMER), Assistant Professor of Physiology, JIPMER, Puducherry.
Dr. Lourdu Jafrin, MD, Associate Professor of Pharmacology, IGMC&RI, Puducherry.
Dr. Mahalakshmy T, MD PSM (JIPMER), Assistant Professor of PSM, JIPMER, Puducherry.
Dr. Melvin George, MD, DM Clin Pharm (JIPMER), Assistant Professor, Cardiac Clinical Trials and Research, Department of Cardiology, SRM Medical College and Hospital, Potheri, Tamil Nadu.
Dr. Naveen Nair, MS Orthopedics (JIPMER), Associate Professor of Orthopedics, IGMC&RI, Puducherry.
Dr. Noyal Mariya Joseph, MD (JIPMER), Assistant Professor of Microbiology, JIPMER, Puducherry.
Dr. Raveendranath, MS Anatomy (St Johns), Assistant Professor of Anatomy, JIPMER, Puducherry.
Dr. Rupa Vani, DNB, Assistant Professor of Obstetrics and Gynecology, IGMC&RI, Puducherry.
Dr. Sindhujha Sekar G, MBBS, DGO (JIPMER), Assistant Surgeon, Puduchatram PHC, Cuddalore, TN.

Sincere Thanks to:
Dr. Zubaida Begum A, MBBS (MGMC&RI), Junior Resident in Pediatrics, IGMC&RI, Puducherry.
Dr. Piyush Singh, MBBS, BMCH, Chitradurga, Karnataka.
Dr. Ezhil Kugan, MBBS, IGMC&RI, Puducherry.
Dr. Raghu Ram, MBBS (IGMC&RI), MD Radiology (Stud), PGI, Chandigarh.
Dr. Pradeep Ravi, MBBS, IGMC&RI, Puducherry.
Dr. Dana Lakshmi, MBBS, IGMC&RI, Puducherry.
Dr. Bindu Monika, MBBS, IGMC&RI, Puducherry.
Dr. Vignesh Raja, MBBS, IGMC&RI, Puducherry.
Dr. Priyadharshini A, MBBS (SVMC&RI), Junior Resident in Pediatrics, IGMC&RI, Puducherry.
Dr. Ramachandran M, MBBS, IGMC&RI, Puducherry.
Dr. Jayaram Saibaba, MBBS, Intern, IGMC&RI, Puducherry.
Dr. Ashok E, MBBS DCH, Salem, Tamil Nadu.
Dr. Anandhasayanan Sriramalu, MBBS, Tirukkoyilur, Tamil Nadu.

Dr. Balamurugan, MBBS, IGMC&RI, Puducherry.
Dr. Nandini Varman, MBBS (MGMC&RI), Junior Resident in Pediatrics, IGMC&RI, Puducherry.
Dr. Jeevitha, MBBS (IGMC&RI), Junior Resident in Pediatrics, IGMC&RI, Puducherry.
Dr. Vignesh Loganathan, MBBS (IGMC&RI), MD PSM (Stud), AIIMS, New Delhi.
Dr. Vijayadevagaran, MBBS, Senior Resident, Department of Pediatrics, IGMC&RI, Puducherry.
Dr. Narayanan, MBBS, MS Anatomy, JIPMER, Puducherry.
Dr. Sandhiya Selvarajan, MD, DM, Senior Resident, Clinical Pharmacology, JIPMER, Puducherry.
Dr. Jude Antonio Raja, MBBS, Senior Resident, Department of Pediatrics, IGMC&RI, Puducherry.
Dr. Priyadarshini, MBBS, Senior Resident, Department of Obs and Gyne, IGMC&RI, Puducherry.
Dr. Vishwas K Vijayadev, MS, DOHNS (Eng.), Commonwealth Fellow–Facial Plastic Surgery, UK.
Dr. Nilesh Rao, MD (JIPMER), Fellow in Neonatology, Vancouver, Canada.
Dr. Anil Kumar, MD (JIPMER), Asscociate Professor of Pediatrics, BMC, Bengaluru, Karnataka.
Dr. Manish Kumar, MD (JIPMER), Resident in Pediatric Neurology, USA.
Dr. Renitha, MD (JIPMER), Resident in Pediatric Neurology, USA.
Dr. Yasser Soliman, Transport Fellow, Neonatal Perinatal Medicine, Sick Kids, Toronto, Canada.
Dr. Arul Parithi, MD (ICH, Chennai), Assistant Professor of Pediatrics, KVMC, Tamil Nadu.
Dr. Shanthi AK, MD, PhD, HOD, Department of Pediatrics, IGMC&RI, Puducherry.
Dr. Tiroumourugane Serane, MD (JIPMER), DNB, MRCPCH, AG Padmavathy Hospital, Puducherry.
Dr. Rajkumar, MS (JIPMER), Assistant Professor of Surgery, JIPMER, Puducherry.
Dr. Pratap Kumar Patra, MD Pediatrics, Assistant Professor, Department of Pediatrics, AIIMS, Patna.
Dr. Barathy C, MBBS (JIPMER), DCH, DNB Pediatrics, Assistant Professor of Pediatrics, IGMC&RI, Puducherry.
Dr. Sharath, MD Physiology (JIPMER), Puducherry.
Dr. Malathi, MD Dermatology (JIPMER), Assistant Professor, Department of Skin and STD, JIPMER, Puducherry.
Dr. Swetha, MBBS, SLIMS, Puducherry.
Dr. Kumaran, MBBS (JIPMER), Puducherry.
Dr. Sathish, MBBS (JIPMER), Puducherry.
Dr. Balachandar, DNB Ped, IGGHPGI, Puducherry.
Dr. Johnson Reddy, DNB Ped, IGGHPGI, Puducherry.
Dr. Joseph, MBBS (JIPMER), Puducherry.
Dr. Kavitha, MBBS (JIPMER), Puducherry.
Dr. Arun Kumar, MBBS (JIPMER), Puducherry.
Dr. Maheswari, MBBS (JIPMER), Puducherry.
Dr. Sunil, MBBS (JIPMER), Puducherry.
Dr. Mugunthan, MD Micro (Stud), AFMC, Pune.
Dr. Madhumitha, MBBS, SVMCH, Puducherry.
Dr. Suvetha, Intern, MGMC&RI, Puducherry.
Mr. Thirunavukkarasu D, Government School English Lecturer (Retd), Puducherry.
Mrs. Sampurnam, Principal (Retd), SSVHSS, Puducherry.
Mr. Vijayan D, Cash Officer (Retd), SBI, Puducherry.
Mrs. Sagoundala, Under Secretary (Retd), Government of Puducherry.
Mr. Srinivasan Babu, PWD, Puducherry.
Mr. Dhinesh Shankar, EC Software, Chennai.
Mr. Rajkumar, System Engineer, Apple, CA, USA.
Mr. Armin Nuhanovic, Calgary, Alberta.
Mr. Chezhian, Glori Offset Printers, Puducherry.

and

Dr. Govindaraj, MD, Director, IGMC&RI, Puducherry.
Dr. Shanthi AK, MD, PhD, HOD, Department of Pediatrics, IGMC&RI, Puducherry.

Write to Us

Any observations, suggestions, criticisms are welcome. Write to the author at babuarun.t@gmail.com

Errata

Please visit *www.drarunbabu.in & www.peepeepub.com*

Follow Author in Facebook: *www.facebook.com/targetjipmerl* **and Dr. Arun Babu's Pediatrics Discussion group (TARGET Pediatrics by Dr. Arun Babu)**

CONTENTS

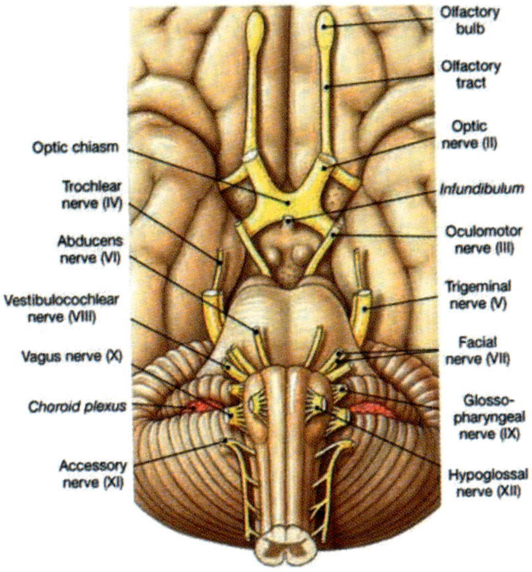

Page 174

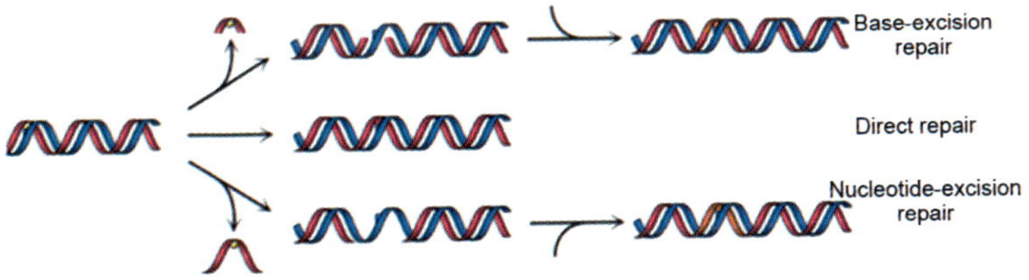

Page 188

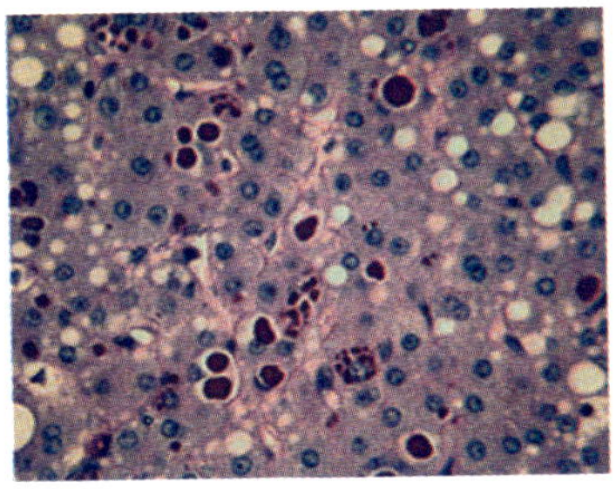

Fig: PAS positive globules in liver
Page 215

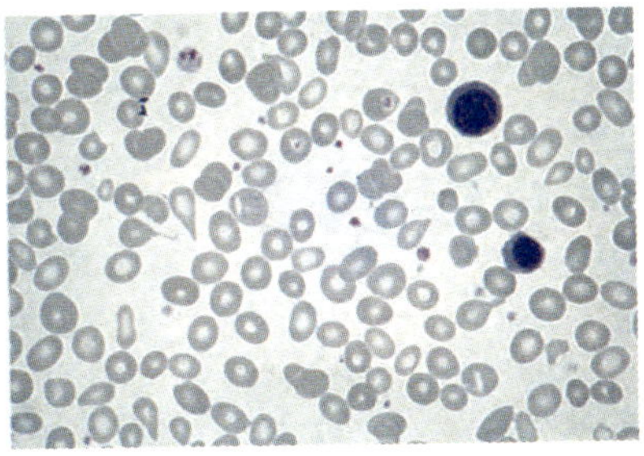

Page 215

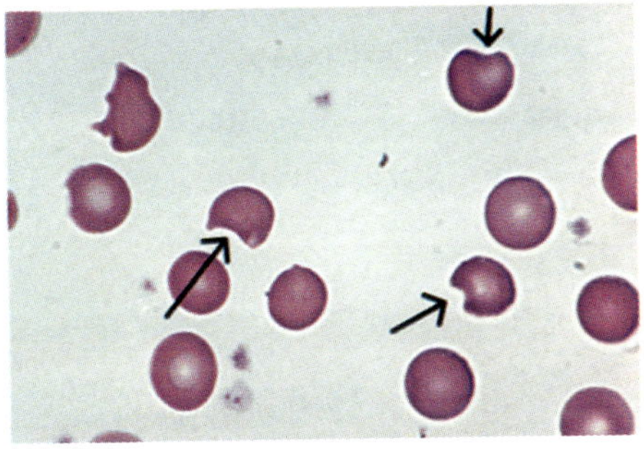

Page 216

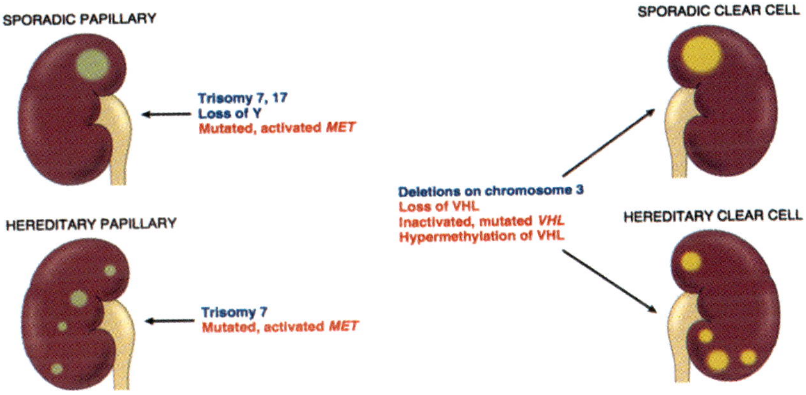

Page 218

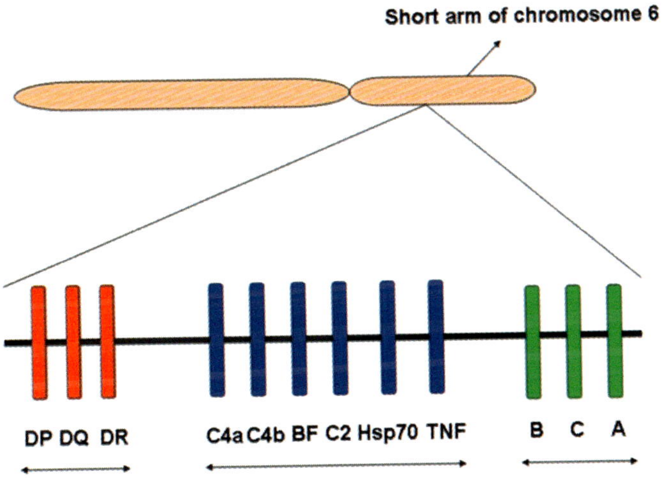

Page 232

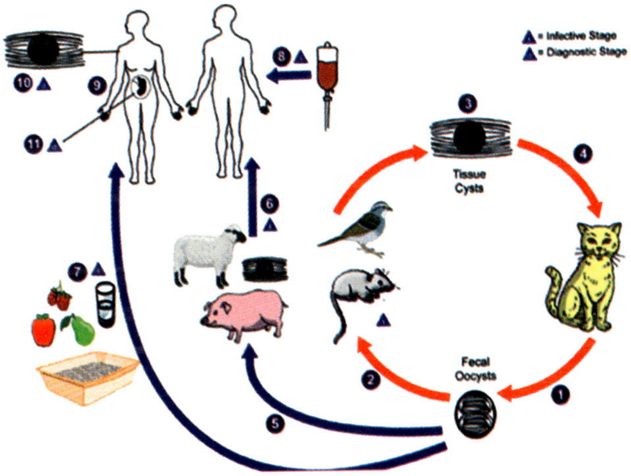

Page 239

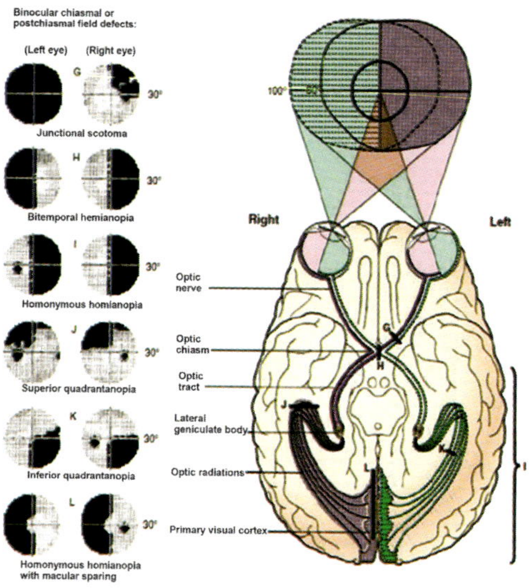

Page 264

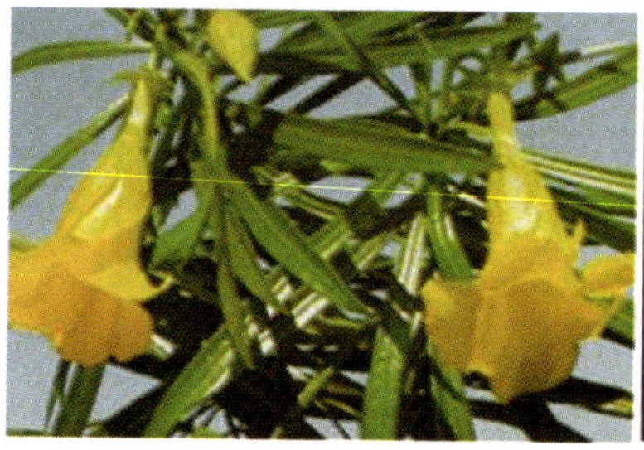

Page 243

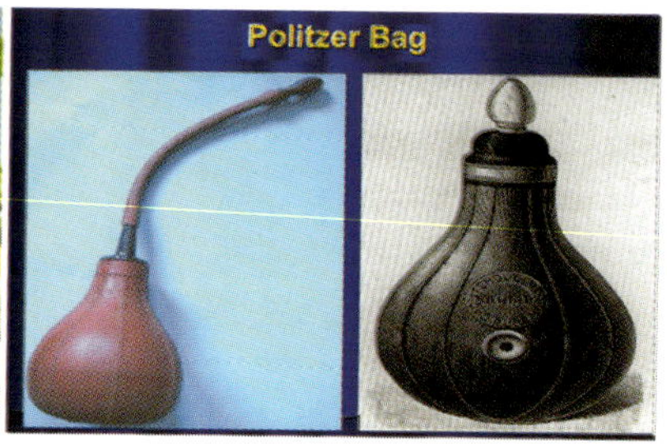

Page 255

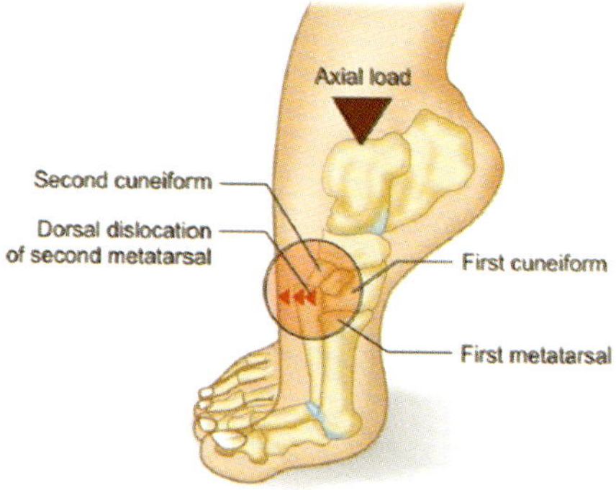

Fig.: Forced hyperflexion injury causing Lisfranc dislocation
Page 305

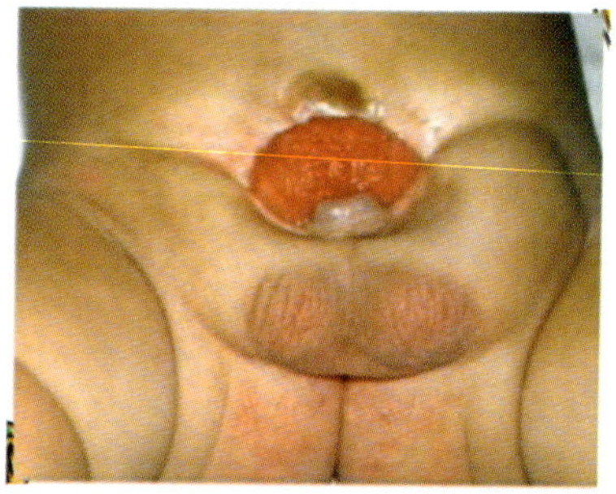

Page 286

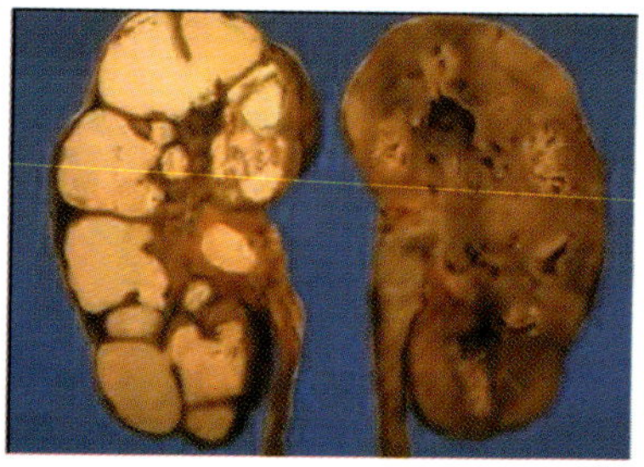

Page 287

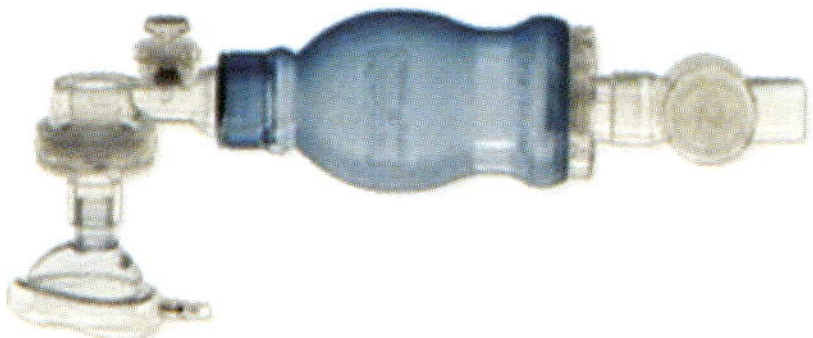

Page 321

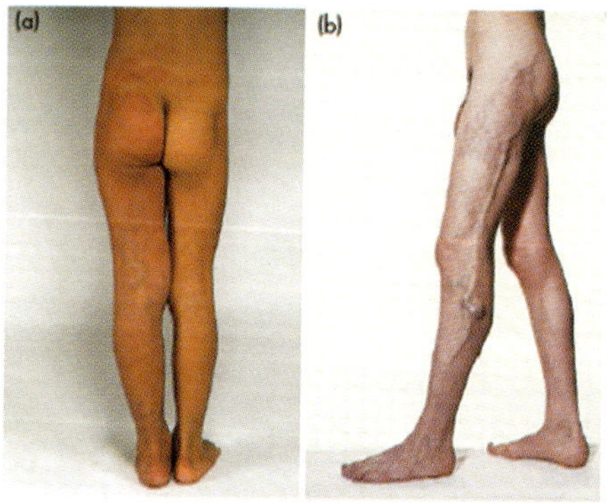

Page 290

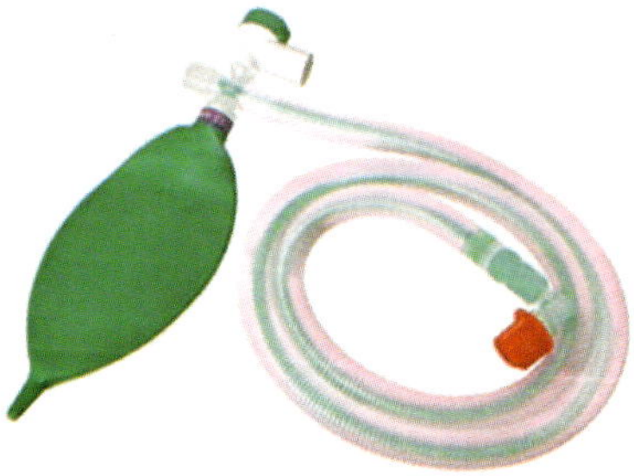

Page 321

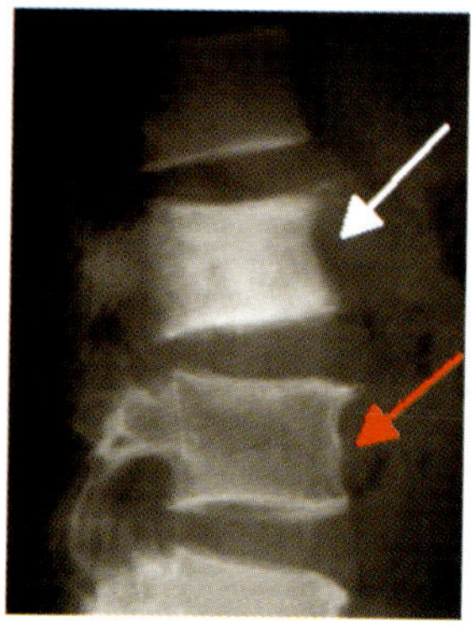

Page 340

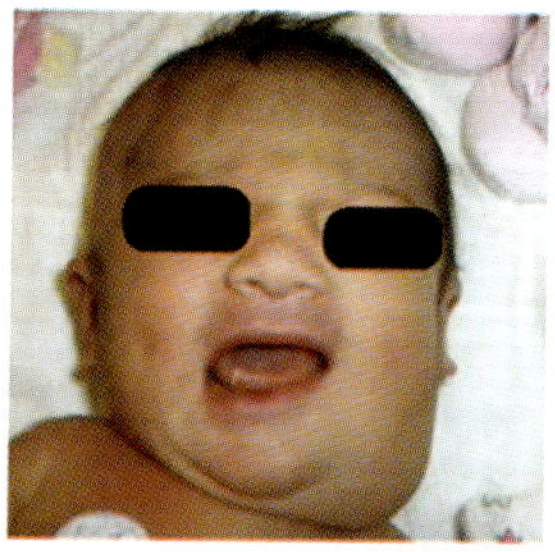

Page 292

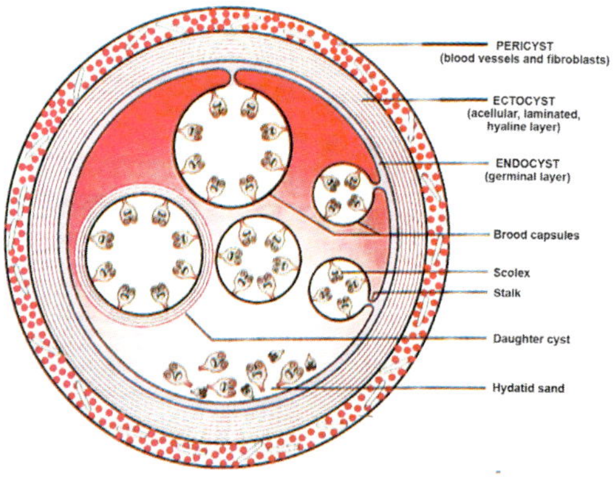

Page 344

JIPMER–MAY 2018

ANATOMY

1. **Gemelli muscles are present in:**

(a) Hip (b) Knee
(c) Elbow (d) Shoulder

Explanation:

Gemelli Muscles

- ***Two** in number*
  - ***Gemellus inferior and gemellus superior***
- *They are **short lateral rotators of hip joint***

	Origin	Insertion	Relation to tendon of obturator internus	Blood supply	Nerve supply	Actions
Gemellus superior	Dorsal surface of ischial spine	Medial surface of greater trochanter	*Above* the tendon of obturator internus	**Internal Pudendal artery**, inferior gluteal artery and sometimes by superior gluteal artery	Nerve to **obturator Internus***	**Rotate** the **extended thigh laterally** and **abduct** the **Flexed thigh**
Gemellus inferior	Upper part of the Lateral surface of the ischial tuberosity	Medial surface of greater trochanter	*Below* the tendon of obturator internus	**Medial circumflex femoral artery**	Nerve to **Quadratus femoris***	**Rotate** the extended **thigh laterally** and **abduct** the **Flexed thigh**

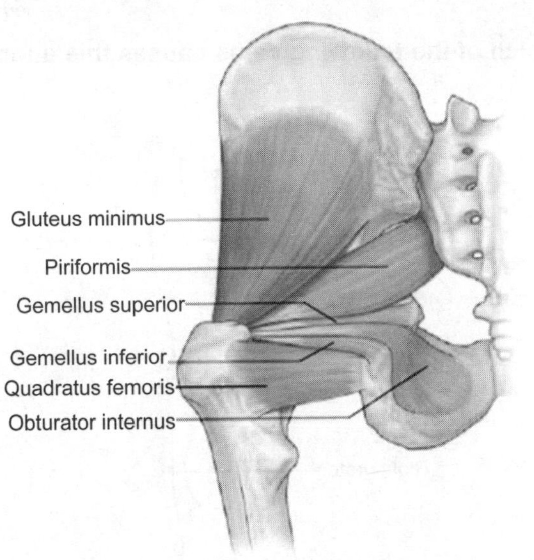

Fig.: Muscles of Hip

Ans: (a) Hip

Ref: Gray's Anatomy, The Anatomical Basis of Clinical Practice, Susan Standring, 41st edition, 2016, Page 1361

2. In peritonsillar abscess, pain is referred to ear due to:

(a) Trigeminal nerve
(b) Glossopharyngeal nerve
(c) Mandibular nerve
(d) Auriculotemporal nerve

Explanation:

- Tonsils and tonsillar fossa are supplied by the ***glossopharyngeal nerve*****.
- The **tympanic branch of the glossopharyngeal (Jacobson's) nerve*** supplies the mucous membrane lining the **tympanic cavity**.
- Infection, malignancy and postoperative inflammation of the tonsil and tonsillar fossa may therefore be accompanied by pain referred to the ear.

Structures related to the tonsillar fossa/tonsillar bed

- ***Muscles*** - Superior constrictor, sometimes by the anterior fibres of palatopharyngeus and styloglossus.
- ***Arteries*** - Tonsillar artery branch of the facial artery, ascending palatine artery and occasionally facial artery.
- ***Veins*** - Paratonsillar vein and venae comitantes accompanying tonsillar artery.
- ***Nerve*** - Glossopharyngeal nerve.
  - o The **internal carotid artery** lies approximately **25 mm** behind and **lateral** to the **tonsil**.
  - o In some individuals, the styloid process may be elongated and deviate towards the tonsillar bed.
  - o The glossopharyngeal nerve lies immediately lateral to the muscular wall of the tonsillar fossa and is commonly temporarily affected by oedema following tonsillectomy.

Points to Remember:

- Because of the nature of the ear's sensory innervations, a wide variety of disorders can produce referred otalgia.
- The ear receives an extensive sensory innervation via **four cranial nerves** (**Trigeminal, Facial, Glossopharyngeal and Vagus**) and **two spinal segments (C2 and C3)**.
- The other causes of referred otalgia (most common causes) are:
  - o **Temporomandibular** joint syndrome
  - o Pharyngitis
  - o Dental disease
  - o Cervical spine arthritis

Ans: (b) Glossopharyngeal nerve

Ref: Gray's Anatomy, The Anatomical Basis of Clinical Practice, Susan Standring, 41st edition, 2016, Page 576 & 577

3. Complete regression of which of the following veins causes this anomaly in the development of IVC (Figure).

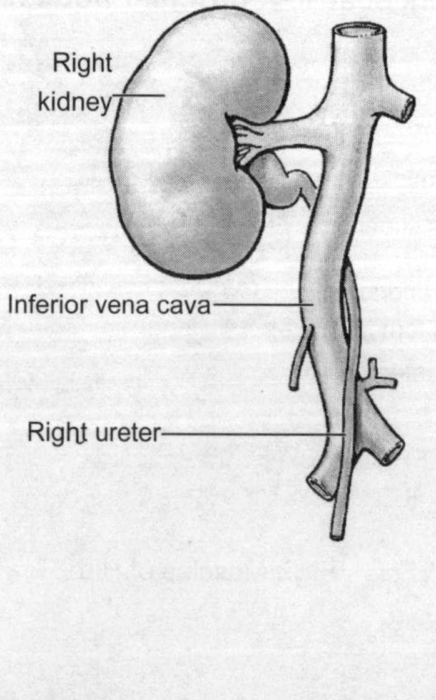

(a) Right vitelline vein
(b) Left vitelline vein
(c) Right supra-cardinal vein
(d) Left supra-cardinal vein

Explanation:

- The anomaly shown in picture is **Retrocaval ureter** (right ureter) passes at first behind the IVC, and then appears in front of it after winding the medial margin of IVC.
- **Retrocaval ureter** occurs when the **post-renal segment** of the **IVC** is developed from the **right posterior cardinal vein** and the **right supra-cardinal vein** regress **entirely**.

Development of IVC

IVC developed from the following sources from below upwards

1. Persistent caudal part of the ***right posterior cardinal vein***
2. ***Right supra-cardinal vein*** (this part receives 3rd and 4th pairs of lumbar veins)
3. ***Anastomosis*** between ***right supra-cardinal and right sub-cardinal veins*** (this part receives the right gonadal vein).
4. Upper part of the ***right sub-cardinal vein*** (this part receives both renal veins and right supra-renal vein).
5. A ***new vessel*** grows dorsal to the liver and **communicates the right sub-cardinal vein with the common *hepatic vein*** (intrahepatic part of IVC).
6. ***Common hepatic vein***–which is developed from the ***suprahepatic part of the right vitelline vein*** (terminal part of IVC).

Anomalies of IVC

1. ***Double IVC*** – IVC persist on both sides below the level of renal veins. This occurs when the **left common iliac vein** fails to develop and the **infra-renal segment** of the **left supra-cardinal vein fails** to **regress**.
2. ***Retro-caval ureter*** (as explained earlier).

Ans: (c) Right supra-cardinal vein

Ref: *Essentials of Human Embryology, A.K.Datta, 5th edition, 2005, Page 205-208*

4. **Tendon of Todaro connects:**

(a) Coronary sinus to tricuspid valve annulus
(b) Ridge of muscle connecting IVC and SVC
(c) Valve in opening of IVC
(d) Raised interatrial ridge

Explanation:

- The **valve of coronary sinus** (**Thebesian valve**) is connected to the central fibrous body (where the tricuspid valve annulus is attached) by tendon **of Todaro.**
- Tendon of Todaro is a palpable, round, collagenous bundle present beneath the endocardium (subendocardial).
- ***Triangle of Koch:*** **Boundaries**:
  - ***Inferiorly*** - septal cusp of the tricuspid valve.
  - ***Basally*** - anteromedial margin of ostium of the coronary sinus.
  - ***Superiorly*** - tendon of Todaro.
- Triangle of Koch is the landmark of **atrioventricular node** and its **atrial connections**.

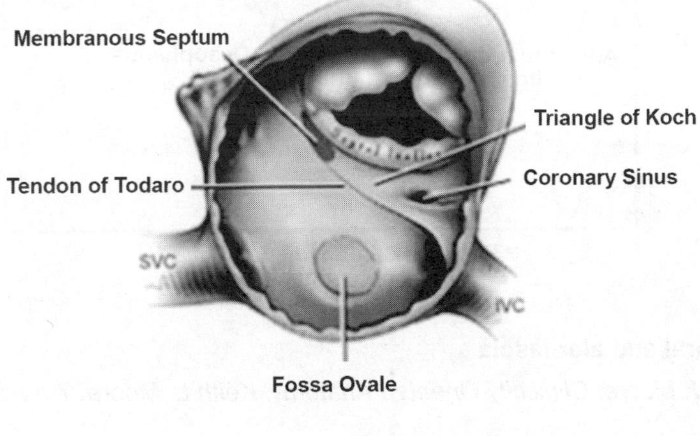

Ans: (a) Coronary sinus to tricuspid valve annulus

***Ref**: Gray's Anatomy, The Anatomical Basis of Clinical Practice, Susan Standring, 41st edition, 2016, Page 1000 &1001*

5. Danger space of neck is situated between:

(a) Buccopharyngeal and prevertebral fascia
(b) Pharyngobasilar and prevertebral fascia
(c) Buccopharyngeal and pharyngobasilar fascia
(d) Prevertebral and alar fascia

Explanation:

Danger space of neck or retropharyngeal space:

- Lies between the **prevertebral layer** (of deep cervical fascia) and the **alar fascia***.
- It is a potential space/dead space consists of loose connective tissue and permits movement of the pharynx, esophagus, larynx and trachea relative to the vertebral column during swallowing.
- This space is closed superiorly by the cranial base and on each side by the carotid sheath. It opens inferiorly into the superior mediastinum.
- **Alar fascia** is nothing but **anterior layer of prevertebral fascia**. Below the prevertebral fascia splits into **anterior (alar fascia) and posterior layer**. Alar fascia blends with the **buccopharyngeal fascia** and posterior layer enters the thorax and blends with **anterior longitudinal ligament**.
- **Buccopharyngeal fascia** is the fascia (areolar coat) covering the constrictor muscles of pharynx.
- **Pharyngobasilar fascia** is the thickened submucous layer of pharynx also called pharyngeal aponeurosis.
- **Retropharyngeal space** also called as **danger space of neck**, because pus may be collected in this space (retropharyngeal abscess) due to acute pyogenic infection may extend to mediastinum of thorax and behind the carotid sheath (appear at the posterior border of sternocleidomastoid).

Note: There is **no space** between **alar fascia and buccopharyngeal fascia**, since the alar fascia blends with **buccopharyngeal fascia**.

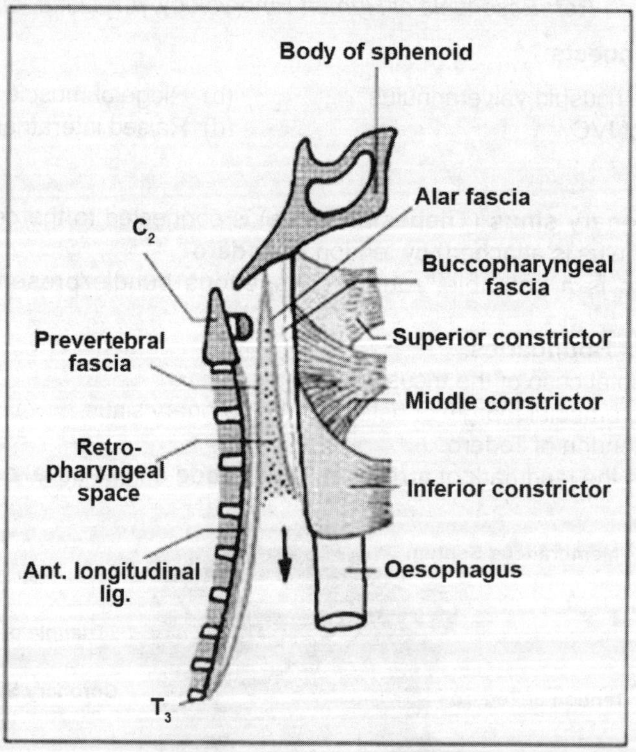

Fig.: Mid-sagittal disposition of Retropharyngeal space

Ans: (d) Prevertebral and alar fascia

***Ref**: Moore, Clinically Oriented Anatomy, Keith L. Moore, 7th edition, 2014, Page 988 & 989*

6. **All the following are true about Chiari network in the heart *except*:**

(a) It is due to incomplete resorption of the left valve of sinus venosus
(b) It originates from the Eustachian valve and connects to the coronary sinus
(c) It is nothing but fenestrated Eustachian valve
(d) It is a network in the Eustachian valve

Explanation:

- Chiari's network – often noticed as ***fenestrated membranous structure*** or ***reticular network like structure*** in the ***valve of inferior vena cava (Eustachian valve) and coronary sinus.***
- It originates from the ***Eustachian valve and connects to*** the different parts of the ***right atrium***, including the ***coronary sinus.***
- It results from ***incomplete resorption of the right valve of sinus venosus*.***
- Often clinically insignificant.
- Chiari's network has been associated with the pathogenesis of thromboembolic disease, endocarditis, arrhythmias, cardiac flow obstructions, heart murmurs, infective endocarditis, cardiac tumours and entrapment of catheters on percutaneous intervention.

Ans: (a) It is due to incomplete resorption of the left valve of sinus venosus

Ref: *Gray's Anatomy, The Anatomical Basis of Clinical Practice, Susan Standring, 41st edition, 2016, Page 1001*

7. **A schematic of interior part of right atrium is shown. The marked area (Fossa ovalis) develops from:**

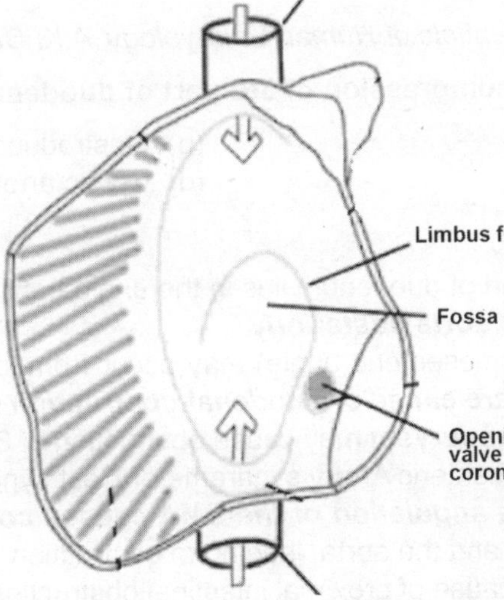

(a) Septum primum
(b) Septum secundum
(c) Septum intermedium
(d) Ostium primum

Explanation:

- The **septum primum** forms the floor of ***fossa ovalis*** (septum primum grows from the roof and dorsal wall of primitive atrium in mid sagittal plane and grows downwards to meet with the septum intermedium).
- The cephalic free edge of septum primum persist as a semilunar fold on the left side of inter atrial septum.
- Septum secundum converts the foramen secundum into a valvular foramen ovale (septum secundum grows on the right side of the septum primum from the intersepto valvular space of right atrium).
- The caudal free edge of septum secundum persist as the ***limbus fossa ovalis.***
- **Foramen ovale** is the gap between the lower margin of the septum secundum on right side and the upper margin of the septum primum on the left side.
- **Septum intermedium** formed by the fusion of ***dorsal and ventral endocardial cushions of the atrioventricular canal***. It divides the atrioventricular canal into right and left atrioventricular orifices.
- **Ostium primum** – appears between the septum primum and septum intermedium.

- **Ostium secundum** – appears in the dorsocephalic part of septum primum following the closure of ostium primum in the 7th week of intrauterine life.

Normal Development of Interatrial Septum:

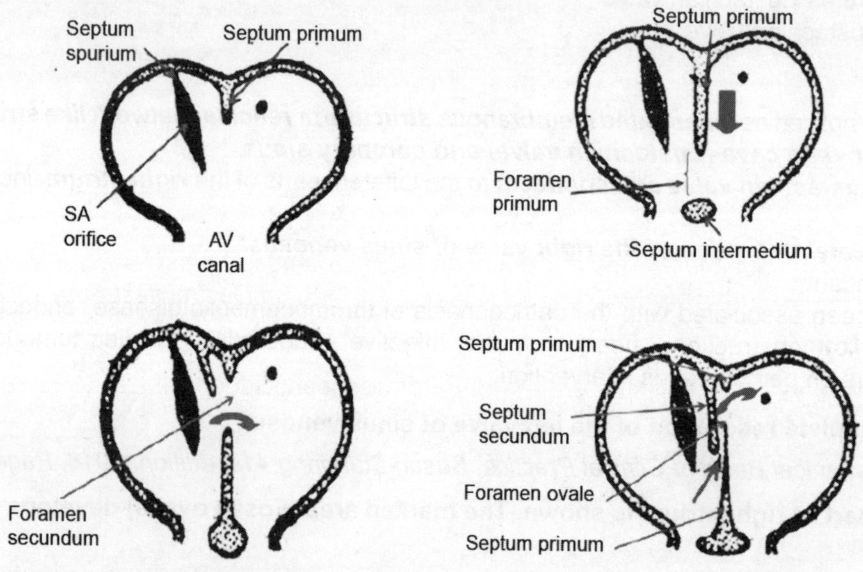

Ans: (a) Septum primum

Ref: *Essentials of Human Embryology, A.K. Datta, 5th edition, 2005, Page 171-175*

8. Which artery dilatation causes compression of 3rd part of duodenum?

(a) Superior mesentric artery
(b) Gastroduodenal artery
(c) Inferior mesenteric artery
(d) Celiac artery

Explanation:

- The mid portion of the third part of duodenum lies in the angle between the ***superior mesenteric artery anteriorly*** and the ***abdominal aorta posteriorly.***
- Narrowing of this angle (aortomesenteric angle) may occur from loss of perivascular adipose tissue or spinal straightening and is a ***rare cause of duodenal obstruction*** (Merrett *et al.* 2009).
- ***Superior mesenteric artery aneurysm*** may cause obstruction of 3rd part of duodenum.

Wilkie's Syndrome or Superior Mesenteric Artery syndrome or Cast syndrome

- ***Rare disorder*** in which ***acute angulation of the SMA causes compression of the third part of the duodenum*** between the SMA and the aorta, leading to obstruction.
- SMA syndrome is an atypical cause of proximal intestinal obstruction, most frequently occurring in young patients who have had an important weight loss.

Normal aortomesenteric angle **Narrow aortomesenteric angle**

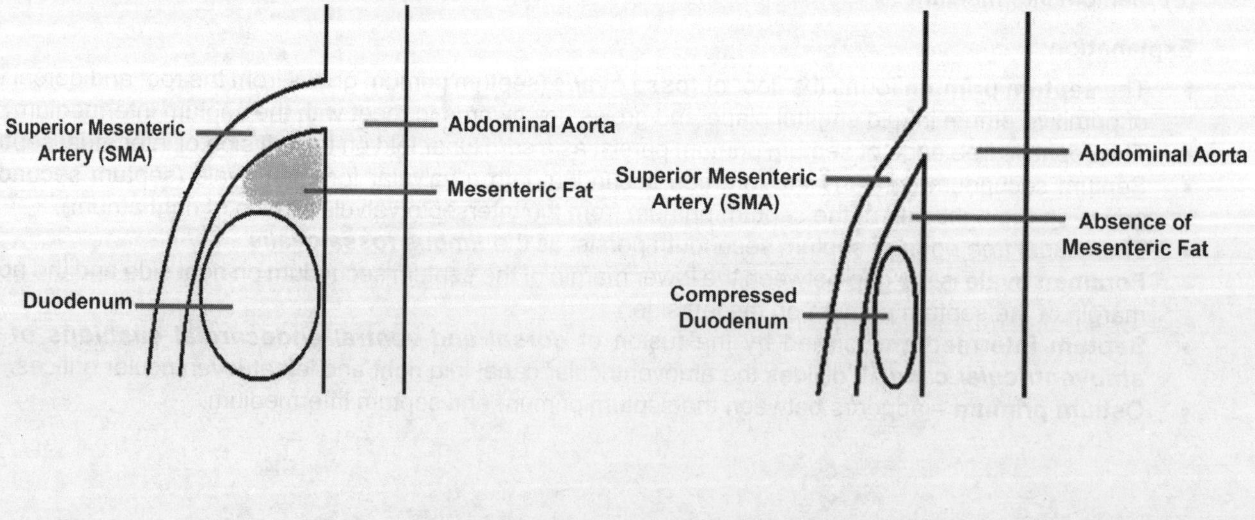

- Surgeries for spinal deformities as well as ***high insertion of the ligament of Treitz*** are other potential ***causes for the occurrence of SMA syndrome***.
- Loss of retroperitoneal fatty tissue as a result of this variety of conditions is believed to be the etiologic factor causing the acute angulation.
- Symptoms vary from postprandial nausea and bilious vomiting to abdominal pain as well as weight loss and can occur acutely or chronically.
- The ***severity of the symptoms*** largely depends on the ***degree of the compression*** as reflected by the ***aortomesenteric angle***.

Ans: (a) Superior mesentric artery

Ref: *Gray's Anatomy, The Anatomical Basis of Clinical Practice, Susan Standring, 41st edition, 2016, Page 1126 and 1135 e-1 and Merrett ND, Wilson RB, Cosman P et al., 2009; Superior mesenteric artery syndrome: Diagnosis and treatment strategies, J Gastrointest Surg 13:287-92*

9. Ejaculatory duct formed from:

(a) Mesonephric duct
(b) Paramesonephric duct
(c) Ureteric bud
(d) Wolffian duct

Explanation:

- In the male, the mesonephric duct itself becomes the **canal of the epididymis**, **vas deferens** and **ejaculatory duct.**

Genital ducts in the female:

Fate of paramesonephric duct in female

- Paramesonephric (**Mullerian duct**) ducts form the **uterine tubes, uterus, cervix and upper vagina.**

Fate of Mesonephric tubules in female

- Some remnants of the cranial and caudal mesonephric tubules in the **mesovarium**, where they form the ***epoophoron*** and ***paroophoron*** respectively.

Fate of Mesonephric duct in female

- The mesonephric duct disappears completely except for a small cranial portion found in the epoophoron.
- Occasionally a small caudal portion that may be found in the wall of the uterus or vagina. Later in life it may form ***Gartner's cyst*.***

Genital ducts in the male:

Fate of Mesonephric tubules in male

- Most of the mesonephric tubules will regress.
- Few ***mesonephric tubules*** (epigenital tubule),establish contact with cords of the rete testis and finally form the ***efferent ductules of the testis.***
- ***Mesonephric tubules*** along the caudal pole of the testis (paragenital tubules) do not join the cords of the rete testis.Their vestiges are collectively known as the ***paradidymis.***

Fate of Mesonephric duct in male

- The most cranial portion of mesonephric duct forms the ***appendix epididymis***.
- The mesonephric ducts persist and form the main genital ducts (vas deferens).
- Immediately below the entrance of the efferent ductules, the mesonephric ducts elongate and become highly convoluted, forming the (ductus) ***epididymis***.
- From the tail of the epididymis to the outbudding of the seminal vesicle, the mesonephric ducts obtain a thick muscular coat and form the ***ductus deferens.***
- The region of the ducts beyond the seminal vesicles is the ***ejaculatory duct.***

Fate of paramesonephric duct in male

- The paramesonephric ducts in the male degenerate except for a small portion at their cranial ends, the ***appendix testis.***

Ans: Mesonephric duct

Ref: *Gray's Anatomy, The Anatomical Basis of Clinical Practice, Susan Standring, 41st edition, 2016, Page 1201*

10. Diagram of bronchopulmonary segment is shown in the picture. Identify the structure 'D':

(a) Bronchial artery (b) Segmental bronchus
(c) Bronchial vein (d) Pulmonary vein

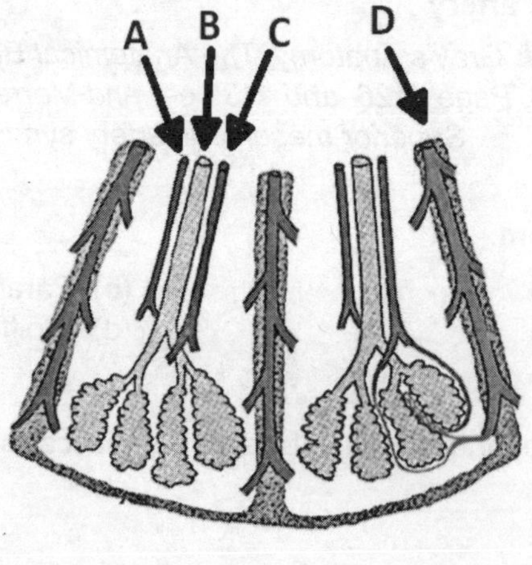

Explanation:

- Each ***bronchopulmonary segments*** is supplied by a ***segmental bronchus***, ***pulmonary arteries*** and ***bronchial artery***.
- But the tributaries of ***pulmonary veins run between segments***, serving adjacent segments.
- So, ***bronchopulmonary segment is not a complete vascular unit*** with an individual bronchus, artery and vein.
- During resection of segments, it is obvious that the planes between bronchopulmonary segments are not avascular but are crossed by pulmonary veins.

Bronchopulmonary segments:

	Right Lung	Left Lung
Upper lobe	Apical (S I)	Apical (S I)
	Posterior (S II)	Posterior (S II)
	Anterior (S III)	Anterior (S III)
		Superior lingular (S IV)
		Inferior lingular (S V)
Middle lobe	Lateral (S IV)	
	Medial (S V)	
Lower lobe	Superior (S VI)	Superior (S VI)
	Medial basal (S VII)	Medial basal (S VII)
	Anterior basal (S VIII)	Anterior basal (S VIII)
	Lateral basal (S IX)	Lateral basal (S IX)
	Posterior basal (S X)	Posterior basal (S X)

Ans: (d) Pulmonary vein

Ref: *Gray's Anatomy, The Anatomical Basis of Clinical Practice, Susan Standring, 41st edition, 2016, Page 959*

11. Superior part of IVC directly develops from:

(a) Right Vitelline vein
(b) Left Vitelline vein
(c) Right umbilical vein
(d) Left umbilical vein

Explanation:

Superior part of IVC (terminal part)* is developed from the *suprahepatic part of the right vitelline vein.

Development of IVC:

IVC developed from the following sources from below upwards:

- Persistent caudal part of the ***right posterior cardinal vein***
- ***Right supra-cardinal vein*** (this part receives 3rd and 4th pairs of lumbar veins).
- ***Anastomosis*** between ***right supra-cardinal and right sub-cardinal veins*** (this part receives the right gonadal vein).
- Upper part of the ***right sub-cardinal vein*** (this part receives both renal veins and right supra-renal vein).
- A ***new vessel*** grows dorsal to the liver and ***communicates the right sub-cardinal vein with the common hepatic vein*** (intrahepatic part of IVC).
- ***Common hepatic vein***–which is developed from the ***suprahepatic part of the right vitelline vein*** (terminal part of IVC).

Ans: (a) Right Vitelline vein

Ref: *Essentials of Human Embryology, A.K.Datta, 5th edition,2005, Page 205-208*

12. Suspensory Lock wood ligament encloses:

(a) Superior oblique and inferior rectus
(b) Inferior oblique and inferior rectus
(c) Superior rectus and inferior oblique
(d) Superior rectus and superior oblique

Explanation

- The suspensory ligament of eyeball (or Lockwood's ligament) forms a hammock stretching below the eyeball between the medial and lateral check ligaments and ***enclosing the inferior rectus and inferior oblique muscles*** of the eye.

Fascial sheath of the eyeball:

- ***Fascia bulbi (Tenon's capsule)-*** thin fascial sheath which envelops the eyeball.
- The fascia bulbi is perforated by the tendons of the extraocular muscles and is reflected on to each as a tubular sheath, the ***muscular fascia (tubular sheath for all orbital muscles).***
- Sheaths of adjacent recti become confluent and form a ***fascial ring.***
- Expansions from the muscular fascia of medial and lateral recti are strong, and are attached to the lacrimal and zygomatic bones, respectively.
- Since they may limit the actions of the two recti, they are termed ***medial and lateral check ligaments.***
- The ***sheath of inferior rectus*** is thickened on its underside and ***blends with*** the sheath of ***inferior oblique***.
- The sheath of inferior rectus and inferior oblique are continuous with the fascial ring formed by medial and lateral recti.
- Since the medial and lateral recti are attached to the orbital walls (lacrimal and zygomatic bones respectively) by check ligaments, a continuous fascial band, the ***suspensory ligament of the eye (Lockwood's ligament)***, is slung like a hammock below the eye, providing sufficient support that even when the maxilla (forming the floor of the orbit) is removed, the eye will retain its position.
    - Injection of local anaesthetics via a cannula into the space between the fascia bulbi and the sclera ***(sub-Tenon's anaesthesia)*** has become a popular technique for many ophthalmic surgical procedures.

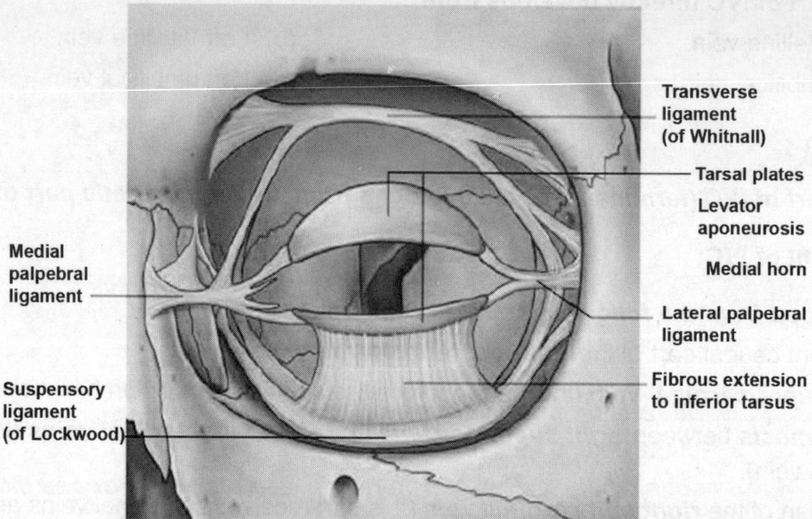

Ans: (b) Inferior oblique and inferior rectus

Ref: *Gray's Anatomy, The Anatomical Basis of Clinical Practice, Susan Standring, 41st edition, 2016, Page 668-681*

13. Vertebral abscess spreads to thigh through which of the following marked nerve tract?

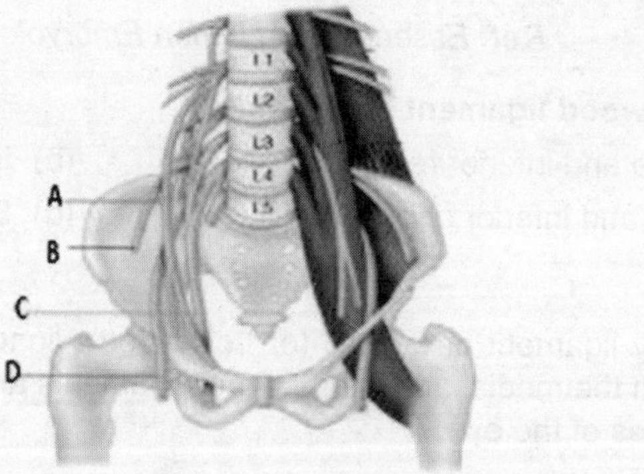

A. A B. B C. C D. D

Key:

(a) Genitofemoral nerve
(b) Lateral femoral cutaneous nerve
(c) Obturator nerve
(d) Femoral nerve

Explanation:

Genitofemoral nerve:

Root value, course and relation (to psoas major):

- ***Ventral rami*** of ***L1 and L2.***
- Formed within the substance of psoas major and descends obliquely forwards through the muscle to emerge on its anterior surface nearer the medial border, opposite the third or fourth lumbar vertebra.
- It then descends beneath the peritoneum on psoas major and divides into genital and femoral branches.
- The ***genital branch enters the inguinal canal*** through the deep ring and accompanies the spermatic cord or round ligament. It exits the superficial inguinal ring.
- The ***femoral branch*** descends to pass behind the inguinal ligament and enter the ***femoral sheath lateral to the femoral artery.***

Lateral femoral cutaneous nerve

Root value, course and relation (to psoas major):

- ***Ventral rami*** of ***L2 and L3.***

- Emerges from the posterolateral border of psoas major and crosses iliacus obliquely towards the anterior superior iliac spine.

Obturator nerve

Root value, course and relation (to psoas major):

- ***Ventral branches*** of the ventral rami of ***L2,L3 and L4.***
- Descends within the substance of psoas major to emerge from its posteromedial border near the L5 vertebra.
- It descends on the lateral wall of the pelvis attached to the fascia over obturator internus and running into the obturator foramen to enter the thigh.

Femoral nerve

Root value, course and relation (to psoas major):

- ***Dorsal branches*** of the ventral rami of ***L2,L3 and L4.***
- ***Under cover of psoas fascia***, runs in a ***groove between psoas major and iliacus*** and emerges on or under its lateral border, about 4 cm above the inguinal ligament.
  - The ***inguinal ligament*** is a ***convergent point of the transversalis fascia*** (fascial sac lining the deep surface of the anterior abdominal wall) and ***iliac fascia*** (fascia covering the posterior abdominal wall).
  - As it passes beneath the inguinal ligament, the ***femoral nerve*** is ***positioned lateral*** and slightly deeper than the ***femoral artery between the psoas and iliacus muscles.***
  - At the femoral crease, the ***femoral nerve*** is on the surface of the iliacus muscle and covered by the fascia iliaca or ***sandwiched between two layers of fascia iliaca.***
  - In contrast, vascular fascia of the femoral artery and vein, a funnel-shaped extension of the transversalis fascia, forms a ***distinctly different compartment*** from that of the ***femoral nerve.***

  Note: Vertebral / psoas abscess spreads to thigh along the psoas fascia. The abscess does not spread to thigh along the femoral nerve but we could trace the abscess along the femoral nerve course.

Ans: (d) Femoral nerve

Ref: *Thieme Atlas of Anatomy, General Anatomy and Musculoskeletal System, 2010 edition, Page 470-475; Gray's Anatomy, The Anatomical Basis of Clinical Practice, Susan Standring, 41st edition, 2016, Page 1091-1096; Hadzic's Peripheral Nerve Block and Anatomy for Ultrasound-Guided Regional Anaesthesia, 2nd edition, 2012, Page 268*

14. Maximum AP diameter of trachea in male and female are__ and__ respectively.

(a) 27 mm and 25 mm (b) 25 mm and 23 mm
(c) 25 mm and 21 mm (d) 20 mm and 15 mm

Explanation:

- The external transverse diameter of trachea is typically **2 cm in adult males and 1.5 cm in adult females**.

Note: Mean transverse diameter is greater than anteroposterior diameter up to the age of 6 years, after that **the two diameters are nearly equal.**

- The lumen of trachea is about 12 mm in diameter (internal transverse diameter).
- In the first postnatal year, the tracheal diameter does not exceed 4 mm.
- Length of trachea : 10–11 cm.
- Trachea consists of 16–20 "C" shaped incomplete rings of hyaline cartilage.

Ans: (d) 20 mm and 15 mm

Ref: *Gray's Anatomy, The Anatomical Basis of Clinical Practice, Susan Standring, 41st edition, 2016, Page 965*

15. Which of the following is involved in auditory pathway?

(a) Inferior colliculus (b) Lateral geniculate body
(c) Inferior olivary nucleus (d) Medial lemniscus

Explanation:

- The ***inferior colliculus*** is part of the ascending ***auditory pathway*** and is the principal site of termination of the lateral lemniscus.

Inferior Colliculus:

Structure

- It has a central, ovoid, main nucleus, which is lateral to the periaqueductal grey matter.
- It is surrounded by a lamina of nerve fibres, many from the lateral lemniscus, which terminate in it.
- The central nucleus has dorsomedial and ventrolateral zones, which are covered by a dorsal cortex.
- Cortex has four cytoarchitectonic layers:
  - Layer I contains small neurones with flattened radial dendritic fields.
  - Layer II, medium-sized neurones with ovoid dendritic fields aligned parallel with the collicular surface.
  - Layer III, medium-sized neurones with spherical dendritic fields.
  - Layer IV, large neurones with variably shaped dendritic fields.

Connections

- Most efferent fibres from the inferior colliculus travel via the ***inferior brachium*** to the ipsilateral ***medial geniculate nucleus.***
- ***Lemniscal fibres relay*** only in the ***central nucleus***, and some pass without relay to the medial geniculate nucleus.
- Ventral division of the medial geniculate nucleus receives a topographic projection from the central nucleus.
- Dorsal division receives a similar projection from the dorsal cortex.
- Some ***colliculogeniculate fibres do not relay in the geniculate nucleus*** but continue, with those that do, via the ***auditory radiation to the auditory cortex.***
- A descending projection from the ***auditory cortex*** reaches ***the inferior colliculus via the medial geniculate nucleus.***
- This descending path may produce effects at levels from the medial geniculate nucleus downwards, and it probably links with efferent cochlear fibres, through the superior olivary and cochlear nuclei.

Superior Colliculus:

Structure

- The superior colliculus is laminated structure.
- It is divided into ***seven layers (***Zonal, Superficial grey, Optic, Intermediate grey, Deep grey, Deep white and Periventricular strata).
- The zonal layer consists chiefly of myelinated and non-myelinated fibres from the occipital cortex (***areas 17, 18 and 19***) which arrive as the external corticotectal tract.
- The superficial grey layer (stratum cinereum) forms a crescentic lamina over the deeper layers and contains many small multipolar interneurons.
- The optic layer consists partly of fibres from the optic tract.
- This arrangement provides a ***retinotopic map of the contralateral visual field***, in which the fovea is represented anterolaterally. Retinal axons terminate in clusters from specific retinotectal neurons and as collaterals of retinogeniculate fibres. ***Efferent fibres to the retina*** are said to start in this layer.
- The intermediate grey and white layers collectively constitute the main receptive zone.

Connections

- The main afferent input is the medial corticotectal path from ***layer V*** neurones of the ***ipsilateral occipital cortex (area 18***), and from other neocortical areas that are ***concerned with ocular movements***.
- Afferent fibres are also received from the contralateral spinal cord (via spinotectal fibres), the inferior colliculus, and the locus coeruleus and raphe nuclei (from noradrenergic and serotoninergic neurones).
- The deep grey and deep white layers adjacent to the periaqueductal grey matter are collectively called the ***parabigeminal nucleus***. They form collicular efferents.
- The superior colliculus receives afferents from many sources including the retina, spinal cord, inferior colliculus and occipital and temporal cortices.
- Collicular efferents pass to the retina, lateral geniculate nucleus, pretectum, parabigeminal nucleus, the inferior, medial and lateral pulvinar, and to numerous sites in the brainstem and spinal cord.
- Fibres passing from the ***pulvinar are relayed to primary and secondary visual cortices and form an extrageniculate retinocortical pathway for visual orientation and attention.***

- The tectospinal and tectobulbar tracts start from neurones in the superior colliculi.
- ***Inferior collicular projections to the brainstem and spinal cord*** appear to traverse the ***superior colliculi*** before they descend. In this way they connect with the origins of the tectospinal and tectotegmental tracts. These projections are relatively small and probably ***mediate reflex turning of the head and eyes in response to sounds.***

Ans: Inferior colliculus

Ref: *Gray's Anatomy, The Anatomical Basis of Clinical Practice, Susan Standring, 41st edition, 2016, Page 325 and 326*

16. If you want to operate on lower medial side of leg, what nerve has to be blocked?

(a) Femoral nerve
(b) Tibial nerve
(c) Common peroneal nerve
(d) Sacral nerve

Explanation:

- The **saphenous nerve**, a branch of the **femoral nerve** supplies the skin on the **anteromedial surface of the leg**.

Distribution of Femoral Nerve Blockade

- Anesthesia of the skin and muscles of the anterior thigh and most of the femur and knee joint.
- The block also confers anesthesia of the skin on the medial aspect of the leg below the knee joint (***saphenous nerve***, a superficial terminal extension of the ***femoral nerve***).

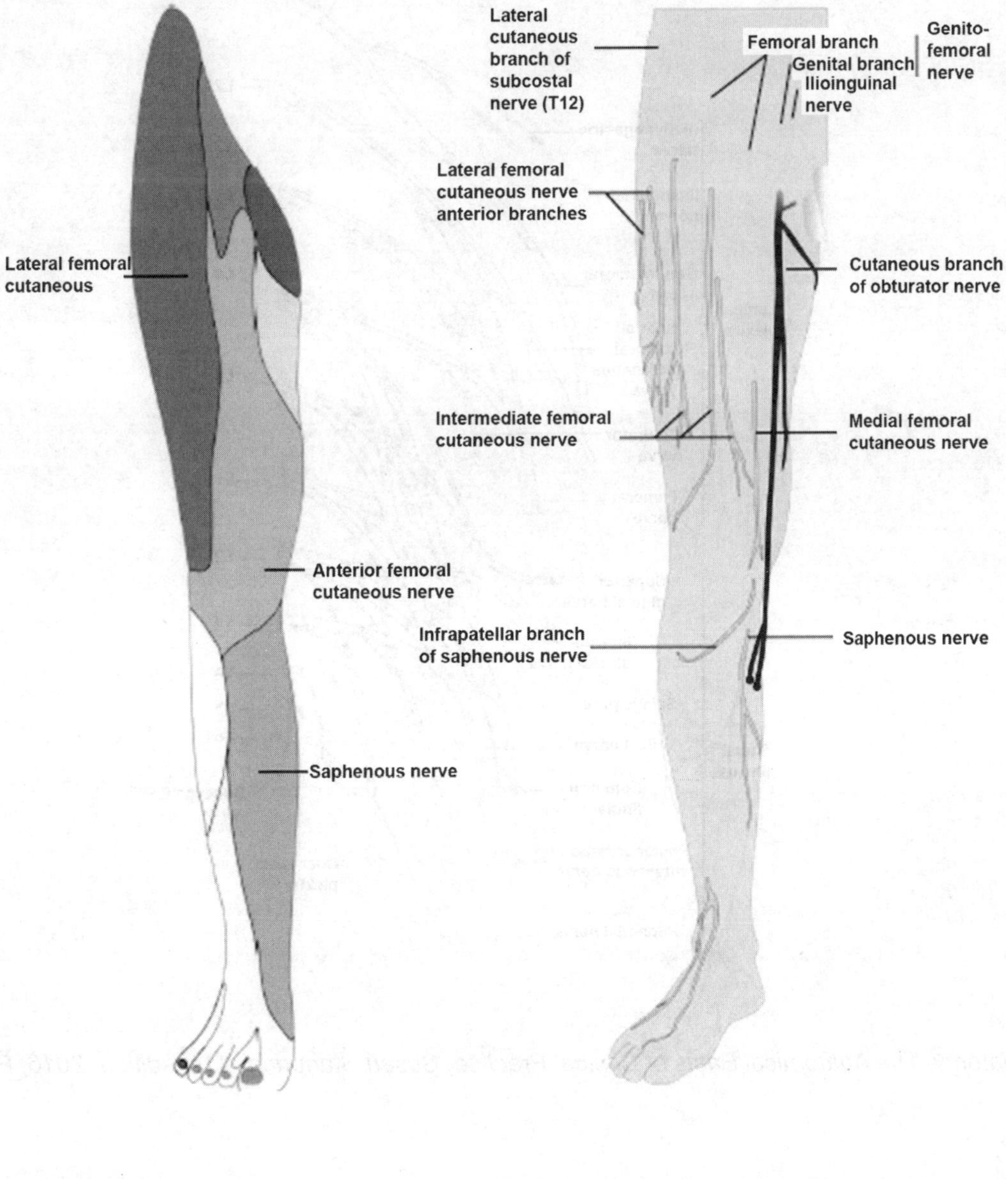

Femoral nerve branches:

Anterior division	Posterior division
• Middle cutaneous nerve of thigh	• ***Saphenous nerve (most medial)***
• Medial cutaneous nerve of thigh	• Muscular branches (individual heads of the quadriceps muscle)
• Muscular (sartorius) branch	• Articular branches (hip and knee)

Ans: (a) Femoral nerve

Ref: *Hadzic's Peripheral Nerve Block and Anatomy for Ultrasound-Guided Regional Anaesthesia, 2nd edition, 2012, Page 269*

17. Nervi Furcalis is related to:

(a) L3 (b) L4 (c) L5 (d) L6

Explanation:

- The furcal nerve is the ***L4 nerve root***.
- The term furcal refers to its ***forked*** nature since it ***links the lumbar and sacral plexuses.***
- The furcal nerve with its own ventral and dorsal rootlets contribute to the **femoral** and **obturator** nerves.
- Occasionally, the furcal nerve arises at the level of the third or the fifth lumbar nerve roots, in which case the sacral plexus is considered prefixed or postfixed, respectively.

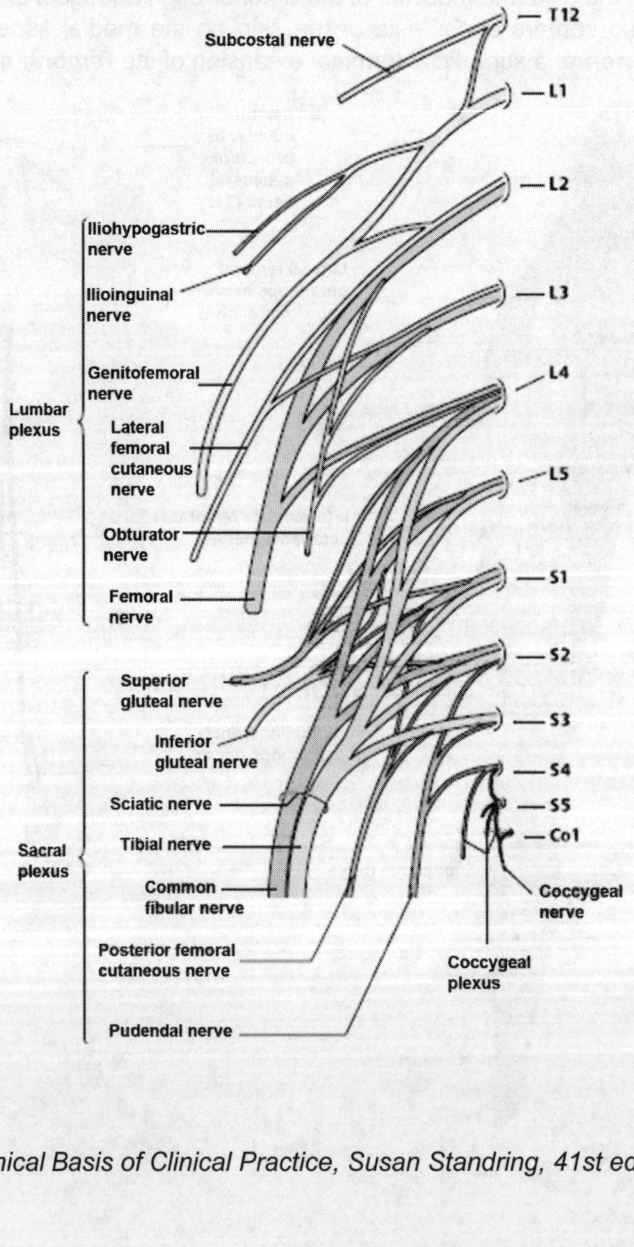

Ans: (b) L4

Ref: *Gray's Anatomy, The Anatomical Basis of Clinical Practice, Susan Standring, 41st edition, 2016, Page 1093*

PHYSIOLOGY

1. **Which of the following is the correct formula to calculate minute volume?**

(a) RR × Tidal volume
(b) RR/Tidal volume
(c) FiO_2/PEEP
(d) FiO_2/PEEP × RR

Explanation:

Minute ventilation

- Also called as **pulmonary ventilation.**
- It is the **volume of air inspired or expired per minute.**
- It is equal to the tidal volume (TV) multiplied by respiratory rate (RR).
- **Minute ventilation = TV × RR.**
- Normal minute ventilation is **6–7.5 L/min*.**

Ans: (b) RR/Tidal volume

Ref: *Ganong, 25th edition, Page 632*

2. **Correct statement regarding the role of vasa recta:**

(a) Regulating Tubulo-glomerular feedback mechanism
(b) Regulating GFR
(c) Concentration of urine
(d) Supplying supra-renal medulla

Explanation:

Countercurrent Multiplier – "Loop of Henle"

- ***Thin descending loop of Henle*** **– "the concentrating segment"**
  - We know that the fluid leaves out of PCT is isosomotic **(300 mosm/kg).**
  - Once it enters the descending loop of Henle (dLOH), water moves out freely leaving the solutes inside. The fluid in the descending limb of the loop of Henle becomes **hypertonic.**
  - The osmolarity reached at the tip of dLOH is around **1200 mosm/kg.**
  - Water moves out of the dLOH through **aquaporin-1.**
- ***Thick ascending loop of Henle*** **– "the diluting segment"**
  - Thick ascending loop of Henle is permeable to solutes and impermeable to water.
  - Sodium, chloride and potassium moves out of the thick ascending limb through Na–K–2Cl co-transporter.
  - Because of selective movement of solutes leaving water inside – fluid inside thick ascending limb becomes hypotonic to plasma.

Countercurrent exchanger – "Vasa recta"

- Vasa recta are straight capillaries that run parallel to loop of Henle.
- Vasa recta serves as countercurrent exchanger–they minimize washout of solutes and maintain the osmolarity gradient developed by loop of Henle.

Ans: (c) Concentration of urine

Ref: *Ganong, 25th edition, Page 685*

3. **Glomerular filtration rate (GFR) will be increased if:**

(a) Increased hydrostatic pressure in bowman capsule
(b) Decreased oncotic pressure in glomerular capillaries
(c) Increased oncotic pressure in glomerular capillaries
(d) Decreased hydrostatic pressure in glomerular capillaries

Explanation:

Determinants of the GFR

- Pressures in the capillaries are the major forces that govern fluid movement in them. Such forces are commonly called Starling forces.
- GFR is determined by:
  - o Hydrostatic and colloid osmotic forces across the glomerular membrane that determines "Net filtration pressure".
  - o Filtration coefficient, K_f.
- **GFR = K_f × Net filtration pressure.**
- Important pressures under consideration are:
  - o Glomerular capillary hydrostatic pressure, **P_G = 60 mm Hg.**
  - o Hydrostatic pressure in Bowman's capsule **(P_B) = 18 mm Hg.**
  - o Colloid osmotic pressure of the glomerular capillary plasma proteins (π_G) = 32 mm Hg.
  - o The colloid osmotic pressure of the proteins in Bowman's capsule (π_B) – In normal individuals, since albumin is not filtered, π_B is zero.
- **Forces Favoring Filtration (mm Hg)**
  - o Glomerular hydrostatic pressure = 60.
  - o Bowman's capsule colloid osmotic pressure = 0.
- **Forces Opposing Filtration (mm Hg)**
  - o Bowman's capsule hydrostatic pressure = 18.
  - o Glomerular capillary colloid osmotic pressure = 32.
- **Net filtration pressure = 60 – 18 – 32 = 10 mm Hg**
  - o Since Glomerular capillary colloid osmotic pressure oppose filtration, its decrease actually increases GFR.

Ans: (b) Decreased oncotic pressure in glomerular capillaries

***Ref:** Ganong, 25th edition, Page 677*

4. **Transthoracic compliance formula:**

(a) C = Vt × RR/PEEP
(b) C= V/Alv p – atmospheric pressure
(c) C = Vt/Pplt - PEEP
(d) C = Vt/Pk - Pplt

Explanation:

- Lungs are elastic structures. Its ability to expand (stretchability) is quantified in terms of compliance.
- Like lung, chest wall is also an elastic structure.
- Compliance is defined as "the change in volume per unit change in the pressure".
- Compliance = **ΔV/ΔP.**
- Here Transthoracic pressure is the difference between alveolar pressure and atmospheric pressure.
- So, **C= V/Alv p – atmospheric pressure.**

Ans: (b) C= V/Alv p – atmospheric pressure

***Ref:** Ganong, 25th edition, Page 631*

5. **Normal dead space to tidal volume ratio is:**

(a) 50 - 70
(b) 10 - 20
(c) 30 - 40
(d) 80 - 90

Explanation:

V_D/ V_T ratio

- This ratio is used to find out the proportion of ventilation remains in dead spaces.
- Normally the ratio is 150/500 which equals **0.3***.
- This means that 30% of the ventilation remains in dead spaces.

- **Dead space** to **tidal volume** ratio is calculated by **PCO_2 of alveolar air** – **PCO_2 of expired air/PCO_2** of **alveolar air.** This equation is called **Bohr's equation.**

$$\textbf{Dead space to tidal volume ratio} = \frac{PCO_2 \text{ of alveolar air} - PCO_2 \text{ of expired air}}{PCO_2 \text{ of alveolar air}}$$

Dead space ventilation

- Dead space ventilation means the ventilation that is not used for gas exchange.
- It can be of three types:
    1. Anatomic dead space.
    2. Alveolar dead space.
    3. Physiologic or total dead space.

Anatomic dead space

- Is the volume of air present in the conducting zone (first 16 generations) which are not used for gas exchange.
- Volume of anatomic dead space (ml) is approximately equal to the body weight in pounds. For a 70 kg man (154 pounds) it is 154 ml.

Alveolar dead space

- Is the volume of air present in those alveoli which do not take part in gas exchange.

Physiologic dead space

- Also called as **total dead space.**
- It is obtained by adding anatomic and alveolar dead space.
- Physiologic dead space = anatomic dead space + alveolar dead space.
- In healthy individuals, physiologic dead space roughly equals anatomic dead space.

Measurement of anatomic dead space

- The technique useful for measuring anatomic dead space is **single-breath Nitrogen method.** This method is also called Fowler's method.

Measurement of physiologic (total) dead space

- Physiologic dead space is measured with the help of an equation termed **Bohr's equation.**

Ans: (c) 30 - 40

Ref: *Ganong, 25th edition, Page 632*

6. A muscular man weighing 70 kg has haematocrit of 45%, what would be his plasma volume?

(a) 2310 ml (b) 2695 ml
(c) 3080 ml (d) 2890 ml

Explanation:

- Blood volume **= Plasma Volume/(1-hematocrit).**
- **So, Plasma volume = Blood volume *(1- hematocrit).**
- Normal blood volume is 8% of body weight. For 70 kg male its 5.6 L.
- **Plasma volume = 5.6 * (1- 0.45).**
- **So, Plasma volume = 3080 ml.**

Ans: (c) 3080 ml

Ref: *Ganong, 25th edition, Page 3*

7. What is the expected mixed venous oxygen tension, in mmHg, in a normal adult after breathing 100% oxygen for 10 minutes?

(a) 150 (b) 740
(c) 45 (d) 573

Explanation:

- Breathing 100% oxygen will not change the oxygen saturation much. In arterial blood its around 97% saturation which corresponds to a PO_2 of 100 mm Hg.
- In venous blood its 75% saturation which corresponds to a **mixed venous oxygen tension of around 40 – 45 mm Hg.**

Ans: (c) 45

Ref: *American Board of Anesthesiology American Society of Anesthesiologists, Book A 1996 Q-67*

8. **Normal value of EPO (U/L) is:**

(a) 10-25 (b) 15-40
(c) 45-55 (d) 55-65

Explanation:

Erythropoietin (Epo)

- Is a glycoprotein hormone whose normal level is **10–25 U/L.**
- Receptor for erythropoietin – **Cytokine receptor** that activates **tyrosine kinase Jak/STAT** signaling cascade.
- Mechanism of action of EPO – **inhibits apoptosis** of **red blood cells.**

Sources of erythropoietin

- **Kidney** is the major source. Approx **85%** of the erythropoietin comes from **peritubular capillary bed** cells of the kidneys.
- Remaining **15%** of erythropoietin comes from **perivenous hepatocytes** in the **liver.**
- Erythropoietin is also found in **brain, uterus** and **fallopian tube.**

Ans: (a) 10-25

Ref: *Ganong, 25th, edition, Page 555*

9. **Regulation of smooth muscle tone is persistently influenced by:**

(a) Calcium release from sarcoplasmic reticulum (b) Beta 1 receptor
(c) Latch bridge mechanism (d) Troponin

Explanation:

Latch Bridge mechanism:

- Smooth muscle can be maintained in a prolonged state of partial contraction (tonus) with very little use of ATP. This is due to latch bridge mechanism in which myosin cross-bridges remain attached to actin for some time after the cytoplasmic Ca^{2+} concentration falls.
- This phenomenon is very important in vascular smooth muscle and intestine.

Ans: (c) Latch bridge mechanism

Ref: *Ganong, 25th edition, Page 118*

10. **Which of the following is true regarding urea?**

(a) Transported through aquaporins (b) Re-absorbed in proximal tubule
(c) No role in concentration of urine (d) Resorption is independent of ADH

Explanation:

- **2/3rd** of filtered **urea** is resorbed in **PCT.**
- Remember that only **50%** of medullary hyperosmolarity is due to **Nacl***. Remaining 50% is contributed by the end product of protein metabolism – **urea***.
- It is for this reason, high protein diet increases the concentrating ability of kidney and low protein diet decreases kidneys' ability to concentrate the urine.
- Under the influence of anti-diuretic hormone (**ADH**), urea is reabsorbed from **medullary collecting tubules** and from there urea diffuses into **ascending loop of Henle** and recirculates.

- Urea transporters in kidney is **UT-A**. It has 4 isoforms namely **UT-A1 to UT-A4.**
- Urea transport in the collecting duct is mediated by **UT-A1 and UT-A3**. They both are regulated by Anti-diuretic hormone (**ADH**).
- **Urea transporter** present in **descending limb** of **vasa recta** is **UT-B**. It is not regulated by **ADH**. **UT-B** is also present in **RBCs.**

Ans: (b) Re-absorbed in proximal tubule

***Ref:** Ganong, 25th edition, Page 686*

11. True regarding properties of dendritic cells:

(a) All cells are same in nature
(b) Are derived from neural crest cells
(c) Are not antigen presenting cells
(d) Active in mucosa and lymph nodes

Explanation:

- **Dendritic cells** are **antigen presenting cells.**
- They are abundant in issues that are in contact with the external environment, such as the skin, intestine and lymph nodes.
- They mainly acts as connecting links between innate and acquired immunity.

Ans: (d) Active in mucosa and lymph nodes

***Ref:** Ganong, 25th edition, Page 554*

12. Normal cardiac index in an adult is:

(a) 5.9 $L/min/m^2$
(b) 2.3 $L/min/m^2$
(c) 3.2 $L/min/m^2$
(d) 4.6 $L/min/m^2$

Explanation:

Cardiac output is the product of heart rate (HR) and stroke volume (SV).
Cardiac output = HR × SV.
Normal cardiac output values:

- Men - 5.6 L/min.
- Women - 4.9 L/min.

Cardiac index:

- Cardiac index is expressing cardiac output per square meter of body surface area.
- **Cardiac index = Cardiac output / Body surface area.**
- Normal cardiac index for adults is **3.2** $L/min/m^2$ of body surface area.

Ans: (c) 3.2 $L/min/m^2$

***Ref:** Ganong, 25th edition, Page 543*

13. In a measurement of cardiac output using the Fick principle, the O_2 concentrations of mixed venous and arterial blood are 16 and 20 ml–100 ml-1, respectively, and the O_2 consumption is 300 ml·min-1. The cardiac output in liters·min-1 is:

(a) 5
(b) 8
(c) 9
(d) 7.5

Explanation:

- The Fick principle states that the cardiac output is equal to the oxygen consumption divided by the arterial-venous oxygen concentration difference.
- Here, its (20 - 16) ml·100 ml-1 or (200 - 160) ml·liter-1.
- Therefore, the cardiac output is equal to 300/(200 - 160) or 7.5 liters·min-1

Ans: (d) 7.5

***Ref:** Ganong, 25th edition, Page 543*

BIOCHEMISTRY

1. **Which decreases affinity of oxygen with hemoglobin?**

(a) Decreased H^+ ions
(b) Reduced 2,3 DPG
(c) Increase in temperature
(d) Decreased sorbitol

Explanation:

- Hb can transport H^+ and CO_2 from the tissues to the lungs, and can carry four molecules of O_2 from the lungs to the cells of the body.
- The oxygen-binding properties of Hb are regulated by allosteric effectors.
- There are four primary regulators, each of which has a negative impact.
  - o CO_2.
  - o Hydrogen ion (H^+).
  - o Temperature.
  - o 2,3-bisphosphoglycerate (2,3-BPG).
- Effect of these allosteric regulators is represented in Oxygen Dissociation Curve (ODC).
- ODC is a plot of % saturation of Hb with O_2 measured at different partial pressures of oxygen (pO_2). Thus O_2 saturation curve for Hb is Sigmoid in shape.
  - o Factors which favor **O_2 unloading (decrease affinity of Hb for O_2)** include: $\downarrow pO_2$ $\uparrow$2,3 BPG, $\uparrow pCO_2$, $\downarrow$pH, $\uparrow$temperature (as shown in the figure below).

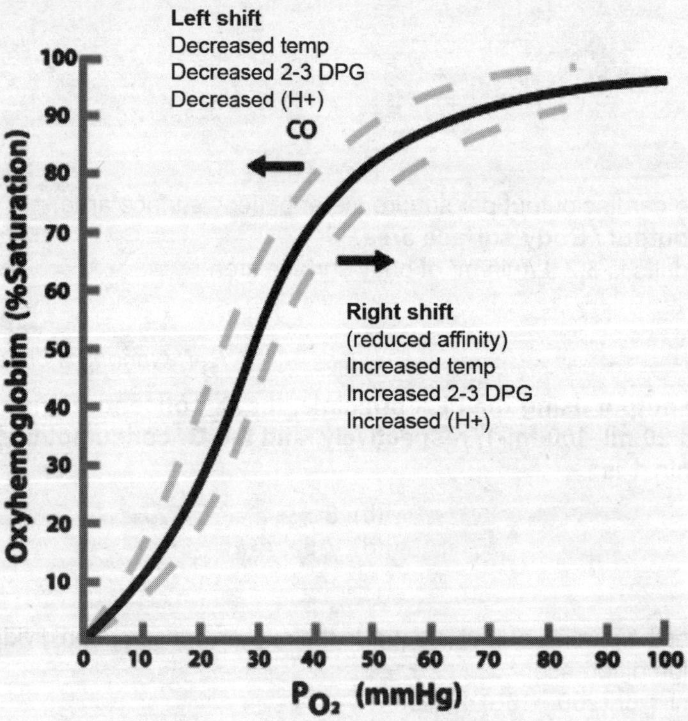

Ans: (d) Decreased sorbitol

***Ref**: Lippincott's Illustrated Reviews, Biochemistry, 4th edition, Chapter 3, Page 29-32*

2. Mutation in hartnup disease:

(a) SLC5A18 (b) SLC6A19 (c) SLC7A9 (d) SLC3A1

Explanation:

Hartnup disease

- Rare autosomal recessive condition.
- Defect of the membrane transport mechanism for **neutral amino acids**, especially **tryptophan**.
- Results in large losses as a result of intestinal malabsorption and failure of renal reabsorption mechanism.
- The defective gene, **SLC6A19*,** encodes a **sodium dependent** and **chloride independent** neutral **amino acid transporter**, which is expressed predominantly in the **small intestine*** and **proximal tubule of kidneys***.
- Tryptophan is abnormally retained in the intestinal lumen and converted to indole compounds that are toxic to **CNS** resulting in **cerebellar ataxia*.**
- Abnormal tryptophan metabolism leads to a **niacin deficiency*** resulting in **pellagra like skin rashes*.**
- **High protein diet** and **nicotinamide** supplements are recommended.

Ans: (b) SLC6A19

Ref: *Harrison's Principles of Internal Medicine, 18th edition, Volume 2, Chapter 284, Page 2365*

3. False statement regarding Schilling test is:

(a) Unlabelled B_{12} is given IM
(b) Labelled B_{12} given orally
(c) Vit B_{12} excreted in urine
(d) Abnormal test rules out primary intestinal malabsorption

Explanation:

Schilling test

- Done in those patients who have **low B_{12} levels** and **negative anti-intrinsic factor antibodies** to determine whether there is B_{12} malabsorption.
- The test is done in two parts, as depicted in the following flowcharts along with the interpretation.
- If the urinary excretion **of radiolabelled B_{12}** is **less than 10%** even with intrinsic factor supplementation, it is implied that B_{12} deficiency is due to gut disease leading to malabsorption.

Part One

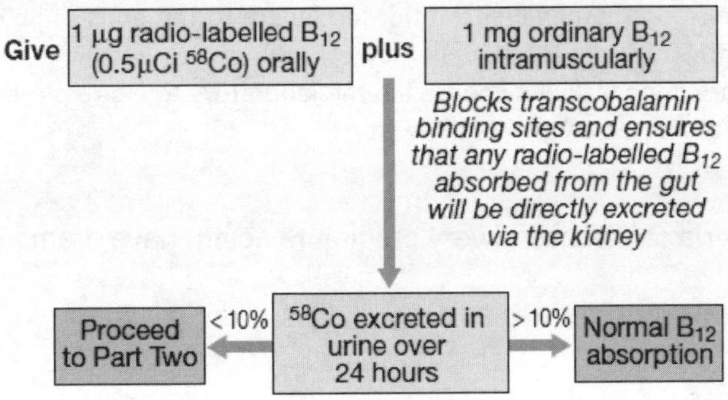

Part Two
(in excretion ↓ in Part One)One

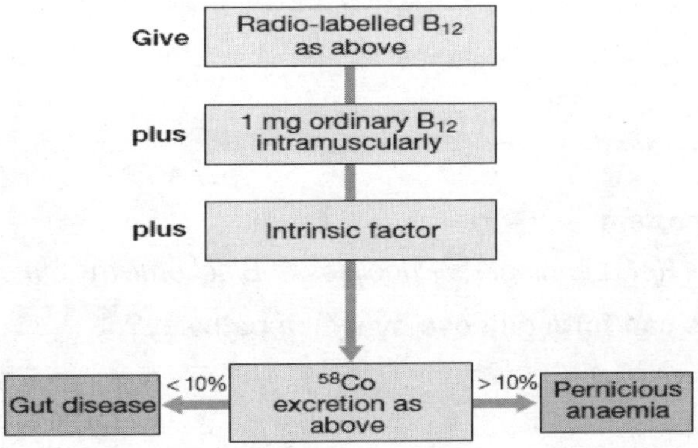

Ans: (d) Abnormal test rules out primary intestinal malabsorption

***Ref:** Davidson's Principles and Practice of Medicine, 21st edition, Chapter 24, Page 1021*

4. **True about telomerase is:**

(a) Ribonucleoprotein
(b) Transcriptional factor activation
(c) Membrane receptor
(d) DNA binding domain

Explanation

Telomeres:

- **Telomeres** are nucleotide sequences at the **ends** of **linear chromosomes** that maintain the **structural integrity** of eukaryotic chromosomes.
- These structures contain multiple repeats of specific **hexanucleotide DNA** sequences.
- The telomeres of normal cells shorten on repeated cell division, which may result in cell death.
- There is a **ribonucleoprotein** called **telomerase** that is involved in **synthesizing** the ends of **DNA.**
- Telomerase contains an **RNA molecule** that serves as the **template** and a protein that has polymerase activity.
- Telomerase is thought of as a **template-bearing reverse transcriptase**, i.e., it synthesizes DNA from an RNA template.
- Human **somatic cells** generally ***lack*** telomerase activity, so the subsequent shortening of DNA that occurs with each division might be related to **aging** (and death).
- The enzyme **telomerase** replicates **telomeres** and is often expressed in **cancer cells**, helping them **to evade cell death**.
- The **telomeres** provide an **innocuous source of DNA** whose decreasing length is of little immediate consequence to the cell. However, once the supply of telomere DNA is exhausted, roughly **100 cell divisions** for humans, **mitosis ceases** and the somatic cell enters a state of **replicative senescence**. As more and more cells within the body enter senescence, it progressively loses the capacity to replace lost or damaged cells.
- Organisms are able to generate progeny that contain full length telomeres thanks to the intervention of the enzyme telomerase.
- Telomerase is a **ribonucleoprotein** that is expressed in **stem cells** and **most cancer cells**, but **not in somatic cells.**
- Using an **RNA template**, **telomerase** adds **GT-rich hexanucleotide** repeat sequences ranging from a few hundred (yeast) to several thousand (humans) nucleotides in length to the ends of linear DNA molecules to restore their telomeres to full length.
- When somatic cells are genetically engineered in the laboratory to express telomerase, they continue to divide in culture long after an unaltered control cell line stops.

Clinical Implications:

- Patients with **progeria** (a disease of very premature aging) have dramatically shortened telomeres at an early age.
- Most cancer cells have **telomerase activity.**

Note:

- Cells with telomerase activity
  - Germinal cells
  - Cancer cells
  - Stem cells
- **Cells without telomerase activity**
  - Somatic cells.

Ans: (a) Ribonucleoprotein

***Ref:** Lehninger's Principles of Biochemistry, 5th edition, Chapter 26, Page1053-1055*

5. **Odd chain fatty acids can form glucose by which pathway?**

(a) By forming Propionyl CoA
(b) By forming Glycerol
(c) Acetyl CoA entering TCA cycle
(d) By Lactic acid formation

Explanation:

- Fatty acids with an odd number of carbon atoms are oxidized by the pathway of β-oxidation, producing acetyl CoA (2C) until a three-carbon (propionyl-CoA) residue remains.
- End product of even chain FA oxidation–acetyl CoA(2C).
- End product of odd chain FA oxidation–acetyl CoA units **+ 1 propionyl CoA**(3C).
- Propionyl CoA is converted to succinyl–CoA (steps mentioned below), a constituent of the citric acid cycle, which after few steps, enters in to gluconeogenesis.

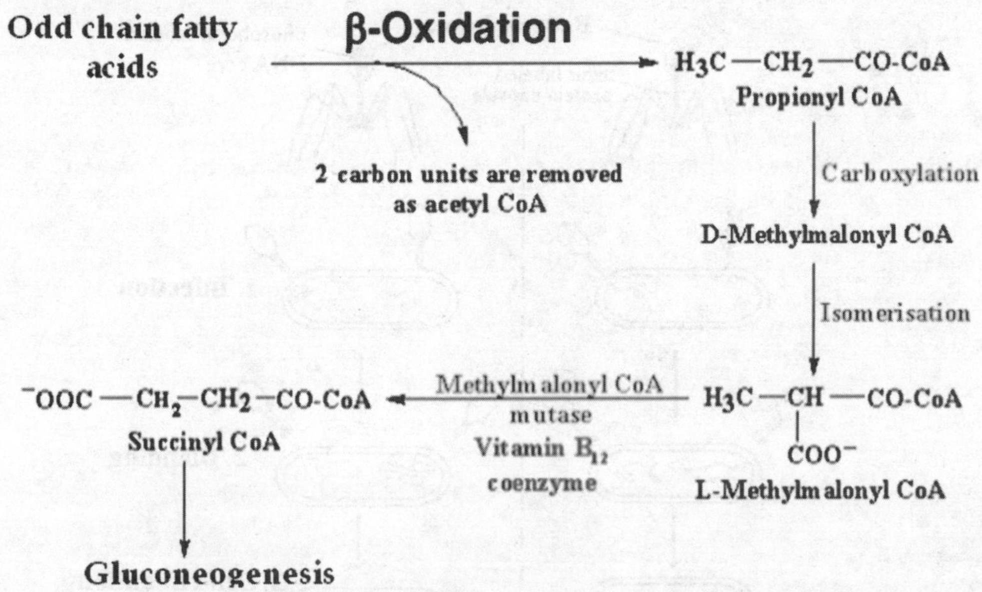

Only 2 enzymes in our body requires **vit B_{12}** as cofactor:

- **Methyl malonyl CoA mutase (AKA methylmalonyl-CoA isomerase).**
- **Methionine synthase** (Synthesis of Methionine by methylation of homocysteine).
    - Hence, **the propionyl residue from an odd-chain fatty acid is the only part of a fatty acid that is glucogenic.**
    - **Even chain fatty acids cannot synthesize glucose, because PDH reaction is irreversible.**
    - Gluconeogenesis is glucose synthesized from **non-carbohydrate** sources like lactate, propionyl CoA and Glucogenic amino acids. **So glucose derived from glycogen break down (carbohydrate source) is NOT gluconeogenesis.**

Ans: (a) By forming Propionyl CoA

Ref: *Harper, Illustrated Biochemistry, 30th edition, Page 225, 558; Styer Biochemistry, 7th edition, Page 650*

6. **Hershey chase experiment was done on:**

(a) Lactobacillus (b) Tuberculous bacteria
(c) Bacteriophages (d) Mycoplasma

Explanation:

- Alfred Hershey and his assistant Martha Chase showed that the DNA, not the protein, of the phage virus contains the phage genes. After a phage particle attaches to a bacterium, its DNA enters through a tiny hole while its protein coat remains outside.
- In 1952, Hershey and Chase infected bacteria with T2 phages that had been radioactively labelled either in their DNA component (with 32P) or in their protein component (with 32S).The infected bacteria were agitated in a blender, and two fractions were separated by centrifugation.

- One contained the empty phage coats that were released from the surface of the bacteria; these consist of protein and therefore carried the 32S radioactive label. The other fraction consisted of the infected bacteria themselves. Most of the 32P label was present in the infected bacteria.
- The progeny phage particles produced by the infection contained 30% of the original 32P label. The progeny received very little less than 1% of the protein contained in the original phage population.
- This experiment therefore showed directly that the DNA of parent phages enters the bacteria and then becomes part of the progeny phages, exactly the pattern of inheritance expected of genetic material.

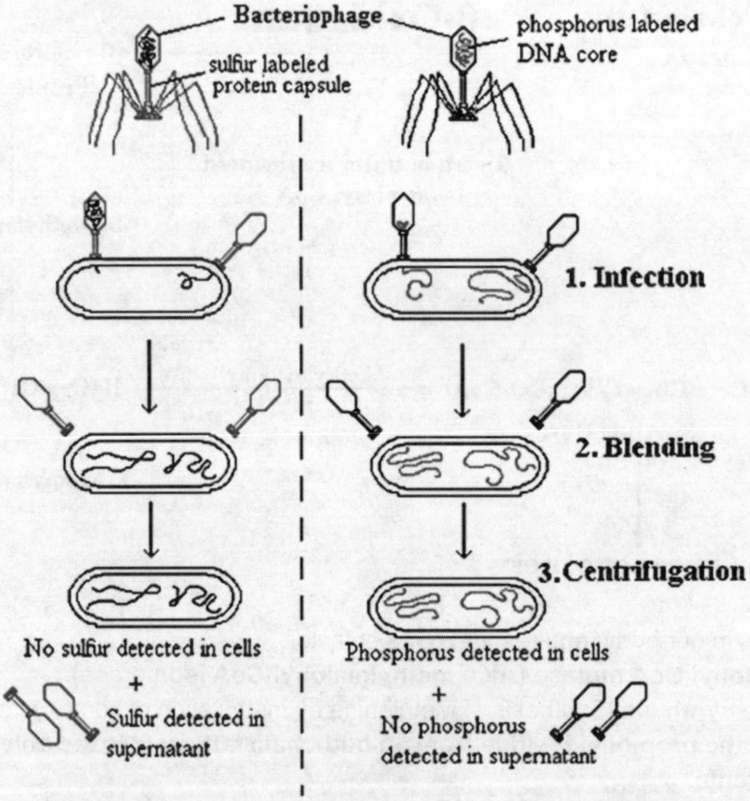

The Hershey-Chase Experiment

Ans: (c) Bacteriophages

Ref: Harper Illustrated Biochemistry, 30th edition

PHARMACOLOGY

1. **A patient comes 6 hours after consuming morphine and presents with pin point pupils and respiratory depression. T ½ of morpine is 3 hours and Volume of distribution (Vd) is 200 L. Plasma concentration is 0.5 microgram/ml. Calculate the initial morphine dose consumed.**

(a) 100 mg
(b) 400 mg
(c) 10 mg
(d) 50 mg

Explanation:

- Vd = 200 L
- T ½ = 3 hours
- Plasma concentration **after 6 hours** = **0.5 microgram/ml**
- T ½ = 3 hours, so Plasma concentration before 3 hours = **1 microgram/ml**
- Plasma concentration at the time of consumption = **2 microgram/ml** = **2 mg/L**
- So, applying the formula
- **Loading dose = Vd × plasma concentration (at time of consumption of morphine)**
- **Loading dose** = 200 × 2 = 400 mg

Ans: (b) 400 mg

Ref: *Goodman and Gillman's, The Pharmacological Basis of Therapeutics,13th edition, Page 28*

2. **False about Bedaquiline is:**

(a) Mycobacterial ATP synthase inhibitor
(b) Food intake decreases bioavailability
(c) It should be given alone
(d) It has cross resistance with clofazimine

Explanation:

Bedaquiline

- Anti-tuberculous drug used in the treatment of MDR TB.
- **MOA**:
  - o Mycobacterial **ATP synthase inhibitor***.
  - o It acts by inhibiting **proton pump activity** of the ATP synthase.
- Clofazimine-resistant Mycobacterium tuberculosis carries a mutation in the gene encoding a transcription repressor for efflux pump MmpL; this is associated with cross resistance to bedaquiline.
- It should **never** be given **alone**. If it is given as single drug it will lead to **resistance.**
- It should only be used in combination with at least 3 other drugs to which the patient's MDR-TB isolate has been shown to be susceptible in vitro.
- Bedaquiline should be taken **with food** to enhance its **oral bioavailability.**
- Interactions.
  - o CYP3A4 enzyme inducers like rifampicin reduces concentration of drug
  - o CYP3A4 enzyme inhibitors like Ketoconazole increases drug levels
- **Side effects:**
  - o Nausea, headache, chest pain
  - o Prolonged QT interval, Arrhythmias

Ans: (c) It should be given alone

Ref: *Goodman and Gillman's, The Pharmacological Basis of Therapeutics,12th edition, Page 1076*

3. **Antibiotics for treatment of Toxic shock syndrome (TSS):**

(a) Linezolid
(b) Clindamycin
(c) Cephalexin
(d) Quinupristin and dalfopristin

Explanation:

Antibiotics for treatment of Toxic shock syndrome (TSS)

- TSS is usually managed in the intensive care setting and the main line of management is **supportive management** along with **appropriate antibiotic therapy** to eradicate Staph. aureus which is mostly the causative organism.
- Because of the increasing frequency of methicillin-resistant Staphylococci in the community, **vancomycin** is often recommended*.
- Beta lactamase resistant penicillins are not very effective due to emerging resistance and they may increase TSST-1 production in vitro probably due to cell lysis. Hence, if they are prescribed they are usually coprescribed with **clindamycin** which inhibits bacterial protein toxin production.
- Other treatment options are a **combination of vancomycin and clindamycin** for suspected serious staphylococcal infections pending culture and sensitivity.
- **Intravenous immunoglobulin** (IVIG; which presumably acts in part via neutralizing antibodies against toxins) has been used and appears to have significant promise. At present, IVIG is used in severe or recalcitrant cases.

Treatment of choice:

- **Vancomycin** (15 mg/kg q12h) plus **Clindamycin** (600 mg q8h).
- If a penicillin or oxacillin-sensitive strain is isolated.
  - o Penicillin or Oxacillin can be given.
- **In severe cases:**
  - o IV immunoglobulins.

Ans: (b) Clindamycin

Ref: *Harrison, 19th edition, Page 780*

4. A hypertensive patient with BP 160/90 mm of Hg presents with increased level of Lipoprotein a. Which Hypolipidemic drug will you prescribe?

(a) Fenofibrate
(b) Pitavastatin
(c) Niacin
(d) Ezetimibe

Explanation:

- **Niacin** is the only drug that lowers lipoprotein (a).
- So, niacin may be preferable for individuals with **lipoprotein (a) elevations.**
- It causes maximum **HDL** increase among drugs used in dyslipidemia treatment.

Other options:

Fenofibrate

- It is a **fibric acid derivative**, acting through **PPAR alpha** receptor and activates **lipoprotein lipase.**
- It reduces **triglycerides.**

Pitavastatin

- **HMG CoA Reductase inhibitor.**
- Causes maximum reduction of **LDL.**

Ezetimibe

- It is a cholesterol ester transport inhibitor, inhibiting transport of cholesterol from intestine to circulation.
- It is used along with statins.

Ans: (c) Niacin

Ref: *SN Narasingan, Newer Lipid Guidelines: Interpretation and Applications for Indians. ttp://www.apiindia.org/pdf/medicine_update_2017/mu_155.pdf*

5. **Beta blocker which increases HDL:**

(a) Celiprolol
(b) Nebivolol
(c) Carvedilol
(d) Bucindolol

Explanation:

Bucindolol

- Third-generation nonselective β adrenergic antagonist with weak α1 adrenergic blocking property.
- **Increases** plasma **HDL cholesterol**, but does not affect plasma **Triglycerides**.

Celiprolol:

- Third-generation cardioselective β blocker.
- Has weak **vasodilating** and **bronchodilating** property.

Nebivolol:

- One more third-generation selective β1 blocker.
- Has **vasodilator** activity which is nitric oxide-mediated.
- Has **antioxidant** property.
- Has neutral to favorable effects on both carbohydrate and lipid metabolism.
- No negative effect on serum lipids.

Carvedilol:

- Third-generation β receptor antagonist.
- Blocks β1, β2 and α1 receptors and has **antioxidant** and **anti-inflammatory** effects.
- Prevents low density lipoprotein (LDL) oxidation, which in turn induces the uptake of LDL into the coronary vasculature.

Ans: (d) Bucindolol

***Ref**: Goodman and Gillman's, The Pharmacological Basis of Therapeutics, 12th edition, Page 329*

6. **Which is true about monoclonal antibodies?**

(a) Tofactinib inhibits JAK1 and JAK3
(b) Tocilizumab used in rheumatoid arthritis
(c) Tofactinib given IV
(d) Tocilizumab given IV and subcutaneous

Explanation:

Tofacitinib

- **Oral JAK inhibitor.**
- JAK inhibitor that primarily inhibits **JAK1 and JAK3** and to a lesser extent, JAK2.
- Approved for use in **rheumatoid arthritis** in adults.
- It has demonstrated efficacy for **psoriasis** in clinical trials and for **atopic dermatitis** in a pilot study.

Tocilizumab

- An **IL-6 receptor antagonist.**
- FDA-approved for treatment of:
  - o **Rheumatoid arthritis.**
  - o Systemic juvenile idiopathic arthritis.
- It is a mab, so need to be given parentally.
- Given as IV and subcutaneous.

Ans: Tofactinib given IV

***Ref:** Goodman and Gillman's, The Pharmacological Basis of Therapeutics, 13th edition, Page 1288*

7. **Which liver enzyme is elevated in Azathioprine toxicity?**

(a) GGT
(b) SGPT
(c) ALP
(d) TPMT

Explanation:

Azathioprine toxicity and liver enzymes:

- Mild serum **aminotransferase** elevations can occur during azathioprine therapy, particularly with high doses during the **first 12 weeks** of therapy.
- These elevations are generally asymptomatic, benign and self-limited, resolving rapidly either with stopping therapy and often even with continuing treatment at a lower dose.
- **ALT(SGPT)** elevations during azathioprine therapy may be due to a **direct toxic effect of the drug.**
- **ALT(SGPT)** elevations as well as **myelotoxicity** have been linked to higher levels of **methyl-mercaptopurine**, a product of one of the metabolic pathways of azathioprine metabolism.
- Azathioprine can also cause an acute, clinically apparent liver injury that is typically **cholestatic.**
  - o The acute cholestatic injury due to azathioprine usually presents with fatigue and **jaundice** after **2 to 12 months** of starting therapy.
- The serum **ALT and alkaline phosphatase** tend to be only mildly or moderately elevated and in a mixed cholestatic-hepatocellular pattern.

Ans: (b) SGPT

Ref: *https://livertox.nih.gov/Azathioprine.htm*

8. **Axicabtagene ciloleucel is used in:**

(a) Relapsed myeloma
(b) T cell lymphoma
(c) Diffuse large B cell lymphoma
(d) Small cell lung Ca

Explanation:

Axicabtagene ciloleucel

- It is a **CD19**-directed genetically modified autologous T cell immunotherapy
- **Chimeric antigen receptor (CAR) T cell therapy**
- **Anti-CD19 CAR T cell therapy**
- Used in the treatment of adult patients with:
  - o **Relapsed or refractory large B-cell lymphoma.**
  - o Diffuse large B-cell lymphoma.
  - o Primary mediastinal large B-cell lymphoma.
  - o High grade B-cell lymphoma.
  - o Diffuse large B-cell lymphoma arising from follicular lymphoma.

Note:

- It is not indicated for the treatment of patients with **primary central nervous system lymphoma.**

Ans: (c) Diffuse large B cell lymphoma

Ref: *https://www.fda.gov/downloads/UCM581226.pdf*

9. **Ibrutinib drug is used in all *except*:**

(a) Mantle cell lymphoma
(b) Chronic lymphocytic leukemia
(c) Waldenström's macroglobulinemia
(d) AML

Explanation:

Ibrutinib

- Kinase inhibitor indicated for the treatment of patients with:
  - o Mantle cell Lymphoma.
  - o Chronic lymphocytic leukemia.
  - o Chronic lymphocytic leukemia with 17p deletion.
  - o Waldenström's macroglobulinemia.
  - o Small lymphocytic lymphoma.

Mechanism of action:

- Small-molecule inhibitor of BTK (**Bruton's tyrosine kinase**).
- Forms a covalent bond with a cysteine residue in the BTK active site, leading to inhibition of BTK enzymatic activity.
- BTK is a signaling molecule of the B-cell antigen receptor (**BCR**) and cytokine receptor pathways.
- BTK's role in signaling through the B-cell surface receptors results in activation of pathways necessary for B-cell trafficking chemotaxis and adhesion.

Ans: (d) AML

Ref: *GG, 13th edition, Page 1232*

10. All adverse effects of theophylline are mediated by A_1 receptor *except*:

(a) Cardiac arrhythmias (b) Diuresis
(c) Seizures (d) GI discomfort

Explanation:

Theophylline

- Belongs to methylxanthines group of drugs.
- It has bronchodilator action and nonbronchodilator effects.
- It has various mechanisms of action:
  - o Inhibition of phosphodiesterases.
  - o Adenosine receptor antagonism.
  - o Interleukin-10 release.
  - o Prevents the translocation of the pro-inflammatory transcription factor NF-kB into the nucleus.
  - o Promotes apoptosis in eosinophils and neutrophils in vitro.
  - o Histone deacetylase activation.
- **Side Effects:**
  - o The most common side effects are headache, nausea and vomiting, abdominal discomfort and restlessness.

Side effects of theophylline and proposed mechanisms

Side effect	Proposed mechanism
Nausea and vomiting	PDE4 inhibition
Headache	PDE4 inhibition
Gastric discomfort	PDE4 inhibition
Diuresis	A1 receptor inhibition
Cardiac arrhythmias	PDE3 inhibition, A1 receptor inhibition
Epileptic seizures	A1 receptor inhibition

Ans: (d) GI discomfort

Ref: *Goodman and Gillman's, The Pharmacological Basis of Therapeutics 13th edition, Page 735*

11. Correct order based on Volume of distribution is:

(a) Haloperidol > Gentamicin > Phenytoin > Heparin
(b) Gentamicin >Haloperidol > Phenytoin > Heparin
(c) Phenytoin > Heparin > Gentamicin >Haloperidol
(d) Heparin < Gentamicin < Phenytoin < Haloperidol

Explanation

Factors affecting volume of distribution (Vd):

- Molecular weight of drug.
- Lipid solubility.
- Plasma protein binding.

- Tissue binding.
- Pathological conditions.
- Large molecular size of drug (remain in vascular compartment).
  - o **Heparin.**
- Low molecular weight drugs have high Vd.
- Plasma protein binding
  - o High plasma protein binding decreases Vd.
  - o Low plasma protein binding increases Vd.
- Tissue perfusion
  - o Decreased tissue perfusion implies decreased Vd.
- Water soluble drugs have low Vd.
  - o **Gentamicin.**
- Lipid soluble drugs have high Vd.
  - o Phenytoin, Haloperidol, Thiopentone.
- Acidic drugs have low Vd.
- In edematous condition, water soluble drugs have high volume of distribution.
- Tissue binding
  - o High Vd with higher tissue binding.
  - o Digoxin.
  - o Choroquine.

Vd of individual drugs:

- Heparin: 0.058 L/Kg.
- Gentamicin: 0.31 L/Kg.
- Phenytoin: 0.64 L/Kg.
- Haloperidol: 18 L/Kg.

Note:

- It is difficult to remember Vd of these drugs, so at least you should know that heparin has lowest Vd because of its molecular size.

Ans: (d) Heparin < gentamicin < phenytoin < haloperidol

Ref: *Goodman and Gillman's, The Pharmacological Basis of Therapeutics, 13th edition, Page 1349*

12. Which is correct among the following?

(a) Rilonacept approved for psoriatic arthritis
(b) Belimumab is used in SLE
(c) Efalizumab acts against IL 1
(d) Ocrelizumab is approved for rheumatoid arthritis

Explanation

Belimumab:

- Monoclonal antibody that inhibits **B cell activating factor (BAFF).**
- **BAFF** is also known as B lymphocyte stimulator (**BLYS**).
- Used in **systemic lupus erythromatosus (SLE).**
- Also tried in **Rheumatoid arthritis and Sjogren syndrome.**

Efalizumab:

- Anti–LFA-1.
- Binds to the **CD11a** subunit of **lymphocyte function-associated antigen 1 (LFA-1).**
- Inhibits lymphocyte activation and cell migration out of blood vessels into tissues.
- Used in **Psoriasis*.**
- **Side effects** – Bacterial sepsis, Viral meningitis, Invasive fungal disease, Progressive multifocal leukoencephalopathy (JC virus).

Ocrelizumab:

- Anti **CD-20** monoclonal antibody.
- Approved for **Multiple sclerosis.**

Rilonacept:

- Anti-IL-1
- Inhibitor of Interleukin-1
- Used in **Rheumatoid arthritis, cryopyrin-associated syndromes**
- Tried in **gout**

Ans: (b) Belimumab is used in SLE

Ref: Goodman and Gillman's, The Pharmacological Basis of Therapeutics, 13th edition, Page 649

13. The drug having higher concentration in the bone:

(a) Piperacillin (b) Vancomycin
(c) Clindamycin (d) Paramomycin

Explanation:

Clindamycin

- Widely distributed in many fluids and tissues.
- **Achieves good concentrations in bone.**
- CSF concentrations are limited even when the meninges are inflamed, but concentrations sufficient to treat cerebral toxoplasmosis are achievable.
- Drug readily **crosses** the **placental barrier.**
- Ninety percent or more of clindamycin is bound to plasma proteins.
- Clindamycin accumulates in polymorphonuclear leukocytes and alveolar macrophages and in abscesses.

Note:

- Beta lactams and vancomycin don't achieve very good concentration in bone.

Paromomycin (aminosidine)

- Aminoglycoside of the neomycin/kanamycin family.
- Used as an oral agent to treat E. histolytica infection, cryptosporidiosis and Giardiasis.
- It doesn't achive good concentration in bone.

Ans: (c) Clindamycin

Ref: Goodman and Gillman's, The Pharmacological Basis of Therapeutics, 13th edition, Page 1056

14. Treatment of ventilator associated pneumonia (VAP) caused by MDR Acinetobacter baumannii is:

(a) Quinupristin and dalfopristim (b) Colistimethate sodium
(c) Lavendamycin (d) Tedizolid

Explanation:

Acinetobacter baumannii

- Non-fermentative, aerobic, gram-negative coccobacilli, non-lactose-fermenting and oxidase negative microorganism.
- Multiple mechanisms have been implicated in the resistance of Acinetobacter species.
- It is considered one of the most virulent MDR pathogens.
- Acinetobacter has been isolated in food and inanimate objects and may colonize humans and survive on dry or moist environment.

Treatment

- Aminoglycosides.
- Carbapenems
  - o Were considered for many years the mainstay of therapy of VAP caused by Acinetobacter spcies.
  - o Due to emergence of carbapenem-resistant Acinetobacter infection.
- For resistant cases.
- **Colistin**
  - o Effective **drug for resistant Ventilator-Associated Pneumonia (VAP) caused by Acinetobacter species.**
  - o Has dose-dependent neurotoxicity and nephrotoxicity.

- **Tigecycline**
  - o Safe broad spectrum tetracycline
  - o It has displayed inhibitory activity against Acinetobacter spp

Lavendamycin:

- Naturally occurring derived from Streptomyces lavendulae.
- Has antibiotic properties and significant anti-proliferative effects against several cancer cell lines.
- Not used now-a-days due to serious adverse effects.

Ans: (b) Colistimethate sodium

Ref: *Garnacho-Montero et al., BMC Infectious Diseases, 2014, 14:135*

15. Warfarin embryopathy is due to action of:

(a) Osteophysin
(b) Osteotensin
(c) Osteocalcin
(d) Osteogenin

Explanation:

Warfarin embryopathy

- The process of **osteocalcin** carboxylation in human bone formation is a **vitamin K-dependent** process and that **circulating osteocalcin** will be altered structurally by **warfarin administration**
- This finding has pathophysiological implications for:
  - o **Fetal warfarin embryopathy syndrome**
  - o Bone disease associated with chronic liver diseases
  - o Osteoporosis
- In all the above conditions vitamin K deficiency has been implicated

Note:

- The similarity between fetal warfarin syndrome and X-linked recessive chondroplasia puntata has suggested a common pathogenesis for these two disorders. Warfarin appears to inhibit arylsulfatase, a genetically determined deficiency which is responsible for chondroplasia puntata.

Ans: (c) Osteocalcin

Ref: *http://memo.cgu.edu.tw/cgmj/2709/270908.pdf*

16. Correctly matched dose of drugs used in gout is:

(a) Febuxostat 40 – 80 mg OD
(b) Probencid – 2000g OD
(c) Sulphinpyrazole 1500 mg OD
(d) Benzbromarone 15 mg OD

Explanation:

Doses of drug used in Gout

Febuxostat:

- 40–80 mg OD.

Probenecid:

- Second line/adjuvant drug to Allopurinol.
- Started at 0.25 g BD and increased to 0.5 g BD.

Sulphinpyrazole:

- The starting dose of sulfinpyrazole is usually 100 mg or 200 mg a day (one-half of a 100 mg tablet two times a day, one 100 mg tablet one or two times a day, or one 200 mg capsule or tablet once a day).
- Then, the dose is usually increased by 100 mg or 200 mg every few days, up to 800 mg a day.

Benzbromarone:

- The usual dose of Benzbromarone is 100 mg per day.
- Doses of 50 – 200 mg per day may be used.

Ans: (a) Febuxostat 40 – 80 mg OD

Ref: *KDT, 7th edition, Page 217*

PATHOLOGY

1. **BCL 2 protein is located in:**

(a) Cell membrane
(b) Mitochondria
(c) Nucleus
(d) Cytosol

Explanation:

BCL 2

- BCL 2 is a human **proto-oncogene** located on **chromosome 18**
- BCL 2 is involved in **apoptosis**
- BCL 2 is involved in the **intrinsic (mitochondrial) phase** of the **initiation pathway**
- It's anti-apoptotic. **BCL 2, BCL-XL, and MCL1** are the principal members of this group
- The normal location of **BCL 2** – in on the **mitochondrial membrane.**
- When cells are deprived of survival signals or their DNA is damaged, or misfolded proteins induce ER stress, the BH3-only proteins "sense" such damage and are activated.
- BH3 only proteins antagonize BCL 2 and the pro-apoptotic factors are activated, which lets the Cytochrome C in the cytosol – activating the apoptotic cascade.

Ans: (b) Mitochondria

Ref: *Robbins Pathology, 9th edition, Page 55*

2. **A 40-year-old woman is on treatment for CLL. Over the past few months she noticed swellings in the neck and axilla which was rapidly increasing in size. She complains of feeling feverish and experiences weight loss. Which of the following is responsible?**

(a) Richter transformation
(b) Progression of CLL
(c) EBV infection
(d) Immunodeficient hemolytic anemia

Explanation:

Richter Syndrome

- Transformation of CLL into an **aggressive lymphoma** (most commonly **diffuse large B-cell lymphoma**) occurs in **5–10%** of all cases.
- The syndrome may be suspected if there are **signs of aggressive disease**, such as:
  - o **Impairment of performance status**
  - o **Presence of B symptoms,** and
  - o **Rapid increase in the size of lymph nodes**

Pro Lymphocytic Leukemia (PLL)

- **CLL** can progress to **PLL** (Pro lymphocytic leukemia)
- PLL generally presents with **Splenomegaly**, more WBC count and low platelet count. Those are the symptoms
- **Elderly men** with **peripheral blood lymphocytosis > 100,000**, marked **splenomegaly**
- 80% are B cell, 20% are T cell
- B-PLL has better prognosis than T-PLL patients, but still considered incurable
- Pro lymphocytes in peripheral blood are large cells with scant to moderate pale blue agranular cytoplasm, round to polygonal nuclei and prominent central nucleoli; may have occasional nuclear grooves
- T pro lymphocytes have very irregular nuclear outlines and cytoplasmic protrusions or blebs

Ans: (a) Richter transformation

Ref: *WHO, 2016, Page 220*

3. **Palatal edema is significant for:**

(a) Alpha heavy chain disease
(b) Gamma heavy chain disease
(c) Mu chain disease
(d) Beta heavy chain disease

Explanation:

- The **heavy chain diseases (HCDs)** are three rare B-cell neoplasms characterized by the production of monoclonal immunoglobulin heavy chains (**IgG in gamma HCD, IgA in alpha HCD and IgM in mu HCD**) and **typically no light chains.**

Gamma Heavy Chain Disease – Also known as Franklin Disease

- The disease involves the **lymph nodes, Waldeyer ring, gastrointestinal tract** predominantly.
- **Clinical Features:**
  - o **Autoimmune manifestations** are reported in **25-70%** of cases.
  - o Involvement of the **Waldeyer ring** – presents with **Palatal Edema*.**
- Cell of origin – A **post-germinal centre B cell** that can differentiate into a plasma cell.
- IHC
  - o The cells express **CD79a** and **cytoplasmic gamma chain** and are **negative for CD5 and CD10.**
  - o **Kappa** and **lambda** light chains are typically **NOT** expressed.

Ans: (b) Gamma heavy chain disease

Ref: *WHO, 2016, Page 235-237*

4. **Gastrin is a marker of which carcinoma?**

(a) Medullary carcinoma of thyroid
(b) GIST
(c) Gastric carcinoma
(d) Pancreatic carcinoma / neuroectodermal tumour

Explanation:

Pancreatic Neuroendocrine Tumour

Insulinoma	**Hypoglycemia**
Gastrinoma	Severe peptic ulceration
VIPoma	Watery diarrhea, hypokalemia, achlorhydria (WDHA syndrome)
Glucagonoma	Glucose intolerance, necrolytic migratory erythema, stomatitis/ glossitis, hypoaminoacidemia
Somatostatinoma	Hyperglycemia, cholelithiasis, steatorrhea, achlorhydria

Gastrinoma:

- Second most common functioning **pancreatic neuroendocrine tumor.**
- Tumour cells secrete **Gastrin.**
- Zollinger-Ellison syndrome (peptic ulcers, gastroesophageal reflux, diarrhea).
- "**Gastrinoma triangle**" (common bile duct, duodenum, pancreatic head).
- **Gastrin** is a serum marker.
- **Duodenum** affected more than pancreas.
- 20 - 30% of gastrinomas are associated with **MEN-1*.**
- Malignant in **80%.**

Ans: (d) Pancreatic carcinoma / neuroectodermal tumour

Ref: *Sternberg Surgical Pathology, Page 1478*

5. **True about single donor platelet transfusion:**

(a) Equal to 6-8 RDP
(b) Stored in 2-6 degree
(c) 10 days shelf life
(d) Bedside leukodepletion done

Explanation:

Random Donor Platelets

- Platelets prepared from whole blood are often referred to as random donor platelet concentrates.
- Platelet rich plasma is separated from red blood cells by centrifugation at a low G force within 4 hours after donation.
- Platelets can be **preserved for 5 days** under these conditions. Platelet concentrates are pooled immediately prior to transfusion and can then be **stored for 4 hours.**
- **Stored at 20 to 24 degree Celsius with continuous agitation.**

Single Donor Platelets

- Apheresis platelets are usually called single donor platelets because they are collected from a single donor with an automated cell separator.
- A single donor platelet concentrate contains a minimum of 3.0×10^{11} platelets suspended in approximately 200 mL of plasma, which is the equivalent of **6 to 8 random donor platelet concentrates RDP**.
- They can be stored **up to 5 days (Shelf life).**
- **Stored at 22 to 24 degree celsius.**
- Leukocyte reduction during collection eliminates the need for bedside filtration.

Ans: (a) Equal to 6-8 RDP

***Ref:** Manual of Blood Transfusion Protocol – ISHTM*

6. **Ring sideroblast in myelodysplastic syndrome is associated with which gene mutation?**

(a) ASXL1 (b) EZH2
(c) TET2 (d) SF3B1

Explanation:

Ring Sideroblast

- **Myelodysplastic syndrome (MOS) with ring sideroblasts (MOS-RS)** is an MOS characterized by:
  - o **Cytopenias**
  - o **Morphological dysplasia**
  - o **Ring sideroblasts** usually constituting $\geq$**15%** of the bone marrow erythroid precursors
- Secondary causes of ring sideroblasts must be excluded.
- There is associated **SF3B1 mutation** in most cases, and in the presence of such mutation, the diagnosis can be made with $\geq$ 5% marrow ring sideroblasts.
- **Myeloblasts** account for **< 5%** of the nucleated bone marrow cells and < 1% of peripheral blood leukocytes.
- **Auer rods are absent**, and the diagnostic criteria for MOS with isolated del (5q) are not fulfilled.

Two categories of MOS-RS are recognized.

- In **MOS** with **ring sideroblasts** and **single lineage dysplasia** (MOS-RS- SLO), patients present with **anaemia and dysplasia is limited to the erythroid lineage.**
- In **MOS** with **ring sideroblasts and multilineage dysplasia** (MOS-RS-MLO), patients present with any number of **cytopenias**, and significant **dysplasia** is present in **two or three haematopoietic lineages.**

Ans: (d) SF3B1

***Ref:** WHO, 2016, Page 109*

7. **Which of the following is correctly matched in RPGN?**

(a) Type 1 IgA nephropathy
(b) Type 2 Anti-GBM antibody
(c) Type 2 – Wegener's granulomatosis
(d) Type 2 – SLE nephritis

Explanation:

TYPE I (ANTI-GBM ANTIBODY)	
• Renal limited • Goodpasture syndrome	**IF findings:** Linear GBM deposits of IgG and C3
TYPE II (IMMUNE COMPLEX)	
• Idiopathic • Post-infectious glomerulonephritis • Lupus nephritis • Henoch-Schönlein purpura (IgA nephropathy)	**IF findings:** "**Lumpy bumpy**" granular pattern of staining
TYPE III (PAUCI-IMMUNE)	
• ANCA-associated • Idiopathic • Wegener granulomatosis • Microscopic polyangiitis	**IF findings:** No immunoglobulin or complement deposits in GBM

Ans: (d) Type 2 – SLE nephritis

Ref: *Robbin's Patholgoy, 9th edition, Page 912*

8. **True regarding 'Bare lymphocytes syndrome':**

(a) Autosomal recessive
(b) Part of SCID
(c) MHC overexpression
(d) MHC non-expression

Explanation:

Bare Lymphocyte Syndrome

- Bare lymphocyte syndrome (BLS) encompasses a series of rare autosomal recessive disorders in which patients display **low or null expression of HLA major histocompatibility proteins**.
- Both the types have **Autosomal Recessive** Inheritance.
- Two types of BLS have been classified, with the severity of these disorders varying both in phenotypic HLA expression and loss of immune function.
    - In **BLS type I**, low or no expression of HLA **class I** molecules are displayed on **peripheral blood cells**. The degree of immunodeficiency is most variable in BLS type I, with some individuals displaying essentially normal immunity.
    - **Type II BLS** is defined as a reduction or complete loss of **HLA class II** protein expression on all cells. This disorder typically manifests as a **severe combined immunodeficiency**.

Ans: (d) MHC non-expression

Ref: *Genetic, Home Reference*

9. **Origin of lymphoplasmacytic lymphoma (Waldenstorm Macroglobulinemia) is from:**

(a) Germinal centre T cell
(b) Germinal centre B cell
(c) Post germinal centre B cell
(d) Pre germinal centre B cell

Explanation:

Waldenstorm Macroglobulinemia [also known as Lymphoplasmacytic lymphoma (LPL)]

- Neoplasm of **plasma cells**, **lymphocytes** and **plasmacytoid lymphocytes**
- **Post germinal centre B cell**
- Often associated with **IgM** paraprotein (not essential for diagnosis)

- **Waldenstorm's macroglobulinemia** = LPL + Bone marrow involvement + IgM monoclonal gammopathy of any concentration
- **Hepatitis C** association seen
- **Hyperviscosity** in 30% patients
- **Coagulopathy** may occur (IgM binding to platelets, clotting factors and fibrin)

IHC

- CD 19, CD 20, CD 22, CD 79a and CD 38 positive
- CD 5, CD 23, CD 10 negative

Treatment

- Alkylating agents are used as a part of **RCD regimen** – Rituximab Cyclophosphamide Dexamethasone

Ans: (c) Post germinal centre B cell

Ref: *WHO, 2016, Page 236*

10. In Alibert bazin syndrome, origin of lymphoma is from:

(a) Eosinophil
(b) B lymphocyte
(c) Monocyte
(d) T lymphocyte

Explanation:

- **Alibert bazin syndrome** is the other name of **Mycosis Fungoides.** Think now, the answer will be much easier.

Mycosis Fungoides (MF)

- Epidermotropic, **primary cutaneous T cell lymphoma** (CTCL).
- Characterized by infiltrates of **small to medium sized T lymphocytes** with **cerebriform nuclei.**

Stages

- **Patch stage**: Superficial band-like or lichenoid infiltrate, mainly lymphocytes and histiocytes but also a few atypical cells (small / medium sized, cerebriform nuclei, halo) usually confined to the epidermis (basal layer).
- **Plaque stage**: More pronounced epidermotropism with occasional characteristic intraepidermal collections of atypical cells (Pautrier microabscesses).
- **Tumor stage:** More diffuse dermal infiltrate, may lose epidermotropism, more size and shape variability of tumor cells, histologic transformation may occur (> 25% large lymphoid cells in the dermal infiltrate).

IHC

- CD 4, CD 3, CD 5 and CD 5 - Positive
- CD 7, CD 8 - Negative

Ans: (d) T lymphocyte

Ref: *WHO, Hematology, Page 385*

11. Vinyl chloride is associated with:

(a) Hemangiosarcoma
(b) Hepatoma
(c) Testicular carcinoma
(d) Thyroid malignancy

Explanation:

Chemical Carcinogens

Chemicals	Associated tumours
Arsenic and arsenic compounds	Lung carcinoma, skin carcinoma
Asbestos	Lung, esophageal, gastric and colon carcinoma; mesothelioma
Benzene	Acute myeloid leukemia
Beryllium and beryllium compounds	Lung carcinoma

Contd.

Contd.

Cadmium and cadmium compounds	**Prostate carcinoma***
Chromium compounds	Lung carcinoma
Nickel compounds	Lung and oropharyngeal carcinoma
Radon and its decay products	Lung carcinoma
Vinyl chloride	**Hepatic angiosarcoma***

Ans: (a) Hemangiosarcoma

***Ref:** Robbins, 9th edition, Page 278*

12. Which antibody is associated with reduced risk of lupus nephritis in SLE?

(a) Anti-ribosomal
(b) Anti-Ro
(c) Anti La
(d) ANA

Explanation:

SLE and Antibodies

- **Most sensitive** antibody – **ANA** (Anti-Nuclear Antibody).
- **Drug** induced Lupus–**Anti-histone antibodies**.
- Most specific antibody in "Neonatal lupus with congenital heart block" is **Anti Ro (SS-A).**
- **Antibody** in SLE predisposes to **photo toxicity – anti-RO (=SS-A) antibody.**
- **Antibody** with decrease risk of **Lupus Nephritis – Anti La (=SS-B) antibody.**
- "**Shrinking lung syndrome**" is characteristically associated with **anti-RO (=SS-A) antibody**.
- **Raynaud's phenomenon** in SLE is associated with **anti-U1 Ribonucleoprotein** (anti-U1 RNP) antibody.

Ans: (c) Anti La

***Ref:** A Compilation from Different Books*

13. Blau syndrome is associated with mutation of:

(a) NOD2/CARD 15 gene
(b) NOD1/CARD 1 gene
(c) NOD2/CARD 10 gene
(d) NOD3/CARD 12 gene

Explanation:

Blau's syndrome

- Caused by mutations in ***CARD15* (also known as *NOD2*)**, which regulates nuclear factor-κB activation.
- The protein produced from this gene helps defend the body from foreign invaders, such as viruses and bacteria, by playing several essential roles in the immune response, including inflammatory reactions.
- Inheritance – **Autosomal dominant.**
- Blau's syndrome is characterized by **granulomatous dermatitis, uveitis and arthritis**; distinct CARD15 variants predispose to **Crohn's disease.**
- Recessive mutations in one or more components of the proteasome lead to excessive interferon signaling and the syndrome of **chronic atypical neutrophilic dermatosis with lipodystrophy and elevated temperature** (**CANDLE**), a severe form of generalized panniculitis.

Ans: (a) NOD2/CARD 15 gene

***Ref:** Harrison, 19th edition, Page 2215 and Genetic Home Reference*

14. BK virus infection – True statement is:

(a) Causes nephropathy in transplant patients
(b) Causes progressive multifocal leukoencephalopathy
(c) 20 – 25% transplant cases associated with BK virus nephropathy
(d) Single stranded DNA virus

Explanation:

BK Virus

- BK virus is a **non-enveloped double-strand DNA virus** which belongs to family **polyoma viridae.**
- Primary BKV infection occurs by the upper respiratory route until age 10 without any obvious symptoms.
- 80% of the population is infected by BKV, and approximately 50% of healthy native kidneys contain latent BKV.
- **After renal transplantation, 35–60%** of patients have BKV viruria, 5–30% of patients have BKV viremia.
- The prevalence of BKV nephropathy is about **10%** of renal transplant patients.
- Progressive multifocal leukoencephalopathy is caused by JC virus (belongs to polyoma viridae).

Ans: (a) Causes nephropathy in transplant patients

Ref: *Harrison, 19th edition*

15. DITRA syndrome is associated with mutation in:

(a) IL - 36 (b) IL - 46
(c) IL - 10 (d) IL - 26

Explanation:

DITRA Syndrome

- DITRA is an **autosomal recessive** disorder due to the genetic deletion of **IL36RN**, the gene encoding the **IL-36 receptor antagonist.**
- **IL-36** has proinflammatory effects in **keratinocytes 78**; loss of the IL-36-receptor antagonist potentiates IL-36-mediated inflammation in keratinocytes.
- IL-36 is a member of the **IL-1 cytokine superfamily.**
- Homozygous or compound heterozygous IL36RN gene mutations are the cause of different clinical features of **psoriasis** including generalized pustular psoriasis, palmoplantar pustular psoriasis, acrodermatitis continua Hallopeau and acute generalized exanthematous pustular eruption.
- DITRA is characterized by intra-epidermal neutrophilic spongiform pustules, acanthosis with elongation of rete ridges, and parakeratosis in the stratum corneum.

The recessively inherited deficiency of the IL-36 receptor antagonist (**DITRA**) presents with episodes of **generalized pustular psoriasis** and **dramatic systemic inflammation.**

Ans: (a) IL-36

Ref: *Harrison's 19th edition, Page 2215, Genetic Home Reference*

16. CNS involvement in DLBCL is not seen with which of the following organ involvement:

(a) Ovary (b) Testis
(c) Kidney (d) Adrenal

Explanation:

CNS Diffuse Large B Cell Lymphoma (DLBCL)

- Primary CNS lymphomas (PCNSLs) account for 2.4-3% of all brain tumours and 4-6% of all extranodal lymphomas.
- Most common location – **Supratentorial region.**
- PCNSL can affect patients of **any age**, with a peak incidence during the fifth to seventh decade of life.
- CNS lymphoma are at increase risk when DLBCL involves **kidney** and **adrenals**, and **testicular** DLBCL is closely linked with CNS DLBCL.
- **MRI** is the **most sensitive** technique to detect PCNSL, which is hypointense on T1-weighted images, isointense to hyperintense on T2-weighted images.
- **Stereotactic biopsy*** is the **gold standard** for establishing the diagnosis and classification of CNS lymphoma.
- PCNSLs are highly cellular, diffusely growing, patternless tumours. Centrally, large areas of geographical necrosis are common, and may harbour viable perivascular lymphoma islands.
- **IHC** - The tumour cells are **mature B cells** with a **PAX5-positive, CD19-positive, CD20- positive, CD22-positive, CD79a-positive phenotype**.

Ans: (a) Ovary

Ref: *WHO, CNS 2017, Page 272*

17. Para proteins are seen in all *except*:

(a) CLL (b) RA
(c) Scleroderma (d) Lymphoma

Explanation:

All of them have paraproteins Sir, this question the recall I got also is the same. Not sure about this. Since all of the above disorders can have paraproteins.

Causes of Paraproteins

A. Malignant B-cell disorders

- Multiple myeloma (IgG, IgA, IgD, IgE, or κ, λ free light chains), Symptomatic myeloma, Asymptomatic myeloma, Plasma cell leukaemia, Non-secretory myeloma, MGUS.
- **POEMS** syndrome–Polyneuropathy, organomegaly, endocrinopathy, M-protein, skin changes.
- Plasmacytoma.

B. Lymphoproliferative disorders

- Chronic lymphocytic leukaemia, Non-Hodgkin lymphomas including lymphoplasmacytic lymphoma (Waldenstrom macroglobulinemia).
- Heavy chain disease γ, α, μ.

C. Non-malignant systemic disease

- Autoimmune disease: Rheumatoid arthritis, Scleroderma, Hashimoto thyroiditis.
- Cutaneous disease: Pyoderma gangrenosum, Necrobiotic xanthogranulomatosis.
- Amyloidosis (AL).
- Liver disease: Hepatitis/cirrhosis.
- Infectious disease: Mycobacterium tuberculosis, Bacterial endocarditis.

Ans: None

18. Which of the following is Autosomal dominant disorder?

(a) Bests disease (b) Laurence-Moon Biedl syndrome
(c) Bassen-Kornzweig syndrome (d) Usher syndrome

Explanation:

- Best Disease – This is an easy question, old repeat question.

Autosomal dominant disorders

System	Disorder
Nervous	**Huntington disease** **Neurofibromatosis** Myotonic dystrophy **Tuberous sclerosis** **Best disease**
Urinary	Polycystic kidney disease
Gastrointestinal	Familial polyposis coli
Hematopoietic	Hereditary spherocytosis von Willebrand disease
Skeletal	**Marfan syndrome*** Ehlers-Danlos syndrome (some variants) Osteogenesis imperfecta **Achondroplasia**
Metabolic	Familial hypercholesterolemia **Acute intermittent porphyria**

Ans: (a) Bests disease

***Ref:** Robbins Pathology, 9th edition, Genetics Chapter*

19. Eosin-5-Maleamide flow cytometry is used for diagnosis of:

(a) G6PD
(b) Hereditary spherocytosis
(c) Sickle cell anemia
(d) Alpha thalassemia

Explanation:

Hereditary Spherocytosis

- AD inheritance
- Most common mutation – **Ankyrin***
- Most severe mutation **Spectrin***
- The spherocytes of HS have 2 defects:
  - o Reduced deformability
  - o Reduced membrane plasticity

Peripheral smear

- Spherocytes
- Howell jolly bodies – post splenectomy
- Hemolysis – Extravascular

Diagnosis

- Peripheral smear
- Osmotic fragility test – Screening
- **Gold standard – Flow cytometry – EMA (Eosin-5-Maleamide) Flowcytometry**

EMA Flowcytometry

- A flowcytometric test based on **eosin-5-maleamide (EMA)** which binds to band 3 of red cell membrane is a sensitive and specific test for diagnosis of HS.
- The mean fluorescence intensity of EMA tagged red cells is lower in HS (MCF < 0.80).
- EMA fluorescence is normal or increased in AIHA (DD for spherocytosis).

Ans: (b) Hereditary spherocytosis

***Ref:** Wintrobe's Hematology, compiled*

20. Most immunogenic RBC blood group system:

(a) Kell
(b) Duffy
(c) Kidd
(d) K antigen

Explanation:

Few High Yield Points Related to Blood Group Antigens (From Harrison)

- **A and B antigens** are secreted by the cells and are present in the circulation.
- Nonsecretors are susceptible to a variety of infections (e.g., Candida albicans, Neisseria meningitidis, Streptococcus pneumoniae, Haemophilus influenzae) because many organisms may bind to polysaccharides on cells.
- Antibodies to Lewis system carbohydrate antigens are the most common cause of incompatibility during pretransfusion screening.
- MNSsU system is regulated by genes on chromosome 4.
- The immunogenicity of **Kell** is third behind the **ABO** and **Rh systems.**
- The absence of the Kell precursor protein (controlled by a gene on X) is associated with acanthocytosis, shortened RBC survival, and a progressive form of muscular dystrophy that includes cardiac defects. This rare condition is called the McLeod phenotype.

- The **Duffy antigens** are codominant alleles, **Fya and Fyb, that** also serve as receptors for **Plasmodium vivax.**
- The naturally occurring anti-A and anti-B antibodies are termed isoagglutinins are IgM.
- Autoantibodies (antibodies against autologous blood group antigens) arise spontaneously or as the result of infectious sequelae (e.g., from Mycoplasma pneumoniae) and are also often IgM.
- IgG antibodies can cross the placenta and bind fetal erythrocytes bearing the corresponding antigen, resulting in hemolytic disease of the newborn, or hydrops fetalis.

Ans: (a) Kell

***Ref:** Harrison, 19th edition, Page 138*

21. Contraindication for platelet transfusion are all *except:*

(a) Flavivirus infection
(b) Thrombotic thrombocytopenic purpura (TTP)
(c) Immune thrombocytopenic purpura (ITP)
(d) Heparin induced thrombocytopenia

Explanation:

Platelet concentrates (PC)
- Same as for whole blood. Replacement of red cells in anaemic patients.

Description:
- PCs are prepared from units of whole blood that have not been allowed to cool below +20°C. A single donor unit consists of 50-60 mL plasma that should contain ≥55 × 109 platelets.

Unit of issue:
- PCs may be supplied as a pooled unit, i.e., platelets prepared from 4-6 donor units containing at least 240 × 10^9 platelets.

Infection risk:
- Bacterial contamination affects about 1% of pooled units.

Storage:
- PCs may be stored for up to 5 days at +20°C to +24°C (with agitation). PCs require continuous agitation during storage, on a platelet shaker and in an incubator that maintains the required storage temperature.

Dosage:
- 1 unit of platelet concentrate/10 kg; for an adult of 60-70 kg, 4-6 single donor units containing at least 240 × 10^9 platelets should raise the platelet count by 20-40 × 10^9/L. Increment will be less if there is splenomegaly, disseminated intravascular coagulation (DIC) or septicaemia.

Indications:
- Treatment of bleeding due to:
  - o Thrombocytopenia.
  - o Platelet function defects.
  - o Prevention of bleeding due to thrombocytopenia as in bone marrow failure.

Contraindications:
- Idiopathic autoimmune thrombocytopenic purpura (ITP).
- Thrombotic thrombocytopenic purpura (TTP).
- Heparin induced thrombocytopenia.
- Congenital IgA deficiency.
- Untreated DIC.
- Thrombocytopenia associated with septicaemia or in cases of hypersplenism.

Ans: (a) Flavivirus infection

***Ref:** WHO, Manual of Blood Transfusion*

22. All of the following are seen in RASopathies *except:*

(a) Hair abnormalities
(b) Craniofacial abnormalities
(c) Keratosis pilaris
(d) Desquamation of skin

Explanation:

- This is an entirely new topic, not for an undergraduate. Know the below and no need to learn anything more for a normal exam. Any further questions of this difficult nature will not be a competition in exams as almost for every student these questions will be a Doosra.

RASopathies include:

- Neurofibromatosis type 1 (NF1)
- Noonan syndrome (NS)
- Noonan syndrome with multiple lentigines (NSML)
- Capillary malformation–ateriovenous malformation syndrome (CM-AVM)
- Costello syndrome (CS)
- Cardio-facio-cutaneous syndrome (CFC)
- Legius syndrome.

Skin Findings

- Ectodermal findings typically consist of sparse, curly hair with sparse eyebrows and eyelashes, hyperkeratosis, keratosis pilaris, hemangioma, ichthyosis and progressively forming nevi.
- Desquamation of skin is not a finding in RAS-o-Pathies.

Ans: (d) Desquamation of skin

***Ref:** Genetic Home Reference*

23. Which of the following is true about Nodular Regenerative Hyperplasia?

(a) Nodule size 0.1 to 1 cm
(b) Fibrosis septa present
(c) Portal hypertension seen in 50% of patients
(d) AST and ALT are markedly elevated

Explanation:

Features of Nodular Regenerative Hyperplasia of Liver

- Nodular hyperplasia diffusely affecting entire liver but with no / minimal fibrous septa
- Develops at all ages but usually symptomatic at age 40+
- Associated with:
  - o Portal hypertension
  - o Connective tissue disease (rheumatoid arthritis, polyarteritis nodosa)
  - o Myeloproliferative disorders
  - o Lymphoproliferative disorders
  - o Vascular disorders
  - o Chemotherapy
  - o Immunosuppressive drugs
- AST – ALT mild elevation or normal
- Presents as non-cirrhotic portal hypertension

Pathology (Gross and Microscopy)

- 1-3 mm diameter nodules
- No fibrosis, only nodules
- On biopsy, apparent lack of central veins and presence of curvilinear areas of congestion are suggestive
- Reticulin stain highlights the fibrous nature

Ans: (c) Portal hypertension seen in 50% of patients

***Ref:** Robbins Pathology, 9th edition*

24. Most common tumor in tuberous sclerosis in females:

(a) Rhabdomyosarcoma
(b) Angiomyolipoma
(c) Pulmonary lymphangiomyositosis
(d) Optic glioma

Explanation:

Tumours in tuberous sclerosis

- **Renal angiomyolipomas** develop in as many as 80% of people with tuberous sclerosis by the age of 10 years.
- **Lymphangioleiomyomatosis** is present in as many as 40% of adult women with tuberous sclerosis. Though the incidence is more common in women than in men, since the question also has angiomyolipoma I personally prefer to go for renal angiomyolipomas.
- If the question comes in future without angiomyolipomas – go for Lymphangioleiomyomatosis – since the overall incidence of it is 1-4% (WHO) and in women it is close to 40% (WHO).

Diagnostic criteria for tuberous sclerosis

Major features • > 3 hypomelanotic macules > 5 mm in diameter • > 3 angiofibromas or fibrous cephalic plaque • > 2 ungual fibromas • Shagreen patch • Multiple retinal hamartomas • Cortical dysplasias (including tubers and cerebral white matter radial migration lines) • Subependymal nodules • Subependymal giant cell astrocytoma • Cardiac rhabdomyoma • Lymphangioleiomyomatosis • > 2 angiomyolipomas
Minor features *Confetti skin lesions* • > 4 dental enamel pits • > 2 intraoral fibromas, Retinal achromic patch, Multiple renal cysts, Non-renal hamartomas
Definitive diagnosis; 2 major features or 1 major feature with > 2 minor features
Possible diagnosis: 1 major feature or 2 minor features

Ans: (b) Angiomyolipoma

Ref: *Robbins Pathology, 9th edition*

25. True about BCR- ABL 'traits' are all *except*:

(a) P190 has an indolent course
(b) P190 is a bad prognostic factor
(c) P230 is positive in chronic neutrophilic leukemia
(d) P230 has an indolent course

Explanation:

Chronic myeloid leukemia (CML) is characterized by the **Philadelphia (Ph) chromosome**, which results from the **t(9;22)(q34;q11) balanced reciprocal translocation.**

- Three breakpoint cluster regions have been characterized to date: **major (M-BCR), minor (m-BCR) and micro (mu-BCR).**
- The smallest of the fusion proteins, **p190BCR-ABL** (m-BCR breakpoint) is principally associated with **Ph-positive ALL.**
- **P190** transcript is associated with a **poor prognosis.**
- **CML** due to a p90-type of BCR-ABL gene have a prominent **monocytic** component, resembling **CMML.**
- CML resulting from a p230 BCR-ABL gene (mu-bcr breakpoint) is associated with the CNL variant and/or with marked thrombocytosis.
- Patients with **p230** positive CML-N have **indolent course**, probably as a result of low **p230** mRNA and protein levels.
- CML – More than 90% have p210 fusion protein.

Ans: (a) P190 has an indolent course

***Ref:** Robbins Pathology, 9th edition*

26. Which is not a feature of Lofgren syndrome?

(a) Uveitis
(b) Erythema nodosum
(c) Polyarthralgia
(d) Bilateral hilar adenopathy

Explanation:

Lofgren Syndrome

- Lofgren's syndrome is an acute form of sarcoidosis.
- Triad comprises:
  - o **Erythema nodosum.**
  - o **Bilateral hilar lymphadenopathy (bhl).**
  - o **Polyarthralgia or polyarthritis.**
- Associated with HLA-DQB1 and HLA-DRB1.
- **Uveitis** and **elevated levels of ACE**, are often **absent** in patients with Lofgren's syndrome (eye involvement, 5%; elevated ACE levels, 50%).
- Lofgren's syndrome was regarded as a **self-limiting disease** that is generally resolved within the first year.

Ans: (a) Uveitis

***Ref:** Robbins Pathology, 9th edition*

27. Secondary hemolytic anemia is seen in all *except*:

(a) CML
(b) CLL
(c) CRRT
(d) ECMO

Explanation:

- Hemolytic anemia is an umbrella term for a huge list of disorders causing them.

Causes of Acquired Hemolysis

A. *Immuno hemolytic anemias*
   - Autoimmune hemolytic anemias
     - o Due to **warm antibodies** – idiopathic, secondary (Neoplasms – **CLL***)
     - o Due to **cold antibodies** – cold agglutinin disease (Neoplasms – **CLL**), **paroxysmal cold hemoglobinuria***
   - Hemolytic disease of the newborn, transfusion reaction

B. *Fragmentation syndromes*
   - Hemolytic uremic syndrome
   - Thrombotic thrombocytopenic purpura
   - Disseminated intravascular coagulation
   - Cardiac hemolytic anemia due to prosthetic cardiac valves

C. *Paroxysmal nocturnal hemoglobinuria*

D. *Drugs* – Quinidine, Methyl dopa, penicillin

E. *Infections*
   - Clostridium perfringens
   - Bartonellosis
   - Cholera
   - Clostridium welchii
   - Septicemia

F. *Misc.*
   - **Burns**
   - **CRRT** (continuous renal replacement therapy)
   - **ECMO** (long-term extracorporeal membrane oxygenation causes hemolysis).

Ans: (a) CML

***Ref:** Robbins Pathology, 9th edition*

28. False about micro satellites is:

(a) Repeat size more than 10 to 15 nucleotides
(b) More prone to variation
(c) Found in colonic carcinoma
(d) DNA repeats present

Explanation:

Micro and Mini Satellites

- **Micro satellites** are usually **less than 1 kilo base** and are characterized by a **repeat size of 2 to 6 base pairs***.
- **Mini satellite** repeats, by comparison, are **larger (1 to 3 kilobases)**, and the repeat motif is usually **15 to 70 base pairs***.
- Number of repeats, both in micro satellites and mini satellites, is extremely variable within a given population.
- Micro satellites and the smaller mini satellites can be readily distinguished by using **PCR primers** that flank the repeat region.
- Patients with **HNPCC syndrome** have defects in the **mismatch repair system**, leading to development of carcinomas of the colon. These patients' genomes show microsatellite instability, characterized by changes in length of short repeats throughout the genome.

Ans: (a) Repeat size more than 10 to 15 nucleotides

Ref: *Robbins Pathology, 9th edition, Page 179*

29. Myeloma associated with good prognosis:

(a) t (11:14)
(b) t (14,18)
(c) del 17
(d) t (14,16)

Explanation:

Prognostic factors in Multiple myeloma

Test	Values Indicating a More Favorable Prognosis
Beta 2-microglobulin (β2-microglobulin or β2-M)	<3 mg/mL
Albumin level	≥3.5 g/dL
Lactate dehydrogenase (LDH) level	Age ≤60 years.: 100-190 U/L Age >60 years.: 110-210 U/L
Serum free light chain assay	Free light chain ratio MGUS: 0.26-1.65 Asymptomatic myeloma:0.125-8.0 Symptomatic myeloma:0.03-32

Molecular Prognostic factors

Gene	Cytogenetic abnormality	Prognosis
FGFR3	T(4,14)	Poor
Cyclin D1	T(11,14)	Good
C-Maf	T(14,16)	Poor
P53	Del (p53)	Poor
13q	Loss of 13q14	Poor prognosis

Ans: (a) t (11:14)

Ref: *WHO, FGT, Page 69*

MICROBIOLOGY

1. **True regarding *H. influenzae* growth:**

(a) Growth in MacConkey and blood agar but not chocolate agar
(b) Growth in MacConkey and chocolate agar but not blood agar
(c) Growth in blood and chocolate agar but not MacConkey medium
(d) Growth in MacConkey, blood and chocolate agar

Explanation:

Haemophilus influenzae:

General characteristics	Cultural characteristics
• **Gram negative coccobacillus** • **Capsulated**, Highly pleomorphic • Growth – **Factor X and V** • **Growth in blood and chocolate agar and not in blood agar**	**Selective media** – Levinthal's medium, Field's agar

- ***H.influenzae, H.haemolyticus*** and ***H.aegyptius***: Requires **both factor X and V.**
- ***H.parainfluenzae***, ***H.parahaemolyticus*** and ***H.paraphrophilus***: Requires only **factor V.**
- ***H.aphrophilus***: Doesn't require both factors.

Ans: (c) Growth in blood and chocolate agar but not MacConkey medium

Ref: *Ananthanarayan and Paniker, 9th edition, Page 327-328*

2. **Selective culture medium to grow Leptospira:**

(a) Thayer Martin medium
(b) Mc Conkey agar
(c) Korthof medium
(d) EMJH

Explanation:

Leptospira spp

General characteristics	Cultural characteristics
• Spirochete – More number of spirals with hooked end; **endoflagella +** • Zoonotic disease • ***Leptospira icterohemorrhagiae***–Weil's disease • ***L.canicola***–Canicola fever • ***L.grippotyphosa***–Marsh fever • ***L.hebdomadis***–Seven-day fever	• Media with rabbit serum: Ellinghausen-McCullough-Johnson-Harris (EMJH) medium • Fatty acid albumin media: Korthof's medium, Stuart's medium, Fletcher medium (can be used for Antigen preparation for MAT)

Ans: (d) EMJH

Ref: *Ananthanarayan and Paniker, 9th edition, Page 381*

3. **True statement about *Clostridium perfringens* are all *except*:**

(a) Gas gangrene – alpha toxin is produced by type A strains and responsible for profound toxemia
(b) Clostridium perfringens is not the major cause of gas gangrene
(c) Present in normal feces
(d) *C.perfringens* type C strains is responsible for necrotizing enteritis

Explanation:

Clostridium perfringens/Cl.welchii

General characteristics	Cultural characteristics
• **Gram positive, spore producing, capsulated anaerobe** • Both saccharolytic and proteolytic • Spores – **oval and sub terminal**	• **Target hemolysis** (Double zone - β surrounded by α hemolysis)
Biochemical reactions	**Virulence factors**
• Litmus milk reaction – **Stormy clot fermentation**	• **α toxin** – lecithinase/phospholipase C • **β and i (iota) toxin** – lethal and necrotizing properties • **θ toxin** – Hemolysin (Perfringolysin O)
Clinical features	
• Most common organism for **gas gangrene** • **Clostridial myonecrolysis** • **Food poisoning** – cytotoxin mediated and induces calcium dependent alteration of permeability • **Necrotizing enteritis** – beta toxin of type C of Cl. perfringens • **Neutropenic Enterocolitis**	
Diagnosis	**Treatment**
• **Naegler reaction** positivity due alpha toxin • **Reverse CAMP test ++** • Frozen section biopsy of muscle	• Gas gangrene – **Clindamycin + Penicillin, Surgery, Hyperbaric O_2** • Food poisoning – No role of antibiotics

Gas gangrene causative agents:

Common	Less pathogenic
• *Cl.perfringens* • *Cl.septicum* • *Cl.novyi*	• *Cl.histolyticum* • *Cl.fallax* • *Cl.tertium*

Ans: (b) Clostridium perfringens is not the major cause of gas gangrene

***Ref:** Ananthanarayan and Paniker, 9th edition, Page 253-259*

4. **Parasites not transmitted through soil:**

(a) Pin worm
(b) Hookworm
(c) Tapeworm
(d) Roundworm

Explanation:

Nematodes based on mode of infection:

Mode of Infection		Organisms
Ingestion	Eggs	**Enterobius , Ascaris , Trichuris (EAT)**
	Larva within intermediate host	*Dracunculus medinensis*
	Encysted larva in muscle	*Trichinella spiralis*
Penetration of skin		**Strongyloides, Ancylostoma ,Necator (SAN)**
Blood sucking insects		Filaria
Inhalation of dust containing eggs		**Ascaris, Enterobius**

Ans: (c) Tapeworm

***Ref:** K.D. Chatterjee, 13th edition, Page 212-222*

5. **Ebola – type that is non-fatal in human beings is:**

(a) Zaire
(b) Reston
(c) Cote de ivory
(d) Bundibugyo

Explanation:

- The virus family Filoviridae includes three genera:
  - Cuevavirus.
  - Marburgvirus, and
  - Ebolavirus.
- Within the genus **Ebolavirus, five species** have been identified: **Zaire, Bundibugyo, Sudan, Reston and Taï Forest (Cote de ivory).**
- The first three, Bundibugyo-Ebolavirus, Zaire-Ebolavirus, and Sudan-Ebolavirus have been associated with large outbreaks in Africa.
- The virus causing the 2014–2016 West African outbreak belongs to the Zaire-Ebolavirus species.

Ans: (c) Cote de ivory

Ref: *http://www.who.int/news-room/fact-sheets/detail/ebola-virus-disease*

6. **True regarding 'Tsetse fly':**

(a) Lays single egg
(b) Lays cluster of eggs
(c) Gives birth to single larvae
(d) Gives birth to multiple larvae

Explanation:

Tsetse Fly:

Scientific Name	• Glossina spp.
Size	• The tsetse is about the size of a housefly: 6-14 mm
Colour	• Yellowish to brown
Description	• Possesses a large, widely spaced eyes, forward-projected mouth parts and wings which in rest cover the whole abdomen horizontally, like closed blades of a pair of scissors. • They are holometaboulos insects, females giving birth to full-grown larvae which rapidly pupate in the soil. • Fold their wings completely when they are resting so that one wing rests directly on top of the other over their abdomen. Have a long proboscis which extends directly forward and is attached by a distinct bulb to the bottom of their head.
Habitat	• Local patches of dense vegetation along banks of rivers • Lakes in arid terrain, and also in dense, wet, heavily forested equatorial rainforest
Lifecycle	• Female tsetse mate just once. After 7-9 days she **produces a single egg which develops into a larva within her uterus.** • About nine days later, the mother produces a larva which burrows into the ground where it pupates. 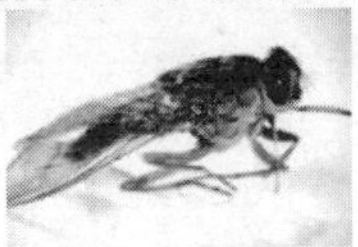 • The mother continues to produce a single larva at roughly nine-day intervals for her entire life. • Eggs hatch in the female and after larval development, the deposited larvae pupates immediately. • The pupal stage lasts about 3 weeks. • The adult fly emerges from the pupa in the ground after about 30 days. • Over a period of 12-14 days it matures, mates and, if it is a female, deposits its first larva. • Thus 50 days elapse between the emergence of one female fly and the subsequent emergence of the first of its progeny. • This lifecycle, with a slow reproductive rate and substantial parental investment in the care of young, is a relatively unusual example of an insect with a so-called 'K-type' life history. • Both sexes are blood feeders and feed on a wide range of hosts, including man. • This fly is a potent vector for several diseases of animals and man including trypanosomiasis. • This slow rate of reproduction means that tsetse populations can be eradicated by killing just 2-3% of the female population per day.
Disease Transmitted	**Sleeping sickness:** Chronic form also called **trypanosomiasis.**

Ans: (a) Lays single egg

***Ref:** http://www.kznhealth.gov.za/environ/vector/tsetsefly.htm*

7. **True about *Campylobacter jejuni:***

(a) 37°C microaerophilic
(b) 42°C microaerophilic
(c) 5 – 10% CO_2
(d) 37°C and 10% capnophilic

Explanation:

Campylobacter jejuni:

General characteristics	Cultural characteristics
• **Motile** with polar flagellum, non-spore forming **curved bacilli** • **Microaerophilic** • Gram negative rods • **Gull wing /seagull/comma shaped** • Thermophilic – **42°C** • **Zoonotic disease** • **Source**: Food of animal origin especially **raw milk,** *C.jejuni* is part of the normal intestinal flora of birds and animals and is **shed in their faeces**	• Selective media – **Campy BAP, Skirrow** and **Butzlers medium** • Transport media: **Cary-Blair medium** • Inoculated plates are incubated at 42°C in **5% O_2, 10% CO_2 and 85% N_2** • **Non-hemolytic, colorless and moist colonies**

Ans: (b) 42°C microaerophilic

***Ref:** Ananthanarayan and Paniker, 9th edition, Page 398-399*

8. **Salmonella like diarrhoea is caused by:**

(a) Entero aggregative E.coli persistent diarrhea
(b) Entero toxigenic E.coli – travellers' diarrhea
(c) Entero pathogenic E.coli – infantile diarrhea
(d) EHEC – HUS

Explanation:

- **ETEC – Traveller's diarrhea** (LT, ST toxins, Fimbrial antigens)
- **EHEC – HUS** (E.coli O157:H7 – sorbitol non fermenter in sorbitol MacConkey)
- **EPEC – Infant diarrhea**
- **EIEC – Dysentery** (Epithelial cell invasion by virulence marker antigen)
- **EAEC – Persistent diarrhea**, traveller's diarrhea

Ans: (d) EHEC – HUS

***Ref:** Ananthanarayan and Paniker, 9th edition, Page 279*

9. **Neisseria vaccine (MCV-4 and MPSV-4) strains are not protective against:**

(a) A
(b) B
(c) C
(d) W135

Explanation:

Classification of Meningococci – Based on capsular polysaccharide:

Group A	Group B	Group C	Group Y	Group W
Most common strain in India Epidemics	Epidemic and Outbreak Most prevalent in **worldwide** **Vaccine not available**	Localized outbreaks	Sporadic	Sporadic and Epidemic in Sub-Saharan Africa

- Monovalent and polyvalent vaccines containing the capsular polysaccharides **of group A, C, W-135 and Y are available except for B.**

Ans: (b) B

***Ref:** Ananthanarayan and Paniker, 9th edition, Page 230*

10. Which of the following is true regarding HPV vaccine strains?/Current WHO recommendations for HPV vaccination is:

(a) Monovalent vaccine 6, 11, 16, 18, 31, 52, 56, 58 strains
(b) Monovalent vaccine 6, 11, 16, 18, 31, 33, 45, 52, 58 strains
(c) 3 doses to girls if initiated prior to 15 years of age
(d) 2 doses recommended irrespective of age, gender, type of vaccine

Explanation:

Vaccine Recommendations

- **HPV vaccine is recommended for routine vaccination** at age 11 or 12 years (Vaccination can be started at age 9).
- **ACIP also recommends vaccination** for females aged 13 through 26 years and males aged 13 through 21 years not adequately vaccinated previously.
- Vaccination is also recommended through age 26 years for gay, bisexual and other men who have sex with men, transgender people, and for immunocompromised persons (including those with HIV infection) not adequately vaccinated previously.
- Ideally, adolescents should be vaccinated before they are exposed to HPV. However, people who have already been infected with one or more HPV types can still get protection from other HPV types in the vaccine.

Dosing Schedules

- **Two doses of HPV vaccine are recommended** for most persons starting the series before their 15th birthday.
  - The second dose of HPV vaccine should be given **6 to 12 months** after the first dose.
  - Adolescents who receive 2 doses less than 5 months apart will require a third dose of HPV vaccine.
- **Three doses of HPV vaccine are recommended for teens** and **young adults** who start the series at ages **15 through 26 years**, and for **immunocompromised persons**.
  - The recommended 3-dose schedule is **0, 1–2 and 6 months.**
  - Three doses are recommended for **immunocompromised persons** (including those with HIV infection) aged 9–26 years.

Contraindications and Precautions

A severe allergic reaction (e.g., anaphylaxis) to a vaccine component or following a prior dose of HPV vaccine is a contraindication to receipt of HPV vaccine.

- Anaphylactic allergy to latex is a contraindication to bivalent HPV vaccine in a prefilled syringe since the tip cap might contain natural rubber latex.
- Quadrivalent and 9-valent HPV vaccines are produced in *Saccharomyces cerevisiae* (baker's yeast) and are contraindicated for persons with a history of immediate hypersensitivity to yeast.

Pregnancy: HPV vaccine is **not** recommended for use during pregnancy.

Clinical spectrum of HPV:

HPV type	Clinical lesion
1, 4	Plantar warts
2, 4, 26, 27, 29	Common warts
3, 10, 28, 41	Flat warts
5, 8	Epidermodysplasia verruciformis
6, 11	Anogenital condylomas Laryngeal papillomas Intraepithelial neoplasia
7	Hand warts

Contd.

9, 12, 14, 15, 17, 19 – 25, 36, 46, 47	Epidermodysplasia verruciformis
13, 32	Oral focal epithelial hyperplasia
16, 18, 30, 31, 33, 35, 39, 45, 51, 52, 56	High grade dysplasia CA genital mucosa CA larynx and oesophagus
34, 40, 42, 44, 53 – 55, 58, 59, 61, 62, 64, 66, 69	Intraepithelial neoplasia
75, 77	Common warts in organ transplant patients
37	Keratoacanthoma

Ans: (d) 2 doses recommended irrespective of age, gender, type of vaccine

Ref: *Ananthanarayan and Paniker, 9th edition, Page 553;*
https://www.cdc.gov/vaccines/vpd/hpv/hcp/recommendations.html

11. True statement regarding HCV diagnosis:

(a) 3 genotype diagnosis is based on IgG HCV
(b) Spreads through feco-oral route
(c) Pegylated INF is treatment of choice
(d) HCV NAT is the molecular diagnostic method of choice

Explanation:

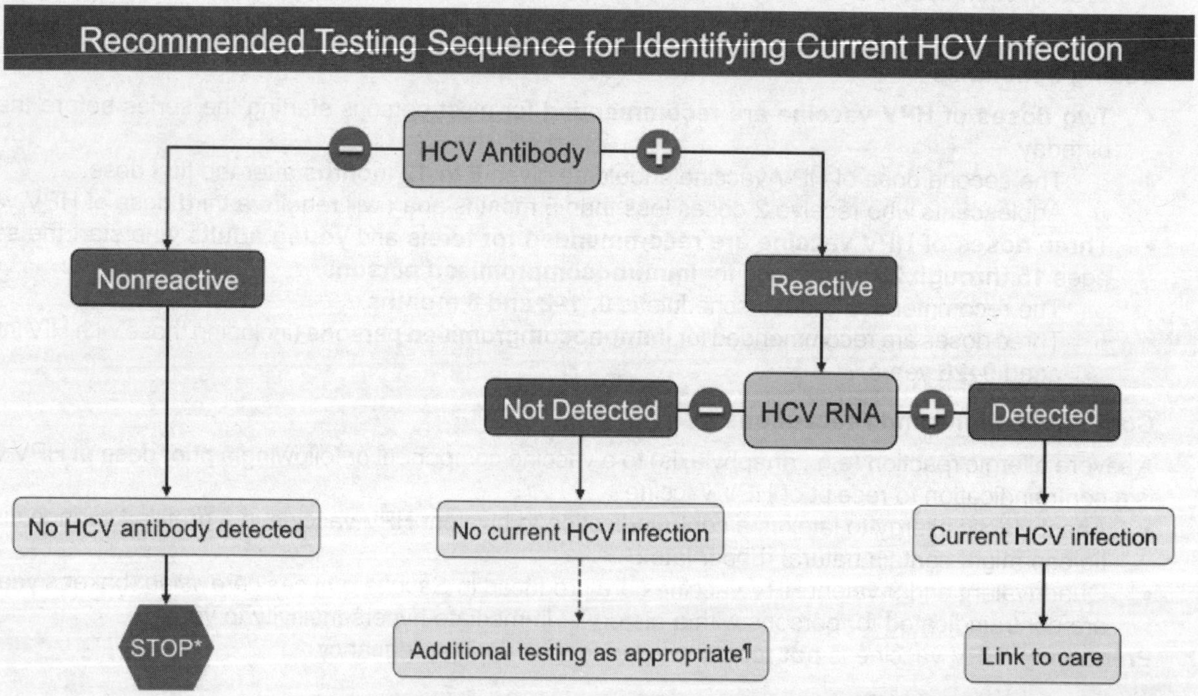

* For persons who might have been exposed to HCV within the past 6 months, testing for HCV RNA or follow-up testing for HCV antibody is recommended. For persons who are immunocompromised, testing for HCV RNA can be considered.

¶To differentiate past, resolved HCV infection from biologic false positivity for HCV antibody, testing with another HCV antibody assay can be considered. Repeat HCV RNA testing if the person tested is suspected to have had HCV exposure within the past 6 months or has clinical evidence of HCV disease, or if there is concern regarding the handling or storage of the test specimen.

- Diagnostic tests for hepatitis C include **serologic assays** that measure human antibodies generated in response to HCV infection and molecular virologic assays that directly detect **HCV RNA.**
- The third-generation **HCV EIA test** is the most frequently used antibody test to initially screen for HCV infection. The test has high sensitivity and specificity, but does not distinguish between current and resolved hepatitis C infection.

- The **OraQuick HCV Rapid Antibody Test** is available as a point-of-care rapid test and this test can be used for initial HCV antibody screening.
- **Quantitative HCV RNA assays** are the preferred supplemental test for persons who have a positive screening HCV antibody test. Testing positive for HCV RNA indicates current (active) HCV infection. Qualitative HCV RNA assays can be used for supplemental testing but do not offer any advantage over the quantitative assay.
- The 2013 CDC recommended testing sequence for identifying current HCV infection consists of initial **HCV antibody testing** (either rapid or laboratory-conducted assay) followed by an **HCV RNA assay** for all positive antibody tests.

Ans: (c) Pegylated INF is treatment of choice

Ref: *Ananthanarayan and Paniker, 9th edition, Page 549;*
https://www.hepatitisc.uw.edu/go/screening-diagnosis/diagnostic-testing/core-concept/al

12. True regarding Metapneumovirus is:

(a) Segmented negative sense single stranded RNA virus
(b) Incidence is 5% of total respiratory infection
(c) Spreads through sexual contact and blood transfusion
(d) Human metapneumovirus contains NS1 and NS2 antigens

Explanation:

Metapneumovirus

- **Virus classification**
  - Group: Group V [(−)ssRNA]
  - Order: Mononegavirales
  - Family: Pneumoviridae
  - Genus: Metapneumovirus
  - Type species: Avian metapneumovirus
- **Species:**
  - Avian metapneumovirus (AMPV).
  - Human metapneumovirus (HMPV).
- HMPV is associated with **6% to 40% of respiratory tract infections in hospitalized and outpatient children**. The virus is distributed worldwide and, in temperate regions, has a seasonal distribution generally following that of RSV and **influenza** virus during late winter and spring.
- The **genomic** organization of HMPV is similar to **RSV**; however, HMPV **lacks the non-structural genes, NS1 and NS2**, and the HMPV antisense RNA genome contains eight open reading frames in slightly different gene order than RSV. HMPV is genetically similar to the avian metapneumoviruses A, B and in particular type C.

Ans: (a) Segmented negative sense single stranded RNA virus

Ref: *Ananthanarayan and Paniker, 9th edition, Page 514*

13. Chandler's index is used for:

(a) Guinea worm
(b) Pin worm
(c) Hookworm
(d) Round worm

Explanation:

Chandler's Index

- It is used to identify the importance of **hookworm infestation** as a public health problem in a community.
- Morbidity and mortality from hookworm infection depend much on the **worm load**.
- **Chandler** worked out an index on the basis of an average number of hookworm eggs per gram of faeces for the entire community.
- It is calculated based on average number of hookworm eggs/gram of stool:
  - **<200: No significance.**

- o **200-250: Potential danger.**
- o **250-300: Minor public health problem.**
- o **>300: Major public health problem.**

- This index is still used in **epidemiological studies** of hookworm disease. By this index, worm loads in different population groups can be compared and also the degree of reduction of egg output after mass treatment.

Ans: (c) Hookworm

Ref: *K.D. Chatterjee, 13th edition, Page 212-222*

14. A HIV positive patient presents with cough for 10 days. Sputum culture by SDA reveals broad budding yeast, diagnosis:

(a) Histoplasma capsulatum (b) Blastomycosis
(c) Coccidiodomycosis (d) Paracoccidiomycosis

Explanation:

Histoplasmosis

- Intracellular infection of the **reticuloendothelial system**
- **Causative agent:** *Histoplasma capsulatum* **(Dimorphic fungus)**
- *H.capsulatum var.capsulatum* **(Darling's disease)** and *H.capsulatum var.duboisii* **(African histoplasmosis)**
- Worldwide distribution and most common in central and eastern states of America
- Fungus is seen more commonly in **the soil**

Clinical Features

- Infection acquired through **inhalation**
- Mostly asymptomatic and heals spontaneously
- Some cases it causes **tuberculate lesions** resembles tuberculosis
- **Disseminated form:** Reticuloendothelial system (Lymphadenopathy, hepatosplenomegaly and anaemia)
- **Cutaneous form:** Granulomatous and ulcerative lesions on skin

Lab Diagnosis

- Blood cultures, sputum and skin biopsies
- Cultured in **glucose-BHI agar and SDA**, incubated **at 37°C and 25°C**–grows as yeast and mycelial forms respectively
- **Mycelial forms** shows spherical spores with tubercles
- **Serology:** Latex agglutination test, CFT and precipitation test
- **Skin tests:** With Histoplasmin antigen (delayed hypersensitivity reaction)

Treatment

- DOC–**Amphotericin B** and Alternative–Itraconazole

Blastomycosis

- Chronic infection of the lungs, also known as **North American Blastomycosis/Gilchrist disease**
- Disseminated Blastomycosis–**immunosuppressed patients** including AIDS
- **Causative agent:** ***Blastomyces dermatitidis*** (Dimorphic fungus)
- **Pathogenesis:** Acquired through inhalation from soil (mycelial fragments and conidia)→ in the alveoli they transforms into yeasts→ acute inflammation (neutrophils and macrophages)→ granuloma formation→ grows intracellular and relatively resistant to phagocytosis

Clinical Features

- **Pulmonary blastomycosis:** Asymptomatic or flu like illness sometimes resembles chronic lung disease
- **Cutaneous blastomycosis:** Primary (direct transcutaneous spread) or secondary (hematogenous spread)
- Disseminated extrapulmonary blastomycosis

Lab Diagnosis

- **Specimens:** Sputum, BAL, CSF, urine, skin and lung biopsy
- **Direct examination with KOH mount:** Thick walled **broad based budding yeasts**

- **Culture:** SDA with or without antibiotics at both **room temperature (mold forms)** and **at 37°C (yeast forms) in BHI glucose agar**
- **Fungal stains:** GMS, LCB mount, H and E–yeast forms: **Broad based budding yeast cells (figure of 8 morphology)** and mold forms: **Thick walled terminal chlamydoconidia**
- **Serology:** CFT, EIA, Immunodiffusion test
- **PCR:** Labeled DNA/RNA hybrid

Treatment: DOC–Amphotericin B

Coccidioidomycosis

- **Causative agent:** *Coccidioides immitis*
- Highly infectious organism, select **agent of bioterrorism**
- **Not seen in India,** reported in **Central and South America**
- **Pathogenesis:** Acquired through inhalation from soil **(arthroconidia)**→ in the alveoli they transforms into spherules filled with **endoconidia** (endospores)→ acute inflammation (neutrophils and macrophages)→ granuloma formation→ grows intracellular and relatively resistant to phagocytosis.

Clinical Features:

- **Primary pulmonary coccidioidomycosis:** Asymptomatic or hilar or parenchymal calcification due to hypersensitivity to coccidioidin and acute febrile illness to residual cavitary lesion
- **Disseminated coccidioidomycosis:** Hematogenous spread of endoconidia from lungs to other organs→Skin, bones, joints, GIT, endocardium and meninges

Lab Diagnosis

- **Specimens:** Sputum, BAL, urine, pleural, pericardial and peritoneal fluids, skin and lung biopsy
- **Direct examination with KOH mount:** Thick walled **spherules with endoconidia**
- **Culture:** SDA with or without antibiotics at both **room temperature** and **at 37°C (yeast forms) in BHI glucose agar, mold forms** seen both at 25°C and 37°C
- **Fungal stains:** GMS, LCB mount, H and E–**spherules with endoconidia and barrel shaped arthroconidia with alternate cells**
  - **Serology:** CFT, EIA, Immunodiffusion test
  - **PCR:** Labeled DNA/RNA hybrid

Treatment: DOC–Amphotericin B

Paracoccidioidomycosis

- **Causative agent:** *Paracoccidioides brasiliensis* **(Dimorphic)**
- Also called as **South American Blastomycosis**
- Increased reports among **immunocompromised and AIDS patients**
- **Pathogenesis:** Acquired through inhalation from soil mycelial fragments **(arthroconidia and aleuroconidia)**→ in the alveoli they transforms **into yeasts**→ acute inflammation (neutrophils and macrophages)→ granuloma formation→ grows intracellular and relatively resistant to phagocytosis

Clinical Features:

- **Pulmonary:** Persistent cough with purulent sputum, fever, chest pain and nodular cavitary lesions
- **Extrapulmonary:** Skin, mucosa, lymph nodes (cervical), adrenals, liver, CNS and bones
- **Cutaneous:** Ulcerative or granulomatous lesions

Lab Diagnosis:

- **Specimens:** Sputum, BAL, CSF, urine, skin and lung biopsy
- **Direct examination with KOH mount:** Presence of multiple buds that are attached to the parent cells
- **Culture:** SDA with or without antibiotics at both **room temperature (mold forms)** and **at 37°C (yeast forms) in BHI glucose agar**
- **Fungal stains:** GMS, LCB mount, H and E–yeast forms: Presence of multiple buds that are attached to the parent cells **(Mickey mouse head/Mariner's wheel/Ship's wheel appearance)** and mold forms: **Intercalary chlamydoconidia**

- **Serology:** CFT, EIA, Immunodiffusion test
- **PCR:** Labeled DNA/RNA hybrid

Treatment: DOC–Amphotericin B

Ans: (b) Blastomycosis

Ref: *Ananthanarayan and Paniker, 9th edition, Page 605-608*

15. Northern blotting used in separation and diagnosis of:

(a) Histones
(b) Proteins
(c) RNA
(d) DNA

Explanation:

- **Southern** blotting – **DNA**
- **Northern** blotting – **RNA**
- **Western** blotting – **Proteins**
- **Mnemonic**: **North India – R**oti; **South India – D**osa; **Western countries– P**izza (R-RNA; D-DNA; P-Proteins).

Ans: (c) RNA

Ref: *Ananthanarayan and Paniker, 9th edition, Page 65*

FORENSIC MEDICINE

1. **Itai-itai disease is caused by:**

(a) Mecury toxicity
(b) Cadmium toxicity
(c) Lead toxicity
(d) Arsenic toxicity

Explanation:

- **Itai-itai / Ouch-ouch disease** is seen in **Cadmium** poisoning which is so named because of sudden muscle cramps causing victim to cry out in pain periodically (In Japan) – *Itai – Painful (Japanese)*
- Anosmia, yellowing of teeth, renal tubular dysfunction
- Bone demineralization with osteomalacia leading to bone lesions and pseudofractures
- Treated with EDTA or DMSA

Trivia

- Outbreak of Itai-Itai disease in Japan occurred in 1945 and was the result of consumption of rice grown in paddy fields which were irrigated by the local Jintzu river containing cadmium contaminated water

Ans: (b) Cadmium Toxicity

Ref: *VV Pillai, Modern Medical Toxicology, 4th edition, Page 103*

2. **Bolam's test is used in:**

(a) Drowning
(b) Arsenic poisoning
(c) Medical negligence
(d) Legal test of insanity

Explanation:

- The judgment given by Mr. Justice Mc Nair in Bolam vs. Friern Hospital Management Committee (1957) is a landmark decision in deciding cases of medical negligence and is known as the "Bolam test".
- It says, "The test is the standard of the ordinary skilled man exercising and professing to have that special skill. A man need not possess the highest expert skill, it is well established law that it is sufficient if he exercises the ordinary skill of an ordinary competent man exercising that particular art (a health care professional), is not guilty of negligence if he has acted in accordance with a practice accepted as proper by a responsible body of medical man skilled in the particular act."
- Bolam test says that to term the act of doctor as negligent we should consider the act of another doctor in the similar circumstances and facilities as existed with the treating doctor. Also the professional knowledge and skill of the treating doctor should be compared with another doctor having same educational background.
- Bolam test has been approved and followed by the courts in India.

Trivia

- Mr Bolam was a voluntary patient at Friern Hospital, a mental health institution run by the Friern Hospital Management Committee. He agreed to undergo electro-convulsive therapy. He was not given any muscle relaxant, and his body was not restrained during the procedure. He flailed about violently before the procedure was stopped, and he suffered some serious injuries, including fractures of the acetabula. He sued the Committee for compensation. He argued they were negligent for (1) not issuing relaxants (2) not restraining him (3) not warning him about the risks involved.

Other important tests in Forensic Medicine (Legal Tests of Insanity)

(a) Mc Naughten Rule – 1843 (The right or wrong test/ legal test)
- *No criminal responsibility if suffering from disease of **M**ind, did not know **N**ature and quality of act and w**R**ongfulness of act*

(b) Durham Rule –1954 (Product test)
- *No Criminal responsibility if unlawful act is pro**D**uct of mental **D**isease or mental **D**efect*

(c) Curren's Rule –1961
- *No criminal responsibility if accused lacked **C**apacity to **C**onform the **C**onduct as per law*

(d) American law Institute test – 1970 (Model penal code test/Brawner rule/Substantial capacity test)
- *No criminal responsibility if lacks capacity to **A**ppreciate criminality of conduct due to mental disease or defect or unable to conform his conduct as per law*

(e) Irresistible impulse test (1887) – New Hemisphere Doctrine
- *No criminal responsibility if unlawful act is due to inability to restrain because of will destroyed by mental disease*

Ans: (c) Medical negligence

***Ref:** Prateek Rastogi, Bolam Test, JIAFM, 2007 (29) 1, Page 7-8*

3. Poroscopy term coined by:

(a) Galton
(b) Edmund Locard
(c) Joseph Bell
(d) Alphonso Bertillion

Explanation:

System of Identification	Devised by
(a) Fingerprint/Dactylography	Sir Francis Galton
(b) Poroscopy	Edmund Locard
(c) Rugoscopy/Palatoprint	Harrison Allen
(d) Anthropometry	Alphonso Bertillion
(e) DNA Fingerprinting	Sir Alec Jaffery

- Edmund Locard is also credited with famous "Locard's Principle of Exchange" which is basis of all crime detection
- "Whenever 2 objects come in contact with each other, there is a mutual transfer of material from one object to the other"

Poroscopy

- Described by Locard (in 1912) – consists of study of microscopic pores of ridges formed by the mouths of ducts of sub-epidermal sweat glands.
- Each mm of a ridge contains 9 to 18 pores.
- Pores are permanent and vary in size, shape, position and no. over a given length in each individual.
- Useful when only fragments of fingerprints are available.

Trivia:

- **Joseph Bell**, a Scottish surgeon is considered a Pioneer in Forensic Pathology, and was one of the first scientists to put an emphasis on close observation, claiming it to be the key to forensics. He is best known as an inspiration for Sir Arthur Conan Doyle's for literary character Sherlock Holmes. He is also said to have identified the infamous serial killer "Jack the Ripper".

Ans: (b) Edmund Locard

***Ref:** Gautam Biswas, Review of Forensic Medicine and Toxicology, 3rd edition, Page 88*

4. A-10-year old girl was admitted in ER with history of ingesting 10 crushed seeds of a plant, she couldn't recall how much she had and her ECG looks like this (Figure). Probable cause Is______.

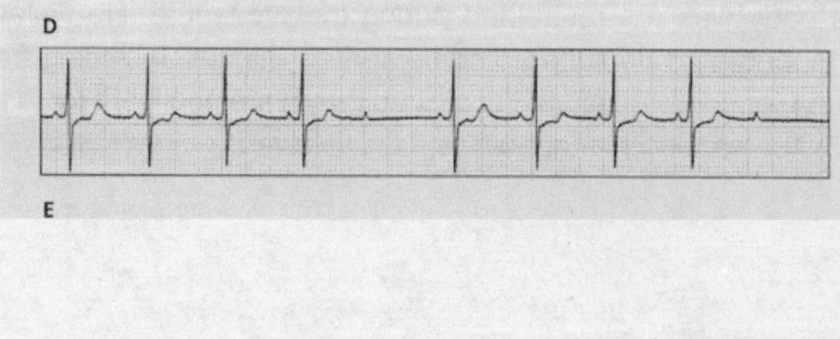

(a) Strychinine seeds
(b) Abrus precatorius
(c) Yellow oleander seeds
(d) Ricinus communis seeds

Explanation:

- ECG is diagnostic of 2:1 AV block which is seen in case of Cerbera thevetia poisoning.

Yellow oleander (Cerbera thevetia)

- A cardiac poison
- All parts – poisonous
- Active principles – Glycosides – Thevetin + thevotoxin = cardiac poison and Cerberin = acts like strychnine

Sign and Symptoms

- GIT – Burning sensation in mouth with tingling of tongue, nausea, vomiting, diarrhea
- CVS – Rapid, weak pulse, low BP, **heart block**, collapse and death to peripheral circulatory failure

Treatment

- Sodium molar lactate transfusion with glucose and 1mg atropine, 2 cc adrenaline and 2 mg noradrenaline (Bisht Regimen)

Trivia

- Bisht Regimen is named by **Dr. D B Bisht**, Former Principal of JIPMER who advocated its use in Cerbera poisoning. So numerous times, questions have come from this topic in JIPMER exams. Must know topic for JIPMER aspirants.

Ans: (c) Yellow oleander seeds

Ref: *VV Pillai, Modern Medical Toxicology, 4th edition, Page 344*

5. **Patient died during surgery/under anesthesia, which section among here applies for the surgeon?**

(a) 174 (3) CrPC
(b) 174 CrPC
(c) 39 CrPC
(d) 176 CrPC

Explanation:

Sections	Explanation
(a) 174(3) CrPC	Investigations in unnatural death of woman within 7 years of marriage
(b) 174 CrPC	Police inquest
(c) 39 CrPC	Information to police about certain offences
(d) 176 CrPC	Magistrate inquest

- All the options are from Criminal Procedural Code, hence it is expecting likely course of action by the Doctor or the Police.
- As per Section 39 CrPC all deaths occurring in due course of surgery and anesthesia should be treated as unnatural deaths and should be reported to the police. Failing of which the doctor can be punished under Section 202 IPC (upto 6 months) for intentional omission to give information of offence to police by the person who is bound to inform.
- Inquest likely to be held in this case would be under Section 174 CrPC, i.e., Police Inquest and Doctor/Anesthetist is likely to be punished if negligent under Section 304A IPC (Upto 2 years).

Ans: (c) 39 CrPC

Ref: *Amit Kumar, Ashok Kumar Srivastava, Bindu Sharma; Anaesthetic Deaths: A Medico-Legal Scenario; JIAFM, 36(3), Page 292-296*

6. **What is the earliest definite site of external putrefaction?**

(a) Epigastric region
(b) Umbilical region
(c) Right iliac fossa
(d) Left iliac fossa

Explanation:

- **Greenish or bluish green discoloration** is a sign of **decomposition.**
- This discolouration is due to formation of **sulphamethemoglobin** from H_2S and hemoglobin.

Sites of occurrence

- **Internally**, it is first seen as Reddish brown discolouration on inner surface of vessels especially **aorta (earliest sign).** It is also seen on **undersurface of liver** where it is in contact with **transverse colon** (along with **external discolouration**).
- **Externally** it is seen as **greenish discolouration** in the **Right iliac fossa** in skin over the **caecum** (as contents of bowel here are more fluid and full of bacteria).

Timeline since death

- Appears **in 12 to 18 hours in summer** and **1 or 2 days in winter.**
- Passage of bacteria through blood vessels results in formation of **sulphamethemoglobin** along route causing greenish or reddish brown liner branching pattern on skin (**marbling**) first on shoulder, roots of limbs, thighs, side of abdomen, chest and neck – prominent in 36 to 48 hours.

Ans: (c) Right iliac fossa

Ref: *NG Rao, Textbook of Forensic Medicine and Toxicology, 2nd edition, Page 150*

7. **Exhumation is done following court order. Only skull bone was found with basiocciput fused with basisphenoid. What is the approximate age?**

(a) 18 – 21 years
(b) 40 – 50 years
(c) 70 – 80 years
(d) 6 – 7 years

Explanation:

- Age estimation in skull is done based on the fusion of the sutures as follows:

2 years	Metopic suture
18-21 years	Baso-occiput Baso-sphenoid suture
30-40 years	Post. 1/3rd of Sagittal suture
40-50 years	Ant. 1/3rd of Sagittal suture
	Inferior ½ of Coronal suture
50-60 years	Middle 1/3rd of Sagittal suture
	Superior ½ of Coronal suture
	Medial ½ of Lamboid suture
60-70 years	Lateral ½ of Lamboid suture

Also Note:

- Fusion of sutures occurs in decades.
- Reliability of suture closure – Sagittal > Lamboid > Coronal.
- Fusion of sutures occurs earlier in males compared to females (C.I. Fusion of long bones occur earlier in females).

Ans: (a) 18 - 21 years

Ref: *Rajesh Bardale, Principles of Forensic Medicine and Toxicology, 1st edition, Page 93*

8. **What is living will?**

(a) Written consent when patient in conscious state
(b) Verbal consent by relatives to do mercy killing
(c) Written consent prior to incapacitation
(d) Verbal consent not to resuscitate

Explanation:

"A **living will** is a legal document that allows you to express your wishes to doctors in case you become **incapacitated.**"

Living will (advance directive)

- Supreme Court Judgment on Passive Euthanasia on **9th March 2018,** laid down the guidelines for Writing Living Will.
- It can be written by terminally ill adult patient or authorized next of kin in presence of 2 witness and countersigned by 1st Class Judicial Magistrate (JMFC).
- JMFC shall preserve one copy of the document in his office (also in digital format) and forward one copy of the document to the Registry of the jurisdictional District Court for being preserved (in digital format).
- It has to be approved by Medical Board set up by hospital (can appeal in HC against Board decision).

Trivia:

- Preparing advance directive is also permitted under Mental Health Care Act 2017.

Ans: (c) Written consent prior to incapacitation

***Ref:** https://supremecourtofindia.nic.in/supremecourt/2005/9123/ 9123_2005_Judgement_09-Mar-2018.pdf*

9. Murder is___________offence.

(a) Cognizable, non-compoundable and non-bailable
(b) Cognizable, compoundable and bailable
(c) Non-cognizable, non-compoundable and non-bailable
(d) Non-cognizable, compoundable and bailable

Explanation:

Cognizable offences

- Cognizable offences are more serious crimes wherein police can arrest the suspect without any warrant.
- Ex. rape, murder, ragging, dowry death etc.

Compoundable offences

- Compoundable offences are those offences where, the complainant (one who has filed the case, i.e., the victim), enter into a compromise and agrees to have the charges dropped against the accused.

Bailable offences

- Bailable offences are less serious crimes wherein the suspect can be released from custody by furnishing a bond on bail.

Ans: (a) Cognizable, non-compoundable and non-bailable

***Ref:** The First Schedule, Classification of Offences, Indian Penal Code*

10. Black powder composition:

(a) 15% potassium nitrate + 10% sulphur + 10% charcoal
(b) 15% potassium nitrate + 8% sulphur + 10% charcoal
(c) 75% potassium nitrate + 8% sulphur + 15% charcoal
(d) 75% potassium nitrate + 10% sulphur + 15% charcoal

Explanation:

- **Black gun powder** is composed of **75% potassium nitrate + 10% sulphur + 15% charcoal.**
- It is designated as Fg, FFg, FFFg based on the size of black powder.

	Black powder	Smokeless powder	Semi-smokeless
Contents	• Potassium nitrate 75% (Oxidiser) • Charcoal 15% (Fuel) • Sulphur 10% (Makes mixture denser and more ignitable)	• **Single base** - nitrocellulose (gun cotton) • **Double base** - nitrocellulose and nitroglycerine • **Triple base** - nitrocellulose, nitroglycerine and nitroguanidine	80% BP + 20% SP
Features	1 gm of BP produces 3000 – 4500 cc of gas Each grain produces 200-250 cc of gas	1 gm of SP produces 12000 – 13000 cc of gas Each grain produces 800-900 cc of gas	

Ans: (c) 75% potassium nitrate + 10% sulphur + 15% charcoal

Ref: *Krishan Vij, Textbook of Forensic Medicine and Toxicology, 5th edition, Page 237*

11. En block dissection and organ separation are done by:

(a) Virchow
(b) Ghon
(c) Rockitansky
(d) Letulle

Explanation:

- **Ghon method** is method of organ block dissection where organs are removed in blocks such as cervical, thoracic

Methods of Organ dissection at Autopsy

Method	Technique	Remarks
(a) M. Letulle	En masse dissection and organ separation + dissection	Ideal since preserves connection between organs
(b) R. Virchow	Individual organ removal + dissection	Most common
(c) A. Ghon	Separate block dissection and organ separation + dissection	
(d) C. Rokitansky	In-situ organ dissection	Preferred in children and infected bodies

Ans: (d) Ghon

Ref: *Gautam Biswas, Review of Forensic Medicine and Toxicology, 3rd edition, Page 103*

PSM

1. **Kayakalp award is given for:**

(a) Hospital administration
(b) Hospital hygiene
(c) Leadership
(d) Environmental sanitation

Explanation:

Kayakalp scheme:

- Launched on15.05.2015 by Ministry of Health and Family Welfare.
- Mainly to promote cleanliness and enhance the quality of public health facilities.

Categories:

- The awards would be categorized as follows:
    - Best two District Hospitals in each state (One Best District hospital in small states).
    - Best two Community Health Centres/Sub District Hospitals (limited to one in small states).
    - One Primary Health Centre in every district.

Parameters:

The parameters on which the performance of the facility would be judged are as follows:

- Hospital/Facility upkeep
- Sanitation and hygiene
- Waste management
- Infection control
- Support services
- Hygiene promotion

Criteria for Application to the Awards Scheme:

Following are the prerequisites for applying for an award:

- Constituted a Cleanliness and Infection Control Committee.
- Instituted a mechanism of periodic internal assessment/peer assessment based on defined criteria.
- Achieved at least 70% score in the criteria during the peer assessment process.

Ans: (d) Environmental sanitation

Ref: *https://www.nhp.gov.in/kayakalp-swacchta-guidelines-for-public-health-facilities_pg*

2. **AIDS day slogan of World AIDS Day 2017 is:**

(a) Unite for HIV
(b) HIV wellness
(c) Right to health
(d) Everyone counts

Explanation:

To complement the global **World AIDS Day 2017** campaign which promotes the **theme "Right to health",** the World Health Organization will highlight the need for all 36.7 million people living with HIV and those who are vulnerable and affected by the epidemic, to reach the goal of universal health coverage.

Under the **slogan "Everybody counts",** WHO will advocate for access to safe, effective, quality and affordable medicines, including medicines, diagnostics and other health commodities as well as health care services for all people in need, while also ensuring that they are protected against financial risks.

Key messages to achieve universal health coverage.

- Leave no one behind.
- HIV, tuberculosis and hepatitis services are integrated.
- High-quality services are available for those with HIV.
- People living with HIV have access to affordable care.
- The HIV response is robust and leads to stronger health systems.

Ans: (d) Everyone counts

Ref: *http://www.who.int/campaigns/aids-day/2017/event/en/*

3. **Triage means:**

(a) First comes first served basis
(b) Treating person with better prognosis
(c) Labelling the death patients
(d) Identifying seriously ill who needs treatment first

Explanation:

- **Triage** is systemic approach to rapidly identifying patients with urgent or life threatening conditions.
- Defined as "A system where by a group of casualties or other patients are sorted according to seriousness of their injuries or illness so that treatment priorities can be allocated between them.
- In emergency situations it is designed to maximize the no. of survivors.
- "First come first treated" is not applicable in mass casualties.

Example of Color Coded Triage System

Priority	Colour
High	Red
Medium	Yellow
Ambulatory	Green
Dead or moribund	Black

Ans: (d) Identifying seriously ill who needs treatment first

Ref: *Emergency Department Leadership and Management by Stehanie Kayden, Page 203*

4. **Most important factor in sewage treatment:**

(a) Bacterial count
(b) Solids
(c) Nitrite and phosphorus
(d) Water content

Explanation:

Sewage:
- Waste water containing solid and liquid excreta.

Sullage:
- Waste water which does not contain human excreta.

Dry weather flow: Average amount of sewage that flows thru sewerage system in 24 hours.

Strength of Sewage

Biochemical oxygen demand (BOD):

- Standard test for indicator of organic content.
- Amount of oxygen absorbed by a sample of sewage during a specified period (5 days), at specified temperature (20 degree), for aerobic destruction or use of organic matter by living organisms.
- Ranges from 1 mg/L for natural water to 300 mg/L for untreated domestic sewage:
  BOD > 300 mg/L – strong.
  BOD < 100 mg/L – weak.

Chemical oxygen demand (COD):

- Oxygen equivalent of that portion of organic matter in a sample which is susceptible to oxidation by strong chemical oxidiser.

Suspended solids:
- Amount of suspended solids may vary from 100 to 500 ppm (mg/L)
  500 mg/L – strong.
  100 mg/L – weak.

Ans: (b) Solids

Ref: *Park, 24th edition, Page 800*

5. **True about Sentinel surveillance of HIV AIDS by NACO are all *except:***

(a) Yearly checkup is done
(b) Pregnant females are included
(c) Reduced antenatal HIV transmission
(d) Target high risk population

Explanation:

Sentinel surveillance is done once in 2 years.

Types of Surveillance in HIV/NACO:

(a) HIV sentinel surveillance
(b) HIV sero surveillance
(c) AIDS case surveillance
(d) STD surveillance
(e) Behavioural surveillance

HIV Sentinel Surveillance:

Objectives of sentinel surveillance:

- To monitor trends in prevalence of HIV infection over time.
- To monitor the distribution and spread of HIV prevalence in different population subgroups and in different geographical areas.
- To identify emerging pockets of HIV epidemic in the country.

Methodology Summary

	High Risk Groups: IDU/ MSM/FSW/TG	**Bridge Population: STD patients/SMM/LDT**	**General Population: Pregnant women attending ANC clinics**
Sentinel Site	Targeted Interventions (TI) Projects	STD clinic; TI Projects	Antenatal clinic
Sample Size	250	250	400
Duration	3 months	3 months	3 months
Frequency	Once in 2 years	Once in 2 years	Once in 2 years
Sampling Method	Consecutive/Random	Consecutive	Consecutive
Age Group	15-49 years	15-49 years	15-49 years
Testing Strategy	Unliked Anonymous with informed consent	Unlinked Anonymous at STD; with Informed consent at T1 Sites	Unlinked Anonymous
Blood Specimen	Dried Blood Spot	Serum at STD; DBS at T1 Sites	Serum
Testing Protocol	Two Test Protocol	Two Test Protocol	Two Test Protocol

Ans: (a) Yearly check up

Ref: *Park, 24th edition, Page 453*

6. **Cronbach alpha is a measure of:**

(a) Criterion validity
(b) Internal consistency
(c) Values are between 1 and 100
(d) Content validity

Explanation:

Cronbach alpha:

- It is a measure of **internal consistency**, that is, how closely related a set of items are as a group.
- It is considered to be a measure of **scale reliability**.
- A "high" value for alpha does not imply that the measure is unidimensional.

- Most widely used measure to assess the **internal consistency**.
- Widely used to evaluate **questionnaires**.

Accuracy Vs Precision

Accuracy and Precision

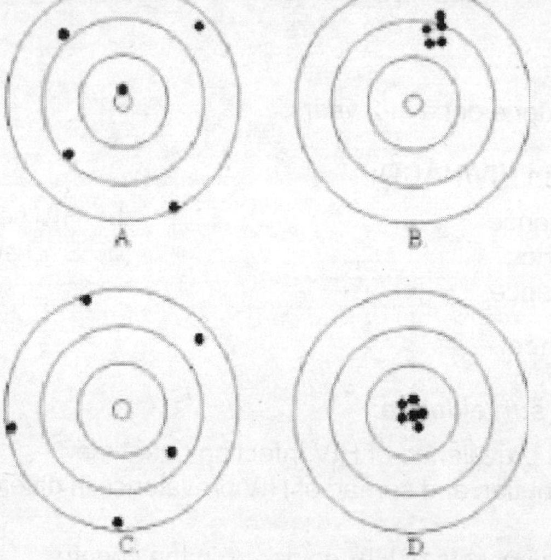

A. Accuracy present no precision
B. Precision present no accuracy
C. No precision and no accuracy
D. Accuracy and precision

- Validity refers to what extent the test measures which it purports to measure.
- Closeness with which measured values agree with true values.
- In simple terms, ability of a test to separate those who have the disease from those who do not.

Ans: (b) Internal consistency

Ref: *Biomedical Research, Page 623*

7. **A newly married husband is diagnosed with Hepatitis B and C infection. What advice should be given to his wife?**

(a) Explaining husband alone is enough
(b) Wife to be informed only after consent obtained from husband
(c) Wife should be informed about this as it is sexually transmitted
(d) Wife should be informed due to familial concern

Ans: (c) Wife should be informed about this as it is sexually transmitted

Ref: *Natl Med J India 2000 Jul-Aug;13(4):207-11*

Explanation:

- This is a grey area as there is no law yet covering this in Indian judiciary system.
- As increasing numbers of persons with HIV and other sexually transmitted infection come under the care of clinicians and community programmes, the questions of breaching confidentiality to warn unsuspecting partners will be faced repeatedly in medical practice.
- Research and clinical experience suggest that many individuals who know that they are infected fail to inform their sexual partners of the fact. Clinicians will be increasingly called upon to notify partners,
- Policy makers will have to decide whether this process of notification should be discretionary, as it is currently, or be made mandatory.
- The moral claim of persons who have been placed at risk entails the correlative moral duty of clinicians to ensure that unsuspecting partners are informed.

8. **Formula for calculating positive predictive value (PPV):**

(a) a/a+b
(b) d/c+d
(c) a/a+c
(d) d/b+d

Explanation:

Basic measures used in evaluation of a diagnostic test are:

a. **Sensitivity** and **specificity**
b. **Predictive values** – positive predictive value and negative predictive value

Sensitivity	Ability of the test to identify **true positives**
Specificity	Ability of the test to identify **true negatives**
Positive predictive value	Probability that a patient with **positive test result truly has the disease**
Negative predictive value	Probability that a patient with **negative test result truly does not have the disease**

Screening test	**Diagnosis**		**Total**
	Diseased	**Non diseased**	
Positive	a (True Positive)	b (False Positive)	a+b
Negative	c (False Negative)	d (True Negative)	c+d
Total	a+c	b+d	a+b+c+d

Using above table

- **Sensitivity** = a/(a + c) × 100
- **Specificity** = d/(b + d) × 100
- **Predictive value of a positive test** = a/(a + b) × 100
- **Predictive value of a negative test** = d/(c + d) × 100
- **Percentage of false negatives** = c/(a + c) × 100
- **Percentage of false positive** = b/(b + d) × 100

Tips to avoid confusions and to be clear of this concept:

Whatever question is asked about these indicators

1. First make the table with disease in columns and test in the rows
2. Remember the rule that sensitivity and specificity are column percentages and predictive values are row percentages.
3. Always, true values in numerator.

In the below tables, concentrate on the shaded areas

Sensitivity

	Diseased	Non-Diseased	Total
Test +	a (True Positives)	b (False Positives)	a+b
Test -	c (False Negatives)	d (True Negatives)	c+d
Total	a+c	b+d	a+b+c+d

Sensitivity = a/a+c *100

Specificity

	Diseased	Non-Diseased	Total
Test +	a (True Positives)	b (False Positives)	a+b
Test -	c (False Negatives)	d (True Negatives)	c+d
Total	a+c	b+d	a+b+c+d

Specificity = d/b+d*100

Positive Predictive Value

	Diseased	Non-Diseased	Total
Test +	a (True Positives)	b (False Positives)	a+b
Test -	c (False Negatives)	d (True Negatives)	c+d
Total	a+c	b+d	a+b+c+d

Positive predictive value = a/a+b*100

Negative Predictive Value

	Diseased	Non-Diseased	Total
Test +	a (True Positives)	b (False Positives)	a+b
Test -	c (False Negatives)	d (True Negatives)	c+d
Total	a+c	b+d	a+b+c+d

Negative predictive value = d/c+d*100

Ans: (a) a/a+b

Ref: *Park, 24th edition, Page 149*

ENT

1. **Vocal cord position when cricoarytenoids are in neutral positions:**

(a) Paramedian (b) Median
(c) Intermediate (d) Abducted

Explanation:

- The **Neutral point** of a joint is the position where there is the **least amount of support** from the **ligaments** and other **non-muscular tissues** around the joint.
- In this position, stress to the joint is minimized, which helps the joint to function well over time.

Cord Position	Location from midline	Position in normal condition	Position in diseased conditions
Median	Midline	Normal phonation	Recurrent laryngeal nerve paralysis
Paramedian	1.5 mm	Strong whisper	Recurrent laryngeal nerve paralysis
Intermediate [Cadaveric] – Neutral position from which abduction and adduction take place	3.5 mm	–	Both superior and recurrent laryngeal nerve paralysis
Gentle abduction	7 mm	Quite respiration	Paralysis of adductors
Full abduction	9.5 mm	Deep respiration	–

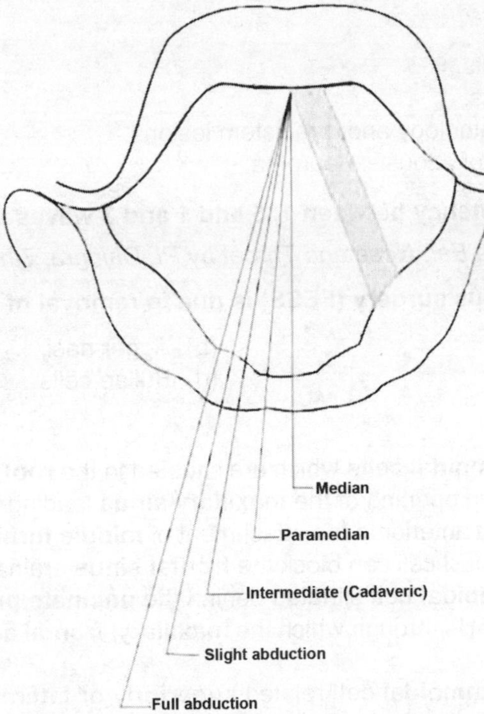

Ans: (c) Intermediate

Ref: *Diseases of the Ear, Nose and Throat by PL Dhingra, 7th edition, 2018, Page 338-339*

2. **Brainstem evoked potential in vestibular schwannoma:**

(a) Flat amplitude
(b) Increased amplitude in 5, 6
(c) Decreased amplitude in 5, 6
(d) Increased amplitude in 1 to 5
(e) Increased inter-wave latency between 1, 5 and 1 and 3 waves

Explanation:

Vestibular Schwannoma or Acoustic Neuroma

- Compresses the VIIIth cranial nerve, thus affecting the central auditory pathway.
- The difference is measured between wave **I** and wave **V** on both sides and a **difference of >0.2 ms in wave V** between two ears is significant.

BERA – Brainstem Evoked Response Audiometry

- Also called **BAER or BAEP or ABR** (auditory brainstem response).
- In this electric potentials are generated in response to several click stimuli or tone bursts and picked up from the vertex by surface electrodes.
- Tests the integrity of central auditory pathway.
- Noninvasive test.
- Normally **7 waves** are seen in the first 10 milliseconds.
- **I, III and V waves** are **most important.**
- Absolute latency, inter wave latency and the amplitude of the waves are measured.
- Site of generation of waves are:
  i. Wave I – distal CN VIII
  ii. Wave II – proximal CN VIII
  iii. Wave III – cochlear nucleus
  iv. Wave IV – superior olivary complex
  v. Wave V – lateral lemniscus
  vi. Wave VI and VII – inferior colliculus

Uses

- Screening for hearing in infants.
- Threshold estimation in infants.
- To diagnose retro cochlear pathology and brainstem lesions.
- Monitor VIII N during surgery of acoustic neuroma.

Ans: (e) Increased inter-wave latency between 1, 5 and 1 and 3 waves

Ref: *Diseases of the Ear, Nose and Throat by PL Dhingra, 7th edition, 2018, Page 28 and 126*

3. **Optic nerve injury following sinus surgery (FESS) is due to removal of which ethmoidal cells?**

(a) Haller
(b) Agger nasi
(c) Onodi cells
(d) Bullae cells

Explanation:

- **Haller cells** are a type of **ethmoidal cells** which are situated in the **roof of maxillary sinus**. Sometimes they may enlarge and block the opening of the **maxillary sinus** leading to maxillary sinusitis.
- **Agger nasi** is an elevation just anterior to the attachment of **middle turbinate** and can contain the **agger nasi cell**. An enlarged agger nasi cell can block the **frontal sinus** drainage and lead to frontal sinusitis.
- **Bula ethmoidalis** is the **ethmoidal cell** situated behind the **uncinate process** and forms the **posterior boundary of hiatus semilunaris** through which the **maxillary, frontal and anterior ethmoidal sinuses drain.**
- **Onodi cell** is the **posterior ethmoidal cell** related **superiorly or laterally to the sphenoid sinus**. The **optic nerve** lies in its **lateral wall** and can be **injured** while operating in this **cell**.

Ans: (c) Onodi cells

Ref: *Diseases of the Ear, Nose and Throat by PL Dhingra, 7th edition, 2018, Page 210*

OPHTHALMOLOGY

1. **A 75-year-old patient who was a known case of diabetes mellitus for the past 25 years presented with sudden painless loss of vision. On fundus examination, flame shaped hemorrhages were seen in retina. Probable diagnosis:**

(a) CRAO
(b) Retinal detachment
(c) Proliferative retinopathy
(d) Cystoid macular edema

Explanation:

The question is not framed with all the information needed to answer it.

- **Retinal detachment** presents with **sudden painless loss of vision** but fundus picture usually shows **detached retina with break or tractional bands**, not with flame shaped hemorrhages alone.
- **Proliferative Diabetic retinopathy (PDR)** alone will not cause loss of vision. Patient can have 6/6 vision even in the presence of PDR.
- If vitreous hemorrhage was given in the option, I would go for it.

Causes of Defective Vision in Diabetic Retinopathy:

- **Diabetic maculopathy** – Macular edema, ischemic maculopathy, clinically significant macular edema (CSME). The most common cause of defective vision in DR.
- **Advanced diabetic eye diseases** like:
  - o Vitreous hemorrhage.
  - o Tractional retinal detachment.
  - o Neovascular glaucoma.

Classification of Diabetic Retinopathy:

- **ETDRS** (Early Treatment Diabetic Retinopathy Study) Classification:
  - o Non-proliferative diabetic retinopathy (NPDR).
  - o Proliferative diabetic retinopathy (PDR).
  - o Diabetic macular edema (DME).

Non-Proliferative Diabetic Retinopathy (NPDR)

Mild	Few microaneurysms Retinal haemorrhage Hard exudates in 1 or 2 quadrants
Moderate	Above findings seen in 2 or 3 quadrants
Severe	**4:2:1 Rule** • Haemorrhages or Microaneurysms or both in all **4 Quadrants** • Venous Beading in **2 Quadrants** • **IRMA** (Intra Retinal Microvascular abnormality – A-V shunts secondary to microvascular occlusion) in atleast **1 Quadrant**
Very severe	Any two of the above 4:2:1 rule

Proliferative diabetic retinopathy:

- Neovascularization of the disc (NVD).
- Neovascularization elsewhere (NVE).

Advanced diabetic eye disease:

- Neovascular glaucoma.
- Tractional retinal detachment.
- Vitreous hemorrhage.

Clinically Significant Macular Edema:

- Retinal edema within **5ooμ from the centre of fovea.**
- **Retinal thickening** that is one disc area or larger, any part of which is within one disc diameter from the centre of fovea.

- **Hard exudates** within **500μ from the centre of fovea**, if associated with **adjacent retinal thickening.**

Ans: (b) Retinal detachment

Ref: *A.K.Khurana's Comprehensive Ophthalmology, 6th edition, Page 277*

2. In common canalicular blockage, which is true about Jones test findings?

(a) First test positive second test negative
(b) First test negative second test positive
(c) Both positive
(d) Both negative

Explanation:

Jones Dye Test

- Indicated **to distinguish functional disorders from the organic blockage**. E.g.: Atony of the sac.
- In atony of the sac, Lacrimal syringing will be normal but watering will be there. Drainage system is patent but lacrimal pump is not functioning properly.

Two Tests

- ***Test 1:*** Instillation of 2% fluorescein dye in the conjunctiva and look for the dye in the nasal cavity after 5 minutes.
- ***Test 2:*** Lacrimal syringing done with saline.

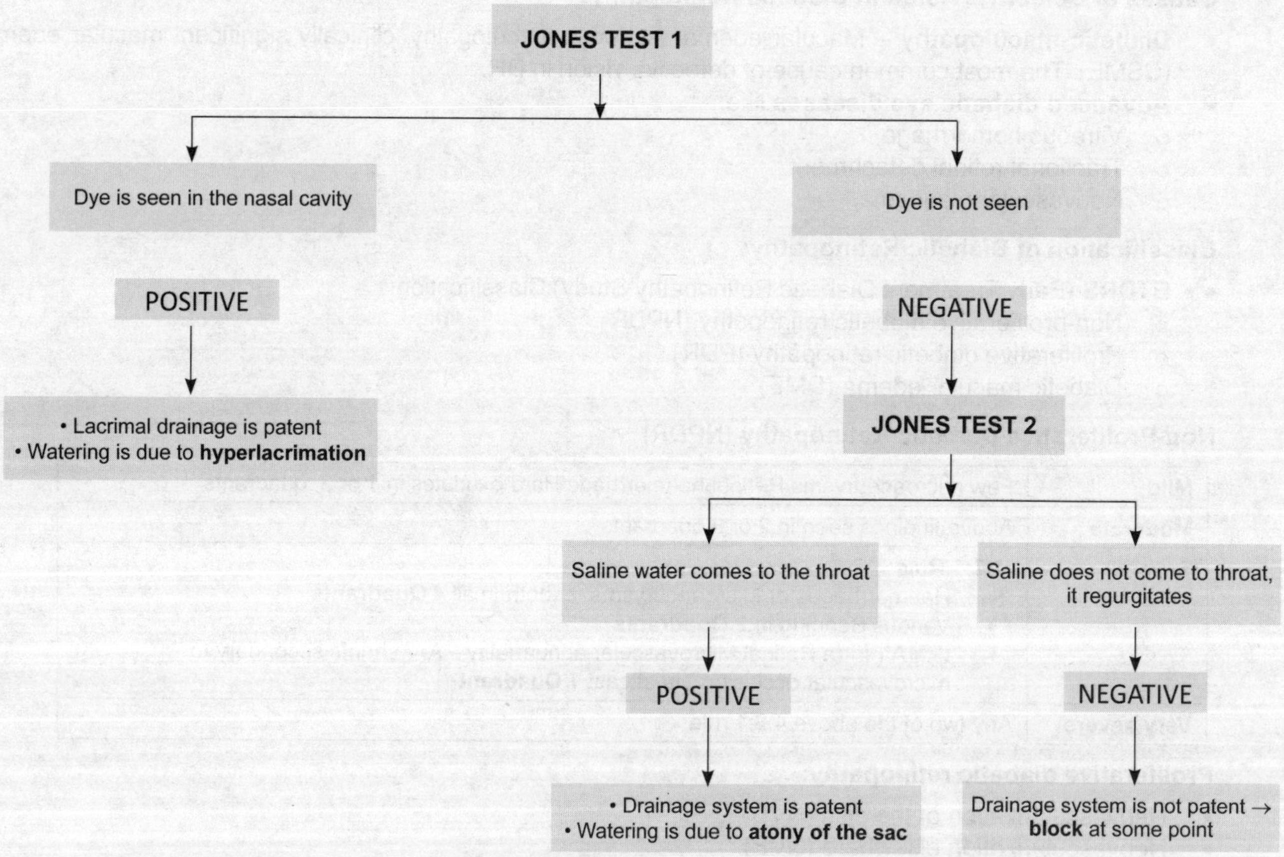

	JONES TEST 1	JONES TEST 2
Block in the drainage system	Negative	Negative
Atony of the sac	Negative	Positive
Normal/hyperlacrimation	Positive	Positive

Ans: (d) Both negative

Ref: *A.K. Khurana's Comprehensive Ophthalmology, 6th edition, Page 392; Parson's Diseases of the Eye, 22nd edition, Page 478*

3. A 60-year-old man who underwent phacoemulsification surgery and placement of foldable intra-ocular lens of left eye a year back has come with complaints of hazy vision now in that eye. There is no associate redness or pain or watering of eye. The most common cause is:

(a) Posterior capsular opacification
(b) Cystoid macular edema
(c) Neovascular glaucoma
(d) Chorioretinits

Explanation:

The causes of defective vision after cataract surgery are:

- **Postoperative astigmatism** due to surgical incision.
- **Wrong IOL power.**
- **Cystoid macular edema.**
- **Posterior capsular opacification.**
- Other associated ocular disorders like glaucoma, retinal diseases.
- Post operative **astigmatism** and wrong IOL power presents with defective vision from day 1 post operative period.
- **Cystoid macular edema** (**Irvin Gauss syndrome**) presents with defective vision **1-3 months** after surgery till then vision will be good.
- Similarly, **PCO (posterior capsular opacification**) usually presents **after 1 year.**

Posterior Capsular Opacification / After Cataract / Secondary Cataract

Causes

- Residual lens matter – when all the cortex is not removed completely during cataract extraction.
- Proliferative type – **germinative zone** of the anterior lens epithelium proliferate → dysplasia → opaque cells (**Waddl cells**).

Types

- When the PCO involves the peripheral capsule, it will not cause defective vision. When it involves the visual axis/Central part of the PC, then the patient will have glare and defective vision which is gradual in onset and painless in nature.
  - **Membranous** – thin/dense.
  - **Sommering's Ring** → Peripheral ring shaped opacity between anterior and posterior lens capsule. So, visual axis clear → Asymptomatic.
  - **Elschnig's Pearls** → Soap bubble like appearance migrating towards the visual axis.

Treatment

- When the visual axis is clear → no need of treatment.
  - **ND YAG laser capsulotomy** (**1064 nm** wavelength and **photodisruption** in action).
  - Discission with cystitome.

Cystoid Macular Edema (Irvin Gauss syndrome)

- Usually presents with defective vision **1-3 months** after **cataract surgery**.
- **Etiology:** Vitreous disturbances during surgery → Prostaglandin release → Accumulation of fluid in the Henle's layer of macula.
- On **Fundoscopy: Honey Comb appearance**.
- **On FFA: Flower Petal appearance**.
- **Prevention: Perioperative and post-operative** use of topical anti-prostaglandins eyedrops.

Treatment

- Topical steroids and anti-prostaglandins.
- Vitrectomy.

Ans: (a) Posterior capsular opacification

Ref: *A.K. Khurana's Comprehensive Ophthalmology, 6th edition, Page 215; Parson's Diseases of the Eye, 22nd edition, Page 285*

4. A 30-year-old male with family history of glaucoma presents with headache. On examination IOP is 22 and 24 in right and left eye respectively. Angles were open on gonioscopy. No visual field defects were noted. True statement regarding the management of this patient is:

(a) Normal tension glaucoma–to be treated
(b) POAG–to be treated
(c) Ocular hypertension–no intervention required
(d) Ocular hypertension–to be treated

Explanation:

OCULAR HYPERTENSION

- **Definition of Ocular Hypertension**
  - ***IOP is 22 mm Hg or more.***
  - ***Normal optic disc.***
  - ***Normal visual fields.***
  - ***Open angle.***
  - ***Absence of any ocular or systemic disorder contributing to elevated IOP.***
- **Risk Factors:**
  - Increasing IOP.
  - Increasing age.
  - Central corneal thickness less than 555 micrometer.
  - Increased vertical C:D ratio.
  - **Myopia, family history of glaucoma, diabetes** are not found to be risk factors for developing **glaucoma in ocular hypertension patients (Ocular Hypertension Treatment Study).**
- **Indications for Management:**
  - IOP > 30 mm Hg.
  - Presence of risk factors.

Ans: (c) Ocular hypertension–no intervention required

Ref: *Kanski, Clinical Ophthalmology, 8th edition, Page 348*

5. A 20-year-old boy came with complaints of sudden pain in the left eye with loss of vision. On examination, left eye cornea was hazy and on looking down, there was a bulging in the lower eyelid. Retinoscopy shows scissoring reflex and oil drop sign was positive in both eyes, what is the diagnosis?

(a) Corneal dystrophy
(b) Keratoconus
(c) Pathological myopia
(d) Keratoglobus

Explanation:

KERATOCONUS

- Defined as non-inflammatory **bilateral ectactic condition** of **cornea** in which the cornea assumes a **conical shape** secondary to **stromal thinning** and **protrusion**.
- The diagnosis is **keratoconus** with **acute hydrops.**

Etiology: Not clear.

Symptoms: Defective vision due to progressive myopia and irregular astigmatism.

Signs:

- Window **reflex** is **distorted.**
- **Slit lamp:**
  - **Thinning and ectasia** of **cornea.**
  - **Fleischer"s ring** at the base of the cone.
  - **Vogt's line** (deep stromal striae due to stretching of cornea).
- **Retinoscopy:** ***Scissoring/Yawning reflex.***
- **Distant direct ophthalmoscopy:** ***Oil Droplet Reflex.***
- **Munson's Sign:** Bulging of **lower lid** on **downward gaze.**

Management:

- **Spectacle correction** in early cases.
- Rigid gas permeable contact lenses.
- Intra corneal ring segments (**INTACS**).
- **Collagen cross linking.**
- Deep anterior **lamellar keratoplasty / penetrating keratoplasty.**

Remember:

- **Acute hydrops** is a complication of **keratoconus** where the **descemet's membrane ruptures** and **aqueous enters** the **cornea**.

Ans: (b) Keratoconus

Ref: *Kanski, Clinical Ophthalmology, 8th edition, Page 218-220;*
A.K. Khurana's Comprehensive Ophthalmology, 6th edition, Page 131

6. **A patient is presenting with c/o itching at the lid and swelling for the past 1 month. On examination, there are crusting, scaling with small ulcers near eyelid margin. If untreated, it can lead to:**

(a) Orbital cellulitis
(b) Ectropion and Epiphora
(c) Chalazion
(d) Orbital abscess formation

Explanation:

The diagnosis is ulcerative blepharitis.

BLEPHARITIS

- Subacute or chronic inflammation of the lid margins.

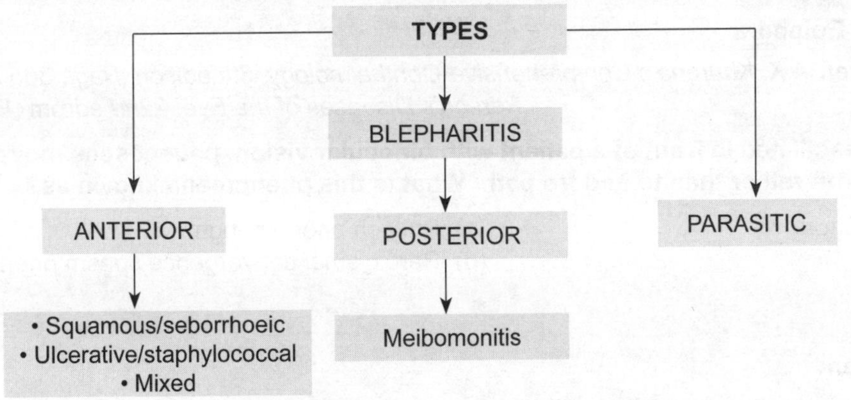

Types	Etiology and pathogenesis	Clinical features	Treatment
Squamous	• Associated with seborrhea of the scalp • Zeiss gland → abnormal excessive neutral lipids which are split by corynebacterium acne into irritating free fatty acids	• **White** dandruff like deposition among the lashes • On removal, **no ulcer**	• Lid hygiene • Treat the seborrhea
Ulcerative / staphylococcal	Due to staphylococcal infection	• **Yellow** crusts at the root of the cilia with matting of lashes • On removal of the crusts, bleeding **small ulcers** are seen • Red, thickened lid margins	• Lid hygiene • Topical and systemic antibiotics

Contd.

Contd.

Posterior/ Meibomianitis	• Associated with acne rosacae • Meibomian gland dysfunction. Bacterial lipases play a role	• **Meibomian Seborrhea*** – **white frothy discharge** at the lid margin • **Toothpaste like** thick secretion on expressing the meibomian gland • Meibomian gland appears like **vertical yellow streaks** due to thick secretion	• Lid hygiene and warm compress • Topical and systemic antibiotics
Parasitic	• **Phthiriasis palpebrum→** Phthirus pubis (crab louse). It is sexually transmitted • **Peduculosis→**pediculus humanis corporis/capitus (head louse). Spill over from the head if severely infested	• **Lice and Nits** anchoring the lashes	• Mechanical removal of the lice and nits with forceps • Yellow mercuric oxide 1% application • Delousing the whole family

Complications of chronic blepharitis:

- Lash abnormalities: Madarosis, trichiasis, poliosis.
- Tylosis.
- **Punctual eversion→ chronic watering of the eyes→ eczema of the surrounding skin →cicatrization → ectropion.**
- Recurrent hordeolum externum.
- Marginal keratitis.
- Dry eyes.
- Chronic inflammatory changes in the cornea and conjunctiva.

Ans: (b) Ectropion and Epiphora

Ref: *A.K. Khurana's Comprehensive Ophthalmology, 6th edition, Page 365 and 368; Parson's Diseases of the Eye, 22nd edition, Page 451*

7. **When a small target is oscillated in front of a patient with binocular vision, patient sees movement of the object in elliptical orbit rather than to and fro path. What is this phenomena known as?**

(a) Oppenheim phenomenon
(b) Pulfrich phenomenon
(c) Uthoff phenomenon
(d) Paroxysmal convergence spasm phenomenon

Explanation:

Oppenheim Phenomenon:

- The great toe dorsiflex when the periostium of the tibia is rubbed with the knuckles.
- Other three options are seen in **multiple sclerosis.**

Uthoff's Phenomenon:

- Seen in **multiple sclerosis.**
- Worsening of neurologic symptoms.
- Transient visual blurring during exercise, during a hot bath or shower, or during emotional stress.

Pulfrich Phenomenon:

- Seen in:
  - **Multiple sclerosis.**
  - **Cataract.**
  - **Optic neuritis.**
- Because optic nerve damage delays transmission of impulses to the visual cortex, patients with unilateral or markedly asymmetric optic neuritis may experience the **Pulfrich effect or stereoillusion**.
- The examiner oscillates a small target in the frontal plane while the patient binocularly observes it. The delay in signal transmission from one eye to the visual cortex creates the illusion that the target appears to move in an elliptical rather than a to-and-fro path.

- This disparity in time, caused by the difference in latency between eyes, is interpreted as a disparity in space that results in the stereoillusion.

Paroxysmal Convergence Spasm:

- Rare but typical symptom in **multiple sclerosis** due to **abnormal excitation** (In MS, not only delay in conduction occurs, sometimes spontaneous excitation occurs).
- Due to demyelination plaque in medial longitudinal fasciculus.

Ans: (b) Pulfrich phenomenon

Ref: *Albert and Jacobie's Principles and Practice of Ophthalmology, 3rd edition, Page 3874*

8. **The lipogranulomatous chronic inflammation of the meibomian gland is called:**

(a) Hordeolum internum (b) Stye
(c) Xanthelasma (d) Chalazion

Explanation:

	Hordeolum externum	Hordeolum internum	Chalazion
Definition	• Acute **suppurative** inflammation of the glands of **Zeis and Moll** • Zeis – modified sebaceous glands and Moll – modified sweat gland. Both open at the root of lash follicles	• Acute **suppurative** inflammation of the **meibomian glands** • Meibomian gland is a modified sebaceous gland situated in the tarsal plate	• Chronic **lipogranulomatous** inflammation of the **meibomian gland**
Etiopathogenesis	• Infective – Staphylococcus aureus	• Infective – Staphylococcus aureus	Low grade infection of the meibomian gland → proliferation of the duct epithelium and infiltration → **blockage of meibomian gland ducts** → retention of lipid secretion (sebum)→ extravasated fatty contents act like irritant → induce chronic non-infective lipogranulomatous inflammation of the gland
Symptoms	Acute painful lid swellings	Acute painful lid swellings	Chronic **painless lid swelling**
Signs	Swelling and pus point seen **at the lid margin** at the root of the lashes	Swelling and pus point seen **away from the lid margin** more on the conjunctival side	Painless swelling – increasing in size Large chalazion may cause defective vision by pressing on the cornea (astigmatism)
Treatment	• Hot fomentation • **Topical and systemic antibiotics** • Systemic anti-inflammatory • Epilation to evacuate pus	• Hot fomentation • **Topical and systemic antibiotics** • Systemic anti-inflammatory • Incision and drainage to evacuate pus	• **Incision and curettage*** • **Intralesional long acting steroids**

* Incision and curettage for chalazion: Incision on conjunctival side is **vertical** over the swelling to prevent injuries to the neighbouring glands since the meibomian glands are **vertically arranged**. If the swelling is more towards the skin side, then incision is done along the skin crease, i.e., horizontal.

Ans: (d) Chalazion

Ref: *A.K. Khurana's Comprehensive Ophthalmology, 6th edition, Page 367-370*

MEDICINE

1. **A patient on warfarin presents with major bleeding and found to have PT INR of 1.5. How much fresh frozen plasma (FFP) is required to treat this situation?**

(a) 15 ml/kg (b) 10 ml/kg
(c) 5 ml/kg (d) 20 ml/kg

Explanation:

Guidelines for reversal of warfarin anticoagulation

INR	Bleeding	Recommendation
<5.0	None	Decrease or omit warfarin dose
	Minor	Discontinue warfarin Consider vitamin K_1 (2.5 mg orally)
	Major	Discontinue warfarin Vitamin K_1 (10 mg by slow intravenous infusion)* Fresh frozen plasma (15 mL/kg) or prothrombin complex concentrate Consider recombinant factor VIIa
5.0-9.0	None	Omit one or two doses of warfarin; resume at lower dose
	Minor	Discontinue warfarin Vitamin K_1 (2.5 to 5.0 mg orally)
	Major	Discontinue warfarin Vitamin K_1 (10 mg by slow intravenous infusion)* Fresh frozen plasma (15 mL/kg) or prothrombin complex concentrate Consider recombinant Factor VIIa
> 9.0	None	Hold warfarin Vitamin K_1 (5 to 10 mg orally)
	Minor	Discontinue warfarin Vitamin K_1 (5 to 10 mg orally) Consider fresh frozen plasma (15 mL/kg)
	Major	Discontinue warfarin Vitamin K_1 (10 mg by slow intravenous infusion)* Fresh frozen plasma (15 mL/kg) or prothrombin complex concentrate Consider recombinant Factor VIIa

Ans: (a) 15 ml/kg

Ref: *Practical Transfusion Medicine edited by Michael F. Murphy, Derwood H. Pamphilon, 2nd edition, Page132; Rossi's Principles of Transfusion Medicine, 5th edition, Page 387*

2. **A 70-year-old patient presents with dizziness and headache followed by left sided hemiparesis with right eye dilatation and ptosis. Most probable blood vessel damaged is:**

(a) Middle cerebral artery (b) Anterior communicating artery
(c) Posterior cerebral artery (d) Basilar artery

Ans: (c) Posterior cerebral artery

Ref: *Adams and Victor's Principles of Neurology, 10th edition, Page 804; Localisation in Clinical Neurology, 6th edition, Chapter 105*

Explanation:

Eponym	Site	Cranial nerves involved	Tracts involved	Signs	Arteries involved
Weber syndrome	Base of midbrain	III	Corticospinal tract	Oculomotor palsy with crossed hemiplegia	Proximal posterior cerebral artery
Claude syndrome	Tegmentum of midbrain	III	Red nucleus, superior cerebellar peduncles after decussation	Oculomotor palsy with contralateral cerebellar ataxia and tremor	Proximal posterior cerebral artery
Benedict syndrome	Tegmentum of midbrain	III	Red nucleus, corticospinal tract superior cerebellar peduncles after decussation	Oculomotor palsy with contralateral cerebellar ataxia, tremor, and corticospinal signs, choreoathetosis	Proximal posterior cerebral artery
Nothnagel syndrome	Tectum of midbrain	Unilateral or bilateral III nerve	Superior cerebellar peduncles	Ocular palsies (IV), paralysis of gaze, nystagmus and ataxia	
Parinaud syndrome	Dorsal midbrain		Supranuclear mechanism for upward gaze and dorsal midbrain, periaqueductal gray matter	Paralysis of upward gaze and accommodation; fixed pupils	
Millard-Gubler syndrome	Unilateral lesion of the ventrocaudal pons	Fascicles of cranial nerves VI and VII	Pyramidal tract, cranial nerve VI, cranial nerve VII	Contralateral hemiplegia, Ipsilateral lateral rectus paresis, Ipsilateral peripheral facial paresis	
Raymond Syndrome	Unilateral lesion of the ventral medial pons	Abducens nerve fascicles and the corticospinal tract but spares cranial nerve VII	Pyramidal tract, cranial nerve VI	Ipsilateral lateral rectus paresis, contralateral hemiplegia	
Locked-in syndrome	Bilateral ventral pontine lesions		Bilateral corticospinal tract involvement in the basal pontis, involvement of the corticobulbar fibers innervating the lower cranial nerve nuclei	Quadriplegia, Aphonia	
Foville syndrome	Dorsal pontine tegmentum	Involvement of the nucleus and fascicle (or both) of cranial nerve VII	Corticospinal tract, involvement of the PPRF or abducens nucleus, or both	Contralateral hemiplegia (with facial sparing), Ipsilateral peripheral type facial palsy, Inability to move the eyes conjugately to the ipsilateral side involvement of the PPRF or abducens nucleus, or both	

Contd.

Contd.

Raymond-Cestan syndrome	Rostral lesions of the dorsal pons		Involvement of the cerebellum, medial lemniscus and the spinothalamic tract, PPRF	Cerebellar signs (ataxia), Contralateral hypoesthesia with reduction of all sensory modalities (face and extremities), contralateral hemiparesis, paralysis of conjugate gaze toward the side of the lesion	
Marie-Foix syndrome	Lateral pontine lesions brachium pontis		Involvement of cerebellar connections, corticospinal tract, spinothalamic tract	Ipsilateral cerebellar ataxia, Contralateral hemiparesis, Variable contralateral hemihypesthesia for pain and temperature	
Wallenburg syndrome	Lateral tegmentum of medulla	Spinal V, IX, X, XI	Lateral spinothalamic tract,spinocerebellar and ollivocerebellar tracts	Ipsilateral V, IX, X, XI palsy, Horner syndrome, -cerebellar ataxia; contralateral loss of pain and temperature sense	Intracranial vertebral artery or posterior inferior cerebellar artery
Medial Medullary syndrome (Dejerine's Anterior Bulbar Syndrome)	Medial medulla	XII	Cranial nerve XII,Corticospinal tract, medial lemniscus	Ipsilateral paresis, atrophy, and fibrillation of the tongue, Contralateral hemiplegia, Contralateral loss of position and vibratory sensation	Vertebral artery, anterior spinal artery, or the lower segment of the basilar artery
Avellis syndrome	Tegmentum of medulla	X	Spinothalamic tract	Paralysis of soft palate and vocal cord and contralateral hemianaesthesia	
Thalamic syndrome of Dejerine and Roussy					Occlusion of thalamogeniculate branches of PCA

3. What is the site of lesion in a patient with Alexia without agraphia?

(a) Fusiform gyrus (b) Inferior occipital gyrus
(c) Psalternum (d) Splenium

Explanation:

Effects of disease of the occipital lobes

Effects of unilateral disease, either right or left

A. Contralateral (congruent) homonymous hemianopia, which may be central (splitting the macula) or peripheral; also **homonymous hemiachromatopsia**
B. Elementary (unformed) hallucinations–usually because of irritative lesions

Effects of left occipital disease

A. Right homonymous hemianopia
B. If deep white matter and **splenium of corpus callosum** is involved, alexia without agraphia
C. Visual object agnosia

Effects of right occipital disease

A. Left homonymous hemianopia
B. With more extensive lesions, visual illusions (**metamorphopsias**) and hallucinations (more frequent with right-sided than left-sided lesions)
C. Loss of topographic memory and visual orientation

Dilateral occipital disease

A. Cortical blindness bilateral hemianopias
B. **Anton syndrome** (visual anosognosia, denial of cortical blindness)
C. Loss of perception of color (**achromatopsia**)
D. **Prosopagnosia** (impaired face recognition, bilateral temporooccipital including fusiform gyrus)
E. **Balint syndrome** (bilateral dorsal parietooccipital)

Contd.

Contd.

Effects of unilateral disease of the parietal lobe, right or left A. Corticosensory syndrome and sensory extinction (or total hemianesthesia with large acute lesions of white matter) B. Mild hemiparesis or poverty of movement (variable), poverty of movement, hemiataxia (seen only occasionally) C. Homonymous hemianopia or inferior quadrantanopia (incongruent or congruent) or visual inattention D. Abolition of optokinetic nystagmus with target moving toward side of the lesion E. Neglect of the opposite side of external space (more prominent with lesions of the right parietal lobe)	**Effects of unilateral disease of the dominant (left) parietal lobe (in right-handed and most left-handed patients);** additional phenomena include: A. Disorders of language (especially alexia) B. **Gerstmann syndrome** (dysgraphia, dyscalculia, finger agnosia, right-left confusion) C. Tactile agnosia (bimanual astereognosis) D. Bilateral ideomotor and ideational apraxia **Effects of unilateral disease of the nondominant (right) parietal lobe** A. Visuospatial disorders B. Topographic memory loss C. Anosognosia, dressing, and constructional apraxias D. Confusion E. Tendency to keep the eyes closed, resist lid opening, and blepharospasm **Effects of bilateral disease of the parietal lobes** A. **Balint syndrome**: Visual-spatial imperception (simultagnosia), optic apraxia (difficulty directing gaze), and optic ataxia
Effects of unilateral disease of the dominant temporal lobe A. Homonymous contralateral upper quadrantanopia B. Wernicke's aphasia (word deafness; auditory verbal agnosia) C. Dysnomia or amnesic aphasia D. Amusia (some types) E. Visual agnosia F. Occasionally, amnesic (Korsakoff) syndrome	**Effects of unilateral disease of the nondominant temporal lobe** A. **Homonymous upper quadrantanopia** B. Inability to judge spatial relationships in some cases C. Impairment in tests of visually presented nonverbal material D. Agnosia for sounds and some qualities of music **Effects of disease of either temporal lobe** A. Auditory, visual, olfactory and gustatory hallucinations B. **"Dreamy" states** with seizure (focal temporal lobe seizure) C. Emotional and behavioral changes D. Delirium-confusional states (usually nondominant) E. Disturbances of time perception **Effects of bilateral disease** A. **Korsakoff amnesic defect** (hippocampal formations) B. Apathy and placidity C. **Kluver-Bucy syndrome**: Compulsion to attend to all visual stimuli, hyperorality, hypersexuality, blunted emotional reactivity
Effects of frontal lobe disease **Effects of unilateral frontal disease, either left or right** A. Contralateral spastic hemiplegia B. Contralateral gaze paresis C. Apathy and loss of initiative or its opposite, slight elevation of mood, increased talkativeness, tendency to joke inappropriately (witzelsucht), lack of tact, difficulty in adaptation D. If entirely prefrontal, no hemiplegia; but grasp and suck reflexes or instinctive grasping may be released E. Anosmia with involvement of orbital parts **Effects of right frontal disease** A. Left hemiplegia B. Changes as in B, C and D above	**Effects of left frontal disease** A. Right hemiplegia B. Broca's aphasia with agraphia, with or without apraxia of the lips and tongue C. Sympathetic apraxia of left hand **Effects of bifrontal disease** A. Bilateral hemiparesis B. Spastic bulbar (pseudobulbar) palsy C. If prefrontal, abulia or akinetic mutism, lack of ability to sustain attention and solve complex problems D. Decomposition of gait and sphincter incontinence

Ans: (d) Splenium

***Ref:** Adams and Victor's Principles of Neurology, 10th edition, Page 466-481*

4. Differential diagnosis for 'Thunderclap headache' are all *except*:

(a) Encephalitis (b) Ischemic stroke
(c) Subarachnoid hemorrhage (d) Meningitis

Explanation:

Causes of Thunderclap Headache

- **Migraine** variant
- **Meningitis/Encephalitis**
- **Subarachnoid hemorrhage***
- Cerebral venous **thrombosis**
- Diffuse cerebral vasculopathy (**Call-Fleming syndrome**)
- Subdural hematoma
- Accelerated **hypertension**
- Pituitary apoplexy
- Cervical arterial dissection
- **Cocaine**
- Serotoninergic drugs
- Perimesencephalic hemorrhage

Ans: (b) Ischemic stroke

Ref: *Adams and Victor's Principles of Neurology, 10th edition, Chapter 10, Headache and Other Craniofacial Pains, Page189*

5. A patient with undulating fever presents with features of encephalitis. He is treated successfully with doxycycline and rifampicin. Probable diagnosis:

(a) Brucellosis
(b) Bordetella pertussis
(c) Francessilea tularensis
(d) Mycoplasma

Explanation:

- Brucellosis is a bacterial zoonosis transmitted directly or indirectly to humans from infected animals, predominantly domesticated ruminants and swine.
- Known colloquially as ***undulant fever*** because of its remittent character.
- Left untreated, the fever of brucellosis shows an undulating pattern that persists for weeks before the commencement of an afebrile period that may be followed by relapse.

Treatment:

- Gold standard for the treatment of brucellosis in adults is **IM streptomycin (0.75–1 g daily for 14–21 days) together with doxycycline (100 mg twice daily for 6 weeks).**
- The usual alternative regimen (and the current WHO recommendation) is **rifampin (600–900 mg/d) plus doxycycline (100 mg twice daily) for 6 weeks.**

Ans: (a) Brucellosis

Ref: *Harrisons, Principles of Internal Medicine, 19th edition,Chapter 194e*

6. Which is not included in Polymyalgia rheumatica criteria (Healey criteria)?

(a) Morning stiffness more than equal to 1 hour
(b) Involvement of neck, shoulder, back for more than 6 months in a year
(c) ESR > 40 mm/hr
(d) Rapid response to prednisolone < 20 mg/day

Explanation:

Diagnostic and Classification Criteria for Polymyalgia Rheumatica

#Diagnostic Criteria of Chuang and Colleagues (1982)
1. Age 50 years or older
2. Bilateral aching and stiffness for 1 month or more and involving two of the following areas: neck or torso, shoulders or proximal regions of the arms, and hips or proximal aspects of the thighs
3. ESR >40 mm/hr
4. Exclusion of all other diagnoses except giant cell arteritis

Contd.

Contd.

#Diagnostic Criteria of Healey (1984)
1. Pain persisting for at least 1 month and involving two of the following areas: neck, shoulders and pelvic girdle
2. Morning stiffness lasting >1 hr
3. Rapid response to prednisone (≤20 mg/day)
4. Absence of other diseases capable of causing the musculoskeletal symptoms
5. Age older than 50 years
6. ESR >40 mm/hr
#For each set of criteria, all the findings must be present for polymyalgia rheumatica to be diagnosed.

Ans: (b) Involvement of neck, shoulder, back for more than 6 months in a year

***Ref:** Kelley and Firesteins, Textbook of Rheumatology,10th edition, Page1521*

7. A patient presents with cough with expectoration. Diagnosis of farmers lung is suspected. True statement regarding this condition:

(a) May to June seasonal
(b) Persistent cough with expectoration
(c) X-ray features upper lobe predominant in chronic HP
(d) Pleural effusions are common

Explanation:

Farmer's Lung

- Results from exposure to moldy hay containing spores of **Thermophilic Actinomycetes** that produce a hypersensitivity pneumonitis
- Most cases of farmer's lung disease occur in cold, damp climates **in late winter and early spring**, when farmers (usually male) use stored hay to feed their livestock
- Manifestations of the disease may be acute, subacute or chronic
- **Acute clinical presentation** includes transient fever, hypoxemia, myalgias, arthralgias, dyspnea, and cough that occur 2 to 9 hours after exposure and resolve in 12 to 72 hours without specific treatment
  - In acute HP, chest radiographs–diffuse poorly defined nodular radiodensities, often with areas of ground-glass radiodensities or occasionally even consolidation, **tend to occur in the lower lobes and spare the apices**
- **Chronic form** is clinically more insidious, and patients may lack a history of acute episodes, but present with a gradual onset of cough, dyspnea, fatigue, and weight loss. Symptoms are usually present for months to years.
  - In chronic HP, chest radiographs – diffuse linear and nodular radiodensities, **with sparing of the bases and upper-lobe predominance, and volume loss**. Pleural effusions and thickening are very unusual

Ans: (c) X-ray features upper lobe predominant in chronic HP

***Ref:** Fishman's Pulmonary Disease and Disorders, 5th edition, Chapter 58*

8. In revised guideline for Behcet's disease, which criterion carries 2 points?

(a) Ocular lesions
(b) Oral ulcers
(c) Vasculitis
(d) Skin lesions

Explanation:

Revised International Criteria for Behçet's Disease

Oral aphthosis	1 point
Skin manifestations (pseudofolliculitis, skin aphthosis)	1 point
Vascular lesions (phlebitis, large vein thrombosis,aneurysm, arterial thrombosis)	1 point
Positive pathergy test	1 point
Genital aphthosis	2 points
Ocular lesions	2 points

*Diagnosis of Adamantiades–Behçet's disease is made with a score of **3 points***

Ans: (a) Ocular lesions

***Ref:** Kelley and Firesteins Textbook of Rheumatology,10th edition, Page1592*

9. Which of the following diseases doesn't cause lung cavitation?

(a) Sarcoidosis
(b) Silicosis
(c) Histoplasmosis
(d) Wegener's

Explanation:

- All the above conditions can present with cavitation. But in sarcoidosis cavitation is a very uncommon manifestation and should suggest superimposed tuberculosis or fungal abscess.

Causes of lung cavitation

Bacterial lung abscess	Most frequently Staphylococcus, Klebsiella, Pseudomonas and Proteus
Pneumatocele	Develops in approximately 50% of children with staphylococcal pneumonia
Mycobacteria	Cavitation (often multiple) tends to be a more prominent feature of atypical mycobacterial disease than of Mycobacterium tuberculosis
Fungal lung abscess	Pleural effusion and extension into the chest wall are common in actinomycosis and nocardiosis. **Histoplasmosis** typically involves the apical and posterior segments of the upper lobes, coccidioidomycosis is characteristically located in the anterior segment
Amebic lung abscess	Almost always in the right lower lobe and associated with a right pleural effusion
Hydatid cyst (Echinococcus granulosus)	Rupture of the cyst into a bronchus results in part or all of its liquid contents being expelled into the bronchial system, producing the characteristic "meniscus sign" and "water lily sign"
Pneumocystis carinii	Primarily seen in patients with AIDS
Bronchogenic carcinoma	Cavitation in 2% to 10% of cases, most commonly in peripheral squamous cell tumors of the upper lobes
Hematogenous metastases	Cavitation in approximately 4% of cases. Most commonly involves squamous cell neoplasms
Hodgkin's disease	Cavitation typically develops in peripheral parenchymal consolidations (most often in the lower lobes)
Septic embolism	Almost always multiple with lower lobe predominance
Silicosis	Cavitation in conglomerate lesions is more often the result of superimposed tuberculosis than ischemic necrosis. Cavitation also occurs in coal-workers' pneumoconiosis
Wegener's granulomatosis	Cavitation eventually occurs in approximately half of patients
Rheumatoid necrobiotic nodule	Often multiple and generally in a peripheral subpleural location
Cystic bronchiectasis	Cavities represent severely dilated segmental bronchi
Traumatic lung cyst	Typically occurs in a peripheral subpleural location immediately underlying the point of maximum injury
Sarcoidosis	Very uncommon manifestation (suggest superimposed tuberculosis or fungal)
Intralobar bronchopulmonary sequestration	
Bronchogenic cyst	
Cystic fibrosis	Ring shadows in this condition can be caused by cystic bronchiectasis, bullae, microabscesses

Ans: (a) Sarcoidosis

***Ref:** Clinical Imaging, An Atlas of Differential Diagnosis, 5th edition, Page 86*

10. Birt-Hogg-Dube syndrome associated with:

(a) Renal cell carcinoma
(b) Lung Ca
(c) Stomach Ca
(d) Ovarian Ca

Explanation:

Birt-Hogg-Dube syndrome

- Characterized by prominent **cutaneous manifestations**, the development of **spontaneous pneumothorax** in association with **lung cysts**
- Predisposition to **kidney neoplasms (chromophobe renal cancers, oncocytomas, or mixed *oncocytic)***
- Affected gene is ***folliculin****
- Characteristic **skin lesions, fibrofolliculomas (hamartomas of the hair follicle**), develop on the skin of the head and neck of patients with the syndrome after age 30

Genetic syndromes associated with renal cell carcinoma

- VHL syndrome–clear cell histology
- *Multiple cutaneous and uterine leiomyomas* (MCUL)
- Hereditary leiomyomatosis and renal cell cancer (HLRCC) syndrome
- Birt-Hogg-Dube syndrome
- Tuberous sclerosis

Ans: (a) Renal cell carcinoma

Ref: *Brenner and Rector's The Kidney, 10th edition, Page 1372*

11. Wavelength highly sensitive to porphyria:

(a) 290 – 320 nm
(b) 400 – 420 nm
(c) 320 – 400 nm
(d) 250 – 290 nm

Explanation:

Sunlight consists of Ultraviolet, Visible and Infrared spectrum

- **Ultraviolet** – 290 - 400 nm, UV A-320-400 nm, UV B-290-320 nm
- **Visible** – 400-700 nm
- **Infrared** – >700 nm
  - **UV B**–produces redness and erythema of the skin, called ***sunburn spectrum***, causes basal and squamous cell carcinoma
  - **UV A**–less efficient in producing skin redness, deeply penetrates the dermis and capable of causing photoaging of chronically sun exposed skin

Porphyrins are endogenous chromophores released into circulation in increased amounts from liver and bone marrow and are transported to the skin where they absorb incident energy both in **Soret band (around 400 nm)** and to a lesser extent in the red portion of visible spectrum **(580-600 nm)**.

Photosensitive porphyrias:

- Erythropoietic porphyria
- Erythropoietic protoporphyria
- Porphyria cutanea tarda—familial and sporadic
- Variegate porphyria
- Hepatoerythropoietic porphyria

Ans: (b) 400 – 420 nm

Ref: *Harrison's Principles of Internal Medicine, 19th edition, Page 386*

12. Which of the following is true about 'relapsing seronegative symmetric synovitis with pitting edema'?

(a) Responsive to steroids
(b) Malignant arthritis
(c) Poor prognosis
(d) Cause deformities

Explanation:

Remitting Seronegative Symmetrical Synovitis with Pitting Edema (RS3PE)

- First described in 1985 by McCarty *et al.*
- RS3PE is a type of benign seronegative polyarthritis that affects older people
- The main characteristics of RS3PE syndrome are:
  - Acute onset
  - Raised acute phase reactants
  - Bilateral diffuse, symmetrical swelling
  - Dorsal pitting oedema of hands
  - **Symmetrical synovitis***
  - **Rheumatoid factor negative***
  - Hand and wrist involvement
  - Human Leukocyte Antigen (HLA) B7 Positive
  - Positive response to low dose corticosteroids
  - X-rays show soft tissue swelling in the absence of erosions
- **Olive *et al.* diagnostic criteria** for this syndrome:
  - Bilateral pitting oedema of both hands
  - Sudden onset of **polyarthritis***
  - Age **more** than **50 years***
  - Seronegative for rheumatoid factor
- Paraneoplastic forms of RS3PE as primary or secondary manifestations of a neoplastic process without response to corticosteroids.
- Associated with **solid tumours** predominantly adenocarcinomas, such as gastric, pancreatic cancers and haematological malignancies such as myelodysplasia and non-Hodgkin's lymphoma.

Ans: (a) Responsive to steroids

Ref: *Kelley and Firesteins Textbook of Rheumatology, 9th edition, Page 1132*

13. A 14-year-old boy with difficulty in walking and behavioural disturbance, recovered from prolonged jaundice recently, has bluish pigmentation over lunula. The next investigation to be done:

(a) Nail fold capillaroscopy
(b) Slit lamp examination
(c) Biopsy of the pigmented area
(d) Ankle-Brachial Pressure Index

Explanation:

WILSON'S DISEASE

- Autosomal recessive disorder caused by mutations in **ATP7B gene**, a membrane bound **copper transporting ATPase** on **chromosome 13**
- Primarily involves **liver, brain, kidney and cornea**
- Also known as **hepatolenticular** degeneration

Clinical Features

- **Hepatic:** Commonly manifest in children of 5 to 6 years of age hepatitis, cirrhosis, hepatic decompensation, associated with hemolytic anemia, hemolysis and liver disease suspect Wilson's disease
- **Neurologic:** Occurs in early twenties; Dystonia mainly of face, incoordination, tremor, autonomic disturbances, abnormal eye movements, no sensory abnormalities and muscular weakness
- **Psychiatric:** Loss of emotional attachment, depression, hyperactivity, schizophrenia
- **Ocular: Sunflower cataracts, Kayser-Fleischer ring** in the descemet's membrane
- **Renal:** Microscopic hematuria, proximal tubular defects like Fanconi's syndrome

Investigations:

- Serum ceruloplasmin - low
- Serum copper level - total decreased free copper increase
- 24 hours urine cu excretion - > 1.6 micromol

- KF rings (slit lamp exam) - 99% in neurological and psychiatric symptoms 30-50% in hepatic presentation
- Liver biopsy - **>250 μg/g** of dry tissue gold standard for diagnosis
- MRI brain - shows damage in basal ganglia

Nail Findings and Associated Systemic Conditions

Nail finding	Associated systemic conditions
Shape or growth change Clubbing	Inflammatory bowel disease, pulmonary malignancy, asbestosis, chronic bronchitis, COPD, cirrhosis, congenital heart disease, endocarditis, atrioventricular malformations, fistulas
Koilonychia	Iron deficiency anemia, hemochromatosis, Raynaud's disease, SLE, trauma, nail-patella syndrome
Onycholysis	Psoriasis, infection, hyperthyroidism, sarcoidosis, trauma, amyloidosis, connective tissue disorders
Pitting	Psoriasis, Reiter's syndrome, incontinentia pigmenti, alopecia areata
Beau's lines	Any severe systemic illness that disrupts nail growth, Raynaud's disease, pemphigus, trauma
Yellow nail	Lymphedema, pleural effusion, immunodeficiency, bronchiectasis, sinusitis, rheumatoid arthritis, nephrotic syndrome, thyroiditis, tuberculosis, Raynaud's disease
Color change Terry's (white) nails	Hepatic failure, cirrhosis, diabetes mellitus, CHF, hyperthyroidism, malnutrition
Azure lunula	Hepatolenticular degeneration (Wilson's disease), silver poisoning, quinacrine therapy
Half-and-half nails	Specific for renal failure
Muehrcke's lines	Specific for hypoalbuminemia
Mees' lines	Arsenic poisoning, Hodgkin's disease, CHF, leprosy, malaria, chemotherapy, carbon monoxide poisoning, other systemic insults
Dark longitudinal streaks	Melanoma, benign nevus, chemical staining, normal variant in darkly pigmented people
Longitudinal striations	Alopecia areata, vitiligo, atopic dermatitis, psoriasis
Splinter hemorrhage	Subacute bacterial endocarditis, SLE, RA, antiphospholipid syndrome, malignancies, oral contraceptive use, pregnancy, psoriasis, trauma
Telangiectasia	Rheumatoid arthritis, SLE, dermatomyositis, scleroderma

Ans: (b) Slit lamp examination

Ref: *Harrison's Principles of Internal Medicine, 19th edition, Page 2519; Nail Abnormalities: Clues to Systemic Disease Am Fam Physician 2004;69:1417-24*

14. Drug to be avoided in chronic lymphocytic leukemia (CLL) with stroke and IC bleed is:

(a) Idelalisib
(b) Ofatumumab
(c) Ibrutinib
(d) Venetoclax

Explanation:

Monoclonal Antibodies in CLL:

- CD52 - **Alemtuzumab**
- CD20 - **Rituximab**, chimeric, murine monoclonal antibody
- Causes transient, severe thrombocytopenia, rituximab should be used with caution in patients with a preexisting thrombocytopenia
- CD20 - **Ofatumumab** fully human, type 1, IgG1 targeting, monoclonal antibody
- CD20 - **Obinutuzumab**
- BCR kinase inhibitors - **Ibrutinib**, minor bleeding and atrial fibrillation observed with ibritinib. It is avoided in Stroke or IC bleed.
- **Idelalisib** - Isoform selective PI3K-δ inhibitor
- **Venetoclax** (ABT-199) - Oral Bcl-2–targeting agent
- **Blinatumomab** - Specific T-cell engaging (BiTE) antibody that has activity in CD19+ B-cell malignancies

Ans: (c) Ibrutinib

Ref: *Williams Hematology, 9th edition, Chapter 92, Page 1535*

15. A patient with Staphylococcal pneumonia develops acute breathlessness. Probable cause is:

(a) Pericarditis
(b) Pneumothorax
(c) Acute respiratory failure
(d) Parapneumonic effusion

Explanation:

Staphylococcal pneumonia is frequently complicated by:

- Cavitation (20%)
- Pneumothorax (10%)
- Jaundice (8%)
- Empyema (5%)
- Acute renal failure (5%)
- Pericarditis (2%).

Ans: (b) Pneumothorax

Ref: *Fishman's Pulmonary Disease and Disorders, 5th edition, Chapter 128*

16. Hypertonic hyponatremia is seen in:

(a) CRF
(b) IV mannitol
(c) Thiazide diuretics
(d) Vomiting

Explanation:

Diagnostic Approach to Hyponatremia

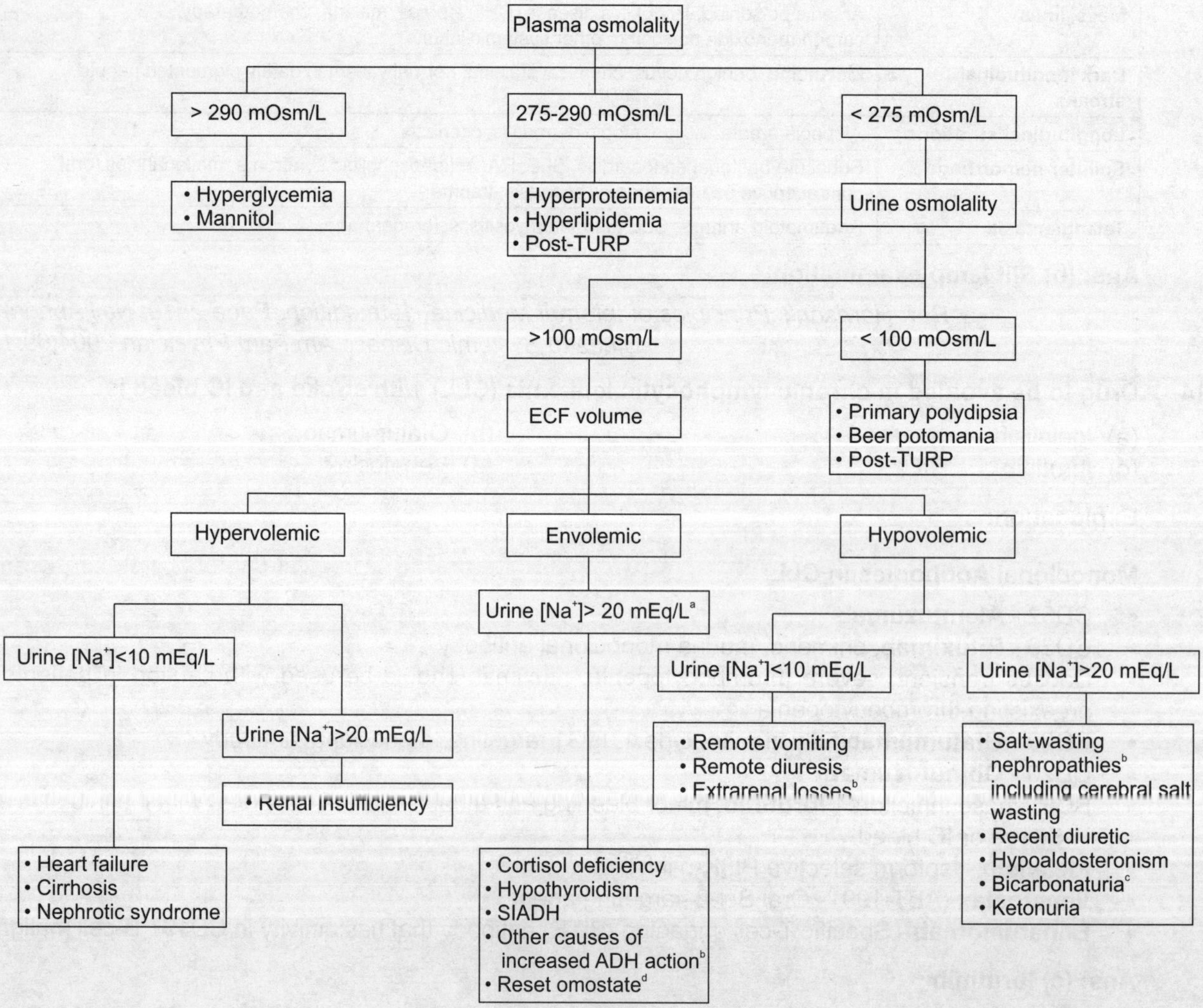

Ans: (b) IV mannitol

Ref: *Washington Manual of Medical Therapeutics, 35th edition, Page 361*

17. ARDS diagnostic criteria:

(a) PaO_2/FiO_2 less than 200 mm Hg
(b) PaO_2/FiO_2 less than 300 mm Hg
(c) PaO_2/FiO_2 more than 200 mm Hg
(d) PaO_2/FiO_2 more than 300 mm Hg

Explanation:

Berlin definition, ARDS is defined as a syndrome characterized by:
(1) Onset within 1 week of a known clinical insult.
(2) Bilateral radiographic opacities, not fully explained by pleural effusions, atelectasis, or nodules.
(3) Respiratory failure not fully explained by cardiac failure or fluid overload, and
(4) Poor systemic oxygenation, with a PaO_2/FiO_2 ≤300 and a PEEP or CPAP ≥5 cm H_2O.

Clinical Variable	Mild ARDS	Moderate ARDS	Severe ARDS
Onset	Onset within 1week of clinical insult known to cause ARDS		
Hypoxemia	PaO_2/FiO_2 ≤ 300 mm Hg PEEP or CPAP ≥ 5 cm H_2O	PaO_2/FiO_2 ≤ 200 mm Hg	PaO_2/FiO_2 ≤ 100 mm Hg
Chest radiograph	Bilateral radiographic opacities, not fully explained by pleural effusions, atelectasis, or nodules		
Non cardiac etiology	Respiratory failure not fully explained by cardiogenic pulmonary edema or fluid overload		

Ans: (b) PaO_2/FiO_2 less than 300 mm Hg

Ref: *Fishmans Pulmonary Disease and Disorders, 5th edition, Chapter 141; Harrison's Principles of Internal Medicine, 19th edition, Page 1736*

18. True about pheochromocytoma are all *except*:

(a) Urinary VMA is least specific
(b) Organ of Zukerkandl is most common extra adrenal site
(c) 10% extra adrenal
(d) Extra adrenal commonly metastasizes

Explanation:

- **Pheochromocytoma** – Occurs in adrenal medulla
- **Paragangliomas** – **Extra adrenal pheochromocytoma** are found where there is chromaffin tissue
  - Along the paraaortic sympathetic chain
  - Within organs of Zuckerkandl (at the origin of inferior mesenteric artery)
  - Along the sympathetic chain in the head and mediastinum (approximately 70% of extra adrenal paragangliomas occur in the head and neck region)
  - In the wall of urinary bladder
- Classic **"Rule of Tens"** for pheochromocytomas states that 10% are bilateral, 10% are extraadrenal, and 10% are malignant
- Approximately 10 percent of pheochromocytomas are malignant compared to 20 to 25 percent of extra-adrenal abdominal and mediastinal paragangliomas
- Risk of malignancy is higher for paragangliomas than for pheochromocytomas, especially if the patient has a mutation in **succinate dehydrogenase subunit B**
- Only reliable clue to the presence of a malignant pheochromocytoma is local invasion or distant metastases

Ans: (b) Organ of Zukerkandl is most common extraadrenal site

Ref: *Williams Endocrinology, 13th edition, Page 559; Robbins and Cotran, Pathologic Basis of Disease, 9th edition, Page 741,1135*

19. Interpret the following ABG values: $PaCO_2$ - 50, HCO_3 - 35, pH - 7.2:

(a) Uncompensated metabolic alkalosis
(b) Mixed respiratory and metabolic acidosis
(c) Combined respiratory and metabolic acidosis
(d) Compensated respiratory acidosis

Explanation:

- **Step 1:** Review the patient
  - o Examine the patient for clues as to the type of disturbance.
- **Step 2:** Analyse the oxygenation
  - o Look for signs of hypoxia, by assessing the PaO_2 and SaO_2.
- **Step 3:** Assess the pH: Is there an acidosis or alkalosis?
  - o pH <7.35 is an acidosis; pH >7.45 is an alkalosis
- **Step 4:** Assess for respiratory disturbance
  - o Consider the state of alveolar ventilation by evaluating the $PaCO_2$.
- **Step 5:** Assess for metabolic disturbance
  - o Examine HCO_3 and BE in relation to pH, to determine metabolic involvement.
- **Step 6:** Establish if the disturbance is compensatory or mixed
  - o Observe the pH to determine if the compensation is appropriate for the primary disturbance (complete or partial)

Disorder	Primary Change	Compensatory Response
Metabolic acidosis	$\downarrow[HCO_3]$	$\downarrow pCO_2$ 1.2 mm Hg for every 1 mEq/L $\downarrow [HCO_3]$ OR pCO_2= last two digits of pH
Metabolic alkalosis	$\uparrow[HCO_3]$	$\uparrow pCO_2$ 0.7 mm Hg for every 1 mEq/L $\uparrow [HCO_3]$
Respiratory acidosis	$\uparrow pCO_2$	
	Acute	$[HCO_3]$ will $\uparrow$ 0.1mmol/L per mm Hg $\uparrow$ in $PaCO_2$
	Chronic	$[HCO_3]$ will $\uparrow$ 0.4 mmol/L per mm Hg $\uparrow$ in $PaCO_2$
Respiratory alkalosis	$\downarrow pCO_2$	
	Acute	$[HCO_3]$ will $\downarrow$ 0.2 mmol/L per mm Hg $\downarrow$ in $PaCO_2$
	Chronic	$[HCO_3]$ will $\downarrow$ 0.4 mmol/L per mm Hg $\downarrow$ in $PaCO_2$

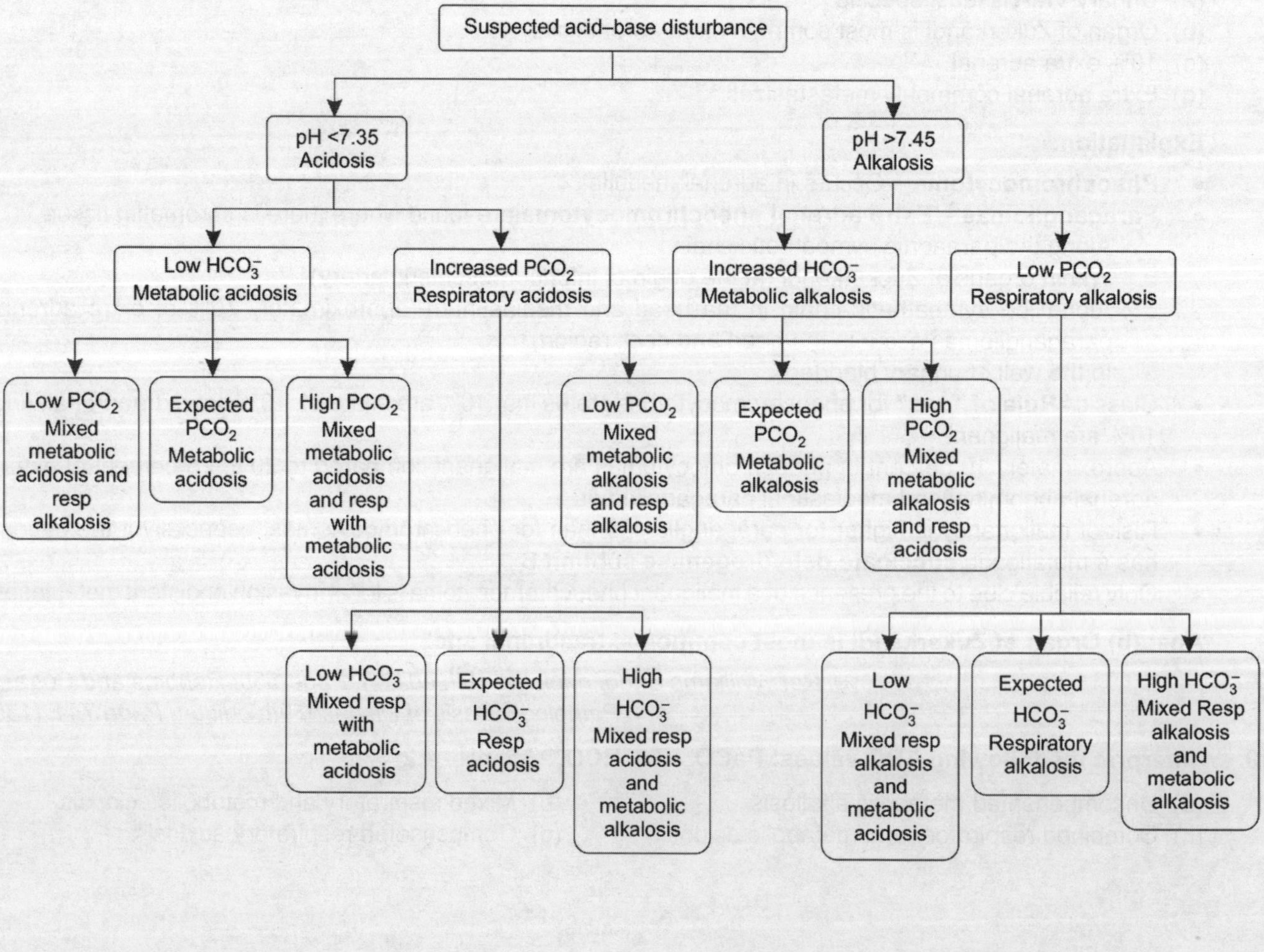

Normal levels of blood pH, pCO_2 and HCO_3

Blood levels criteria	Venous	Arterial
pH	7.35–7.40	7.38–7.45
pCO_2	45–50 torr	35–45 torr
HCO_3	24-25 mEq/L	23–27 mEq/L

Normal ABG values

H^+ (35–45 nmol/L) <35 = alkalemia, >45 = acidemia
pH (7.35–7.45) <7.35 = acidemia, >7.45 = alkalemia
PO_2 (>10.6 kPa or > 80 mm Hg in arterial blood on room air)
PCO_2 (4.7–6.0 kPa or 35–45 mm Hg in arterial blood)
SpO_2 (>96% on room air)
HCO_3 (22–28 mmol/L)
BE (–2 to +2)
Lactate (0.4–1.5 mmol/L)

Stepwise approach for acid-base disorders

pH < 7.35 = acidosis; pH > 7.45 = alkalosis
Primary change in HCO_3→metabolic If the change in HCO_3 is in keeping with the pH (i.e., acidosis + decreased HCO_3), the problem is metabolic If the change in HCO_3 is opposite with the pH (i.e., acidosis + increased HCO_3), the problem is compensatory metabolic
Primary change in CO_2→respiratory If the change in **CO_2** is in keeping with the pH (i.e., acidosis + increased **CO_2**), the problem is respiratory If the change in **CO_2** is opposite with the pH (i.e., acidosis + decreased **CO_2**), the problem is compensatory respiratory

Mixed acid-base disorders

- Present when compensation is not appropriate
- Compensation never overcorrects the primary disturbance

	Expected compensation	Limit of compensation
Metabolic acidosis	$PCO_2 = 1.5 \times [HCO_3^-] + 8 \pm 2$	PCO_2 does not fall below 10 mm Hg
Metabolic alkalosis	PCO_2 increases by 7 mm Hg for each 10 mEq/L increase in serum $[HCO_3^-]$	PCO_2 does not rise above 55 mm Hg
Acute respiratory acidosis	$[HCO_3^-]$ increases by 1 for each 10 mm Hg increase in PCO_2	HCO_3 does not rise above 30 mEq/L
Chronic respiratory acidosis	$[HCO_3^-]$ increases by 3.5 for each 10 mm Hg increase in PCO_2	HCO_3 does not rise above 45 mEq/L
Acute respiratory alkalosis	$[HCO_3^-]$ falls by 2 for each 10 mm Hg decrease in PCO_2	HCO_3 does not fall below 18 mEq/L
Chronic respiratory alkalosis	$[HCO_3^-]$ falls by 4 for each 10 mm Hg decrease in PCO_2	HCO_3 does not fall below 12 mEq/L

Ans: (d) Compensated respiratory acidosis

Ref: *Harrison's Principles of Internal Medicine, 19th edition,Chapter 66*

20. Interpret the following ABG values $PaCO_2$ - 40, HCO_3 - 55 mEq/L and pH - 7.7:

(a) Uncompensated metabolic alkalosis
(b) Mixed respiratory and metabolic acidosis
(c) Combined respiratory and metabolic acidosis
(d) Compensated respiratory acidosis

Explanation:

Refer previous explanation.

Ans: (a) Uncompensated metabolic alkalosis

Ref: *Harrison's Principles of Internal Medicine, 19th edition,Chapter 66*

21. Interpret the following ABG values $PaCO_2$ - 65, HCO_3 - 15mEq/L and pH - 7.21:

(a) Uncompensated metabolic alkalosis
(b) Mixed respiratory and metabolic acidosis
(c) Combined respiratory and metabolic acidosis
(d) Compensated respiratory acidosis

Explanation:

Refer previous explanation.

Ans: (c) Combined respiratory and metabolic acidosis

Ref: *Harrison's Principles of Internal Medicine, 19th edition, Chapter 66*

22. True statement regarding hepatitis C infection:

(a) Most patients have severe symptoms when infected for first time
(b) Highly likely to cause chronic ongoing infection
(c) Transmitted by eating raw oysters
(d) It is DNA virus

Explanation:

- Acute hepatitis C is rarely seen in clinical practice, because nearly all cases are asymptomatic.
- Chronic hepatitis C follows acute hepatitis C in 50-70% of cases
- 20-25%of patients with chronic hepatitis C progress to cirrhosis

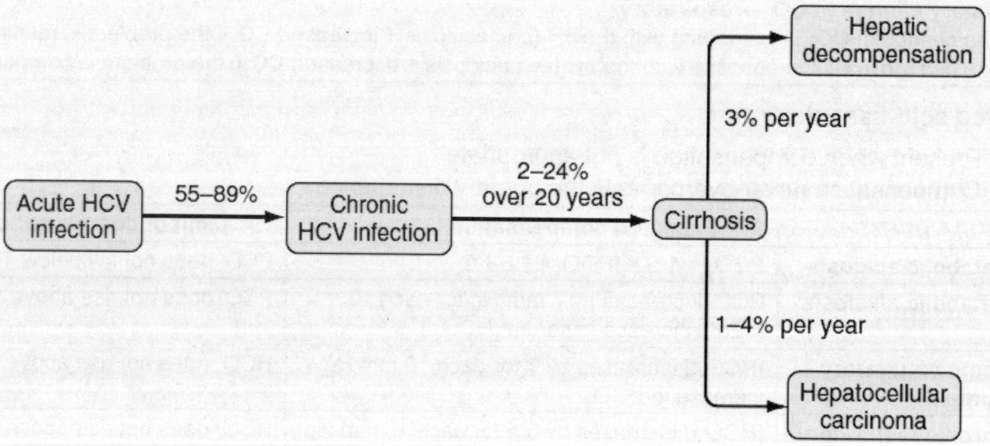

Progression of liver disease depends on:

- Age
- Longer duration of infection – most important factor
- Concomitant other liver disease
- Obesity
- HIV infection
  - Long-term prognosis for chronic hepatitis C in a majority of patients is relatively benign
  - The **best prognostic indicator in chronic hepatitis C is liver histology**
  - Aminotransferase levels tend to fluctuate more (**the characteristic episodic pattern of aminotransferase activity)**
  - Interesting and occasionally confusing finding in patients with chronic hepatitis C is the presence of autoantibodies

Anti LKM

- Drugs used in the treatment of hepatitis C infection: PEG IFN-α plus ribavirin

Agent	Genotype(s)	Dose	Comment
Protease Inhibitors			
Boceprevir	1	800 mg three times daily	Used in combination with pegylated interferon and ribavirin; no longer recommended
Telaprevir	1	1125 mg twice daily	Used in combination with pegylated interferon and ribavirin; no longer recommended
Simeprevir	1 and 4	150 mg once daily	Used in combination with pegylated interferon and ribavirin or with sofosbuvir
Paritaprevir	1 and 4	150 mg once daily	Used in combination with ombitasvir and dasabuvir; ritonavir boosted
Asunaprevir	1 and 4	200 mg twice daily	Used in combination with daclatasvir or with daclatasvir and BMS-791324
Grazoprevir	1, 2, 4-6	100 mg once daily	Used in combination with elbasvir
Non-nucleos(t)ide Polymerase Inhibitors			
Dasabuvir	1 and 4	250 mg twice daily	Used in combination with paritaprevir and ombitasvir
BMS-791325	1	75 mg twice daily	Used in combination with daclatasvir and asunaprevir
Nucleos(t)ide Polymerase Inhibitor			
Sofosbuvir	1-6	400 mg once daily	Used in combination with pegylated interferon and ribavirin (all genotypes) or with ribavirin alone (genotypes 2 and 3) or with simeprevir (genotypes 1 and 4) or with declatasvir (all genotypes) or with ledipasvir (genotypes 1,3 and 4) or with GS-5861 (under study)
NS5A Inhibitors			
Daclatasvir	1-6	60 mg once daily	Used in combination with sofosbuvir (genotypes 1-6) or with pegylated interferon and ribavirin (genotype 4) or with asunaprevir (with or without BMS-791325; under study)
Ledipasvir	1, 3 and 4	90 mg once daily	Used in combination with sofosbuvir
Ombitasvir	1 and 4	25 mg once daily	Used in combination with paritaprevir and dasabuvir
Elbasvir	1-6	50 mg once daily	Used in combination with grazoprevir
GS-5816	1-6	100 mg once daily	Used in combination with sofosbuvir

Ans: (b) Highly likely to cause chronic ongoing infection

Ref: Harrison's Principles of Internal Medicine, 19th edition, Page 2040; Sleisenger and Fordtran's Gastrointestinal and Liver Disease, Page 1332

23. False regarding restrictive lung disease:

(a) FEV-1/FVC decreased (b) FVC decreased
(c) TLC decreased (d) FeV1 increased

Explanation:

How to Interpret Spirometry?

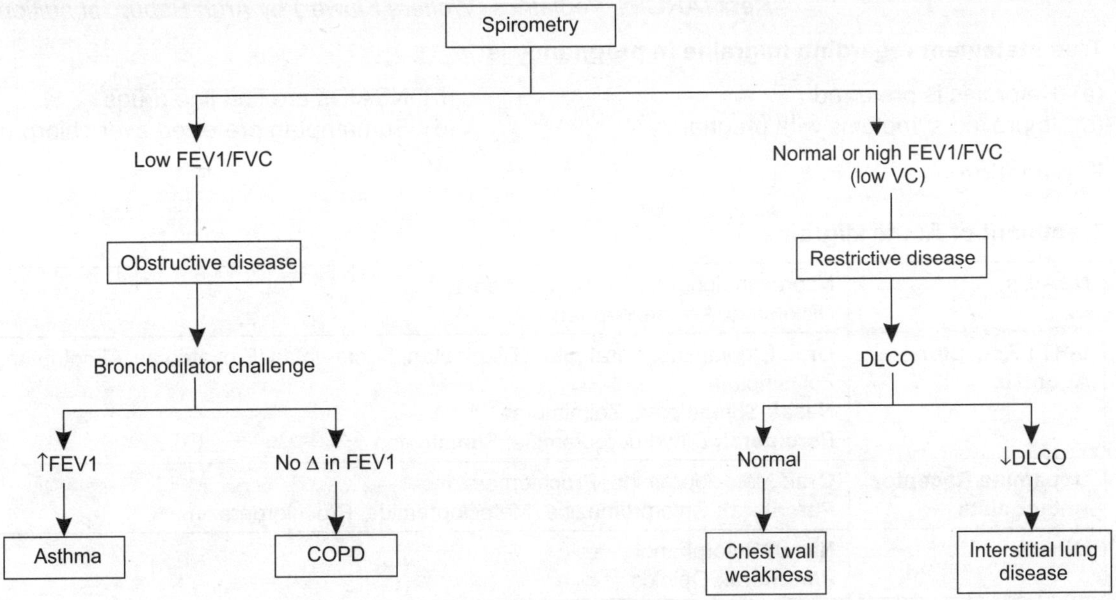

Spirometry	COPD	Restrictive Lung Diseases
FEV1	Low ++	Low+
VC	Low+	Low ++
FEV1/FVC	Low	Normal / high
RV	High	Low
FRC	High	Low

- **TLC:** Volume of air in the lungs following maximal inspiration **(N= 5-6 L)**
- **FVC:** Maximum amount of air exhaled following maximal inspiration **(N= 4.8 L)**
- **VT:** Volume of air entering and leaving lungs during normal respiration **(N= 500 ml)**
- **RV:** Volume of air remaining in the lungs after maximal expiratory effort **(N= 1.2 L)**
- **FRC:** Volume of air within the lungs at the end of normal respiration **(N= 2.5-3 L)**
- **FEV:** Volume of air exhaled in a given time during a forced vital capacity effort
- **FEV1/FVC:** Proportion of a person's vital capacity that they are able to expire in the first second of expiration **(N= 80%)**

Restrictive Lung Disease:

- **FVC is reduced** because of reduction in intra-thoracic air volume.
- **Normal or Increased FEV1/FVC**
- Examples are:
  - ***Interstitial lung disease***
  - ***Neuromuscular disorders***
  - Mechanical compression like ***obesity, kyphoscoliosis***, ***pneumothorax***.
- **TLC and RV** are reduced in all except in **neuromuscular disorders**

Obstructive Lung Disease

- Two major types:
  - COPD
  - Bronchial asthma
- Both show **reduced FEV1/FVC**.
- **FEV1** is used for follow up of asthma and COPD and in evaluation of bronchodilator response.
- **Reversal of obstruction** with bronchodilators (**Improvement of FEV1 >12%** and minimum **of >200 ml)** is characteristic of asthma
- A post-bronchodilator forced expiratory volume in one second (FEV1/FVC) **less than 0.7** confirms COPD.

Ans: (a) FEV-1/FVC decreased

Ref: *TARGET Pediatrics (Wolters Kluwer) by Arun Babu, 1st edition, Page 378*

24. True statement regarding migraine in pregnancy is:

(a) Ketorolac is preferred
(b) NSAIDs are first line drugs
(c) Improved symptoms with pregnancy
(d) Sumatriptan preferred over chlorpromazine

Explanation:

Treatment of Acute Migraine

NSAIDs	Naproxen, Ibuprofen,Tolfenamic acid Diclofenac, Acetominophen
5-HT1 Receptor Agonists	**Oral:** Ergotamine, Naratriptan, Rizatriptan, Sumatriptan, Frovatriptan, Almotriptan, Eletriptan, Zolmitriptan **Nasal:** Sumatriptan, Zolmitriptan **Parenteral:** Dihydroergotamine, Sumatriptan
Dopamine Receptor Antagonists	**Oral:** Metoclopramide, Prochlorperazine **Parenteral:** Chlorpromazine, Metoclopramide, Prochlorperazine
Others	**Nasal:** Butorphanol **Parenteral:** Opioids

Migraine During Pregnancy

- Improvement in 'migraine without aura'
- Worsening of 'migraine with aura'
- **Ergot derivatives** are **contraindicated** due to possibility of uterine hypertonicity and vascular disruption leading on to miscarriage
- Safety of **Triptans during pregnancy is not fully confirmed.** Can be used only if other drugs are not effective
- **Treatment**
  - First line: NSAIDs and paracetamol
  - Triptans are avoided
- **Prophylaxis**: Magnesium, Metoprolol

Ans: (b) NSAIDs are first line drugs

***Ref**: Harrison's Principles of Internal Medicine, 19th edition, Page 2592*

SURGERY

1. **In carcinoma head of pancreas, nausea and vomiting is due to:**

(a) External compression of duodenum
(b) Portal vein infiltration
(c) Proliferation infiltration of tumor into duodenum
(d) Chemotherapy related

Explanation:

Pancreatic adenocarcinoma

- Develops in the **ductal cells** and are called **Ductal Adenocarcinoma**.
- They most commonly occur on the **Right side**, i.e., **Head** and **Uncinate Process (60-70%)** than left side, i.e., Body and Tail of pancreas (20-25%)
- Features of carcinoma head of pancreas are:
  - Jaundice 75%
  - Weight loss 51%
  - Abdominal pain 39%
  - Nausea/vomiting 13%
  - Pruritus 11%
  - Fever 3%
  - Gastrointestinal bleeding 1%
- For tumors at the **body and tail of pancreas**, **Pain** (most common) and **weight loss** are the presenting features as they present at a late advanced stage
- Regarding **Nausea and vomiting**, they occur due to **tumor extrinsic compression** of **duodenum C loop** presenting a state of **Gastric outlet obstruction**.
- In unresectable cases, these patients should be offered Endoluminal duodenal metal stent as palliation.

Ans: (a) External compression of duodenum

Ref: *Blumgarts 6th edition, Page 979; Sabiston, 20th edition, Page 1544*

2. **According to AJCC 8th edition, staging of 2 cm size pancreatic cancer if it involves portal vein is:**

(a) T1
(b) T2
(c) T3
(d) T4

Explanation:

AJCC 8th edition has brought the following changes with regard to **carcinoma pancreas:**

- T1 is subdivided into T1a, T1b and T1c based on size
- T2 and T3 are categorized based on size and not on extrapancreatic involvement any more
- T4 is a radiological staging done by the relationship to vessels
- Nodal staging has N1 and N2 subdivisions unlike before N1 alone

Tx	No primary tumor could not be assessed	**Nx**	Regional nodes cannot be assessed
T0	No evidence of primary tumor	**N0**	No regional nodes
Tis	Carcinoma in situ includes Pan-IN 3, IPMN with high risk features		
T1	Tumor < or = 2 cm in greatest dimension T1a – < or = 0.5 cm T1b – 0.5 to 1 cm T1c – 1.0 to 2.0 cm	**N1**	One to three regional lymph nodes
T2	Tumor > 2 cm but < or = 4 cm	**N2**	Four or more lymph nodes
T3	Tumor > 4 cm in greatest dimension	**M0**	No distant metastases
T4	Tumor any size involvement of celiac axis, superior mesenteric artery and common hepatic artery	**M1**	Distant metastases

- **Portal vein or SMV involvement will not change the staging as per AJCC 7th and AJCC 8th edition**. Staging decided based on the tumor size only.
- Borderline resectable lesion is lesion involvement > 180 degrees of PV/SMV or <180 degree involvement of coeliac axis/SMA.

Ans: (a) T1

Ref: *AJCC, 8th edition, Manual, Page 340-344*

3. **Liver tunneling procedure not done for which segment?**

(a) I (b) IV

(c) V (d) VIII

Explanation:

This is difficult question even for MCh entrance exams.

- In short, there are several difficulties in planning resections in liver.
- Criteria for liver resection based on size alone is not sufficient. Finer details like its proximity to secondary and tertiary portobiliary radicles and hepatic vein is necessary to guide liver resection.
- Common liver resections are Right and Left hepatectomy and its extended versions based on the segments removed.

New Terminologies and their removed segments

Procedure Name	**Removed Liver Segments**
Right hemihepatectomy	Segments 5, 6, 7 and 8
Left hemihepatectomy	Segments 2, 3 and 4
Right trisectionectomy	Segments 4, 5, 6, 7 and 8
Left lateral sectionectomy	Segment 2 and 3
Left trisectionectomy	Segments 2, 3, 4, 5 and 8

- High Level Resections or Named liver resections with limitations to specific conditions based on the extent of involvement in Hilar cholangiocarcinoma and Colorectal metastases and certain forms of HCC in unusual locations like involving caudal lobe.

Taj Mahal Resection **For Hilar Cholangiocarcinoma**	Segments IVa, V and I (caudate lobe) removed (hence the shape of Taj Mahal dome)
Dumbbell Form Resection **For Cholangiocarcinoma**	Segments IVb, I (caudate lobe) and partial Segment V resection about the right hepatic pedicle
Mini-Mesohepatectomy (MMH)	For lesions involving the Middle hepatic vein at caval confluence (not involving caudate lobe)
Liver Tunnel Procedure (if caudate lobe involved as in above condition)	Segments I, IV and VIII are removed as part of parenchymal preserving liver surgery for selected liver tumors which are involving middle hepatic vein along with caudate lobe
Liver Hanging Manoeuvre (LHM)	It uses a tape between the anterior surface of retrohepatic IVC and liver surface to help in better lifting of the liver and efficient vascular control if anterior approach for liver resection is planned (it is the preferred procedure nowadays as it is a no-touch technique)

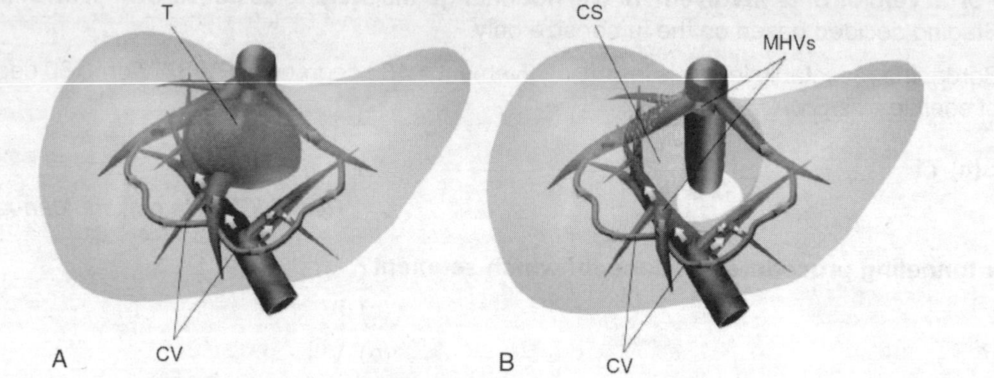

Figure A represents the **typical lesion needing Liver Tunnel Procedure** (CV–Communicating veins)
Figure B represents the **post-operative resection** including MHV.

Ans: (c) V

Ref: *Blumgart's 6th edition, Page 1705*

4. **When to do surgery in Pancreatic ascites?**

(a) Symptomatic
(b) Recurrent ascites following abdominal drainage
(c) Not responding to medical therapy
(d) Leak from the stented duct

Explanation:

Pancreatic Ascites

- It is a rare entity occurs due to **complete disruption of the pancreatic duct** leading to significant accumulation of fluid
- Common causes include:
  - Following **acute pancreatitis** with duct disruption
  - **Chronic pancreatitis** with **ductal obstruction** with **pseudocyst rupture**
  - **Trauma causes.**
- Features include **abdominal distension** due to **free fluid abdomen.**
- **Diagnostic paracentesis** shows **elevated amylase** and **lipase** levels suggesting **pancreatic duct leak.**
- Initial management includes **therapeutic paracentesis** and endoscopic placement of **pancreatic stent** across the disruption.
- Failure of this stenting, mandates **surgical exploration** which involves **distal pancreatectomy** and **closure of the proximal stump.**

Ans: (d) Leak from the stented duct

Ref: *Sabiston, 20th edition, Page 1531*

5. **Best graft for infra-inguinal approach bypass:**

(a) Dacron
(b) PTFE
(c) Polyester
(d) Autologous vein

Explanation:

- **Bypass surgeries** are done for **peripheral arterial occlusive diseases** which are several enough (i.e., more than rest pain) and not eligible for Endovascular approaches (i.e., TASC C or D lesions meaning long segment occlusive disease or occlusion at trifurcation or bifurcation of vessels).
- Another important criteria for bypass is, there should be **sufficient length of normal distal vessel** to allow for **bypass anastomoses.**
- For bypass, two most common conduits used are:
  - **PTFE (Polytetrafluroethylene)** – Synthetic graft, used for larger vessels like iliac and axillary vessels

- **Autologous vein (**most commonly saphenous vein) – Autograft, so innate antithrombotic properties, most preferred for infrainguinal bypass as they size match well, better patency rates than PTFE
- Other graft is **Dacron** (polyethylene terephthalate or polyester) used in aortic aneurysm repair

- **Saphenous vein** used should be reversed, as they have valves which allow unidirectional flow. So saphenous vein should be reversed (turned upside down) for bypass to allow any interruption to blood flow (Reversed saphenous vein graft).

Ans: (d) Autologous vein

Ref: *Sabiston, 20th edition, Page 1774-1775*

6. **Best graft for aortic dissection:**

(a) Dacron
(b) Autologous vein
(c) Autologous artery
(d) PTFE

Explanation:

- **Aortic dissection** occurs when there is a defect in the **intimal layer** which permits blood to create false channel within the aortic wall between media and adventitia.
- **Stanford classification*** is most commonly used:
  - **Type A** (any involvement of ascending aorta) – surgical emergency
  - **Type B** dissection mostly treated with hypertensive control followed by endovascular stenting called TEVAR (thoracic endovascular aneurysm repair)
- As mentioned above, all aortic surgeries are replaced with a **synthetic graft** – **Dacron** (woven/knitted polyester) sutured with 2-0 polypropylene.

Ans: (a) Dacron

Ref: *Sabiston, 20th edition, Page 1730*

7. **True about Splenunculi:**

(a) It is encapsulated
(b) Most common site is tail of pancreas
(c) Often single
(d) Have more red pulp than spleen

Explanation:

Splenunculi or Accessory Spleen

- **Most common of all splenic anomalies** accounting for 10-30% of population
- Formed due to **incomplete fusion of embryologic splenic tissue** during **5th week** leading to the formation of **accessory spleen**, which is more common or always on the left side of abdomen.
- It is encapsulated just like the normal spleen and contains normal splenic tissue and are more commonly identified during radiological investigations and intraoperatively for other conditions
- They are mostly multiple, located in the hilum of spleen (50%), tail of pancreas (30%)
- They are more prone for torsion and needs emergency resection in such cases.

Ans: (a) It is encapsulated

Ref: *Bailey and Love, 27th edition, Page 1178*

8. **False statement regarding subdural hematoma:**

(a) Occurs on both sides
(b) X-ray not visible
(c) Surgery can be done
(d) Unilateral surgery

Explanation:

Subdural hematoma

- Collection of blood between the **dura and arachnoid layers** of the meninges
- Causes being **Trauma** leading to acute subdural hematoma and in elderly, even trivial trauma causes bleed who are on anticoagulation
- Usually diagnosed with **non-contrast CT brain** which differentiates acute from chronic subdural hematoma

- Acute subdural hematoma have characteristic finding of **hyperdense concavo-convex lesion** on side of the brain with or without midline shift.
- In acute conditions, urgent surgical evacuation is needed in the form of craniotomy or craniectomy.
- Those presenting with chronic subdural hematomas, **anticoagulation** should be reversed by **Vitamin K** and **steroids** as conservative options. If severe, can undergo burr hole procedure to evacuate the clot.

Ans: (a) Occurs on both sides

Ref: *Bailey and Love, 27th edition, Page 334-335*

9. **Not a temporary embolization agent is:**

(a) Collagen (b) Gelfoam

(c) Thrombin (d) Onyx

Explanation:

- **Embolization** is an intentional endovascular occlusion of either an artery or vein and it is an interventional radiological procedure.
- There are several agents discovered and each has its own merits and limitations based on the nature of the agent, and the need for occlusion.
- General categorization of embolic agents are:

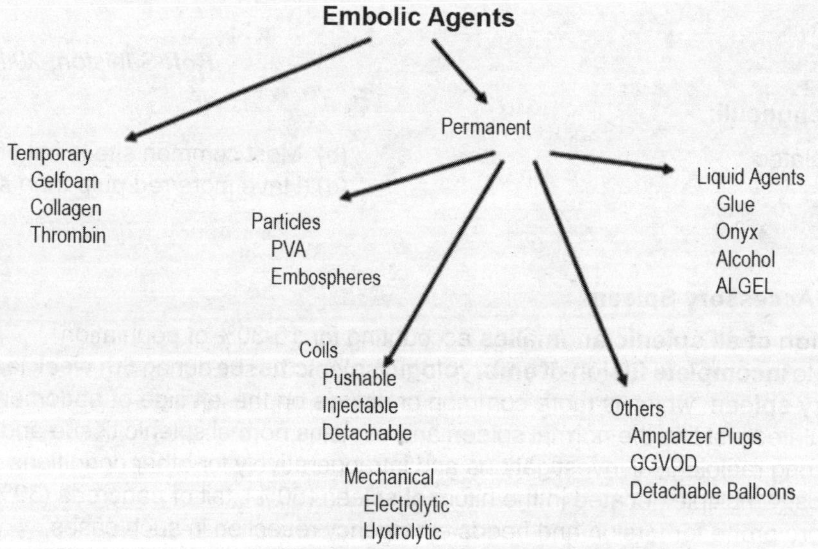

- Temporary embolization agents are used only for temporary occlusion of bleeding vessels which allows recanalization in weeks, so not used in fistulas or tumors. They are used in traumatic parenchymal bleeds from liver or spleen
- Permanent embolization agents are commonly used. Uses are:
- Mechanical embolic agents like coils and plugs used for focal vascular abnormalities like traumatic bleeds or aneurysms
- Flow directed embolic agents are liquid agents, particulate agents which are used in AV malformations, tumors etc.

Ans: (d) Onyx

Ref: *Interventional Radiology Journal*

11. False about Pseudomyoxma peritonei is:

(a) Recurrence after surgery
(b) Refractory to drugs
(c) Hyperthermic intraperitoneal chemotherapy is treatment option
(d) Most commonly associated with appendiceal tumour

Explanation:

Pseudomyxoma Peritonei

- Rare condition which describes **mucinous ascites** arising from a **ruptured ovarian or appendiceal carcinoma.**
- First described by Fraenkel, condition typically has progressive peritoneal tumor deposits, mucinous ascites, omental cake and ovarian involvement in females
- Most commonly associated with **appendiceal tumor**
- Occurs most commonly in patients who are **40 to 50 years** of age and occurs in equal frequency in both males and females
- Risk of developing **pseudomyxoma peritonei** following removal of **appendix** harbouring epithelial tumor is 9%, non mucinous neoplasm is 3% and 30% with mucinous adenocarcinoma
- Current accepted treatment is **Cytoreductive surgery** with **Heated or Hyperthemia Intra Peritoneal Chemotherapy (CRS + HIPEC)** which includes **omentectomy**, **stripping of involved peritoneum**, **resection** of **involved organs and appendicectomy**.
- The survival rates after CRS + HIPEC increased from **20 to 30% to 55%** now-a-days.

Ans: (b) Refractory to drugs

Ref: *Sabiston, 20th edition, Page 1080 and Bailey, 27th edition, Page 1316*

12. True about visceral aneurysm:

(a) Splenic artery is commonly involved
(b) Hepatic aneurysm is operated irrespective of symptoms
(c) Splenic artery aneurysm is most commonly followed by trauma
(d) True aneurysms are more common nowadays with increasing abdominal trauma

Explanation:

Splenic artery aneurysm	Hepatic artery aneurysm
Most common visceral aneurysm 60%	Second most common 20%
Female predominance 1:4	Male predominance 2:1
Associated with Cirrhosis, Portal hypertension and pancreatitis	Associated with congenital or acquired factors
Mean age at presentation 62 years	Mean age at presentation 60 years
	Majority are solitary, extrahepatic 80% and true aneurysms
Pseudoaneurysms occur following trauma	Pseudoaneurysms occur following trauma, iatrogenic procedures
Risk of rupture: Females Pregnant women Aneurysms > 2 cm	Most common site is common hepatic 63% > right hepatic 28% and then left hepatic HAAs have the highest risk of rupture – false aneurysm, multiple aneurysm, more than 2 cm
All aneurysms > 2 cm even if asymptomatic needs intervention	
Most common site of rupture – Intraperitoneal rupture	Most rupture intraperitoneally, but intrahepatic aneurysms rupture – Quincke's triad – pain, jaundice and hemobilia

Contd.

Contd.

Proximal lesions – Resection of aneurysm and end to end anastomoses Distal lesions – Laparoscopic splenectomy	Extrahepatic aneurysm: Proximal to GDA – ligated Distal to GDA – aneurysmectomy and revascularization Intrahepatic aneurysm Percutaneous angioembolization

Ans: (a) Splenic artery is commonly involved

Ref: *Blumgarts 6th edition, Page 1905 and Maingot's Abdominal Operations, Page 1245*

13. Increase in D-dimer levels are noticed in immediate post-operative period. Most appropriate cause is:

(a) DVT
(b) Pulmonary embolism
(c) DIC
(d) Normal

Explanation:

- **D-dimer** is a degradation product of a cross linked fibrin blood clot.
- Increased levels are typically elevated in patients with **acute thromboembolism.**
- D-dimer will increase only if **thrombus** has occurred and also with **fibrinolysis.**
- Presence of D-dimers in the circulation may serve as a **marker of thrombosis** or other conditions in which a significant activation of the fibrinolytic system is present.
- Elevated D-dimer should be followed by **Venous Duplex ultrasound** of the extremities for **diagnosing DVT.**
- If there is a **homogenous hypoechoic clot, without compressibility of the vein** and **absence of flow** across it confirms the diagnosis.
- Initial treatment is with **Low molecular weight heparin Enoxaparin 1.5 mg/kg/day** subcutaneous twice daily along with **Warfarin 5 mg on day 1, 5 mg on day 2 and then 10 mg** thereafter.
- Heparin overlap to be given for 5 days, as the anticoagulant action of warfarin takes 5 doses.
- Maintain INR 2.5 for DVT for 3 months, once recanalization of vein occurs, anticoagulants can be withheld.

Ans: (a) DVT

Ref: *Sabiston, 20th edition, Page 295*

14. All are management options for carcinoma breast in 2nd trimester *except*:

(a) Chemotherapy Doxorubicin + Cyclophosphamide + 5FU
(b) Mastectomy
(c) Focal 3D
(d) Breast conservative surgery is a valid option

Explanation:

Breast Cancer and Pregnancy

- Radiotherapy definitely avoided
- Chemotherapy avoided in first trimester, risk of teratogenicity is 10 to 25% and in second and third trimesters its 1.3%
- After first trimester, sentinel node biopsy can be done safely
- Breast conserving therapy is becoming option nowadays in late 2nd trimester and 3rd trimester, where neoadjuvant chemotherapy is given to downsize tumor and BCS done in third trimester along with C section followed by RT after delivery

First trimester	Mastectomy with axillary dissection
Second trimester	Mastectomy with axillary dissection or sentinel node axillary staging Neoadjuvant chemotherapy followed by Breast conservation surgery and RT post delivery
Third trimester	Mastectomy or BCS followed by RT post delivery

- **Important considerations:**
  - Trastuzumab avoided in pregnancy
  - Methotrexate is avoided
  - Chemotherapy drugs should not be given after 35 weeks of gestation – cause myelosuppression in newborn

Ans: (c) Focal 3D

Ref: *Sabiston, 20th edition, Page 2059-2060*

15. A 50-year-old lady presented with lump in the left breast which has developed suddenly in weeks. Perimenstrual symptoms are present. No associated family history. On examination, the lump is well circumscribed, fluctuant, 1.5 cm oval in shape. Most likely diagnosis:

(a) Breast cyst
(b) Galactocele
(c) Fibroadenoma
(d) Breast cancer

Explanation:

Breast Cyst

- Occur most commonly in the **last decade of reproductive life**
- Results from a non-integrated involution of stroma and epithelium.
- Cavities lined by epithelium
- Common after the age of **35 years** up to **menopause**. Uncommon after menopause
- **Hormone replacement** can cause **cyst** formation in **old women**
- Cyst **size varies with menstruation** due to influence of **ovarian hormones**

Clinical Features

- Often **multiple**, may be **bilateral** and can **mimic malignancy**.
- Typically present **suddenly and cause great alarm**; prompt **diagnosis** and **drainage** provides immediate **relief**.
- Multiple cysts seen is **50%**. Often **bilateral**.
- Risk of breast **cancer** in breast cyst is **very less (0.1%)**
- **Clinically**—smooth, soft, fluctuant often transilluminating well-localised swelling

Diagnosis

- Diagnosis can be confirmed by **aspiration** and/or **ultrasound**.
- **On USG – Smooth margins and echofree center**

Treatment

- Aspiration for **Solitary cyst:** If they resolve completely, and if the fluid is not blood-stained, no further treatment is required
- 30% will recur and require **reaspiration**
- **Core biopsy** or **local excision**: If there is a residual lump or if the fluid is blood-stained, for histological diagnosis (exclude cystadenocarcinoma, which is more common in elderly women)

Note:

- **Fibroadenoma** – usually between the ages of 15 and 25 years
- **Galactocele** – generally occurs after the cessation of location or when feeding frequency has curtailed significantly

Ans: (a) Breast cyst

Ref: *Bailey and Love's Short Practice of Surgery, 26th edition*

16. A 67-year-old chronic heavy smoker presents with 2 weeks history of frank hematuria. USG pelvis shows a filling defect. Most probable diagnosis:

(a) Bladder diverticula
(b) Adenocarcinoma of bladder
(c) Squamous cell carcinoma of bladder
(d) Transitional cell carcinoma of bladder

Explanation:

Bladder Cancer

- **Urothelial/Transitional cell cancer – most common type**
- **Squamous cell carcinoma** (most prevalent form in Schistosomiasis endemic areas)
- **Adenocarcinoma** (usually arise in the fundus of the bladder at the site of urachal remnant)

Risk Factors

Transitional cell cancer	Squamous cell cancer
• **Smoking** • Chemical carcinogens: **naphthylamine, benzidine, aniline** • **Schistosomiasis (Bilharziasis)** • Long term use of analgesics • **Long time Cyclophosphamide exposure** • Pelvic irradiation	• **Schistosomiasis (Bilharziasis)** • Chronic bladder infection • Irradiation • Bladder diverticula

Carcinoma in situ or Flat urothelial carcinoma – Pagetoid spread

Staging and Treatment

- **Superficial bladder cancers** (does not invade the detrusor muscle)
  - **pTa – no lamina propria invasion**
  - **pT1 – lamina propria invasion**
- The most common site of superficial tumors are the **trigone and the lateral walls of bladder**

Clinical Features

- **Painless gross hematuria** is the most common symptom
- Frequency, urgency and dysuria are common symptoms

Metastasis: **Most common primary to metastasize to penis – bladder cancer**

Investigations

- *New tests:* Detection of antigens such as **nuclear matrix proteins (NMP22)** or **mini-chromosome maintenance (MCM)** in urine, which may be able to detect new or recurrent tumors
- The most common radiological sign is a **filling defect**
- For staging **contrast-CT**
- **MRI** can demonstrate LN metastases and muscle invasion
- **Cystourethroscopy** is the mainstay of diagnosis

Treatment

- **Superficial bladder cancers**
  - Solitary papillary lesions, no CIS: **Endoscopic transurethral resection** (TURT)
  - CIS, recurrent disease, T1 disease, > 40% bladder surface involvement: TURT followed by **intravesical therapy**
  - Standard intravesical therapy: **Bacille-Calmette-Guerin (BCG)** 6 weeks instillations; followed by monthly instillations for 1 year
  - Other agents: **Mitomycin C, Interferon, gemcitabine**
  - For persistent disease after BCG, immediate cystectomy
- Muscle invasion cancers **(pT2-pT3):** Radical cystectomy with pelvic lymphadenectomy; neo-adjuvant chemotherapy **(M-VAC:** Cisplatin, methotrexate, doxorubicin and vinblastine or **GC:** gemcitabine and cisplatin)

Ans: (d) Transitional cell carcinoma of bladder

Ref: *Bailey and Love's Short Practice of Surgery, 26th edition*

17. True statement regarding hypertrophic scar:

(a) Usually occurs across the flexural areas
(b) Does not improve with time
(c) Overgrows its boundaries
(d) Develops months after surgery

Explanation:

Features	Hypertrophic scar	Keloid
Genetic	**Not familial**	May be **familial**
Race	**Not race related**	**Black** >white
Sex	Female = male	**Female** >male
Age	**Children**	**10–30 years**
Border	Remains **within woundQ**	**Outgrows** wound area
Natural History	**Subsides** with time	**Rarely subsides**
Site	**Flexor surfaces**	**Sternum (Most common),** shoulder, face
Etiology	Related to **tension**	Unknown
Develop	Within 4 weeks	3 months to year after trauma

Hypertrophic Scar	Keloid
• Develop within 4 weeks after trauma • Proliferation of **mature fibroblasts** • No proliferation of blood vessels • Does not become worse after 12 weeks • Young individuals • Scars crossing Langer's lines • Does **not extend beyond the boundary of original wound** • No claw like process • No itching • Sites: anywhere on the body, common in **flexor surfaces** • Gradually **regress after 6 months** • Does not recur after excision	• Occur 3 months to years after the initial insult • Proliferation of **immature fibroblasts** • Proliferation of **immature blood vessels** • Proliferation **continues after 12 weeks** • Females, negroes, family history, tuberculosis patients, incision across Langer's line • Encroachment of surrounding tissues **claw like process** • **Itching** and blanching • Slightly warm and slightly tender • Sites: Chest wall, upper arm, lower neck, ear • Occasionally malignant change **(Marjolin's ulcer)** • Recurrence after excision common

Ans: (a) Usually occurs across the flexural areas

__Ref:__ Bailey and Love's Short Practice of Surgery, 26th edition

18. What is modified radical gastrectomy?

(a) Spleen and pancreas removed
(b) Gastrectomy with N1 nodes removed
(c) Gastrectomy with N2a nodes removed
(d) 2a node except splenic hilum

Explanation:

- The surgery for stomach cancer evolved during years on constant study of the embryology of the stomach and its peritoneal relations and coverings.
- The **standard surgery** that is being done for all gastric cancers nowadays is **D2 Gastrectomy with Gastrojejunal anastomoses/esophagojejunal anastomoses** depending on the amount of stomach resected.
- **D2 lymphadenectomy** means the removal of **N1 and N2 group of nodes** depending on the location of the tumor in the stomach.
  - N1 group of nodes is the nodes that are present within **3 cm from the primary tumor**
  - N2 group of nodes are the nodes **along the major arteries**.
- **Modified radical Gastrectomy** is an old terminology where the **stomach**, along with **greater** and **lesser omentum** and **omental arcades** with **first part of duodenum** and the **nodes** along it are **removed**. **Spleen** is actually **preserved**.

Ans: (c) Gastrectomy with N2a nodes removed

__Ref:__ Journal

OBSTETRICS AND GYNECOLOGY

1. Labour is said to be prolonged when the first and second stage extend arbitrarily beyond:

(a) 12 hours
(b) 18 hours
(c) 24 hours
(d) 6 hours

Explanation:

First Stage of Labor

- Two phases of **cervical dilatation** are defined:
  - ***Latent phase***
  - ***Active phase***
- The ***latent phase*** corresponds to the **preparatory division**, and the ***active phase***, to the **dilatational division.**
- **Friedman** subdivided the **active phase** into the:
  - **Acceleration phase**
  - **Phase of maximum slope**
  - **Deceleration phase**
- **Latent Phase**
  - The onset of latent labor, as defined by **Friedman** (1972), is the point at which the **mother perceives regular contractions**. The latent phase for most women ends at between **3 and 5 cm of dilatation**.
- **Prolonged Latent Phase**
  - Friedman and Sachtleben (1963) defined this by a **latent phase exceeding 20 hours in the nullipara and 14 hours in the multipara.**
- **Active Labor**
  - *Cervical dilatation of **3 to 5 cm** or **more**, in the presence of **uterine contractions**, can be taken to reliably represent the threshold for active labor*
- **Protraction** as a ***slow rate*** **of cervical dilatation** or **descent:**
  - For **nulliparas** was **less than 1.2 cm dilatation per hour** or **less than 1 cm descent per hour.**
  - For **multiparas**, protraction was defined as **less than 1.5 cm dilatation per hour** or **less than 2 cm descent per hour.**

Second Stage of Labor

- This stage begins when **cervical dilatation is complete** and **ends with fetal delivery**.
- The **median duration** it is highly variable but is approximately:
  - **50 minutes for nulliparas**
  - **20 minutes for multiparas**
- The **mean length of first- and second-stage labor** was approximately:
  - **9 hours in nulliparous women** without regional analgesia, and that the **95th percentile** upper limit was **18.5 hours.**
  - Corresponding times for **multiparous women** were a mean of **6 hours** with a 95th percentile maximum of **13.5 hours.**

Prolonged Labour

- Labour is said to be prolonged when the combined duration of first and second stage is **more than 18 hours**
- **Causes:**
  - Abnormal uterine action
  - Malposition
  - Malpresentation
  - Macrosomia
  - Fetal malformation

  - Contracted pelvis
  - Cephalopelvic disproportion
- **Prolonged latent phase**–in primi more than 20 hours and in multi more than 14 hours
- **Prolonged active phase**–this is the most common. Cervical dilatation less than 1.2 cm/hour in nullipara and less than 1.5 cm/hour in multipara
- **Secondary arrest of dilatation**–there is arrest in cervical dilatation for atleast 2 hours
- **Arrest of descent**–there is arrest of descent of fetal head for atleast one hour

Ans: (b) 18 hours

***Ref:** Williams' Obstetrics, 24th edition*

2. **A pregnant patient comes at 34 weeks gestation with leaking. What examination will reliably confirm premature rupture of membranes in this patient?**

(a) Speculum examination (b) USG
(c) Non stress test (d) Amnisure

Explanation:

PREMATURE RUPTURE OF MEMBRANES (PROM)

- Spontaneous rupture of membranes anytime **beyond 28th week but before the onset of labour is called prelabour rupture of the membranes.**
- When it occurs **before 37 completed weeks** it is called **preterm PROM (PPROM)**

Causes:

- **Polyhydramnios**
- **Cervical incompetence**
- **Multiple pregnancy**
- **Chorioamnionitis**
- **Low BMI**

Confirmation of diagnosis:

- **Speculum examination–Most confirmatory**
- Vaginal pool for pH–6-6.2, **ferning pattern**, **orange blue discoloration of exfoliated cells**
- Amnisure radioimmunoassay
- Ultrasound

Investigations

- Complete blood count, C reactive protein, urine routine and culture
- High vaginal swab for Group B streptococcus
- Vaginal pool for estimation of phosphatidyl glycerol and L:S ratio
- USG for fetal biophysical profile, cardiotocography

Complications:

Obstetric	**Neonatal**
• Chorioamnionitis	• Neonatal sepsis
• Cord prolapse	• RDS
• Dry labour	• IVH
• Placental abruption	• NEC

Note:

How to diagnosis ruptured membranes?

- **Sterile speculum** examination–ruptured membranes are diagnosed if amniotic fluid pools in the posterior fornix or clear fluid flows from cervical canal.

- **Litmus test**–PH of vaginal secretions normally ranges from **4.5 to 5.5** whereas that of amniotic fluid is usually **7.0 to 7.5**. Therefore red litmus paper turns **blue**
- **Microscopic ferning.**
- **Nitrazine test**–yellow nitrazine paper turns blue
- **Arborization or ferning of vaginal fluid**–Amniotic fluid crystallizes to form **fern like pattern** due to relative concentrations of sodium chloride, proteins and carbohydrates.
- **Detection of alphafetoprotein** in vaginal vault has been used to identify amniotic fluid.
- **0.1% Nile blue sulfate test** (orange coloured cells seen)
- **USG** will show **oligohydramnios**
- **False positive test** results may occur with **coexistent blood, semen, or bacterial vaginosis** where results may occur due to scant fluid.

Ans: (a) Speculum examination

Ref: *DC Textbook of Obstetrics, 8th edition, Page 369*

3. All are risk factors for endometrial carcinoma *except*:

(a) Smoking
(b) Nulliparity
(c) Infertility
(d) Tamoxifen

Explanation:

Predisposing factors for endometrial carcinoma:

- **Hormone replacement therapy** after **menopause**
- **Chronic non ovulatory cycles** in DUB
- **Familial predisposition**–familial lynch II syndrome
- **Tamoxifen** given for breast cancer
- **Corpus cancer syndrome**–Obesity, diabetes and hypertension–30%
- **PCOD**
- **Fibroid** (3%)
- **Feminising ovarian tumor**
- **Older age**
- **Early menarche and Late menopause**
- **Pelvic irradiation**
  - **OCPs** have **a protective effect** and reduces the risk by **40-50%** and also adding progestogens for 12 days each cycle to oestrogen in HRT reduces its risk to 2%
  - **Cigarette smoking** was found to be significantly associated with a reduced risk of endometrial cancer, especially among postmenopausal women.

Ans: (a) Smoking

Ref: Shaw's Textbook of Gynecology, 15th edition, page 416 and Am J Med. 2008 Jun;121(6):501-508

4. Progesterone release rate in Progestasert is:

(a) 25 μg/day
(b) 40 μg/day
(c) 65 μg/day
(d) 80 μg/day

Explanation:

INTRAUTERINE CONTRACEPTIVE DEVICES

A. Biologically inert devices: Lippe's loop and Saf-T-coil.

B. Copper carrying devices: Copper T 200, Copper 7, Multiload Copper 250, Copper T 380, Copper T 220 and nova T.
  - About 50 μg of copper is eluted daily.
  - Nova-T has silver added to the copper wire.

C. Hormonal IUCD's

Progestasert	*Levonova*
o 38 mg progesterone o Release **65 μg/day** o Expensive and Effective for 1 year o 40% reduction of menorrhagia and dysmenorrhea	o 60 mg of levonorgestrel o Releases the hormone in very low doses **(20 μg/day)** o Incidence of ectopic pregnancy more o Safe during lacation o Longer acting (5 years)

MIRENA: Emerging as a better alternative to tubectomy in a young woman

MIRENA
o 52 mg Levonorgestrel o Releases 20 μg/day, from 15 mins following insertion o Less systemic side effects o Does not suppress ovulation, mainly acts on the endometrium and cervical mucus o Used in DUB, endometrial hyperplasia, HRT, and with tamoxifen for Ca. Breast, to counteract endometrial hyperplasia o Lasts for 5 years with fewer incidences for Ectopic gestation.

Patient selection for IUCD: • Low risk of PID/STD • Multiparous woman • Monogamous relationship • Desirous of long-term reversible method of contraception • Unhappy or unreliable users of oral contraception or barrier contraception	**Uses of IUCD:** • As a contraceptive • Post coital contraception (emergency contraception) • Following excision of uterine septum, Asherman's syndrome • Hormonal IUCD in menorrhagia and dysmenorrhea and hormonal replacement therapy in menopausal women • In a woman on tamoxifen for Ca. Breast, to counteract endometrial hyperplasia
Contraindications: • Suspected pregnancy • Pelvic inflammatory disease (PID), lower genital tract infection • Presence of fibroids–because of misfit • Menorrhagia and dysmenorrhea • Severe anemia • Diabetic women who are not will controlled–because of slight increase in pelvic infection • Previous ectopic pregnancy • Scarred uterus and uterine anomalies • In unmarried nulliparous because of the risk of PID and subsequent tubal infertility • Levonorgestrel IUCD in breast cancer	**Complications:** ***Immediate:*** • Difficulty in insertion • Vaso vagal attack and Uterine cramps ***Early:*** • Expulsion (2-5%) • Perforation (1-2%) • Spotting, menorrhagia (2-10%) and Dysmenorrhea (2-10%) • Vaginal infection (Actinomycosis) ***Late:*** • PID-2 to 5%, occurs in the 4th week • Does not prevent transmission of HIV • Pregnancy –1 to 3 per 100 women years (failure rate) • Ectopic pregnancy • Perforation • Menorrhagia and dysmenorrhea

Insertion technique:

- ***Cu T*** – withdrawal method
- ***Lippe's*** – push in method

Lifespan:

- Cu 380A (Para guard) : 10 years
- Cu T 200 : 3-4 years
- Multiload Cu 250 : 3 years
- Cu 375 : 5 years
- Nova T : 5 years
- Cu T 380 Ag and Cu T 380 S : 3-4 years

Recent advances:

- Frameless IUCD and fibroblast releasing 14 µg/day for 3 years.
- Frameless IUCD contains several copper cylinders tied together on a string and it is anchored 1 cm deep in the fundus.

Ans: (c) 65 µg/day

Ref: *Shaw's Textbook of Gynecology, 15th edition*

5. **Milky white watery discharge with fishy odour from vagina along with minimal itching is due to:**

(a) Bacterial vaginosis (b) Gonorrhoea
(c) Trichomonas (d) Candida

Explanation:

GARDNERELLA VAGINOSIS

- Alteration in normal vaginal flora
- **Decrease in number of lactobacilli in vaginal discharge** – lactobacilli reduce pH and release hydrogen peroxide toxic to other bacteria
- 100 fold increase in anerobic bacteria
- **Hemophilus vaginalis, Gardnerella, Mobiluncus and Mycoplasma hominis**–cause
- Vaginal discharge without discharge
- White, milky non-viscous discharge, **pH** of discharge more than **4.5**
- **Whiff Test–Fishy odour** when vaginal discharge is mixed with 10% KOH–due to release of amino metabolites from various organisms
- Presence of **Clue Cells**–epithelial cells with granular cytoplasm caused by gram negative bacilli adhering on the surface
- Wet smear, gram stain and culture are investigations
- **Treatment:**
  - **Metronidazole** 500 mg bd for 7 days
  - Ampicillin 500 mg or cephalosporin 500 mg bd for 7 days
  - Tetracycline 500 mg 4 times a day
  - Doxycycline 100 mg bd
  - Sulphafurazole 1g 4 times daily for 10-14 days
  - Clindamycin 300 mg daily for 7 days
  - Clindamycin 2% cream locally
  - Ornidazole 500 mg vaginal tablet for 7 days
  - **Lacteal** is protein free acidifying lactate gel neutralises vaginal ph 5 ml applied for 7 days.

AMSEL CRITERIA FOR DIAGNOSING BACTERIAL VAGNINOSIS

- Thin, white, yellow, homogeneous discharge
- Clue cells on microscopy
- pH of vaginal fluid >4.5
- Release of a fishy odor on adding alkali—10% potassium hydroxide (KOH) solution.
- **At least three of the four criteria** should be present for a confirmed diagnosis.

Ans: (a) Bacterial vaginosis

Ref: *Berek and Novak's Gynecology, 14th edition, Page 542-544*

6. Spiegelberg criteria is used in:

(a) Ovarian pregnancy
(b) Abdominal pregnancy
(c) Cervical pregnancy
(d) Tubal pregnancy

Explanation:

SPIEGELBERG CRITERIA

- The four criteria used to identify **ovarian ectopic**
- Named after **Otto Spiegelberg**.

Description

Four criteria for differentiating ovarian from other ectopic pregnancies:

1. The **gestational sac** is located in the region of the **ovary**.
2. The **ectopic pregnancy** is attached to the **uterus** by the **ovarian ligament**.
3. **Ovarian tissue** in the **wall** of the gestational sac is proved **histologically**.
4. The **tube** on the **involved side** is **intact**.

Note:

- **Studdiford's criteria** – for diagnosis of abdominal ectopic pregnancy
- **Rubin's criteria** – for diagnosis of cervical ectopic pregnancy

Ans: (a) Ovarian pregnancy

Ref: *Berek and Novak's Gynecology, 15th edition*

7. True about 'capacitation' of sperm:

(a) Takes about 6-8 hours
(b) Acrosomal reaction occurs
(c) Zona pellucida reaction occurs
(d) Capacitation takes place in testis

Explanation:

- Capacitation is the physiochemical change in the **sperm by which it becomes hypermotile and is able to bind and fertilize a secondary oocyte**
- **Capacitation takes place in the female genital tract and takes about 2-6 hours**
- The changes involve cyclic AMP dependent phosphorylation with increase in intracellular pH
- **Activation of acrosomal membranes** causes release of hyaluronidase, hydrolytic enzymes, proacrosin, acrosin, that help the sperm to digest the zona pellucida and enter the oocyte
- **Acrosomal reaction is fusion of sperm plasma membrane and outer acrosomal membrane**
- The sperm with acrosomal membrane bind with the zona protein
- Acrosome sperm penetrate the zona pellucida fuse with the oocyte plasma membrane
- The sperm head swells and the fused membrane vesiculates
- Gamete fusion occurs
- After 3-6 hours of insemination, one polar and two pronuclear bodies are visible and they migrate to the center of the oocyte

Ans: (b) Acrosomal reaction occurs

Ref: *Dutta Textbook of Obstetrics, 8th edition, Page 22*

8. All of the following sling operations are done for uterine prolapse *except*:

(a) Khanna
(b) Shirodkar
(c) Abdominocervicopexy
(d) Manchester

Explanation:

Sling surgeries provide a substitute for the weakened supports of the uterus by using nylon or Dacron tapes as slings to support the uterus.

Indications: 2nd or 3rd degree uterine prolapse in women who are desirous of retaining their child bearing and menstrual functions.

The various sling operations are:

A. Purandare's sling

- The tape is fixed **anteriorly** to the uterine isthmus and lateral edges brought between leaves of broad ligament and **fixed to the rectus sheath** on either side

- Plication of round ligament
- **Moschowitz's repair** – abdominal correction of enterocele

B. Shirodkar's sling operation

- Mesilene tape (originally fascia lata) is fixed to posterior aspect of the cervix and to the **anterior longitudinal ligament of the sacral promontory.**
- Sling taken through the **Psoas loop on the left side** due to the presence of sigmoid colon

C. Khanna's sling operation

- Merseline tape fixed to the isthmus of cervix posteriorly and fixed to **anterior superior iliac spine** on either sides.

D. Abdominocervicopexy

MANCHESTER OPERATION

Indications

- Suitable for women less than 40 years, completed their family with the intention of preserving menstrual function
- II or III degree uterine prolapse with cystocele / rectocele with or without supravaginal elongation of cervix

Principal Steps

- Preliminary D & C
- Amputation of cervix
- Shortening of Mackenrodt's and anchoring in front of cervix.
- Anterior colporrhaphy
- Posterior colpoperineorrhaphy

Disadvantages is mainly due to cervical amputation:

- Cervical incompetence leading to:
  - Habitual abortions
  - Preterm deliveries
- Cervical stenosis leading to
  - Dystocia during labor
  - Hematometra
- **Hence usually preferred in women who have completed family**

Ans: (d) Manchester

***Ref**: Berek and Novak's Gynecology, 14th edition, Page 994*

9. **Call exner bodies are seen in:**

(a) Granulosa cell tumor (b) Yolk sac
(c) Dysgerminoma (d) Embryonal carcinoma

Explanation:

WHO classification of ovarian tumours

Common epithelial tumors	**Sex cord (gonadal stroma) tumors**	**Germ cell tumors**
• Serous tumors • Mucinous tumors • Endometrioid tumors • Clear cell (mesonephroid tumors) • Brenner tumors (Transitional cell tumor) • Mixed epithelial tumors • Undifferentiated carcinoma • Unclassified epithelial tumors	• Granulose-stromal cell tumors, theca cell tumors • Androblastomas: Sertoli-Leydig cell tumors • Gynandroblastomas • Unclassified **Gonadoblastoma** • Pure • Mixed with dysgerminoma or other germ cell tumors.	• Dysgerminoma • Endodermal sinus tumors (yolk sac tumour) • Embryonal carcinoma • Polyembryoma • Choriocarcinoma • Teratoma • Mixed forms **Lipid (lipoid) cell tumors** **Soft tissue tumors not specific to ovary** **Unclassified tumors**

- Familial ovarian cancers: HNPCC (LYNCH-2), BRCA 1 and BRCA 2

NOTE:

- **Ovarian cancers are the most common cause of death among all gynecological malignancies.**
- **Ovarian cyst adeno carcinoma is most common malignant tumor** of ovary (33-50% of epithelial cancers)
- Most common benign tumour of ovary: Dermoid cyst
- Most common benign epithelial tumor: Serous cystadenoma
- Largest benign ovarian tumor: Mucinous cyst adenoma
- Most common ovarian tumour in < 20 years of age group – **germ cell tumour**
- Most common germ cell tumour (GCT): Mature teratoma
- Most common malignant germ cell tumour (GCT): Dysgerminoma
- Ovarian tumor whose incidence is increased during pregnancy: Dermoid cyst
- Most common ovarian tumor to undergo torsion in pregnancy: Dermoid cyst
- Most common ovarian tumour to involve opposite side: Granulosa cell tumour
- ***Serous cyst adenoma is overall most common tumour of ovary.***
- Of all the malignant tumors, 90% are epithelial in orgin, 80% are in primary in the ovary and 20% secondary from breasts, gastrointestinal tract and colon.
- Mucinous cyst becomes malignant in 5% but papillary cystadenoma becomes malignant in 50% if left untreated.
- Most common **ovarian tumor associated with pseudomyxoma peritoni: Mucinous cystadeno Ca.**
- **Most common ovarian tumor associated with hyperthyroidism: Germ cell tumour with struma ovarii (struma ovarii is a teratoma with thyroid tissue).**
- Ovarian tumors with calcification:
  - Cystic teratoma / dermoid cyst (bone + teeth)
  - Gonadoblastoma
  - Fibroma
- Torsion of ovarian cyst in the most common complication and seen in teratoma/dermoid cyst most commonly.
- Tumors with lymphocytic infiltration: Dysgerminoma
- **Ovarian serous tumors, both low- and high-grade, have a propensity to spread to the peritoneal surfaces and omentum and are commonly associated with the presence of ascites.**
- ***Meig's syndrome:*** Combination of ovarian Fibroma + Ascites + right sided hemothorax
- ***Pseudo Meig's syndrome:*** *Brenner's tumor, Granulosa Cell tumor, Thecoma*

Risk factors	Protective factors
• Repeated ovulation • Old age • Nullipara • Early menarche, late menopause • White race • Late marriage, infertility • Perineal exposure to talc	• OC pills • Pregnancy • Breastfeeding • Chronic anovulation • Bilateral salpingo oophorectomy • Tubal sterilization • Hysterectomy

Age Group:

Malignant epithelial tumors	40-60 years
Benign cystic teratoma	10-20 years
Dysgerminoma	<20 years
Endodermal sinus tumour	15-20 years
Granulose cell tumour	Post menopausal
Sertoli leydig cell	20-30 years
Thecoma	Post menopausal

GERM CELL TUMOURS

- Account for 15-20% of all ovarian tumors.
- 95% are benign cystic teratoma, also called as dermoids.

- Below the age of 20 years, 60% of the tumors are of germ cell origin.
- < 10 years: 85% belong to this group and are malignant.

Tumour markers of ovarian cancer:

- **CA-125:** > 35U/ml indicates malignant and residual ovarian tumour. It is also raised in abdominal tuberculosis and endometriosis.
- **CEA:** >5 mg/dl seen in Mucinous ovarian tumour.
- **Endodermal sinus tumors produce AFP.**
- **α fetoprotein and alpha-1-antitrypsin:** Endodermal sinus tumor
- **AFP and HCG:** Embryonal carcinoma
- **HCG:** Choriocarcinoma
- **Dysgerminomas and other germinomas:** No markers, but **secrete LDH**

Krukenberg's Tumour

- Primary site: **Stomach (70%), large intestine (15%) and breast (6%), spread by retrograde lymphatics.**
- Characteristic features: **Signet ring cells**
- Involvement of ovary by: **Retrograde lymphatics.**
- Always bilateral with smooth surface, slightly bossy and freely mobile over the pelvis.
- Maintains the shape of ovary and has a peculiar solid waxy consistency.
- No tendency of adhesion and no infiltration of nearby tissues.

Ovarian Tumours and Their Specific Features

- **Schiller Duval bodies** – Endodermal sinus tumour
- **Signet ring cells** – Krukenberg's tumour
- **Coffee bean cells/Call Exner bodies** – Granulosa cell tumour
- **Sertoli and Leydig cells** – Arrhenoblastoma
- **Psammoma bodies** – Papillary Serous Cystadenoma
- **Rokitansky's protuberance** – Dermoid cyst (Mature teratoma)
- **Hobnail cells** – Clear cell Ca (mesonephroid Ca)
- **Reinke's crystal** – Hilus cell tumour
- **Walthard cell nest** – Brenner tumour

Ans: (a) Granulosa cell tumor

Ref: *Berek and Novak's Gynecology, 14th edition*

10. **Single most important feature to diagnose fetal aneuploidy:**

(a) Increased nuchal translucency (b) Absent nasal bone
(c) Cystic hygroma (d) Abnormal ductus venosus flow

Explanation:

Ultrasound markers of fetal aneuploidy:

- **Nuchal translucency is the single most powerful tool.** More than **3 mm** needs evaluation
- Absence of nasal bone
- Absence or reversal of flow in the ductus venosus on Doppler
- Tricuspid regurgitation
- Increase in frontomaxillary angle more than 85 deg

Ans: (a) Increased nuchal translucency

Ref: *Current Progress in Obstetrics and Gynecology, John Stud, Volume 1, Page 17*

11. **An obese diabetic woman presents with menorrhagia. Curette from endometrium demonstrates endometrial carcinoma. Most probable gene associated with this carcinoma? (Repeat)**

(a) PTEN (b) TP53
(c) CDH4 (d) C-myc

Explanation:

- The **most frequently altered gene in estrogen-dependent endometrioid endometrial carcinoma is PTEN.**
- In contrast, **p53 mutations or Her2/neu overexpression are more frequent in non-endometrioid tumors**.
- K-ras mutations are detected in approximately 15–30% of endometrioid carcinomas
- A beta-catenin mutation was detected in about 20% of endometrioid carcinomas
- **Lynch syndrome,** which is an autosomal dominant inherited disorder of cancer susceptibility and is characterized by a MSH2/MSH6 protein complex deficiency, is associated with the development of **non-endometrioid carcinomas.**

Also Know:

The genetic mutations most commonly associated with **endometrioid adenocarcinoma** are in the genes:

- **PTEN**, a tumor suppressor gene*
- **PIK3CA**, a kinase
- **KRAS**, a GTPase that functions in signal transduction
- **CTNNB1,** involved in adhesion and cell signaling. The CTNNB1 (beta-catenin) gene is most commonly mutated in the squamous subtype of endometrioid adenocarcinoma

PROGNOSTIC VARIABLES IN ENDOMETRIAL CA

- **Age:**
  - Younger women with endometrial cancer have better prognosis than older women.
- **Histologic Type:**
  - Non-endometrioid histologic subtypes account for about 10% of endometrial cancers and carry an increased risk for recurrence and spread
- **Histologic grade**
- **Tumour size:**
  - Significant prognostic factor for **lymph node metastasis** and survival in patients with endometrial CA
- **Hormone receptor status:**
  - **Estrogen** and **progesterone** receptor levels are prognostic indicators
  - Patients whose tumours are positive for one or both receptors have **longer survival times.**
  - Progesterone receptors levels appear to be stronger predictors of survival.
- **DNA ploidy and proliferative index:**
  - The proportion of nondiploid tumours increases with **stage, lack of tumour differentiation and depth of myometrial invasion.**
- **Myometrial invasion:**
  - Increasing depth of invasion is associated with increasing likelihood of extrauterine spread and recurrence.
- **Lymph-vascular Space invasion**
- **Isthmus and cervix extension:**
  - Involvement of ishmus and cervix is associated with increased risk for extrauterine disease, lymph node metastasis and recurrence
- **Peritoneal cytology:**
  - Seems to have adverse effect on survival only if the endometrial cancer has spread to adnexa, peritoneum, or lymph nodes and not if the disease is otherwise confined to uterus
- **Lymph node metastases**
- **Intraperitoneal metastases**
- **Molecular aberration:**
  - Inactivation of **PTEN tumor suppressor ge**ne is one of the earliest aberrations observed and most common genetic defect in **TYPE 1 cancer**.
  - Most frequent genetic alteration is **TP53 mutation** found in **type 2 endometrial cancer**.

Ans: (a) PTEN gene

Ref: *https://www.hindawi.com/journals/ogi/2010/984013/genetics of endometrial carcinoma*

Version – 2

A 50-year-old woman who was obese and hypertensive, came with complaints of bleeding and abdomen pain, diagnosed to be endometrial cancer. Which of the following gene is mutated?

(a) P53
(b) PTEN
(c) Beta catenin
(d) CHD4

Explanation:

- Going with PTEN because it's the most common one mutated (***Ref:*** WHO - >50%). P53 mutation is seen only in type 2 carcinomas, incidence of which is less. PTEN is seen in both type 1 and type 2 carcinomas.

Features	Type 1	Type 2
Prototypic form	Endometrioid carcinoma	Uterine (papillary) serous carcinoma
Typical patient	Perimenopausal or early postmenopausal women	Elderly women
	Background of endometrial hyperplasia	Background of atrophic endometrium
	Low-grade	High-grade
	Estrogen-dependent	Not estrogen-dependent
Estrogen receptor	Usually positive; high grade cases may be negative	Negative
MIB1 proliferation index (ki-67)	Low	High
p53	Negative; high grade cases may be positive	Diffuse positivity

Ans: (b) PTEN

Ref: *WHO, FGT, Page 29-34*

12. Drug of choice in postpartum hemorrhage (PPH) resistant to Oxytocin and Ergometrine:

(a) Carboprost
(b) Dinoprostone
(c) Dinoprost
(d) Misoprostol

Explanation:

- **Carboprost** is the alternative drug for control of **PPH unresponsive to ergometrine and oxytocin.**

MANAGEMENT OF PPH:

- **First line of Therapy**
  - **Uterotonic agents**: **Oxytocin**.
  - **Ergot-alkaloids** (Ergometrine, Methyl Ergonovine).
  - **Prostaglandins** (Dinoprostone, Misoprostol)

Oxytocin

- It stimulates the **upper segment of the myometrium** to contract **rhythmically**, which **constricts spiral arteries** and **decreases blood flow** through the **uterus**.
- Clinical response is **rapid** and occurs within **3 and 5 minutes.**
- Side effects are very **rare**, but occasional causes **nausea and vomiting.**
- The only serious side effect is **dilutional hyponatremia**, which may happen with prolonged use.
- **Rapid IV infusion** is associated with **hypotension and tachycardia.**
- Oxytocin is dosed at **10 to 40 U/L.**

Carboprost

- It is **synthetic prostaglandin analogue of PGF2α**
- Enhances **uterine contractility** and cause **vasoconstriction**
- **IM dosing**, initial: **250 mcg**; if needed, may repeat at **15- to 90-minute** intervals; maximum total dose, **2 mg (8 doses).**
- In **75%** of cases, a successful clinical response is reached **within 30 min.**

- The reported side effects include **nausea, vomiting, diarrhea, bronchospasm and hypertension**.
- The recommendation is that the drug be given with caution to patients with **hepatic or cardiovascular disease, asthma, or hypersensitivity to the drug.**
- Clinical response may be enhanced with concomitant use of **oxytocin**.

Methylergonovine Maleate:

- It is a semisynthetic ergot alkaloid.
- It causes **generalized smooth-muscle contraction** in which the upper and lower segments of the **uterus contract tetanically**.
- It is available **as 0.2 mg/ml ampoule for IV/IM use.**
- Side effects are very rare, but occasional causes **nausea and vomiting**.
- This drug should be used with extreme caution in patients with **hypertension or preeclampsia**.
- Onset of action (tablet) is within **5 to 10 minutes.**
- **Used 0.2 mg 3 to 4 times/day** in the puerperium for **2 to 7 days.**
- Onset of the IM dose is **2 to 5 minutes.**

Misoprostol:

- Synthetic prostaglandin **E1 analogue**
- Initially developed for oral use
- Other routes of administration **Sub-lingual, Rectal, Vaginal and Buccal**

Ans: (a) Carboprost

Ref: *DC Dutta Textbook of Gynecology, 8th edition, Page 474; KD Tripathi, Textbook of Pharmacology, Page 189*

13. **Least likely complication in a pregnant mother with Hypothyroidism:**

(a) Polyhydramnios
(b) Recurrent abortions
(c) Preterm labor
(d) Hypertension

Explanation:

HYPOTHYROIDISM IN PREGNANCY

- **Most common** endocrine disorder of pregnancy
- **1-2%** in pregnancy
- Pregnancy may modify the course of disease
- **Increased thyroxine requirement** in **pregnancy**

Normal values in pregnancy

Serum	Units	1st Trimester	2nd Trimester	3rd Trimester
TSH	mU/L	0.03 – 2.3	0.03 – 3.7	0.13 – 3.4
FT_4	ng/dl	0.86 – 1.77	0.63 – 1.29	0.66 – 1.12
FT_3	pmol/L	3.5 – 7	2.8 – 4.2	2.4 – 4.1

Ratio of FT_4:FT_3= 4:1

Effect of untreated hypothyroidism on pregnancy

On Pregnancy	On Fetus
• Early pregnancy failure • Pre-eclampsia (5–10%) • Placental abruption (1%) • Preterm delivery (10–15%) • Malpresentation • Low birthweight • Stillbirth • Post partum hemorrhage • Abortion	• Neurodevelopmental delay • Deafness • Stunted growth • Peripartum hypoxia • Increased risk of neonatal mortality • Congenital anomalies • Prematurity

Etiology

- Lack of iodine
- Diseases of the thyroid gland – autoimmune disease, aplasia, enzyme defect
- Insufficiency following surgical excision, irradiation, drug treatment for hyperthyroidism
- **Lithium and amiodarone** therapy
- Primary hypothyroidism in pregnancy is **mostly related to autoimmune thyroid disease (Hashimoto's thyroiditis).**

Treatment

- **Levothyroxine** is the most widely prescribed treatment
- **Safe for mother and fetus – Category A**
- Available dosage–**25-300 mcg**
- **Dose–30% increase** from non-pregnant value if **already hypothyroid**
- **TSH goal** is **0.5 to 2.5 mIU/ml**
- Newly diagnosed hypothyroid in pregnancy dose is **1-2 mcg levothyroxine/day**

HYPERTHYROIDISM IN PREGNANCY

Etiology

- **Autoimmune hyperthyroidism (Graves' disease)** due to thyroid stimulating antibodies–**Most common cause**
- Nodular thyroid disease
- Sub-acute thyroiditis
- Hyperemesis gravidarum and trophoblastic disease.

Effects of untreated hyperthyroidism

Maternal	Fetal/Neonatal
• Abortion • Preeclampsia • Preterm delivery • Placental abruption • Congestive cardiac failure • Thyroid storm	• IUGR • Prematurity • Stillbirth • Hyperthyroidism • Hypothyroidism • Increased perinatal morbidity and mortality Thyroid stimulating antibodies can cross the placenta producing neonatal thyrotoxicosis and increased neonatal death

Ans: (a) Polyhydramnios

***Ref:** DC Dutta's Textbook of Obstetrics, Page 288*

14. Most common cause of occipito-posterior presentation:

(a) Deflexed head
(b) Android pelvis
(c) Gynecoid pelvis
(d) Multiparity

Explanation:

OCCIPITO-POSTERIOR (OP) PRESENTATION

Incidence–10% at onset of labor.

Right occipito-posterior (ROP) is more common than left occipito-posterior (LOP) because the left oblique diameter is reduced by the presence of sigmoid colon.

Aetiology

- **The shape of the pelvis: Anthropoid and android pelvis are the most common cause of occipito-posterior due to narrow fore-pelvis.**
- **Fetal factors: Marked deflection of the fetal head**, often favors posterior position of the vertex.
- **Uterine factor: Abnormal uterine contraction** which may be the cause or effect, leads to persistent deflexion and occipito-posterior position.

Mechanism of Labor in OP Position

- **Engaging diameter – Occipito-frontal diameter (11.5 cm)**
- **The degree of deflexion determines the mechanism of labor**
- **Normal mechanism (90%)–Long anterior rotation**
- Deflexion is corrected and complete flexion occurs. The occiput meets the pelvic floor first, long anterior rotation 3/8 circle occurs bringing the occiput anteriorly and the fetus is delivered normally.
- **Abnormal mechanism (10%).**

Abnormal mechanism	Mechanism of labor	Further course of labor
Deep transverse arrest	**In mild deflexion**, the occiput rotates 1/8 circle anteriorly and the head is arrested in the transverse diameter	No further progress occurs and labor is obstructed as the head cannot be delivered spontaneously. Delivered by CS
Persistent occipito-posterior	**In moderate deflexion**, the occiput and sinciput meet the pelvic floor simultaneously, no internal rotation and the head persists in the oblique diameter	No further progress occurs and labor is obstructed as the head cannot be delivered spontaneously. Delivered by CS
Direct occipito-posterior (face to pubis)	**In marked deflexion**, the sinciput meets the pelvic floor first, rotates 1/8 circle anteriorly and the occiput becomes direct posterior	**The head can be delivered as face to pubis delivery by flexion** if uterine contractions are strong and there is no contracted pelvis. **Perineal lacerations are more liable to occur** as: • The perineum is distended by the large occipito-frontal diameter 11.5 cm. • Is overstretched by the large occiput.

Factors favoring long anterior rotation

- Well flexed head.
- Good uterine contractions.
- Roomy pelvis.
- Elastic recoil of the pelvic floor.
- No premature rupture of membranes.

Ans: (b) Android pelvis

***Ref**: Dutta's Textbook of Obstetrics, Page 366*

15. **A pregnant woman with HELLP syndrome suddenly developed hypotension, right hypochondriac pain, ascites, pleural effusion and sudden onset of breathlessness. What is your diagnosis?**

(a) Abruptio placentae
(b) DIC
(c) Rupture of hepatic hematoma
(d) Part of pre-eclamptic toximia
(e) Side effect of anti-hypertensive drug

Explanation:

Complications of Preeclampsia

Maternal

During pregnancy	During labor	Puerperium
• Eclampsia • Abruption • Oliguria and anuria • Dimness of vision and even blindness • Preterm labor • HELLP syndrome • Cerebral hemorrhage • Acute respiratory distress syndrome (ARDS)	• Eclampsia • Postpartum hemorrhage	• Eclampsia – usually occurs within 48 hours • Shock • Sepsis – due to increased incidence of induction, operative interference and low vitality

Fetal

- Intrauterine death
- Intrauterine growth restriction
- Asphyxia
- Prematurity

Remote Complications

- Recurrent pre-eclampsia: **25% chance of pre-eclampsia to recur** in subsequent pregnancies.
- Residual hypertension.

HELLP Syndrome – Characterized by Hemolysis (H), Elevated Liver enzymes (EL) and Low Platelet count (LP) (<100,000/mm^3).

- A rare complication of pre-eclampsia (10–15%).
- This syndrome is manifested by **nausea, vomiting, epigastric or right upper quadrant pain, along with biochemical and hematological changes**.
- Parenchymal necrosis of liver causes **elevation in hepatic enzymes (AST and ALT >70 IU/L, LDH >600 IU/L) and bilirubin (>1.2 mg/dL).**
- **Subcapsular hematoma formation (diagnosed by CT scan) can occur and eventually liver may rupture to cause sudden hypotension**, due to hemoperitoneum.

Management of HELLP

- Anti-seizure prophylaxis with **Magnesium sulphate** started
- Careful assessment of maternal and fetal status followed by **termination of pregnancy**
- Administration **of corticosteroids** improves perinatal (↑ pulmonary maturity, ↓ IVH and ↓ necrotizing enterocolitis) and maternal (↑ thrombocyte count, ↑ urinary output) outcome.
- **Cesarean section is the common mode of delivery**. Epidural anesthesia can be used safely if the platelet count is >1,00,000/mm^3).
- Platelet transfusion is given **if the count is <50,000/mm^3.**
- Patient should be managed in an ICU until improvement in platelet count, urine output, BP and liver enzymes.
- **Recurrence risk** of HELLP syndrome is 3–19%.

Risks associated with HELLP syndrome

Maternal	Perinatal
• Abruptio placenta • DIC • Acute renal failure • Severe ascites • Pulmonary edema • Pleural effusion • Cerebral edema • Retinal detachment • Subcapsular liver hematoma • ARDS, sepsis and death.	Morbidity and mortality are significantly increased due to prematurity, RDS and sepsis

Ans: (c) Rupture of hepatic hematoma

Ref: DC Dutta's Textbook of Obstetrics, Page 223

16. Pregnant mother with known case of hypothyroidism. Which of the following is correct regarding management?

(a) Increase thyroxine dose and TSH should be maintained at 2.5
(b) Check every 2-4 weeks
(c) Elective delivery
(d) Continue same dose

Explanation:

Investigations and diagnosis of hypothyroidism in pregnancy

- **Subclinical hypothyroidism** is characterized **by elevated TSH and normal FT4**
- **Overt hypothyroidism** is characterized by **elevated TSH and low FT4**
- Serum **thyroid peroxidase antibodies (anti TPO) or anti-microsomal antibodies** are elevated in **autoimmune thyroiditis.**

Treatment

- Therapy is started with **Levothyroxine 50-100 mcg/day and increased by 25 mcg/week** until the patient is euthyroid.
- If the patient is on substitution therapy before pregnancy, the **dose of levo-thyroxine need to be increased in pregnancy**.
- Serum TSH should be **repeated at an interval of 6-8 weeks** as there is increased demand of thyroid hormone in the second half of pregnancy.
- **After delivery, dose** has to be **reduced** as necessary.
- **Recommendations for TSH levels during pregnancy**–American thyroid association guidelines 2011

Period	Recommended TSH levels
Non pregnant state	**0.3-4.5**
First trimester	**< 2.5 with a range of 0.1-2.5**
Second trimester	0.2-3.0
Third trimester	0.3-3.0

Investigations and diagnosis of hyperthyroidism in pregnancy

- **Free T4–high**
- **Free T4 index–high**
- **FT3–high**

- **TSH – suppressed**
- Antithyroglobulin, antimicrosomal antibodies and thyroid stimulating immunoglobulin are measured.
- **Radioactive iodine uptake and scans are C/I during pregnancy** as it crosses the placenta and can damage the fetal thyroid gland permanently.

Treatment

- The main stay of treatment – antithyroid **drugs Propylthiouracil (PTU) or Carbimazole/Methimazole**
- **PTU is the preferred drug during pregnancy**, especially in I trimester as:
  - o It has lower risk of birth defects
  - o It crosses the placenta less readily
- **Both the drugs may cause fetal goitre and hypothyroidism.**
- **Methimazole embryopathy–characterized by esophageal or choanal atresia, aplasia cutis of the neonate.**
- **The drugs are not contraindicated during breastfeeding.**
- **Cord blood should be taken for TSH and free T4 at the time of delivery to detect neonatal hyper-thyroidism.**
- **Preconceptional–Radioactive iodine therapy should not be given to patients wanting pregnancy within one year.** If pregnancy occurs inadvertently, termination should be done.

Ans: (a) Increase thyroxine dose and TSH should be maintained at 2.5

Ref: *DC Dutta's Textbook of Obstetrics, Page 288; Holland and Brew's Manual of Obstetrics, 4th edition, Page 139*

17. A patient presents with postmenopausal bleed. Endometrial biopsy will be done if endometrial thickness is:

(a) 3 mm (b) 5 mm
(c) 7 mm (d) 8 mm

Explanation:

Causes of postmenopausal bleeding

Benign conditions	Malignant conditions
• Senile endometritis • Atrophic endometrium • Dysfunctional uterine bleeding • Uterine polyp • Tubercular endometritis • Cervical erosion and polyp • Senile vaginitis • Decubitus ulcer • Retained and forgotten pessary or IUCD • HRT • Urethral caruncle, polyp	Endometrial hyperplasia Genital malignancy–Carcinoma of the cervix, endometrium, vagina, vulva and Fallopian tube Granulosa cell tumor of the ovary Sarcoma uterus

- **One-third of the cases of PMB are due malignancy, commonly due to endometrial and cervical carcinoma.**
- Abnormal perimenopausal and postmenopausal bleeding should always be taken seriously and be properly investigated.
- Invasive tumors of the cervix, vagina and vulva are usually evident on **local and Speculum examination** and any lesion identified should be biopsied.
  - o If any visible cervical growth → biopsy is taken for histology.
  - o If cervix apparently looks normal → cervical and endocervical smear to exclude dysplasia or CIN.
- **The possibility of uterine source of bleeding must always be eliminated.**

Uterine Causes of Postmenopausal Bleeding

Cause of Bleeding	Percentage %
Endometrial atrophy (Most common)	**60–80**
Estrogen replacement therapy	15–25
Endometrial polyps	2–12
Endometrial hyperplasia	5–10
Endometrial cancer	**10**

DIAGNOSIS OF UTERINE PATHOLOGY

- **Office endometrial aspiration biopsy is the accepted first step in evaluation of perimenopausal AUB or PMB**
  - Diagnostic accuracy is 90 - 98%.
  - **Endocervical curettage** is performed at the time of endometrial biopsy if cervical pathology is suspected.
- **Hysteroscopy and D&C**
  - Reserved for cases of cervical stenosis, patient intolerance for OPD aspiration biopsy, bleeding recurs after a negative endometrial biopsy or if the specimen obtained is inadequate.
  - Hysteroscopy is **more accurate in identifying polyps and submucous myomas.**
- **Transvaginal sonography (TVS) is a useful adjunct to endometrial biopsy for selecting patients for further evaluation**
  - TVS +/- SIS (saline infusion sonography) – helps to distinguish between patients with postmenopausal atrophic endometrium and those with significant amount of endometrial tissue or polyps who need further evaluation.
  - The finding of **ET > 4 mm, a polypoid endometrial mass, or collection of fluid within the uterus requires further evaluation.**
- Pap smear–Only **30% to 50% of patients with endometrial cancer have abnormal Pap test** results.

Ans: (b) 5 mm

***Ref**: DC Dutta's Textbook of Gynecology, Page 561; Berek and Novak's Gynecology, Page 1978*

ORTHOPEDICS

1. X-ray of a 10-year-old child with fracture is shown. Which of the following is incorrect? (Image)

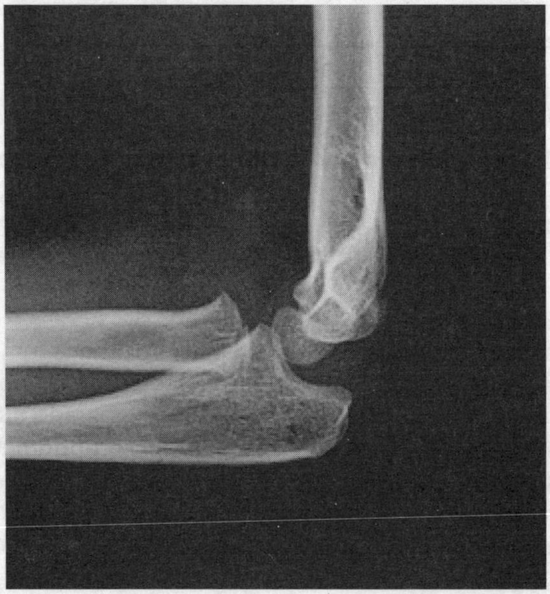

(a) Anterior pad of fat sign present
(b) Fracture of radius head
(c) Radius head articulation is seen
(d) And grade type 4 epiphyseal fracture salter harris

Explanation:

- **Fat Pad signs** are X-ray findings that help to diagnose **undisplaced** and **impacted** fractures of **distal humerus** (**supracondylar area**).
- Fracture in and around the olecranon fossa pushes the olecranon and coronoid fat pads out that cast a "black" shadow on X-ray in front (coronoid/anterior fat pad) and back (olecranon/posterior fat pad) of distal humerus, visible clearly in the posted X-ray.

Ans: (b) Fracture of radius head

Ref: *Fundamentals of Orthopedics by Mohindra and Jain, 2nd edition, Jaypee Publishers, Page 77-78 and Fig 4.29*

2. A-12-year-old boy presents with chronic knee pain for 2 years. Knee X-ray is shown. Probable diagnosis:

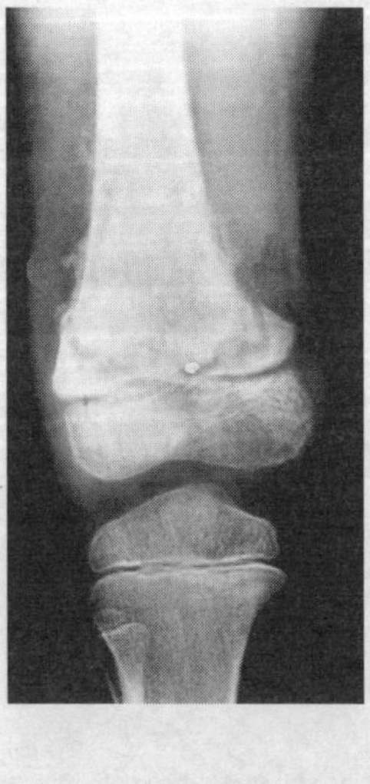

(a) Chronic osteomyelitis
(b) Osteosarcoma
(c) Rickets
(d) Hyperparathyroidism

Explanation:

- X-ray shows **periosteal reaction** around **distal femur.**
- Going by the site (**distal femur**) and age group (2nd decade), answer is **osteosarcoma** > **chronic osteomyelitis** (seen in relatively older age group).
- In osteosarcoma **periosteal reaction** (bone formation under the periosteum) may take the form of sunray appearance (bone formation along **sharpey's fibers**) or **codman's triangle**.
- The X-ray in question seems to depict **sun ray appearance**.

X-ray Appearance in Osteosarcoma

- The X-ray appearances are variable.
- Hazy **osteolytic areas** may alternate with unusually dense **osteoblastic areas**.
- The **endosteal margin** is **poorly defined**.
- Often the cortex is breached and the tumour extends into the adjacent tissues; when this happens, streaks of new bone appear, radiating outwards from the cortex – the so-called '**sunburst**' effect.
- Where the tumour emerges from the cortex, reactive new bone forms at the angles of periosteal elevation (**Codman's triangle**).
- While both the **sunburst appearance** and **Codman's triangle** are typical of osteosarcoma, they may occasionally be seen in other rapidly growing tumours.

Ans: (b) Osteosarcoma

Ref: *Fundamentals of Orthopedics by Mohindra and Jain, 2nd edition, Jaypee Publishers, Page 325 and Figs. 11.34-35*

3. **Peak incidence of osteosarcoma occurs at:**

(a) 2nd decade
(b) 3rd decade
(c) 5th decade
(d) 6th decade

Explanation:

- There are two peaks in incidence of osteosarcoma.
- The first peak is around **10-14 years** i.e., **second decade** (**Pubertal spurt).** Another peak (**relatively smaller**) is seen in **4th to 6th decades** age group.

OSTEOSARCOMA

Risk Factors for Osteosarcoma

(a) Familial cases where the deletion of chromosome '13q14' inactivates the retinoblastoma gene is associated with a high risk of osteosarcoma development.

(b) Bone dysplasias, including Paget's disease, fibrous dysplasia, enchondromatosis, and hereditary multiple exostoses, increase the risk of osteosarcoma.

(c) Li-Fraumeni syndrome (germline TP53 mutation) is a predisposing factor for osteosarcoma development.

(d) Rothmund-Thomson syndrome (i.e., autosomal recessive association of congenital bone defects, hair and skin dysplasias, hypogonadism and cataracts) is associated with increased risk of this disease.

(e) Bone irradiation.

Ans: (a) 2nd decade

Ref: *Fundamentals of Orthopedics by Mohindra and Jain, 2nd edition, Jaypee Publishers, Page 325*

4. **Examine knee X-ray carefully. Diagnosis:**

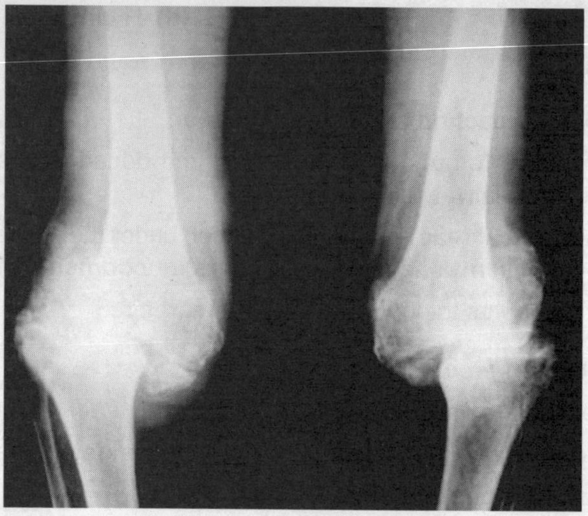

(a) TB
(b) Gout
(c) Charcot
(d) RA

Explanation:

Classical X-ray signs of Charcot arthropathy include:

- **Marked destructive changes***
- **Joint space narrowing***
- **Osteophyte formation***
- **Subchondral sclerosis***
- **Loose body formation***

All of these can be seen on the above X-ray.

Ans: (c) Charcot

Ref: *Fundamentals of Orthopedics by Mohindra and Jain, 2nd edition, Jaypee Publishers, Page 440, Fig. 16.31*

5. **True statement regarding Mseleni joint disease is:**

(a) Should, elbow wrist involvement is characteristic
(b) Elderly males are commonly involved
(c) Height is unaffected
(d) Endemic to northern Kwazulu Natal area in South Africa

Explanation:

MSELENI JOINT DISEASE (MJD)

- Type of crippling **chondrodysplasia** (short stature) endemic in the **Mseleni population** in northern **Kwazulu Natal, South Africa.**
- Commonly involving elderly women, over the age of **50.**
- It **symmetrically** involves multiple joints leading to **pain**, **stiffness** and **decreased range** of **motion.**
- **Hip joints*** are most noticeably involved and **hip dysplasia** and **protrusion acetabuli** are two distinct features.

Ans: (d) Endemic to northern Kwazulu Natal area in South Africa.

Ref: *Fundamentals of Orthopedics by Mohindra and Jain, 2nd edition, Jaypee Publishers, Page 443*

6. **Ankle X-ray image (lower end of Tibia) of an adolescent boy is shown. Probable diagnosis:**

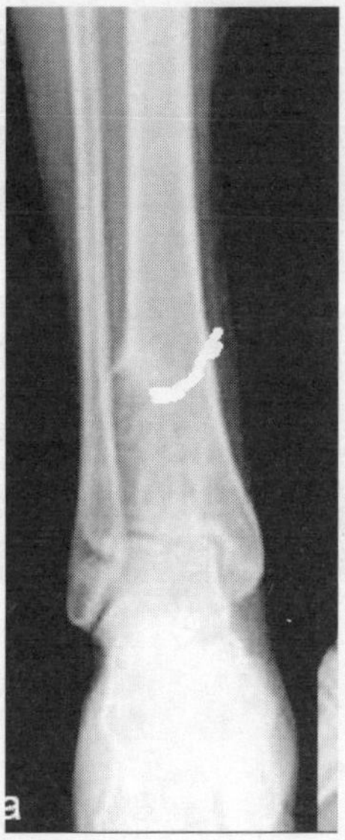

(a) Chondromyxoid fibroma (b) Osteosarcoma
(c) Bone cyst with fracture (d) Fibrosis cystica

Explanation:

- **Well circumscribed** lesion with a **rim of sclerosis** in the **metaphysis** of a long bone having a **bubbly/ lobulated appearance** (mimicking a **non-ossifying fibroma**) is classical of **Chondromyxoid fibroma.**
- In contrast to other cartilaginous lesions, radiographic evidence of **intralesional calcification** usually is **absent**.

Aneurysmal Bone Cysts (ABC)

- Benign expansile tumour-like bone lesions composed of numerous blood-filled channels, and mostly diagnosed in children and adolescents.
- Aneurysmal bone cysts are primarily seen in children and adolescents, with 80% occurring in the patients less than 20 years of age.
- Patients may present with pain, which may be of insidious onset or abrupt due to pathological fracture, with a palpable lump or with restricted movement.
- They are typically eccentrically located in the metaphysis of long bones, adjacent to an unfused growth plate.
- Most common locations are:
  - Long bones: 50-60%, typically the metaphysis
  - Lower limb: 40%
- Radiographs demonstrate sharply defined, expansile osteolytic lesions, with thin sclerotic margins
- MRI shows fluid-fluid levels in aneursymal bone cysts
- Simple/Unicarmel bone cyst shows fluid fluid levels

Non-Ossifying Fibromas (NOF)

- Most common of non-neoplastic fibrous bone lesions.
- NOFs are very common in children and adolescents, with a peak incidence at 10-15 years old.
- NOFs are typically a multiloculated lucent lesion with a sclerotic rim. They are located eccentrically in the metaphysis, adjacent to the physis. As the patient ages, they seem to migrate away from the physis, they are generally asymptomatic and do not require any treatment or biopsy. They are usually found incidentally.

Ans: (a) Chondromyxoid fibroma

Ref: *Fundamentals of Orthopedics by Mohindra and Jain, 2nd edition, Jaypee Publishers, Page 321 and Fig. 11.24*

7. **A patient presents with swelling in right sole (Figure). Probable diagnosis:**

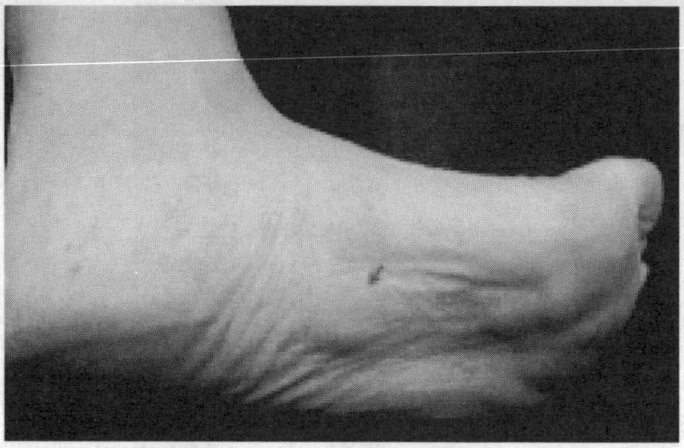

(a) Ganglion
(b) Dupuytren's contracture
(c) Fibromatosis
(d) Rheumatoid nodule

Explanation:

- The above picture shows a plantar nodule in the concavity of the arch of the foot.
- This rules out Ganglion, Rheumatoid nodule and Dupuytren's disease which are associated with hand.
- Plantar fascial fibromatosis or Ledderhose disease is similar to dupuytren's disease in the hand.
- Both are fibrosing diseases causing fibrosing contracture of the plantar aponeurosis (as in Ledderhose) leading to formation of nodules, which are painless.
- After a period of time, this hinders with gait as it is situated most commonly at the height of arch of foot.
- Needs excision before tendon shortening occurs.

Ans: (c) Fibromatosis

***Ref:** Apley's Orthopedics, 10th edition*

PEDIATRICS

1. **In children with classical galactosemia all are true *except*:**

(a) E. coli neonatal sepsis is common
(b) Elimination of galactose in diet will not reverse cataract
(c) Galactose converts to galactitol which is toxic to brain and liver
(d) Duarte variant of galactosemia were asymptomatic

Explanation:

Galactosemia

- Inborn error of galactose metabolism caused by a deficiency of the enzyme:
  - **Galactose-1-phosphate uridyl transferase (GLAT)**
  - **Galactokinase**
  - **Uridine Diphosphate Galactose-4-Epimerase**
- Results in ***accumulation – galactitol and galactose-1-phosphate (toxic to brain and liver)***

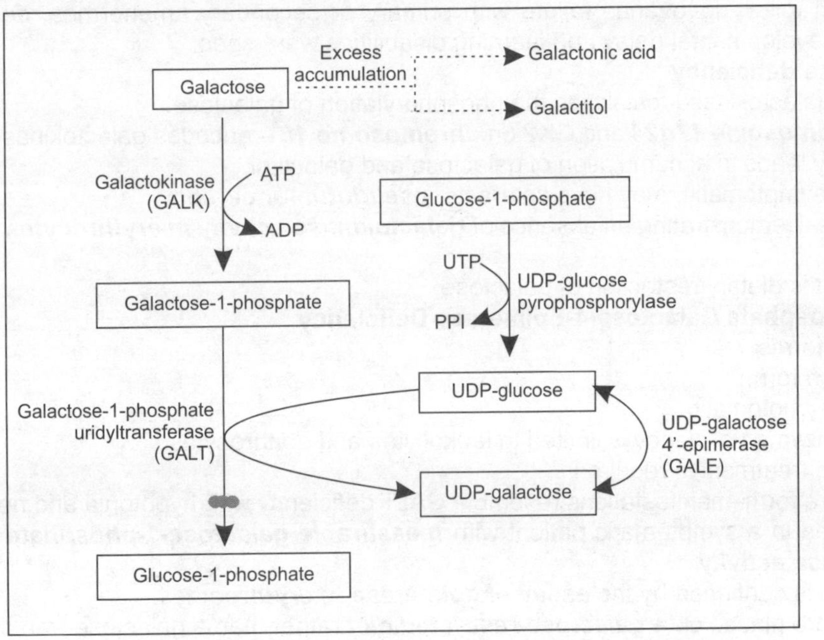

A. **Galactose-1-Phosphate Uridyl Transferase Deficiency:**
Two forms of the deficiency: Complete GALT deficiency (**classic Galactosemia)** and partial GALT deficiency. ***Duarte variant*** – Diminished red cell (GALT) enzyme activity with no clinical significance.

Complete GALT deficiency – Classic Galactosemia

- Autosomal recessive disorder with incidence of ***1/60,000***.
- Onset of symptoms – by the 2nd half of the ***1st week of life***.
- Infant is unable to metabolize galactose-1-phosphate (accumulates in kidney, liver and brain).
- ***Prenatal injury*** – by transplacental galactose derived from the diet of the heterozygous mother or by endogenous production of galactose by the fetus.

Clinical Features

- ***Jaundice***, ***hepatomegaly***, vomiting, hypoglycemia, convulsions, lethargy, irritability, feeding difficulties.
- Poor weight gain or ***failure to regain birth weight***, aminoaciduria, nuclear cataracts, vitreous hemorrhage.

- Hepatic failure, liver cirrhosis, ascites, splenomegaly, or mental retardation and risk for ***Escherichia coli neonatal sepsis***.

Symptoms improve when ***milk is temporarily withdrawn and replaced by lactose-free nutrition.***

Partial GALT deficiency – asymptomatic

- More frequent than classic galactosemia.
- Light and electron microscopy of hepatic tissue–fatty infiltration, the formation of pseudoacini, and eventual macronodular cirrhosis.

Diagnosis

- Demonstrating–***reducing substance*** in urine (collected while the child is receiving lactose containing feeds) or chromatography or enzymatic test specific for galactose.
- ***Enzyme assay*** using erythrocytes (Deficient activity of galactose-1-phosphate uridyl transferase is demonstrable in hemolysates of erythrocytes) ***establishes the diagnosis***.

Blood transfusion before the collection of the blood sample may alter the test result.
Carrier testing and prenatal diagnosis–direct ***enzyme analysis*** of amniocytes or chorionic villi.

Treatment and Prognosis

- Milk substitutes–casein hydrolysates, soybean-based formula, dextrine maltose (if erythrocyte galactose-1-phosphate concentration is ***>10 mg/dL*** and erythrocyte GALT enzyme activity ***is ≤10% of control activity***).
- Elimination of galactose from the diet - ***reverses*** Cataracts, growth failure and renal and hepatic dysfunction.
- Long-term follow-up–ovarian failure with primary or secondary amenorrhea, decreased bone mineral density, developmental delay and learning disabilities were seen.

B. Galactokinase deficiency

- Enzyme galactokinase–catalyzes the phosphorylation of galactose.
- GK1 ***chromosome 17q24*** and GK2 on ***chromosome 15*** – encodes galactokinase.
- Deficiency leads to accumulation of galactose and galactitol.
- Usually asymptomatic, may have cataracts, ***pseudotumor cerebri.***
- Diagnosis–Demonstrating an absence of ***galactokinase activity in erythrocytes*** (While GALT activity is normal).
- Treatment is dietary restriction of galactose.

C. Uridine Diphosphate Galactose-4-Epimerase Deficiency

- 2 distinct forms
  - o Benign form:
    - Asymptomatic
    - Enzyme deficiency is limited to leukocytes and erythrocytes.
    - No treatment is required.
  - o Severe form–manifestations resemble GALT deficiency with hypotonia and nerve deafness.
- Considered in a symptomatic patient with ***measurable galactose-1-phosphate but who has normal transferase activity.***
- Diagnosis is confirmed by the ***assay of epimerase in erythrocytes***.
- Children are placed on a ***galactose-restricted diet*** rather than a galactose-free diet.

Ans: (b) Elimination of galactose in diet will not reverse cataract

Ref: *Nelson Textbook of Pediatrics, 20th edition, Page 726*

2. A 10-year-old girl present with polyuria and polydipsia with hypokalemia, hypercalciuria and metabolic alkalosis. What is the probable diagnosis?

(a) Gitelmann syndrome
(b) Liddle syndrome
(c) Bartter syndrome
(d) Alport's syndrome

Explanation:

BARTTER SYNDROME (AUTOSOMAL RECESSIVE)

Clinical Subtypes:

Antenatal Bartter syndrome (Hyperprostaglandin E syndrome):

- Mutations–genes that encode the sodium potassium 2 chloride transporter NKCC2 (the site of action of furosemide) **or**

- The luminal potassium channel ROMK – cause neonatal Bartter syndrome.
- Present with polyhydramnios, salt wasting and severe dehydration.

Classic Bartter syndrome:

- Defects–genes that produce the basolateral chloride channel ClC-Kb
- Presents milder in childhood with failure to thrive and a history of recurrent episodes of dehydration.

Pathogenesis

- Defect in sodium, chloride and potassium transport in the ascending loop of Henle
- ***Hypokalemic metabolic alkalosis with hypercalciuria*** (similar to chronic loop diuretic use)
- The loss of sodium and chloride, with resultant volume contraction, stimulates the renin/angiotensin II/aldosterone axis.
- Aldosterone promotes sodium uptake and potassium secretion, exacerbating the hypokalemia.
- It also stimulates hydrogen ion secretion distally, worsening the ***metabolic alkalosis.*** Hypokalemia stimulates prostaglandins, which further activate the renin/angiotensin II/aldosterone axis.

Clinical Manifestations

In Smaller Children

- Consanguinity with history of polyhydramnios.
- Triangular facies, protruding ears, large eyes with strabismus and drooping mouth.

In Older Children

- History of recurrent episodes of dehydration, failure to thrive, Hypokalemic metabolic alkalosis, Urinary calcium, potassium and sodium levels – elevated
- ***Serum renin, aldosterone and prostaglandin E levels – elevated*** (antenatal form)
- Blood pressure is usually normal, except in antenatal form – have severe salt wasting
- Renal function is typically normal, Ultrasound shows Nephrocalcinosis, due to hypercalciuria.

Diagnosis – Based clinical presentation + laboratory findings.

(Severe hypokalemia, usually <2.5 mmol/L, with metabolic alkalosis. Hypercalciuria is typical)

Differential Diagnosis:

1. Diuretic abuse.
2. Chronic vomiting – **Measurement** of **urinary chloride** (elevated – Bartter syndrome and low in patients – chronic vomiting).

Treatment and Prognosis

- Prevent dehydration and maintaining nutritional status.
- Correcting hypokalemia (at very high doses)
- Sodium supplementation – Infants and young children.
- Indomethacin, a prostaglandin inhibitor, may also be effective.
- Long-term prognosis is generally good.
- Chronic hypokalemia, nephrocalcinosis and chronic indomethacin therapy can lead to chronic interstitial nephritis and chronic renal failure.

GITELMAN SYNDROME (AUTOSOMAL RECESSIVE)

- Causes hypokalemic metabolic alkalosis, ***hypocalciuria*** and hypomagnesemia.

Pathogenesis

- Defects – in sodium chloride co-transporter NCCT, present in the distal convoluted tubule (resembles chronic thiazide diuretic use).

Clinical Manifestations

- Present late in childhood with history of recurrent muscle cramps and spasms due to **hypomagnesemia.**
- ***No history of recurrent episodes of dehydration***.

- Biochemical abnormalities include hypokalemia, metabolic alkalosis and hypomagnesemia.
- The ***urinary calcium level is usually very low and urinary magnesium level is elevated.***
- Prostaglandin E secretion, Renin and aldosterone levels – normal.

Diagnosis - Adolescent - with hypokalemic metabolic alkalosis, hypomagnesemia and hypocalciuria.
Treatment - Correcting hypokalemia and hypomagnesemia.

Liddle Syndrome:

- In collecting duct – gain of function mutations of the gene coding (epithelial sodium channel)
- Causes an inherited form of hypertension **with** hypokalemia and suppressed aldosterone
- Loss of function mutations – pseudo hypoaldosteronism (severe sodium wasting and hyperkalemia).

X (RECESSIVE)**-linked nephrolithiasis (Dent disease)**

- Mutations in the gene - voltage-gated chloride channel CLN5 (present throughout the nephron)
- Characterized by recurrent stone formation and progression to Fanconi syndrome.
- In loop of Henle - activating (severe hypoparathyroidism) and inactivating mutations (hyperparathyroidism) in the calcium receptor gene (which mediates parathyroid hormone–induced calcium uptake).

ALPORT SYNDROME (AS) – (HEREDITARY NEPHRITIS)

- X-linked disease (85%) – Mutations in the genes coding for type IV collagen (*COL4A5* gene - major component of basement membranes).
- Autosomal recessive - mutations in the *COL4A3* and *COL4A4* genes on chromosome 2
- Autosomal dominant form also occurs.

Clinical Manifestations

Renal manifestations:

- ***Asymptomatic intermittent microscopic hematuria***.
- Recurrent episodes of gross hematuria occurring 1–2 days after an upper respiratory infection
- ***Proteinuria*** - frequently seen in males but may be absent in females.
- Progressive proteinuria can be severe enough to cause ***nephrotic syndrome***.

Extra renal manifestations:

- Bilateral sensorineural hearing loss (***never congenital***)
- Ocular abnormalities - anterior lenticonus (***pathognomonic***), macular flecks and corneal erosions.
- Rarely - Leiomyomatosis of the esophagus, tracheobronchial tree, and female genitals and platelet abnormalities.

Diagnosis

- A careful family history **+** a screening urinalysis of first-degree relatives + an audiogram + ophthalmologic examination.
- Likely in the patient with hematuria and at least two of the following
- Macular flecks, recurrent corneal erosions, GBM thickening and thinning, and sensorineural deafness.
- Absence of epidermal basement membrane staining for the α5 chain of type IV collagen in male hemizygotes and discontinuous epidermal basement membrane staining in female heterozygotes is pathognomonic for X-linked AS.

Treatment:

- Progressive renal dysfunction leading to end-stage renal disease.
- ***Risk factors for progression*** – gross hematuria during childhood, nephrotic syndrome and prominent GBM thickening.

Table for Different Electrolyte Imbalance:

- Combination of metabolic alkalosis, hypokalemia (high urinary losses of potassium and chloride, despite a state of relative volume depletion with secondary hyperaldosteronism), a high urine chloride level, and normal blood pressure is characteristic of **Bartter syndrome, Gitelman syndrome and current diuretic use.**
- **Bartter syndrome** is usually associated with **hypercalciuria**, and often with **nephrocalcinosis**.
- Children with **Gitelman syndrome** have **low urinary calcium** losses but **hypomagnesemia** as a consequence of urinary magnesium losses.

Ans: (c) Bartter syndrome

Ref: *Nelson Textbook of Pediatrics, 20th edition, Page 2534*

3. **Which of the following is not true in assessing skin fold thickness?**
   (a) Measured at the triceps level
   (b) Measured to the nearest of 1 cm
   (c) Tanner's chart contains the normal values
   (d) Indirectly indicates the caloric reserve of the body

Explanation:
- Skin fold thickness - indicator of availability of caloric stores in the form of subcutaneous fat.
- Sites of measurement - triceps and sub scapular region
- Measured using Harpenden and Best type calipers to the nearest of 0.1 cm
- Its normal value is present in Tanners' chart (for both triceps and sub scapular area) and measurements below 90% of the standard are considered subnormal.

Ans: (b) Measured to the nearest of 1 cm

Ref: *Nutrition and Child Development, KE Elizabeth, 4th edition, Page 170*

4. **All are true about anthropometric measurements *except*:**
   (a) Birth weight triples by 1 year
   (b) Skinfold thickness is measured in sub scapular region
   (c) Weight is measured to the nearest 100 gram
   (d) Standing height is about 1.7 cm less than recumbent length

Explanation:

Weight: It is recommended to weigh children using a scale with the following features:
- Solidly built and durable
- Electronic (digital reading)
- Measures up to 150 kg
- Measures to a precision of 0.1 kg (100 g)
- Allows tared weighing

"Tared weighing" means that the scale can be re-set to zero ("tared") with the person just weighed still on it. Thus, a mother can stand on the scale, be weighed, and the scale tared. While remaining on the scale, if she is given her child to hold, the child's weight alone appears on the scale.

Tared weighing has two clear advantages:
- There is no need to subtract weights to determine the child's weight alone (reducing the risk of error).
- The child is likely to remain calm when held in the mother's arms for weighing.
  - Bathroom scales are not recommended as they tend to be unreliable.
  - Hanging scales are also not reliable when weighing agitated babies.
  - Precision describes the smallest exact unit that the scale can measure.

Points to Remember:
- Birth weight of Indian children 2.8 Kg
- Term neonate regains lost birth weight by 7 to 10 days, preterm by 10 to 14 days

Birth weight double by 6 months, triples by 1 year, quadruples by 2 years and increases 5 times by 3 years.

Age in months	Rate of weight gain (gm/day)
10 days to 3 months	25 - 30
4 to 6 months	20
7 to 9 months	15
10 to 12 months	12

Formula for calculating expected weight:

- ***Infants of age 3 to 12 months*** ***weight (Kg) = (Age in months + 9)/ 2***
- ***For 1 to 6 years*** ***weight (Kg) = (Age in years × 2) + 8***
- ***For 7 to 12 years*** ***weight (Kg) = [(Age in years) × 7 - 5] / 2 or Age in years × 3***

Length:

- If a child is less than 2 years old, measure recumbent length.
- If the child is aged 2 years or older and able to stand, measure standing height.
- In general, standing height is about 0.7 cm less than recumbent length.
- If a child less than 2 years old will not lie down for measurement of length, measure standing height and add 0.7 cm to convert it to length.
- If a child aged 2 years or older cannot stand, measure recumbent length and subtract 0.7 cm to convert it to height.
- Equipment needed to measure length is a length board (sometimes called an infantometer) which should be placed on a flat, stable surface such as a table.
- To measure height, use a height board (sometimes called a stadiometer) mounted at a right angle between a level floor and against a straight, vertical surface such as a wall or pillar.

Child should directly look forwards (in stadiometer) or child should be looking straight up (in infantometer) so that the head is positioned in line with ***FRANKFURT PLANE*** (the line joining the floor of external auditory meatus to the lower margin of orbit)

Expected height between 2 and 12 years in cm (***Weech formula***) = *(Age in years × 6) + 77*

Mid-Parental Target Height

- In girl (cm) = (mother's height in cm + father's height in cm - 13) / 2
- In boy (cm) = (mother's height in cm + father's height in cm + 13) / 2

Expected adult height (cm) = Mid-Parental target height ± 8

Ans: (d) Standing height is about 1.7 cm less than recumbent length

Ref: *Pediatrics for Medical Graduates, Arun Babu T, 1st edition, Page 3*

5. **True regarding congenital rubella (CRS) syndrome are all *except*:**

(a) Infants of congenital rubella syndrome can shed virus in respiratory secretions upto 1 year of age
(b) Risk of developing diabetes mellitus is considerably higher in congenital rubella syndrome
(c) Cataract in CRS is always bilateral
(d) Risk of congenital defects is high when fetus is infected during the first trimester

Explanation:

CONGENITAL RUBELLA SYNDROME (CRS)

RNA virus (the toga virus family)

Maternal Infection (in gestation)	Rate of fetal infection	Occurrence of fetal anomalies
First 12 weeks of gestation	81%	100% of the infected fetuses had cardiac defects and deafness
In 13 to 16 weeks	54%	Deafness was found in one-third of fetuses
In 31 to 36 weeks	60%	No abnormalities were found when fetal infection occurred beyond the 20th week of gestation
Beyond 36 weeks	100%	

Clinical Features:

- Cataracts (can be ***both unilateral or bilateral***), ***sensory neural hearing loss (single most common finding among the CRS infants)***, and congenital heart disease (***patent ductus arteriosus and pulmonary artery stenosis***).

- Common early features – IUGR, retinopathy (salt and pepper retinopathy), microphthalmia, meningo-encephalitis, hypotonia, electroencephalographic abnormalities, dermatoglyphic abnormalities, hepatosplenomegaly, thrombocytopenic purpura, ***radiographic bone lucencies***, and ***diabetes mellitus***.
- Rare complications – myocarditis, ***glaucoma***, microcephaly, chronic progressive panencephalitis, hepatitis, anemia, hypogammaglobulinemia, ***thymic hypoplasia***, thyroid abnormalities, cryptorchidism and polycystic kidney disease.

Antenatal Diagnosis:

1. Determination of specific IgM in fetal blood obtained by PUBS.
2. Direct detection of rubella antigen and RNA in a chorionic villus biopsy specimen.

Postnatal Diagnosis: The diagnosis of congenital infection is made by one of the following:

i. **Isolation of rubella virus** (oropharynx, urine).
ii. **Detection of rubella-specific** IgM in cord or neonatal blood.
iii. **Persistent rubella-specific titers over time** (i.e., no decline in titer as expected for transplacentally derived maternal IgG).

If, in addition, there are congenital defects, the diagnosis of CRS is made.

Treatment:

- ***No*** specific therapy for either maternal or congenital rubella infection.
- Maternal disease is almost always mild and self-limiting.
  1. Primary maternal infection occurs during the first 5 months of pregnancy-termination options should be discussed with the mother.
  2. Infection is known to have occurred beyond the 20th week of gestation, its unlikely to develop anomalies
- Individuals with ***postnatal infection typically shed virus for 1 week before and 1 week after the onset of rash***.
- Infants with ***congenital infection may shed virus for many months***, and contact should be avoided during the first year.
- Conception also should be avoided for 3 months following immunization.
- Immunization during pregnancy is not recommended because of the theoretical risk to the fetus. Inadvertent immunizations during pregnancy have occurred – reassurance of little risk to the fetus can be given.

Maternal Infection:

- **Symptoms -** begin 2 to 3 weeks after exposure and include malaise, low-grade fever, headache, mild coryza, ***posterior cervical lymphadenopathy, arthralgias and conjunctivitis***.
- Occurring 1 to 5 days before the onset of rash (salmon-pink macular or maculopapular ***exanthem that begins on the face and behind the ears and spreads downward*** over 1 to 2 days and disappears in 5 to 7 days from onset).
- **Confirmation** - demonstrating a fourfold or higher rise in serum IgG titers when measured at the time of symptoms and approximately 2 weeks later.
  - o If a woman exposed to rubella is known to be seropositive, she is immune, and the fetus is considered not to be at risk for infection.
  - o If the exposed woman is known to be seronegative, a serum sample should be obtained 3 to 4 weeks after exposure for determination of titer.
  - o A negative titer indicates that no infection has occurred, whereas a positive titer indicates infection.

Ans: (c) Cataract in CRS is always bilateral

Ref: *Manual of Neonatal Care, John P. Cloherty, 7th edition, Page 619*

6. **A child with pigment dilution of skin and eyes, hemorrhagic diathesis, ceroid depositions within the reticuloendothelial system has:**

(a) Bloom syndrome
(b) Hermansky Pudlak syndrome
(c) Alezzandrini syndrome
(d) Vogt-Koyanogi syndrome

Explanation:

SYNDROMES ASSOCIATED WITH ALBINISM / VITILIGO

- **Cross-McKusick-Breen syndrome**
  - Tyrosinase-positive albinism with ocular abnormalities
  - Mental retardation
  - Spasticity
  - ***Athetosis***
- **Hermansky-Pudlak syndrome**
  - ***Autosomal recessive***
  - Oculocutaneous albinism
  - ***Ceroid accumulation in lysosomes***
  - ***Prolonged bleeding***
- **Chédiak-Higashi syndrome**
  - ***Hypopigmentation*** of the skin, eye, and hair
  - ***Prolonged bleeding times*** and easy bruising
  - Recurrent infections
  - Abnormal natural killer cell function
  - ***Peripheral neuropathy***.
- **Waardenburg syndrome**
  - Localized areas of depigmented skin and hair.
  - **Type 1** - ***white forelock***, deafness, ***heterochromia iridis***, unibrow (synophrys) and ***dystopia canthorum*** (lateral displacement of the inner canthi of the eyes, giving an appearance of a widened nasal bridge)
  - **Type 2** (similar to type 1) ***except lack dystopia canthorum***
  - **Type 3 / Klein-Waardenburg syndrome** (similar to type 1) with some ***limb abnormalities***.
  - **Type 4** (**Shah-Waardenburg syndrome**). ***Hirschsprung disease and dystopia canthorum is rare***.
- **Vogt-Koyanogi-Harada syndrome**
  - Vitiligo
  - Uveitis
  - ***Dysacusia***
  - ***Meningoencephalitis***
  - Depigmentation of the skin, scalp hair, eyebrows and eyelashes.
- **Alezzandrini syndrome** – Vitiligo with ***tapetoretinal degeneration and deafness***.

SYNDROMES ASSOCIATED WITH PHOTOSENSITIVITY

- **Cockayne Syndrome**
  - ***Facial erythema*** in a butterfly distribution, loss of adipose tissue and atrophic, hyperpigmented skin over the face.
  - Associated with dwarfism; ***large, protuberant ears; long limbs; large hands and feet (cool and cyanotic***); unsteady gait with tremor; limitation of joint mobility; deafness; cataracts; retinal degeneration; and premature graying of the hair.
  - Die of atheromatous vascular disease before the 3rd decade.
- **Rothmund – Thomson Syndrome: Also known as *Poikiloderma congenitale***
  - Plaques of erythema and edema appear on the cheeks, forehead, and are replaced gradually by reticulated, atrophic, hyperpigmented, telangiectatic plaques.
  - Light sensitivity is present, short stature; small hands and feet; sparse eyebrows, eyelashes, and pubic and axillary hair, and sparse, fine, prematurely gray scalp hair or alopecia; bony defects; and hypogenitalism are common.
- **Bloom syndrome**
  - Erythema and telangiectasia in a butterfly distribution on the face after exposure to sunlight.
  - ***Bullous eruption on the lips and telangiectatic erythema on the hands and forearms*** may develop.
  - ***Café-au-lait spots***, short stature and facies (prominent nose and ears).
  - ***Immunodeficiency*** in all patients (recurrent ear and pulmonary infections).
  - Tendency to develop both ***solid tumors and lymphoreticular malignancies***.

Ans: (b) Hermansky Pudlak syndrome

Ref: *Nelson, Textbook of Pediatrics, 20th edition, Page 3138*

7. **A 14-year-old boy was brought in a collapsed state with history of 2 episodes of vomiting and had feeble pulse and cold, clammy limbs. ECG is given (Figure). What is the diagnosis?**

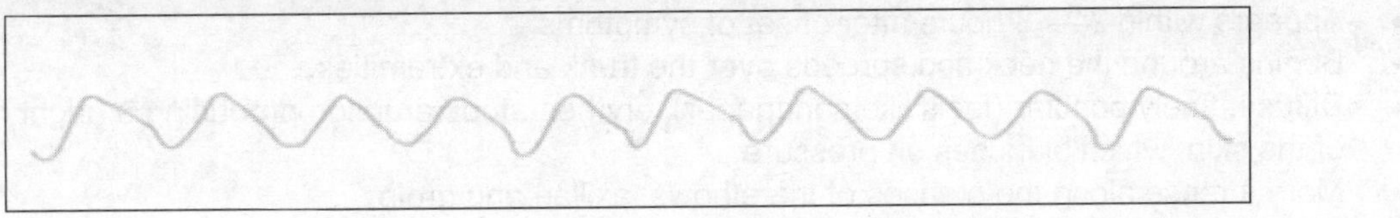

(a) Hypokalemia
(b) Hyperkalemia
(c) Hypocalcemia
(d) Hypomagnesemia

Explanation:

- ECG shows classical **'sine wave pattern'** associated with **hyperkalemia.**

Electrolyte abnormality	**ECG findings**
Hypokalemia (< 2.5 meq/L)	Prolonged PR interval Reduction in T wave amplitude / flattening / inversion ST depression Appearance of U wave
Hyperkalemia	
Mild (5.5 to 6.6 meq/L)	Peaked T waves Prolonged PR segment
Moderate (6.5 to 8 meq/L)	Loss of P wave Prolonged QRS complex ST segment elevation Ectopic beast and escape rhythm
Severe (> 8.0 meq/L)	Progressive widening of QRS complex ***Sine wave*** Ventricular fibrillation Asystole
Hypocalcemia	Prolonged QTc segment (secondary to lengthening of ST segment)
Hypomagnesemia	ST segment depression Tall, peaked T waves Flat T waves or depression in the precordium U waves Loss of voltage PR prolongation Widened QRS complex

Ans: (b) Hyperkalemia

Ref: *Nelson Textbook of Pediatrics, 20th edition, Page 360*

8. **Symptoms suggestive of Scarlet fever are all *except*:**

(a) Gooseflesh like rash
(b) Nagayama spots
(c) Desquamation of palms
(d) Strawberry tongue

Explanation:

SCARLET FEVER

Upper respiratory tract infection + characteristic rash, which is caused:

- **Pyrogenic exotoxin (erythrogenic toxin -** A, B and C**)** – producing Group A streptococcus (GAS) in individuals who do not have antitoxin antibodies.

- **Erythrogenic toxin –** A strongly associated with scarlet fever and confers specific immunity only to that toxin

Scarlet Fever can occur up to three times.

Characteristics of Rash:

- Appears within 24–48 hours after onset of symptoms.
- Begins around the neck and spreads over the trunk and extremities.
- Diffuse, finely popular (feels like sandpaper), erythematous eruption producing a bright red discoloration of the skin, which blanches on pressure.
- More intense along the creases of the elbows, axillae and groin.
- Skin has a ***goose-pimple appearance*** and feels rough.
- Cheeks may be erythematous with pallor around the mouth.
- After 3–4 days:
    - The rash begins to fade and is followed by desquamation.
    - 1st on the face, progressing downward, and often resembling that seen subsequent to mild sunburn.
    - ***Sheet like desquamation may occur around the free margins of the fingernails, the palms and the soles***.
- Staphylococcal infections are occasionally associated with a scarlatiniform rash.

Examination of the Pharynx

- The tongue is usually coated and the papillae are swollen
- After desquamation - the reddened papillae are prominent, giving the tongue a strawberry appearance
- A history of recent exposure to a GAS infection or identification of GAS in the pharynx helps in diagnosis.
- Rapid clinical response to penicillin therapy–differentiates Scarlet fever from Kawasaki disease in a child who is a group A streptococcal carrier
    - **Nagayama Spots -** In Asian countries, ulcers at the uvulopalatoglossal junction (**Nagayama spots**) are common in infants with roseola caused by Human Herpesviruses 6 and 7
    - **Filatov-Dukes disease** (an atypical Scarlet fever)

Ans: (b) Nagayama spots

Ref: *Nelson Textbook of Pediatrics, 20th edition, Page 1328*

9. Which statement regarding Measles is false?

(a) Koplik's spots cannot be seen in conjunctival or vaginal mucosa
(b) Vitamin A administration is part of management of clinical measles
(c) CD150 and PVRL4 are receptors for measles virus
(d) Pneumonia is the common cause of death in children with measles

Explanation:

MEASLES (RUBEOLA)

- High fever, an enanthem, cough, coryza, conjunctivitis and a prominent exanthema
- Caused by single-stranded lipid enveloped RNA virus of the genus Morbillivirus in the family Paramyxoviridae.
- ***Only one serotype*** is known.
- 6 major structural proteins - hemagglutinin (H) protein and the fusion (F) protein (important in inducing immunity)
- Portal of entry - ***respiratory tract or conjunctivae*** in contact with virus suspended droplets
- Virus is shed in nasopharyngeal secretions, blood and urine - 3 days before the rash up to 4–6 days after its onset
- ***Face-to-face contact is not necessary*** - viable virus may be suspended in air up to 1 hour after a source case leaves a room.
- Viruses remain viable for 34 hours at room temperature.
- Mechanism of infection - attachment to ***the PVRL4 receptor (Nectin4)*** that is expressed on cells in the trachea, oral mucosa, nasopharynx and lungs.
- ***CD150 and PVRL4***, account for the lymphotropic and epitheliotropic nature of natural measles virus infection.

Pathology:

- Necrosis of the respiratory tract epithelium and an accompanying lymphocytic infiltrate.
- Small vessel vasculitis - skin and on the oral mucous membranes.
- Histology of the rash and exanthem - intracellular edema and dyskeratosis associated with formation of epidermal syncytial giant cells with up to 26 nuclei.
- Lymphoid hyperplasia is prominent.
- Fusion of infected cells results in multinucleated giant cells, the ***Warthin-Finkeldey giant cells that are pathognomonic (up to 100 nuclei).***

Clinical Features: Incubation period – 8 to 12 days.

4 phases:

- ***Incubation period:*** virus migrates to regional lymph nodes
  - Primary viremia - disseminates the virus to the reticuloendothelial system
  - Secondary viremia - spreads virus to body surfaces
- ***Prodromal illness:***
  - Begins with a mild fever followed by the onset of conjunctivitis with photophobia, coryza, a prominent cough and increasing fever
  - Features increase in intensity for 2–4 days until the 1st day of the rash
- ***Exanthematous phase:***
  - Enanthem, **Koplik spots (bluish white spots on the** inner aspects of the cheeks at the level of the premolars**) also in the** lips, hard palate, gingiva, conjunctival folds and in the vaginal mucosa
  - Is the ***pathognomonic sign of measles and appears 1 to 4 days prior to the onset of the rash***
  - Rash begins around the forehead (around the hairline), behind the ears, and on the upper neck as a red maculopapular eruption
  - Then spreads downward to the torso and extremities, reaching the palms and soles
  - Becomes confluent on the face and upper trunk
  - With the onset of the rash, symptoms begin to subside and the rash fades over about 7 days in the same progression as it evolved, often leaving a fine desquamation of skin in its wake
  - Virus shedding begins with onset of the rash
- ***Recovery:***
  - Cough lasts the longest, often up to 10 days
  - Generalized lymphadenopathy may be present, with cervical and occipital lymph nodes especially prominent.

Inapparent Measles Infection:

- Rash may be indistinct, brief, or, rarely absent
- Individuals with passively acquired antibody
  - Infants, recipients of blood products, received vaccine
  - They do not shed measles virus and do not transmit infection to household contacts.
- Recipient of formalin-inactivated measles vaccine - develop (**atypical measles** - severe form)
- Caused by the development of circulating immune complexes that formed due to an abnormal immune response to the vaccine
- Onset of high fever, headache, maculopapular rash (petechial or purpuric) complicated by pneumonia and pleural effusions.

Hemorrhagic or "Black Measles"

- Hemorrhagic skin eruption and was often fatal.
- Keratitis and Thrombocytopenia are seen.

Diagnosis by Clinical and Epidemiologic Findings:

- Lab findings - Leukopenia, Absolute neutropenia, normal erythrocyte sedimentation rate and C-reactive protein levels (in uncomplicated cases)
- Serologically - immunoglobulin M (IgM) antibody in serum. IgM (Appears 1–2 days after the onset of the rash and remains detectable for about 1 month).

- By demonstration of a 4-fold rise in IgG antibodies in acute and convalescent specimens taken 2–4 week later.
- Viral isolation from blood, urine, or respiratory secretions can be accomplished by culture.

Complications:

- Due to pathogenic effects of the virus on the respiratory tract and immune system
- Factors that make complications more likely.
    - Crowding – attributable to a larger inoculum dose following household exposure
    - Severe malnutrition – suboptimal immune response
    - Low serum retinol levels
    - Common cause of death – Pneumonia
- **Respiratory Complication:**
    - Otitis media, pneumonia/Interstitial pneumonia - by the measles virus (***giant cell pneumonia***), superimposed bacterial infection (**S. pneumoniae, H. influenzae and S. aureus**), laryngitis, tracheitis and bronchitis.
    - May exacerbate underlying Mycobacterium tuberculosis infection.
    - Temporary loss of hypersensitivity reaction to tuberculin skin testing
- Gastrointestinal complications: Diarrhea, vomiting and Appendicitis
- Nervous system complication:
    - Febrile seizures
    - Encephalitis: Greater numbers occurring in adolescents with unfavorable outcome
    - Postinfectious immunologically mediated process rather than due to a direct effect by the virus
    - Begins during the exanthem and presents with seizures, lethargy, coma and irritability.
    - In cerebrospinal fluid - lymphocytic pleocytosis and elevated protein concentration
    - Majority suffer from long-term sequelae like mental retardation, motor disabilities and deafness.
- Other complications: Myocarditis, cellulitis and toxic shock syndrome, fetal wastage and stillbirths, and congenital malformations.

Vitamin A in Measles:

- Hyporetinemia is present in more than 90% of cases of measles
- There is an apparent inverse correlation between retinol concentration and measles severity.
- Treatment with oral vitamin A reduces morbidity and mortality in children with severe measles in the developing world.

Recommended regimen is 2 doses, 24 hours apart

1. 100,000 IU orally for children 6 months to 1 year, and
2. 200,000 IU for children 1 year of age or older.

Subacute Sclerosing Panencephalitis (SSPE)

- Fatal, delayed onset, neuro degenerative and chronic complication of measles (slow virus infection).
- Higher prevalence among children of Hispanic origin.
- Persistent infection with an altered measles virus that is harbored intracellularly in the CNS for several years.
- After 10 years the virus apparently regains virulence and attacks the cells in the CNS that offered the virus protection.

Pathogenesis:

- Defective measles virus (missing 1 of the 6 structural proteins, M protein - responsible for assembly, orientation, replication and alignment of the virus) and
- Its interaction with a defective or immature immune system.

Clinical Features: After 10 years of primary infection.

- 1st stage - Subtle changes (behavior or school performance, irritability, reduced attention span, or temper outbursts).
    a. Fever, headache, or other signs of encephalitis are absent.
- 2nd stage - Massive myoclonus (hallmark) begin in single muscle groups then massive spasms both axial and appendicular muscles
    a. Consciousness is maintained.

- 3rd stage - Involuntary movements are replaced by choreoathetosis, immobility, dystonia and lead pipe rigidity.
    a. Sensorium deteriorates into dementia, stupor, then coma.
- 4th stage - Loss of critical centers that support breathing, heart rate and blood pressure. Death soon ensues.

Diagnosis

- Documentation of a compatible clinical course and at least 1 of the following supporting findings:
    - Measles antibody detected in CSF (elevated IgG and IgM antibody titers in dilutions of >1:8).
    - Characteristic electroencephalographic findings (suppression-burst episodes), or
    - Typical histologic findings and/or isolation of virus or viral antigen in brain tissue obtained by biopsy or postmortem examination.

Management - Primarily Supportive

- Oral **inosiplex** and intraventricular interferon-α2b has been used with some benefit.
- Die within 1–3 years of onset from infection or loss of autonomic control mechanisms.
- Prevention of SSPE - prevention of primary measles infection through the use of vaccine.

Ans: (a) Koplik's spots cannot be seen in conjunctival or vaginal mucosa

Ref: *Nelson Textbook of Pediatrics, 20th edition, Page 1542*

10. True regarding CMV in children:

(a) Ganciclovir resistance is due to mutation in UL97 gene, DNA polymerase
(b) CMV is not detected in the breast milk of mother with CMV infection
(c) Ganciclovir is indicated in CMV infection in Immunocompetent children
(d) Ganciclovir resistant CMV strains do not show cross resistance to Foscarnet.

Explanation:

CYTOMEGALO VIRUS (CMV)

- Most common cause of congenital infection
- Double-stranded DNA - largest of the herpesviruses.
    a. **Primary infection** - in a seronegative, susceptible host.
    b. **Recurrent infection** - reactivation of latent infection or reinfection of a seropositive immune host (more severe than primary infection)
- Risk for fetal infection is greatest with maternal primary CMV infection (30%) and much less likely with recurrent infection (<1%).
- Transmission - saliva, breast milk, cervical and vaginal secretions, urine, semen, stools, blood and tissue or organ transplants.
- Important perinatal sources of virus - ***genital tract secretions at delivery and breast milk.***
- In CMV seropositive mothers - virus is detectable in breast milk (96%) and ***postnatal transmission in*** **38**% of infants.
- **Infected infants *excrete virus for years in saliva and urine.***
    - **Childcare centers** contributing to rapid spread of CMV among children.
    - 2nd peak occurs in adolescence as a result of sexual transmission.

Pathogenesis:

- Depressed cellular immunity, uncontrolled viral replication , multiorgan involvement, and end-organ disease secondary to direct viral cytopathic effects.
- CMV infects placental ***cytotrophoblasts*** and can be transmitted to the fetus.
- Infected cells - large intranuclear and smaller ***intracytoplasmic inclusions (pathognomonic).***

Clinical Manifestations

- Infants and young children - primary infection causes pneumonitis, hepatomegaly, hepatitis and petechial rashes.

- Older children, adolescents–mononucleosis-like syndrome characterized by fatigue, malaise, myalgia, headache, fever, hepatosplenomegaly, elevated liver enzymes, and atypical lymphocytosis, lasting 2–3 weeks.

Immunocompromised Persons

- Primary infection - ***pneumonitis (most common),*** hepatitis, chorioretinitis, gastrointestinal disease, or fever with leukopenia - severe and progressive
- Risk is greatest in ***bone marrow transplant recipients and in patients with AIDS.***

Congenital Infection

- Congenitally infected infants (5% have severe cytomegalic inclusion disease, 5% have mild involvement, and 90% are subclinical, chronic, CMV infection).
- Manifestation - intrauterine growth restriction, ***prematurity, hepatosplenomegaly*** and jaundice, ***blueberry muffin–like rash***, thrombocytopenia and purpura, and microcephaly and intracranial calcifications.
- Other neurologic problems include chorioretinitis, sensorineural hearing loss, and mild increases in cerebrospinal fluid protein.

Perinatal Infection

- Infections - maternal genital tract at delivery or in breast milk (despite the presence of maternally derived antibody).
- Present like pneumonitis and ***sepsis-like syndrome***.
- Premature and ill full-term infants may have neurologic sequelae and psychomotor retardation.
- No increase in risk of hearing loss, chorioretinitis and microcephaly.

Diagnosis

- Active CMV infection is best confirmed by virus isolation from urine, saliva, bronchoalveolar washings, breast milk, cervical secretions, buffy coat, and tissues obtained by biopsy.
- Rapid quantitative detection of CMV antigens, and quantitative polymerase chain reaction (PCR) assays are also available.
- Primary infection is confirmed by seroconversion or the simultaneous detection of immunoglobulin M (IgM) and IgG antibodies with low functional avidity.
- 1st weeks after primary infection, the functional avidity of IgG class antibodies is very low and rises to a peak in 4–5 months.
- IgM antibodies can be demonstrated transiently in both symptomatic and asymptomatic infection at 4–16 weeks, which is during the acute phase of symptomatic disease.

Congenital Infection

- Definitive diagnosis - virus isolation (Urine and saliva are the best specimens for culture) or PCR (performed at or shortly after birth).
- IgG antibody test - little diagnostic value (reflects maternal antibodies).
- IgM tests - lack sensitivity and specificity (***unreliable for diagnosis of congenital CMV infection***).
- Fetal infection can be confirmed by viral isolation / PCR from amniotic fluid (excellent ***sensitivity after the 22nd week of gestation***).

Treatment

- **Not indicated for *immunocompetent persons***, but is ***recommended for immunocompromised persons***, and remains controversial for infants with symptomatic congenital infection.
- **Ganciclovir** combined with immune globulin (IVIG or hyperimmune CMV IVIG) to treat life-threatening CMV infections in immunocompromised hosts.
- CMV retinitis and gastrointestinal disease respond to therapy but ***recur on cessation***.
- Toxicity with ganciclovir - neutropenia, thrombocytopenia, liver dysfunction, reduction in spermatogenesis, and gastrointestinal and renal abnormalities.
- ***Foscarnet*** is an alternative antiviral agent (limited information on its use in children).
- Prophylaxis with ganciclovir or acyclovir reduces the risk for morbidity in solid organ transplantation.
- Oral valganciclovir, the orally bioavailable prodrug of ganciclovir.
- Ganciclovir, cidofovir and foscarnet are the systemic antiviral drugs that are currently licensed for treatment of human cytomegalovirus (CMV) infection:
- All 3 drugs, in their active forms, target the viral ***DNA polymerase (pol) (CMV gene UL54)***

- Resistance to ganciclovir - due to a mutation in the ***viral UL97 phosphotransferase gene***.
- DNA polymerase mutant isolates ***are cross-resistant to ganciclovir, foscarnet and cidofovir.***

Prevention:

- The use of CMV free blood products, especially for premature newborns.
- The use of organs from CMV free donors for transplantation.
- Pregnant women who are CMV seropositive are at low risk for delivering a symptomatic newborn.
- Pregnant women who are CMV seronegative should be counseled regarding ***good handwashing*** and other hygienic measures and avoidance of contact with oral secretions of others.
- Pregnant women with primary CMV who receive CMV hyperimmune globulin may have a reduced risk for delivering a congenitally infected infant.
- The use of IVIG or CMV IVIG for prophylaxis of infection in solid organ and bone marrow transplant recipients reduces the risk for symptomatic disease but does not prevent infection.

Ans: (a) Ganciclovir resistance is due to mutation in UL97 gene, DNA polymerase

Ref: *Nelson Textbook of Pediatrics, 20th edition, Page 1590*

11. A forceps delivered premature baby develops fever, abnormal behaviour, bulging fontanelle 5 days after birth. What is the likely causative organism?

(a) Neisseria meningitidis
(b) Listeria monocytogenes
(c) Staph aureus
(d) Pneumococcus

Explanation:

Etiology of Neonatal Meningitis

In India and Developing countries	In Western countries
Most common causes • **Klebsiella*** • E.coli • Staph aures **Less common** • Listeria monocytogenes • Enterobacter • Citrobacter • Serratia	**Most common cause** • **Group B streptococcus*** • E.coli • Listeria **Less common** • Enterococci • Staph aureus

Ans: (c) Staph aureus

Ref: *IAP Textbook of Pediatrics, 5th edition*

12. Which of the following features of rheumatic fever is not due to molecular mimicry?

(a) Myocarditis
(b) Polyarthritis
(c) Valvulitis
(d) Pericarditis

Explanation:

- Molecular mimicry is definitely the current accepted hypothesis regarding pathogenesis of acute rheumatic fever.
- It is strongly related to presence of cross-reacting antigens in heart, brain, skin and joints.
- In heart, anti-streptococcal antibodies reacting with 'Cardiac myosin' and subsequent T cell activation is proposed. This response is mainly seen in myocardium and Endocardium (Valves).

Ans: (d) Pericarditis

DERMATOLOGY

1. **Darier's sign is seen in:**

(a) Smooth muscle hamartoma
(b) Lichen planus
(c) Psoriasis
(d) Urticaria pigmentosa

Explanation:

- **Darier's sign–**If firm stroking of skin overlying a lesion like papule or macule with a blunt instrument results in exaggerated triple response of Lewis (weal formation over the lesion after stroking) persisting for more than 5 min, Darier's sign positive
- Seen in **urticaria pigmentosa** – type of mastocytosis
- Due to histamine release from mast cells
- **Pseudo Darier sign*–Smooth muscle hamartoma**
- **Dermographism–skin writing–**stoking of normal skin produces exaggerated triple response of Lewis lasting more than 5 min.

Urticaria Pigmentosa

- Firmly rubbing or stroking cutaneous lesions of mastocytosis (Urticaria pigmentosa) often causes urtication (**Darier's sign**); this is generally more pronounced in children.
- **Cutaneous mastocytosis** is also called as Urticaria pigmentosa.
- Mastocytosis is the spectrum of disorders caused by proliferation and accumulation of mast cells in the skin and/or other tissues.
- The onset of cutaneous mastocytosis is before 2 years of age in ~60%.
- Childhood-onset mastocytosis usually has a benign course with spontaneous remission prior to puberty, whereas adult-onset mastocytosis typically persists and may be associated with systemic involvement.
- Patients frequently experience pruritus and may have episodic urtication (redness and swelling) of mastocytosis lesions.
- Lesions in infants and preschool-aged children can blister due to release of proteases from densely packed mast cells.

Smooth Muscle Hamartoma

- Congenital or acquired, skin-colored to hyperpigmented plaque on the trunk > proximal extremities
- Follicular prominence and hypertrichosis may be present.
- May be confused with a congenital melanocytic nevus.
- Is on a clinicopathologic spectrum with Becker's nevus.

Pseudo-Darier's sign

- It is a transient piloerection and elevation or increased induration of a lesion induced by rubbing and is observed in **congenital smooth muscle hamartomas**. A positive pseudo-Darier's sign can be helpful in clinically distinguishing congenital smooth muscle hamartoma from congenital hairy nevus.

*(**Ref:** Surjushe A, Jindal S, Gote P, Saple DG, Darier's Sign, Indian J Dermatol Venereol Leprol 2007;73:363-364)*

Lichen Planus:

- **Violaceous polygonal pruritic papules** more on the **flexural aspects**.
- The lesions show **minimal scaling**.
- **Wickham's striae** may be seen.
- The **mucosa may be involved. White streaks**, often forming a **lacework**, on the buccal mucosa are highly characteristic.
- **Hair and nails** also can be involved.
- Linear lesions often appear along scratch marks or in scars (**Koebner phenomenon).**

Psoriasis:

- In Psoriasis there are erythematous plaques with silvery white plaques which are seen more on the extensor aspects.
- **Auspitz sign** will be positive.
- Scalp scaling is commonly seen.
- Palms and soles may show scaling and fissuring. Nails may be involved.
- Psoriatic arthropathy may affect the joints.

Ans: (d) Urticaria pigmentosa

***Ref:** Bolognia's Textbook of Dermatology, 4th edition*

2. **Most severe type of malignant melanoma mostly arises from:**

(a) Junctional nevus
(b) Arising de novo
(c) Lentigo
(d) Dermal nevus

Explanation:

Most severe type is **Nodular melanoma**. It often arises de novo and carries the worst prognosis.

MALIGNANT MELANOMA – SUBTYPES

- **Superficial spreading melanoma** is by far the **most frequent** type of melanoma.
- **Most common sites: In female - leg** and the In **males - back.**
- If the melanoma is developing in a **pre-existing naevus**, which occurs in approximately **50%** of lesions, the irregular appearance of the growing melanoma may contrast strikingly with the more regularly pigmented and outlined residual naevus component.
- All patients with suspected malignant melanoma should have an **excision biopsy** of the lesion carried out with a **margin of 1–2 mm** of clinically normal skin.
- **Incisional or punch biopsies should NOT be performed** in suspected melanoma because of sampling error, because an inaccurate tumour thickness may be obtained due to biopsy trauma, and also because the overall shape and symmetry of the whole lesion is important to the diagnosis of melanocytic lesions. There is a theoretical risk of displacing melanoma cells deeper into the dermis.
- The essential pathological features of superficial spreading melanoma are the presence of a **focus of malignant melanoma cells invading the dermis** with areas of ***in situ* malignant change** in the adjacent epidermis.

MELANOCYTE DIFFERENTIATION MARKERS

- ***S100***
- ***gp100/HMB-45***
- ***Tyrosinase***
- ***MART-1/Melan-A***
- ***HMW_MAA***

S100 is less specific than the other three, but highly sensitive and therefore is usually used in combination with at least one of the others.

- **Invasive melanomas up to 2 mm thick** may be safely treated with a **minimal excision margin of 1 cm**.
- In patients with **thicker tumours**, the recommended **excision margin is 2 to 3 cm**.

TYPES OF MELANOMA

A. **Superficial spreading melanoma**
   - **Most common subtype**
   - Accounts for **70%** cases
   - Presents as **flat** or slightly **elevated brown lesion**
   - **Variegate** pigmentation (Black, blue or pink discolouration)
   - Prognosis is **worse** than lentigo maligna melanoma type

B. Nodular melanoma

- Presents as a **dark brown to black papule** or **dome shaped** nodule
- **Ulcerates** and **bleeds** with minor trauma
- **Rapid growth** over weeks to months
- **Carries Worst Prognosis***

C. Lentigo maligna melanoma (Hutchinson's freckle)

- **Slowly grows** over 5 – 20 years
- Arises in only a small percentage of the intra-epithelial precursor lesion, the lentigo maligna
- **Malignant Melanoma in situ**
- **Good prognosis**

D. Acral lentiginous melanoma

- **Least common** subtype
- Occurs on the **palms, soles**, beneath the nail plate (**Subungual variant**)
- **Pigment** spread to the **proximal or lateral nailfolds** (**Hutchinson sign**) – Hallmark of this subtype
- Prognosis is worse than superficial spreading melanoma subtype

E. Amelanotic melanoma

- Nonpigmented
- Pink or flesh colored
- Mimics **basal cell carcinoma** or **Squamous cell carcinoma**
- Most commonly occurs in the setting of melanoma **metastasis to the skin**
- Inability of the poorly differentiated cancer cells to synthesize melanin pigment

Ans: (b) Arising de novo

Ref: *Rook's Dermatology and Essentials in Dermatology*

3. Ollendroff sign in which stage of syphilis?

(a) Primary syphilis (b) Secondary syphilis
(c) Latent syphilis (d) Tertiary syphilis

Explanation:

Buschke-Ollendroff sign:

- This is a sign to be elicited in case of **secondary syphilis** and **cutaneous vasculitis**, where there is deep dermal tenderness on pressing the lesion (e.g., papular lesions of syphilis) with a pinhead.

Primary syphilis: Chancre is seen.
Latent syphilis: No skin lesions. Only serological positivity.
Teritary syphilis: Gumma may be seen on the skin.

Ans: (b) Secondary syphilis

Ref: *Madke B, Nayak C, Eponymous Signs in Dermatology, Indian Dermatol Online J 2012;3:159-165*

4. Chiclero's ulcer caused by:

(a) Leishmania mexicana (b) Leishmania braziliense
(c) Leishmania aethiopica (d) Leishmania donovani

Ans: (a) Leishmania mexicana

Ref: 1. *Moyano E G, Blanca M A, Oñate F J, Pilar L M, Painful ulcer of the pinna in an immunocompromised patient. Indian J Dermatol Venereol Leprol 2018;84:369-372*
2. *CDC website https://www.cdc.gov/parasites/leishmaniasis/health_professionals/index.html*

Explanation:

CHICLERO ULCER

- Endemic, zoonotic form of **New World cutaneous leishmaniasis.**
- Found mainly in forest workers in southeastern Mexico, Belize and Guatemala.
- It is caused by **Leishmania mexicana, transmitted by Lutzomyia olmeca.**

- There are usually just a few lesions, self-limited and healing within six months; sometimes the **pinna of the ear** is involved, and lesions are chronic, lasting many years and slowly destroying the cartilage of the ear.

LEISHMANIASIS

- The term **leishmaniasis** encompasses multiple clinical syndromes, the
    - o **Cutaneous form (**infection of macrophages in the dermis)
    - o **Mucosal form (**infection of macrophages in the naso-oropharyngeal mucosa)
    - o **Visceral forms (**infection of macrophages in the reticuloendothelial system)
- The infection can range from asymptomatic to severe.
- Cutaneous and mucosal leishmaniasis can cause substantial morbidity, whereas visceral leishmaniasis can be life threatening.
- **Cutaneous leishmaniasis*** is most common form of leishmaniasis.
- Different Leishmania species cause **Old World versus New World (American) cutaneous leishmaniasis.**
- In the **Old World (the Eastern Hemisphere),** the etiologic agents include **Leishmania tropica, L. major, and L. aethiopica, as well as L. infantum and L. donovani.**
- The main species in the **New World (the Western Hemisphere)** are either in the **L. mexicana species complex (L. mexicana, L. amazonensis and L. venezuelensis)** or **the subgenus Viannia (L. [V.] braziliensis, L. [V.] guyanensis, L. [V.] panamensis and L. [V.] peruviana)**. The Viannia subgenus is also referred to as the **L. (V.) braziliensis species complex.**

Mucosal Leishmaniasis:

- Traditionally refers to a **metastatic sequela of New World cutaneous infection**
- Also known as **Espundia***
- Results from dissemination of parasites from the skin to the naso-oropharyngeal mucosa.
- Caused by species in the **Viannia subgenus** (especially L. [V.] **braziliensis** but also L. [V.] **panamensis** and sometimes L. [V.] **guyanensis**); it also can be caused by L. (Leishmania) **amazonensis.**

Visceral Leishmaniasis:

- Encompasses a broad spectrum of severity and manifestations.
- Caused by the species **L. donovani and L. infantum** (L. chagasi generally is considered synonymous with L. infantum)
- Affects internal organs (particularly, spleen, liver and bone marrow).
- The stereotypical manifestations of clinically manifest visceral infection include:
    - o Fever, weight loss (cachexia; wasting)
    - o Hepatosplenomegaly (usually, the spleen is more prominent than the liver)
    - o Pancytopenia—i.e., anemia, leukopenia and thrombocytopenia
    - o High total protein level and a low albumin level, with hypergammaglobulinemia

Kala azar

- The term **kala azar**—which means black (kala) fever (azar) in Hindi—often is reserved for severe (advanced) cases of **visceral leishmaniasis.**
- Some patients develop **post kala azar dermal leishmaniasis (PKDL),** a syndrome characterized by **skin lesions**
    - o Erythematous or hypopigmented macules, papules, nodules and patches
    - o Typically first noticed and most prominent on the face
    - o Develop at variable intervals after (or during) therapy for visceral leishmaniasis.

5. **Herald patch is seen:**

(a) Psoriasis (b) Pityriasis rosea
(c) Lichen planus (d) Pityriasis rubra pilaris

Explanation:

PITYRIASIS ROSACEA

- **Also known as Gilbert's disease, six-week disease**

- **Papulosquamous disorder** with **pruritic or asymptomatic** lesions
- Common in **adolescents and young adults**
- **Risk factors**
  - **Viral**–HHV-6, HHV-7
  - **Drugs**–Metronidazole, Captopril, Gold
- **Initial 'herald or mother' patch* 1-2 cms oval plaque** on trunk followed by **daughter patches two weeks later**
- **Christmas tree pattern*** along lines of **cleavage** with a **peripheral collarette** of scale producing the **Hanging curtain sign** when stretched.
- **No oral lesions.**
- Self-limiting.

OTHER OPTIONS

- **Pityriasis rubra pilaris**
  - Circumscribed follicular keratoses
  - Branny scale
  - Orange-red erythema
  - Palmoplantar keratoderma
  - If erythroderma develops there will be islands of normal uninvolved skin.
- **Lichen planus**
  - **Violaceous polygonal pruritic papules** more on the **flexural aspects.**
  - The lesions show **minimal scaling.**
  - **Wickham's striae** may be seen.
  - The **mucosa may be involved.**
  - **Hair and nails** also can be involved.
- **Psoriasis**
  - **Erythematous plaques** with **silvery white plaques** which are seen more on the **extensor aspects.**
  - **Auspitz sign** will be positive.
  - **Scalp scaling** is commonly seen.
  - **Palms and soles may show scaling and fissuring.**
  - **Nails** may be involved.
  - **Psoriatic arthropathy** may affect the joints.

Ans: (b) Pityriasis rosea

Ref: *Rook's Textbook of Dermatology, 8th edition, Page 33.78*

6. Dermatitis herpetifomis is associated with:

(a) HLA DR4 (b) HLA DQ2 and HLA DQ8
(c) HLA CW6 (d) HLA DR2

Explanation:

HLA Associations in Bullous Disorders

Disease	Autoantibodies	HLA Association
Pemphigus vulgaris	Dg III	**HLA DR4*** HLA DR6 HLA DQ8 HLADR14
Pemphigus foliaceus	Dg I	**HLA DR1*** HLA DR4 HLADR14
Epidermolysis bullosa acquisita	Collagen type VII	**HLA DR2***
Dermatitis herpetiformis	Unknown	**HLA DQ2*** **HLA DR3*** **HLA DQ8*** HLA DR7

DERMATITIS HERPETIFORMIS (DH)

Epidemiology

- Age–**20 to 40** years, **M=F,** Whites > Blacks/Asians

Etiology

- Genetics: **HLA B8, DRw17 and DQw2**
- External factors: **Gluten containing diet** like **wheat**, **barley**, **oats** and **rye**
- Antigen: Gut epithelial antigen that cross reacts with skin
- Antibodies: **IgA directed** against **gliadin** and autoantigens like **reticulin** and **endomysium**

Pathogenesis

- Gluten or its fragments are taken up by antigen presenting cells like lymphocytes
- Activation of cytokines and inflammatory cells
- Plasma cells release **IgA2** directed against **gliadin**
- Cross-reacts with autoantigens of skin and gut like reticulin, endomyosium

Clinical Features

- Intensely pruritic
- Most vesicles have been scratched away
- Chronic recurrent grouped **papulo vesicles**, **symmetrically**
- Most common on **extensor surfaces, back of neck and sacrum, buttocks**
- Associated with **gluten-sensitive enteropathy**

Diagnosis

- **Tzanck smear**: Plenty of **neutrophils**
- Histopathology: Neutrophilic **microabscesses** at the tips of dermal papilla with **sub-epidermal** vesicle
- Immunopathology: Clinically normal skin on forearm or **buttock** shows granular **IgA deposits** in the **dermal papilla**.

Treatment

- Strict **gluten free diet**
- **Systemic steroids** not the mainstay of therapy
- **Dapsone** 100-200 mg/day
- **Sulphapyridine** 1.5 g/day
- **Tetracycline with nicotinamide**
- **Colchicine** when the above drugs are contraindicated

Ans: (b) HLA DQ2 and HLA DQ8

7. **Xanthoma disseminatum is associated with:**

(a) Downs syndrome (b) Diabetes insipidus
(c) Lymphoma (d) Ca pancreas

Explanation:

Xanthoma Disseminatum

- Rare, **normolipemic, histiocytic** proliferative disorder that affects the **skin**, **mucous membranes** and frequently, the **hypothalamus** and **pituitary gland**, leading to transient **diabetes insipidus**.
- Key features
- Classic triad of **cutaneous xanthomas, mucous membrane xanthomas and diabetes insipidus**
- **Symmetric** distribution of lesions
- Favors **flexural** areas and **intertriginous** zones
- **Corneal** and **conjunctival** lesions can threaten vision

Dermatological findings in Down syndrome:

- Atopic dermatitis

- Seborrheic dermatitis
- Alopecia areata
- Vitiligo
- Milia-like calcinosis cutis
- Syringomas
- Elastosis perforans serpiginosa

Ans: (b) Diabetes insipidus

Ref: *Goodman WT, Barrett TL, Histiocytoses, In: Bolognia JL, Schaffer JV, Cerroni L, editors. Dermatology, 4th edition, United States: Elsevier 2018, Page 1614–1632*

8. In pemphigus, split occurs at the level of:

(a) Intra-epithelial
(b) Sub-epithelial
(c) Inter-epithelial
(d) Endothelial

Explanation:

PEMPHIGUS VULGARIS (PV)

Clinical Features

- Mucosal erosions
- Thin-walled, relatively flaccid, easily ruptured bullae
- Bullae leave denuded areas that don't heal spontaneously.
- Common sites of involvement:
  - Oral cavity, scalp, groins, face, neck, axillae and genitals.
- **Nikolsky sign** and **Bulla spread sign** (**Asboe-Hansen sign**) are usually positive.
- Widespread involvement may be fatal because of sepsis, fluid and electrolyte imbalance.
- Pemphigus is due to IgG antibodies directed against epidermal cell adhesion molecules **(desmoglein 3).**

Pathology

- Disruption of intercellular cementing substance
- Loss of adhesion between epidermal cells (acantholysis)
- **Intraepidermal blistering.**
- **Tzanck smear from** the floor of the blister shows **acantholytic cells.**
- Acantholytic cell is a large, rounded epidermal cell with a large nucleus, perinuclear halo and peripheral condensation of cytoplasm.
- Histopathological examination of a blister shows a supra-basal, intra-epidermal blister.
- The basal keratinocytes remain attached to the basement membrane but are separated from each other and stand like a '**row of tombstones'***.
- **Direct Immunofluoresence**: Done shows deposition of intercellular IgG throughout the epidermis in a **'fish-net' or 'chicken-wire' pattern*.**
- Indirect immunofluorescence done in the sera of the patients shows circulating intercellular IgG, the levels of which correlate with disease activity.
- The mainstay of treatment is systemic steroids given in a conventional manner or as a pulse steroids.

Diseases with Subepidermal Blistering

- Bullous Pemphigoid
- Cicatricial Pemphigoid
- Dermatitis Herpetiformis
- Epidermolysis Bullosa Acquisita

There cannot be any interepithelial or endothelial splitting in any of the diseases.

PEMPHIGUS

- Pemphigus is an autoimmune blistering disorder characterized by ***autoantibody formation*** against the intercellular cementing substance called ***desmogleins***

- The mechanism of cell separation is called ***acantholysis***–loss of intercellular substance causing separation of the epidermal keratinocytes which become rounded→ result in intraepidermal blister
- These large rounded keratinocytes with large nucleus, perinuclear halo and peripheral condensation of cytoplasm are called the ***acantholytic cells*** – seen in Tzanck smear
- **Types of Pemphigus:**
  - o Pemphigus vulgaris (variant-pemphigus vegetans)–Most common type
  - o Pemphigus foliaceus (variant-pemphigus erythematosus; endemic pemphigus or fogoselvagem)
  - o Paraneoplastic pemphigus
  - o Drug induced pemphigus
  - o IgA pemphigus
  - o Neonatal pemphigus
- **Clinical Features:**
  - o Fluid filled bullae→rupture→painful erosions with no tendency to spontaneous healing
  - o Painful mucosal erosions–oral (most common; almost in all cases in pemphigus vulgaris); genital mucosa, pharynx, larynx, conjunctiva, urethra
  - o ***Bulla spread sign/Asboe Hansen sign–positive***
  - o ***Nikolsky sign***–peeling of skin leaving behind erosions when tangential pressure applied over areas of normal looking skin or over bony prominences (other conditions–staphylococcal scalded skin syndrome, toxic epidermal necrolysis)
- **Diagnosis:** Tzanck smear–acantholytic cells; histopathology; direct and indirect immunofluoresence
- **Treatment:** ***Systemic steroids*** are mainstay of treatment
- **Adjuvants:** Cyclophosphamide, azathioprine, methotrexate, mycophenolate mofetil, dapsone, plasmapheresis, IV immunoglobulins; biological agent–Rituximab (anti CD20)

Characteristics of Various Pemphigus Disorders (High Yield Table)

Features	Pemphigus vulgaris	Pemphigus foliaceus	Bullous pemphigoid	Dermatitis herpetiformis
Antigen	Desmoglein 3	Desmoglein 1	BP 180, BP 230	Unknown
Level of split	Intraepidermal - suprabasal	Intraepidermal-subcorneal	Subepidermal	Subepidermal
Mechanism of blister	Acantholysis	Acantholysis	Basement membrane zone disruption	Basement membrane zone disruption
Age	40-60 years	40-50 years	>60 years	20-55 years
Symptoms	Pain	Pain (less severe)	Pruritus	Intensely pruritic
Type of blister	Flaccid bullae on normal or erythematous skin	Transient blisters	Tense bullae on normal or erythematous or urticated skin	Grouped erythematous papules and papulovesicles; vesicles excoriated
Nature of erosion	Painful erosions with no tendency to spontaneous healing	Crusted moist scaly erosions	Erosions heal spontaneously	–
Distribution	Scalp, face, trunk, axilla, groins, pressure sites	Seborrheic distribution	Flexural aspect of limbs, lower abdomen, groin, axilla	Extensor aspect of limbs (elbows, knees), buttock, nasal cleft, shoulder, upper back, face, scalp
Bulla spread sign	+	Transient vesicles	+/-	Vesicles not seen as excoriated
Nikolsky sign	+	+	-	-

Contd.

Contd.

Mucosal involvement	Almost in all patients; may be presenting or the only feature (80-90%)	Uncommon	Rare; never presenting feature; desquamative gingivitis (40%)	Common but asymptomatic
Tzanck smear	Acantholytic cells	Acantholytic cells	Eosinophils	Neutrophils
HPE	Suprabasal cleft with row of tomb stone appearance	Subcorneal split	Subepidermal blister with eosinophils	Neutrophilic microabscess at tips of dermal papillae
DIF	**Intercellular IgG** deposits throughout the *epidermis* in fish net pattern	**Intercellular IgG** deposits in upper *epidermis*	**Linear IgG** and **C3** deposits in *basement membrane zone*	**Granular IgA** deposits in *dermal papilla*
IIF	Antibody titres correlate with disease severity	Antibody titres correlate with disease severity	Antibody titres do not correlate with disease severity	Negative or anti basement membrane zone or dermal autoantibodies. Antithyroid or antigliadin antibodies present
Associations	Thymoma, myasthenia gravis, lymphoma, bronchogenic carcinoma	-	Gastric carcinoma, diabetes, rheumatoid arthritis, psoriasis	Gluten sensitive enteropathy
Mainstay of treatment	Steroids + adjuvants	Steroids + adjuvants	Steroids + adjuvants	Dapsone Gluten free diet

Ans: (a) Intra-epithelial

Ref: *Andrews' Diseases of the Skin, 11th edition, Page 448-451*

9. **Cayenne Pepper stippling due to hemosiderin is found in:**

(a) Erythroplasia of Queyrat
(b) Paget's disease
(c) Plasma cell balanitis of zoon
(d) Bowen's disease

Explanation:

Plasma Cell Balanitis of Zoon

- Presents as single or multiple well-circumscribed, orange-red, shiny, moist, glistening macular to slightly raised plaque.
- Multiple pinpoint, brighter red spots may be speckled on the background of this orange-red plaque, called as "**cayenne pepper spots**" due to **microhemorrhage** and **hemosiderin deposition**. Sometimes, prepuce may display "**kissing lesion**" on areas that is in direct contact with the lesions. Subsequently, these may erode and leave behind a "**rusty stain**".
- Two distinct clinical variants of ZB have been reported, which include:
    - **Erosive type** with **bleeding**, particularly on the inner surface of prepuce
    - **Vegetative type**.

Erythroplasia of Queyrat

- Presents as a well-demarcated, velvety erythematous plaque on the glabrous skin of the penis, vulva or perianal region
- Histologically is a **High grade Squamous Intraepithelial Lesion**.

Bowen Disease

- Can present as a solitary patch or plaque, sometimes scaly, of the vulva or penis.
- Most often in older individuals.

Extramammary Paget Disease (EMPD)

- Can be primary, arising as an intraepithelial adenocarcinoma, or secondary, due to pagetoid spread of an adjacent or contiguous in situ or invasive neoplasm.
- It may become invasive and metastasize via the lymphatic system.
- The most commonly involved sites are the vulva in women and the perianal region in men. The symptoms may be itching or burning.
- They can be asymptomatic also at times.
- A slowly expanding erythematous plaque is classical.
- There is a sharp demarcation between normal and involved skin.
- Scattered areas of white scale and erosion can give rise to a "**strawberries and cream**" appearance.

Ans: (c) Plasma cell balanitis of zoon

Ref: *Cooper SM, Wojnarowska F. Anogenital (non-venereal) Disease. In: Bolognia JL, Jorizzo JL, Schaffer JV, editors, Dermatology, 3rd edition, United States: Elsevier; 2012, Page 1171–86*

ANESTHESIOLOGY

1. **Anesthetic agent known to cause pain on intravenous injection:**

(a) Ketamine (b) Etomidate
(c) Thiopentone (d) Propofol

Explanation:

- **Propofol:** Causes pain on intravenous injection due to presence of egg lecithin in its commercial preparation.
- **Etomidate** – Pain and venous irritation has been virtually eliminated with the use of lipid emulsion vehicle and avoid in propylene glycol.
- **Ketamine** and **Thipenthol Na** are not emulsion preparations and do not cause pain on IV injection.
- **Composition of 1% Propofol Emulsion:**
  - o 1% propofol
  - o 10% soyabean oil
  - o 2.25% Glycerol
  - o 1.2% egg lecithin
  - o 0.005% di sodium edetate (to prevent bacterial growth)
- **Prevention of pain duration IV injection of Propofol:**
  - o Should be given in large bore cannula and in running fluid
  - o Add 1% lidocaine with 10 ml of propofol before injection
  - o Give fentanyl before propofol injection
  - o Use lipid based formulation of propofol
- **Fospropofol (Aquavan):** Is a phosphorylated prodrug of propofol
  - o No pain on IV injection
  - o Longer shelf half life
  - o Slight longer peak effect and more prolong duration of action
  - o 1 mg Fospropofol = 0.54 mg propofol

Ans: (d) Propofol

Ref: *Stoelting's Pharmacology and Physiology in Anesthetic Practice, 4th edition*

2. **Anesthectic agent with least minimum alveolar concentration (MAC):**

(a) Nitrous oxide (b) Isoflurane
(c) Desflurane (d) Xenon

Explanation:

MAC (MINIMUM ALVEOLAR CONCENTRATION)

- MAC is the concentration of inhalational agent in **alveoli at 1 atm** that **prevents skeletal muscle movement in response to a supra-maximal painful stimulus** (surgical skin incision) in **50% of patients.**
- It is used to **measure potency** of inhalational agents
- **MAC $\propto$ 1/Potency**
- **Potency** is a measure of **drug activity** expressed in terms of the amount required to produce an effect of given intensity.
- Lesser amounts of drug required to produce maximum effect is called as more **potent drug**.
- For inhalational anaesthetic agents potency are measured by **MAC value**
- Lesser the **MAC** more is the **potency (MAC $\propto$ 1/Potency)**
- Inhalational agents order from maximum potent to minimum potent
- ***Methoxyflurane > Trilene > Halothane > Chloroform > Isoflurane > Enflurane > Sevoflurane > Ether > Sevoflurane > Xenon > N2O****

MAC of Common Inhalational Agents:

Inhalational agents	MAC
Methoxyflurane	0.16
Trilene	0.2
Halothane	0.75
Chloroform	0.8
Isoflurane	1.17
Enflurane	1.63
Sevoflurane	1.8
Ether	1.9
Desflurane	6.6
Xenon	71
N2O	104

Factor Affecting MAC:

Increase of MAC	Decrease of MAC	No Change of MAC
• Hyperthermia • Hypernatremia (↑ Na) • Sympathomimetic drugs • Cyclosporine • Excessive pheomelanin production (red hair)	• Hypothermia • Increasing age (6% per decade) • Alpha 2 agonist agents • Acute alcohol ingestion • Pregnancy and postpartum upto 72 hours • Lithium • Lidocaine • Hyponatremia • Ketanserine • Adrenergic antagonist agents • BP <40 mm Hg • PaO_2 <38 mm Hg	• Chronic alcohol abuse • Gender • Duration of anaesthesia • $PaCO_2$ 15 - 95 mm Hg • PaO_2 >38 mm Hg • BP > 40 mm Hg • Hyper or Hypokalemia • Thyroid dysfunction • Anaesthetic metabolism

Ans: (b) Isoflurane

Ref: *Stoelting's Pharmacology and Physiology in Anesthetic Practice, 4th edition*

3. **Inhalational agent with lowest blood gas coefficient is:**

(a) Isoflurane
(b) N_2O
(c) Xenon
(d) Enflurane

Explanation:

- **Blood gas partition coefficient (BG coefficient):** It is ratio of solubility of a gas (inhalational agent) in blood and in the air (alveolar air)
- ***"Low the BG coefficient = Lesser the solubility of gas in blood => Rapid onset of action"***
- **BG coefficient** can be affected by:
  - Serum lipid content
  - Serum protein content
  - Hematocrit
  - Age

Inhalational agents	BG coeficient	Vapour pressure (mm Hg)	Boiling point (degree celsius)
Xenon	0.115	-	-
Desflurane	0.42	673	23.5
Nitrous oxide	0.46	5200	-88
Sevoflurane	0.69	162	58.5
Isoflurane	1.46	238	48.5
Enflurane	1.90	174	56.5
Halothane	2.54	243	50
Chloroform	8	160	60
Trilene	9	60	87
Ether	12	425	36
Methoxyflurane	13	23	103

Ans: (c) Xenon

***Ref**: Stoelting's Pharmacology and Physiology in Anesthetic Practice, 4th edition*

4. **Regarding Neuraxial Anesthesia, which of the following statement is true?**

(a) Aspirin should be stopped 7 days before surgery
(b) Unfractionated heparin should be stopped 7 days before surgery
(c) Fondaparinux should be stopped 7 days before surgery
(d) Clopidrogrel should be stopped 7 days before surgery

Explanation:

Drug Therapy During Neuraxial Anesthesia

Anticoagulants	When to stop before neuraxial block	When to start after neuraxial block
IV heparin	6 hours (APTT < 40 sec)	2-4 hours
SC heparin	12 hours (APPT < 40 sec)	2-4 hours
LMWH (Enoxaparin)	24 hours	12 hours
Aspirin	No need to stop	No restriction
Clopidogrel	7-10 days	2 hours
Warfarin	4-5 days (INR < 1.4)	2 hours
Fondaparinux	72 hours	12 hours
Rivaroxaban	24 hours	6 hours (24 hours if Traumatic puncture and Major risk of bleeding)
Aoixaban	48 hours	
Thrombin inhibitor (desirudin, lepirudin, bivalirudin)	**5 days (wait upto APTT <40 sec)**	**2 hours**
Fibrinolytics–Streptokinase, Alteplase, Reteplase, Tenecteplase	10 days	10 days
Glycoprotein IIb/IIIa inhibitors–Abciximab, Eptifibatide and Tirofiban	**48 hours** **8 hours**	**2 hours**

Ans: (d) Clopidrogrel should be stopped 7 days before surgery

***Ref:** ASRA, Guidelines 2017*

5. **A resident at the emergency department is preparing for a lumbar puncture in a 26 years old female with suspected subarachnoid bleeding. Although she presented with altered sensorium, CT brain was found to be normal. During LP, which structure is pierced after the spinal needle crosses interspinous ligament?**

(a) Ligamentum flavum
(b) Arachnoid membrane
(c) Areolar tissue
(d) Subarachnoid space

Explanation:

STRUCTURES PIERCED BY SPINAL NEEDLE DURING LP

1. Skin
2. Subcutaneous tissue
3. Supraspinous ligament
4. Interspinous ligament
5. Ligamentum flavum
6. Dura mater
7. Arachnoid membrane

Lumbar Puncture

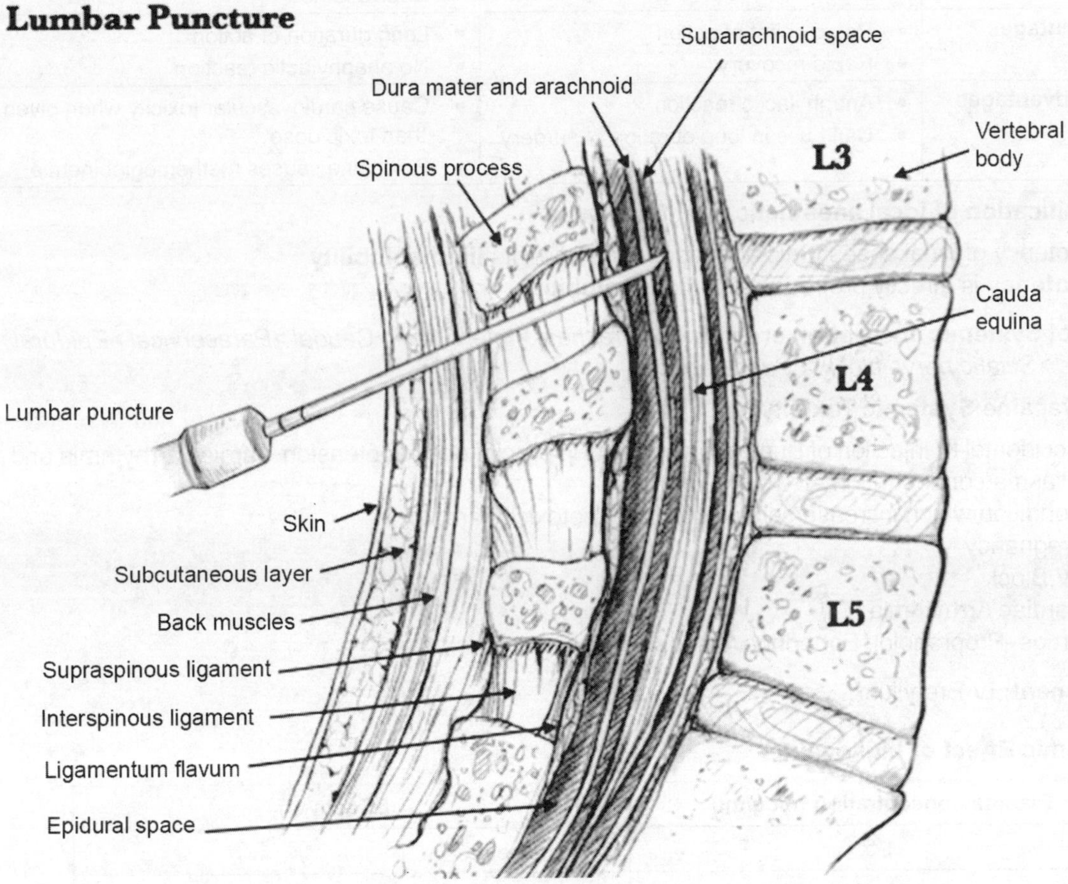

Ans: (a) Ligamentum flavum

Ref: *Morgan's Clinical Anesthesiology, 5th edition, Chapter 16*

6. **Local anesthetic acts by:**

(a) Blocking sodium gated channel
(b) Blocking calcium gated channel
(c) Blocking potassium gated channel
(d) Blocking chloride gated channel

Explanation:

LOCAL ANAESTHETIC AGENTS

Mechanism of LA

- Na channel (membrane bound protein) made up of 1 Alpha and 2 beta units, exits in 3 states–resting, activated (open) and inactivated.
- **LA** binds with **alpha unit** and block **voltage gated Na channel** from inside which prevents subsequent channel activated activation.
- It will not alter the RMP but threshold potential no longer generated.
- Nerve sensitivity for local anaesthetic are **Autonomic> sensory> motor.**

Type	Esters	Amides
Examples	• Procaine • Chloroprocaine • Cocaine • Tetracaine	• Lidocaine • Bupivacaine • Etidocaine • Mepivacaine • Prilocaine • Ropivacaine
Advantages	• Rapid onset of action • Rapid recovery	• Long duration of action • No anaphylactic reaction
Disadvantages	• Anaphylactic reaction • Can't use in long duration of surgery	• Cause cardiovascular toxicity when given more than toxic dose • Prilocaine causes methemoglobinemia

Classification of local anesthetic agents: 2 types

- Potency of local anaesthetic agent depends upon its **lipid solubility**.
- **Potency** is directly proportional to **lipid solubility**.

Rate of Systemic absorption order is: *IV> Tracheal >Intercostal >Caudal >Paracervical >Epidural >Brachial plexus >Sciatic nerve block > Subcutaneous.*

Bupivacaine Systemic Toxicity:

- Accidental IV injection of Bupivacaine results in precipitous hypotension, cardiac arrhythmia and AV block. (Plasma concentration >8-10 mcg/ml).
- Condition which increase sensitivity for cardiotoxicity are:
- Pregnancy
- AV Block
- Cardiac Arrhythmia
- Drugs–Propranolol, Ephedrine, Phenylephrine

Treatment: IV Bretylium

Systemic Effect of Lignocaine:

Plasma concentration (mcg/ml)	Effects
1-5	• Analgesia
>5-10	• Circumoral numbness, tinnitus • Sketetal muscle twitching • Systemic hypotension • Myocardial depression
>10-15	• Seizures • Unconsciousness
>15-25	• Apnea • Coma
>25	• Cardiac arrest

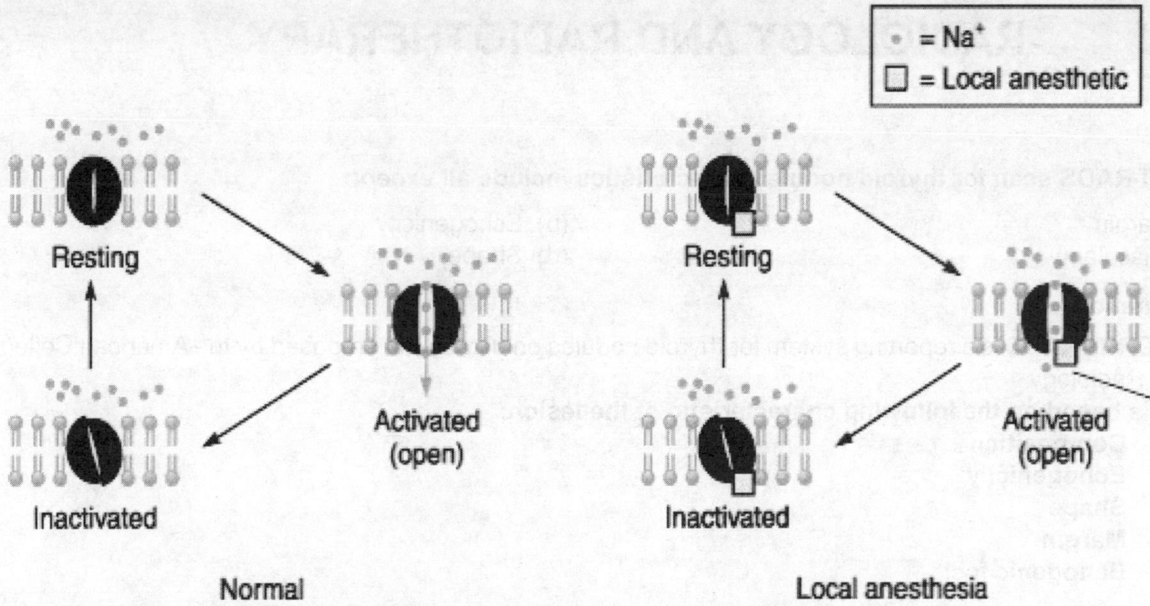

Treatment of Lignocaine Toxicity:

1. Maintain airway and give 100% oxygen
2. Control seizures with benzodiazepine (thiopental)
3. Treat hypotension–Dopamine infusion
4. If cardiac arrest–CPR with standard protocol
5. Injection 'Intra Lipid' emulsion

Though intravenous injection of lignocaine can cause systemic hypotension, it is more common with bupivacaine.

* Ropivacaine is not cardiotoxic.

Ans: (a) Blocking sodium gated channel

Ref: *Stoelting's Pharmacology and Physiology in Anesthetic Practice, 4th edition*

RADIOLOGY AND RADIOTHERAPY

1. ACRTI-RADS scan for thyroid nodule characteristics include all *except*:

(a) Margin
(b) Echogenicity
(c) Vascularity
(d) Shape

Explanation:

- **ACR TI-RADS** is a reporting system for thyroid nodules on ultrasound proposed by the American College of Radiology.
- **It is based on the following characteristic of the lesion:**
  - **Composition**
  - **Echogenicity**
  - **Shape**
  - **Margin**
  - **Echogenic foci**

ACR TI-RADS

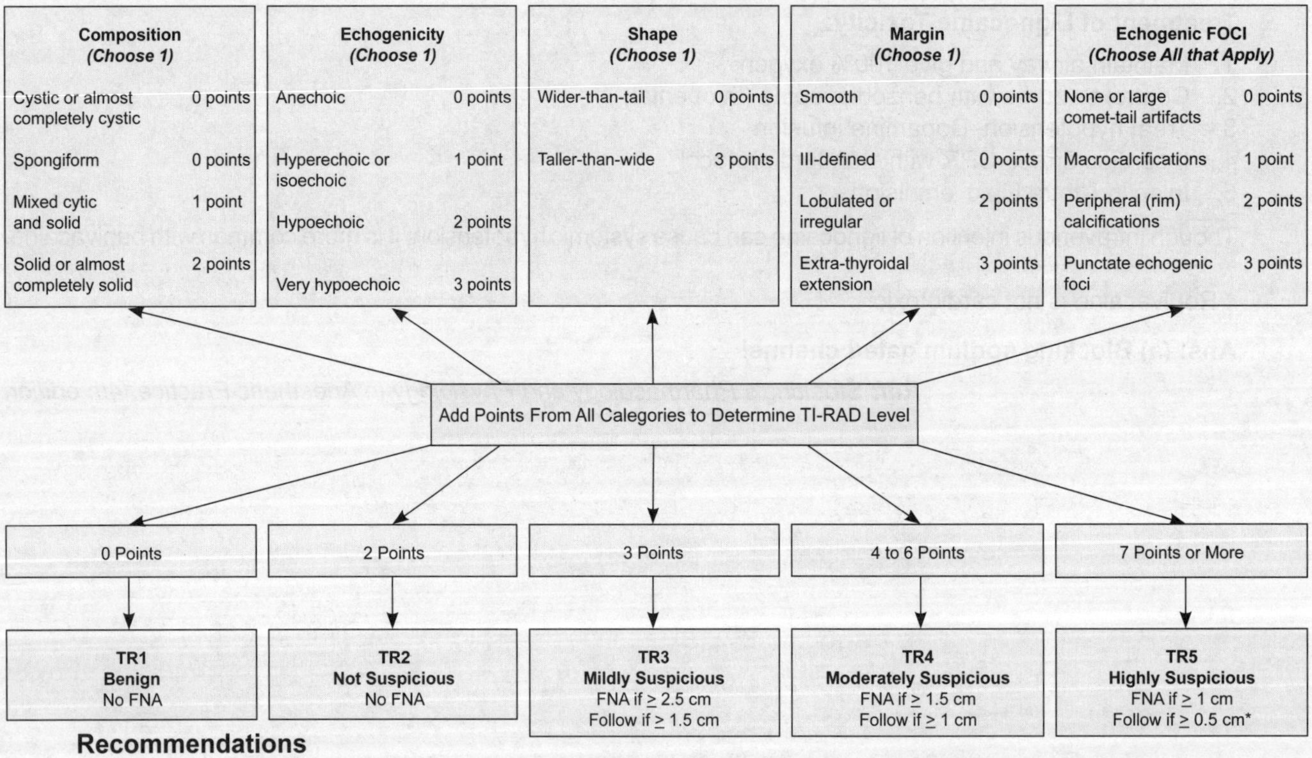

Recommendations

- **TR1**: No FNAC required
- **TR2**: No FNAC required
- **TR3**: ≥1.5 cm follow up, ≥2.5 cm FNAC
  - Follow up: 1, 3 and 5 years
- **TR4**: ≥1.0 cm follow up, ≥1.5 cm FNAC
  - Follow up: 1, 2, 3 and 5 years
- **TR5**: ≥0.5 cm follow up, ≥1.0 cm FNAC
  - Annual follow up for up to 5 years

Ans: (c) Vascularity

Ref: *J Am Coll Radiol 2017 May,14(5), Page 587-595*

2. Imaging modality employed in PI-RAD reporting scheme for prostate glands is all *except*:

(a) MR spectroscopy
(b) Dynamic contrast enhancement
(c) Diffusion weighted MRI
(d) T2W imaging

Explanation:

PI-RADS (Prostate Imaging Reporting and Data System)

- Refers to a structured reporting scheme for evaluating the prostate for prostate cancer
- The score is calculated from evaluation of a prostate specific MRI. Images are obtained using a multiparametric technique including T2 weighted imaging, Dynamic contrast enhancement study (DCE) and Diffusion Weighted imaging (DWI)/**ADC SCORE**
- T2W is the primary determining sequence for the transition zone
- DWI is the primary determining sequence for the peripheral zone
- A score is given according to each variable. The scale is based on a score from 1 to 5 (which is given for each lesion), with 1 being most probably benign and 5 being highly suspicious of malignancy:
  - **PI-RADS 1**: Very low (clinically significant cancer is highly unlikely to be present)
  - **PI-RADS 2**: Low (clinically significant cancer is unlikely to be present)
  - **PI-RADS 3**: Intermediate (the presence of clinically significant cancer is equivocal)
  - **PI-RADS 4**: High (clinically significant cancer is likely to be present)
  - **PI-RADS 5:** Very high (clinically significant cancer is highly likely to be present)

Ans: (a) MR spectroscopy

Ref: *J Urol. 2017 Sep;198(3):583-590; Radiopedia*

3. Winking owl sign is seen in:

(a) Vertebral tuberculosis
(b) Vertebral metastasis
(c) Vertebral fracture due to cervical traction
(d) Vertebal mass

Explanation:

- The **winking owl sign**, also called **absent pedicle sign** occurs on plain film when a pedicle is absent on AP view of thoracic or lumbar spine.
- The term, winking owl sign, where the missing pedicle corresponds to the closed eye, the contralateral pedicle to the other open eye, and the spinous process to the beak of the owl on AP views of the thoracic or lumbar spine, it usually occurs almost always due to a **vertebral bony metastasis*** causing destruction of the pedicle (closed eye).

Ans: (b) Vertebral metastasis

Ref: *Radiology Review*

4. A MRI contrast used for imaging liver is:

(a) Gadoterate
(b) Gadoxetate
(c) Gadoteridol
(d) Gadopenate

Explanation:

Hepatobiliary MRI contrast agents are specialised agents used to aid diagnosis in MRI.

They are separated into three categories: gadolinium-based agents, manganese-based agents and superparamagnetic iron oxide particles.

Gadolinium-based Agents

- Hepatobiliary specific gadolinium agents include two of the high relaxivity agents: **gadobenate disodium (Gd-BOPTA) and gadoxetate disodium (Gd-EOB-DTPA)**
- **Gadoxetate disodium (Gd-EOB-DTPA):** has almost equal biliary and renal excretion (~50% each). Compared to gadobenate, it has more intense liver parenchymal enhancement.

Manganese-based Agents

- **Mangafodipir trisodium (Mn-DPDP)** is specifically taken up by hepatocytes due to its chemical similarity to Vitamin B_6. This property results in the increase in signal intensity of normal hepatic parenchyma, giving high lesion-liver contrast.

- Unlike the gadolinium agents, mangafodipir trisodium readily dissociates to yield free manganese ions. This in vivo instability of the chelate rose concerns about potential toxicity.
- Free manganese, in chronic exposure, causes a parkinsonism-like syndrome due to accumulation in the brain, other neurological features and cardiac suppression.
- Hence, mangafodipir trisodium was effectively withdrawn from the market.

Superparamagnetic Iron Oxide Particles

- Superparamagnetic iron oxide particles do not leak into the interstitium. They, therefore, act as intravascular contrast agents or blood pool agents as long as the vessel endothelium is intact and unaltered by any pathological process. Their elimination from the blood is by uptake into the reticuloendothelial system cells in liver, spleen, bone marrow and lymph nodes and are phagocytosed by macrophages throughout the body.
- The superparamagnetic iron oxide particles agents are preferentially entrapped by the Kupffer cells in the liver and spleen and reduce their T2 relaxation time. Thus, normal liver appears dark on T2 weighted images. Most liver tumours which are usually deficient in Kupffer cells, do not exhibit superparamagnetic iron oxide particles agent uptake and appear relatively hyperintense.

Ans: (b) Gadoxetate

Ref: *J Magn Reson Imaging, 2012 Nov; 36(5):1060-71*

5. **X-ray spine of a child is shown. What is the probable diagnosis?**

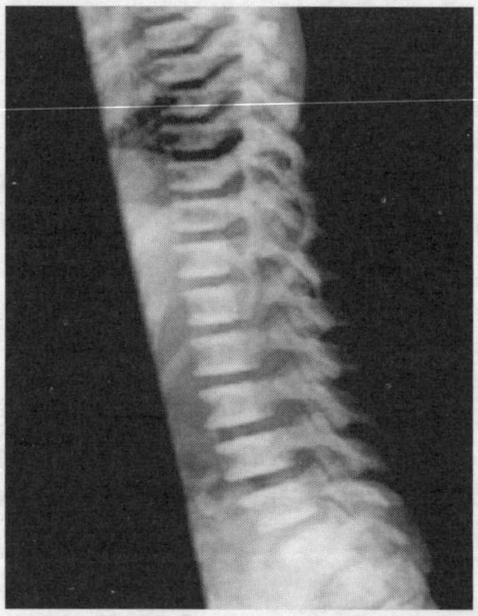

(a) Bamboo spine (b) Rugger Jersey spine
(c) Normal spine (d) Ivory spine

Explanation:

RUGGER JERSEY SPINE

- The sclerotic bands on the superior and inferior endplates of the vertebral bodies represent accumulations of excess osteoid and appear opaque because of their increased volume when compared to normal bone.
- **Rugger jersey spine** describes the prominent subendplate densities at multiple vertebral levels to produce an alternating sclerotic-lucent-sclerotic appearance. This mimics the horizontal stripes of a **rugby jersey**, seen with **secondary hyperparathyroidism*** associated with **Renal Osteodystrophy*** and **Osteopetrosis***.
- **Bamboo spine** is feature of **ankylosing spondylitis***.
- **Ivory spine** is feature of **Paget's disease***.

RENAL OSTEODYSTROPHY

- CRF leading on to hyperparathyroidism.
- **Signs of chronic renal failure:**
  - o Findings of osteomalacia
  - o Hyperparathyroidism
  - o Bone sclerosis

- ***Rugger jersey spine***
- ***Rotting fence post appearance***: Due to Rickets + Hyperparathyroidism
- In children, **metaphyseal** changes resembling rickets are seen, which together with **cortical** erosibons can give rise to the so-called 'rotting fence-post' appearance, particularly at the **femoral neck**.
- ***Looser's zone.***

Ans: (b) Rugger jersey spine

Ref: *Radiology Review*

6. **A 2-year-old child with lump in abdomen, abdominal pain, USG - Hydronephrotic Right kidney with thin cortical parenchyma. Best imaging method to assess functional status of kidney:**

(a) Doppler Ultrasonography
(b) Contrast Ultrasonography
(c) 99mTc DMSA scintigraphy
(d) NCCT

Explanation:

Preferred isotope study for functional status of kidney is 99mTc **DMSA Scan.**

- **Tc99m DMSA scan** is a static or anatomical imaging suitable for imaging **renal morphology** and **cortical function.**
- It is the agent of choice for evaluation of **scar in the kidney** and for **differential renal cortical function/ split renal function.**
- **99m Tc dimercaptosuccinic acid (99m Tc-DMSA)** is an agent that is actively taken up by the proximal and distal renal tubular cells, directly from the peritubular vessels, and accumulates in the renal cortex.
- This modality is primarily used for imaging **functioning cortical mass** and indi**vidual renal function.** It is the most reliable method for assessing chronic cortical scarring.

IMAGING STUDIES IN CHRONIC KIDNEY DISEASE

- The most useful imaging study is a **renal ultrasound.**
- If the kidney size is normal, it is possible that the renal disease is acute or sub-acute.
- The exceptions are **diabetic nephropathy** (when kidney size is increased at the onset of diabetic nephropathy before CKD with loss of GFR supervenes), **amyloidosis, and HIV nephropathy, where kidney size may be normal in the face of CKD.**
- Polycystic kidney disease that has reached some degree of renal failure will almost always present with enlarged kidneys with multiple cysts.
- The diagnosis of renovascular disease can be undertaken with different techniques, including Doppler sonography, **nuclear medicine studies,** or CT or MRI studies.
- If there is a suspicion of reflux nephropathy (recurrent childhood urinary tract infection, asymmetric renal size with scars on the renal poles), a voiding cystogram may be indicated.
- However, **in most cases by the time the patient has CKD, the reflus has resolved, and even if still present, repair does not improve renal function.**
- **Radiographic contrast imaging studies are not particularly helpful in investigation of CKD**
- **Intravenous or intra-arterial dye should be avoided** where possible in the CKD patient, especially with diabetic nephropathy, because of the risk of radiographic contrast dye-induced renal failure.
- When unavoidable, appropriate precautionary measures include avoidance of hypovolemia at the time of contrast exposure, minimization of the dye load, and choice of radiographic contrast preparations with the least nephrotoxic potential.
- Additional measures thought to attenuate contrast-induced worsening of renal function include judicious administration of **sodium bicarbonate-containing solutions and *N*-acetyl-cysteine.**

Radionuclide techniques for studying the function of the renal tract:

Problem	Method used
Total renal function	^{51}Cr-EDTA blood clearance or total renal uptake of ^{99m}Tc-DTPA ^{99m}Tc-DMSA
Divided renal function	^{99m}Tc-DTPA uptake at 2 min or ^{99m}Tc-DMSA uptake at 3 hours
Intrarenal distribution of function	^{99m}Tc-DMSA at 3 hours, multiple views with or without SPECT

Contd.

Contd.

Differential renal blood flow	First-pass phase of ^{99m}Tc-DTPA dynamic renal scan
Renovascular hypertension	^{99m}Tc-DTPA captopril stress test
Renal transit time	^{99m}Tc-DTPA dynamic scan with deconvolution analysis
Outflow tract kinetics	^{99m}Tc-DTPA dynamic scan with furosemide washout analysis
Vesico-ureteric reflux	^{99m}Tc-DTPA dynamic scan with voiding study *(indirect)*
	^{99m}Tc-DTPA pertechnetate filling and voiding study *(direct)*
Residual urine volume	^{99m}Tc-DTPA dynamic scan with quantitative bladder emptying
Urinary tract infection	^{67}Ga-citrate or ^{111}In autologous white cell localization

DTPA (Renogram)	DMSA (Isotope scanning)
• DTPA is useful for evaluating **perfusion** and **function** of each kidney • Indications: 1. Measurement of relative renal function in each kidney. 2. Urinary tract obstruction 3. Diagnosis of renovascular cause of hypertension 4. Investigation of renal transplant	• Tc 99 DMSA is used for Renal **morphological imaging** • This compound gets fixed in renal tubules and images may be obtained after 1-2 hours of injection-Lesions such as tumors and being lesions as shown filling defect • Used to assess cortical function of kidney

Ans: (c) 99mTc DMSA scan

Ref: *Radiology Review*

7. **Half life of radioactive fluorine 18:**

(a) 110 mins
(b) 110 days
(c) 110 secs
(d) 110 hours

Explanation:

- Half life of **18F** is **110 minutes***
- Half life of **99mTc=6 hours***
- Half life of **iodine 123=13 hours***

ISOTOPES USED IN MEDICINE

- **Reactor Radioisotopes (Half life indicated within brackets)**
- **Bismuth-213 (46 min):** Used for targeted alpha therapy (TAT) as it has a high energy (8.4 MeV).
- **Chromium-51 (28 d):** Used to label red blood cells and quantify gastrointestinal protein loss.
- **Cobalt-60 (5.27 yr):** Formerly used for external beam radiotherapy.
- **Dysprosium-165 (2 h):** Used as an aggregated hydroxide for synovectomy treatment of arthritis.
- **Erbium-169 (9.4 d):** Use for relieving arthritis pain in synovial joints.
- **Holmium-166 (26 h):** Being developed for diagnosis and treatment of liver tumours.
- **Iodine-125 (60 d):** Used in cancer ***brachytherapy (prostate and brain***), also diagnostically to evaluate the ***filtration rate of kidneys*** and to diagnose ***deep vein thrombosis*** in the leg. It is also widely used in ***radioimmunoassays*** to show the presence of ***hormones*** in tiny quantities.
- **Iodine-131 (8 d):** Widely used in ***treating thyroid cancer*** and in ***imaging the thyroid***; also in diagnosis of ***abnormal liver function***, ***renal (kidney) blood flow*** and ***urinary tract obstruction***. A strong gamma emitter, but used for ***beta therapy.***
- **Iridium-192 (74 d):** Supplied in wire form for use as an ***internal radiotherapy*** source for cancer treatment (used then removed).
- **Iron-59 (46 d):** Used in studies of ***iron metabolism in the spleen***.

- **Lead-212 (10.6 h):** Used in TAT for cancers, with decay products Bi-212, Po-212, Tl-208.
- **Lutetium-177 (6.7 d):** Lu-177 is increasingly important as it emits just enough ***gamma*** for imaging while the beta radiation does the therapy on ***small (e.g., endocrine) tumours***. Its half life is long enough to allow sophisticated preparation for use.
- **Molybdenum-99 (66 h):** Used as the 'parent' in a generator to produce technetium-99m.
- **Palladium-103 (17 d):** Used to make brachytherapy permanent implant seeds for early stage ***prostate*** *cancer*.
- **Phosphorus-32 (14 d):** Used in the treatment of polycythemia vera (excess red blood cells).
- **Potassium-42 (12 h):** Used for the determination of ***exchangeable potassium in coronary blood flow.***
- **Rhenium-186 (3.8 d):** Used for ***pain relief in bone cancer***.
- **Rhenium-188 (17 h):** Used to ***beta irradiate coronary arteries*** from an ***angioplasty balloon***.
- **Samarium-153 (47 h):** Sm-153 is very effective in ***relieving the pain*** of ***secondary cancers*** lodged in the ***bone***. Also very effective for ***prostate and breast cancer***.
- **Selenium-75 (120 d):** Used in the form of selenomethionine to study the production of ***digestive enzymes.***
- **Sodium-24 (15 h):** For studies of ***electrolytes*** within the body.
- **Strontium-89 (50 d):** Very effective in reducing the pain of ***prostate and bone cancer***.
- **Technetium-99m (6 h):** Used in to image the **skeleton** and **heart muscle** in particular, but also for ***brain, thyroid, lungs (perfusion and ventilation), liver, spleen, kidney (structure and filtration rate), gall-bladder, bone marrow, salivary and lacrimal glands, heart blood pool, infection*** and numerous specialised medical studies.
- **Xenon-133 (5 d):** Used for **pulmonary** (lung) **ventilation** studies.
- **Ytterbium-169 (32 d):** Used for ***cerebrospinal fluid studies*** in the brain.
- **Yttrium-90 (64 h):** Used for ***cancer brachytherapy*** and as silicate colloid for the relieving the pain of arthritis in larger synovial joints.

CYCLOTRON RADIOISOTOPES

- **Carbon-11, Nitrogen-13, Oxygen-15, Fluorine-18: These** are **positron** emitters used in PET for studying brain physiology and pathology, in particular for localising epileptic focus, and in dementia, psychiatry and neuropharmacology studies. They also have a significant role in cardiology. ***F-18 in FDG (fluorodeoxyglucose)*** has become very important in detection of cancers and the monitoring of progress in their treatment, using PET.
- **Cobalt-57 (272 d):** Used as a marker to ***estimate organ size*** and for in-vitro diagnostic kits.
- **Copper-64 (13 h):** Used to study genetic diseases affecting ***copper metabolism***, such as **Wilson's** and **Menke's** diseases, and for PET imaging of tumours and therapy.
- **Copper-67 (2.6 d):** Beta emitter, used in therapy.
- **Fluorine-18 as FLT (fluorothymidine), F-miso (fluoromisonidazole), 18F-choline:** tracer.
- **Gallium-67 (78 h):** Used for tumour imaging and localisation of ***inflammatory lesions*** (***infections***).
- **Gallium-68 (68 min):** Positron emitter used in **PET and PET-CT** units. Derived from germanium-68 in a generator.
- **Germanium-68 (271 d):** Used as the 'parent' in a generator to produce Ga-68.
- **Indium-111 (2.8 d):** Used for specialist diagnostic studies, e.g., brain studies, infection and colon transit studies.
- **Iodine-123 (13 h):** Increasingly used for diagnosis of ***thyroid function***, it is a gamma emitter without the beta radiation of I-131.
- **Krypton-81m (13 sec) from Rubidium-81 (4.6 h):** Kr-81m gas can yield functional images of ***pulmonary ventilation***, e.g., in asthmatic patients, and for the early diagnosis of lung diseases and function.
- **Rubidium-82 (1.26 min):** Convenient **PET agent** in **myocardial perfusion** imaging.
- **Strontium-82 (25 d):** Used as the 'parent' in a generator to produce Rb-82.

- **Thallium-201 (73 h):** Used for ***diagnosis of coronary artery disease*** other heart conditions such as heart muscle death and for location of low-grade lymphomas.

Ans: (a) 110 minutes

Ref: *Radiology Review*

8. **Iodine isotope used for radio ablation of thyroid in Graves' disease is:**

(a) I-125 (b) I-123
(c) I-131 (d) I-124

Explanation:

Iodine-125

- Half life–60 days
- Commonly used in **brachytherapy** in the treatment of cancer especially in **prostate cancer**, enclosed in an implanted **titanium capsule**
- It is also widely used in **Radioimmunoassay** to show presence of **hormones** in **tiny quantities**

Iodine-123

- Half-life -13 hours
- Has **no beta activity only gamma activity**
- More suitable as nuclear imaging tracer to evaluate the anatomic and physiologic function of the **thyroid** (**thyroid scintigraphy/functional scan/radioactive iodine uptake/RAIU**)
- Abnormal results may be caused by disorders such as **Graves' disease** or **Hashimoto's thyroiditis.**
- **Tc99m pertechnetate** is also used for **functional imaging of thyroid** (used in India due to **nonavailability** of I^{123}).

Iodine-131

- Half life–8 days
- Preferred for **Radioablation of thyroid gland** in **Graves' disease** and systemic **Radiotherapy**
- Widely used for localizing and treating **thyroid cancer** and **thyroid metastasis**
- Also used in **Imaging the thyroid**
- I -131 has **both a beta and gamma decay**
- Destruction of thyroid tissue by Iodine -131 is due to emission of **Beta Rays**
- Iodine -131 is also used in **tissue targeting** radiopharmaceutical agents such as **MIBG**.
- The high energy **beta radiation** from I-131 causes it to be the **most carcinogenic** of the **iodine isotopes.**

Iodine-124

- Iodine-124 is a proton-rich isotope of iodine.
- Half life-4.18 days.
- Its modes of decay are: 74.4% electron capture, 25.6% positron emission.
- Iodine-124 can be made by numerous nuclear reactions via a **cyclotron**.
- Iodine-124 as the **iodide salt** can be used to directly **image** the **thyroid** using **positron emission tomography (PET).**

	I^{125}	I^{131}	I^{123}	I^{124}
t1/2	60 days	8 days	13 hours	4.2 days
Emission	Gamma	Gamma	Gamma	Gamma
Energy	35keV	364 keV	159 keV	606 keV
Use	RIA	Imaging/ablation	Imaging e.g. MIBG	PET imaging
Relatively long half life and low energy photon emission are main criteria for preference towards I^{125} for Radio-immunoassay				

Ans: (c) I-131

Ref: *Magdy Khalil, Basic Sciences of Nuclear Medicine, Page 34*

9. Mushroom cap sign in MRI is seen in:

(a) Ileocaecal TB
(b) Pulmonary endometriosis
(c) Ovarian endometriosis
(d) Rectal endometriosis

Ans: (d) Rectal Endometriosis

Explanation:

- **Mushroom cap sign** is an important signs of deep **rectosigmoid endometriosis** seen on T2 weighted MRI sequence. It indicates the **submucosal involvement** in rectosigmoid region.
- Heterogeneous low signal intensity of the hypertrophic muscularis propria, covered with high signal intensity of the mucosa and submucosa on T2-weighted MR images, looked like a "**mushroom cap"** with the pattern of intraluminal endophytic growth.

10. Investigation not useful in myeloma:

(a) MRI
(b) Bone scan
(c) PET
(d) Low dose CT

Explanation:

MULTIPLE MYELOMA

- Most common primary malignant bone neoplasm in adults.
- It arises from red marrow due to monoclonal proliferation of plasma cells and manifests in a wide range of radiographic abnormalities.
- Four main patterns are recognised:
  - **Disseminated form**: Multiple well-defined "punched out" lytic lesions: predominantly affecting the axial skeleton
  - **Disseminated form: Diffuse skeletal osteopenia**
  - **Solitary plasmacytoma:** A single large/expansile lesion most commonly in a vertebral body or in the pelvis
  - *Osteosclerosing myeloma*

Radiographic Features

- Numerous, well-circumscribed, lytic bone lesions (more common)
  - Punched out lucencies
    - **Raindrop skull***
  - Endosteal scalloping
- Generalised osteopenia (less common)
  - Often associated with vertebral compression fractures/vertebra plana
- **Plain radiograph**
  - A skeletal survey is essential not only for the diagnosis of multiple myeloma but also in pre-emptying potential complications (e.g., pathological fracture) and assessing response to therapy. A typical skeletal survey consists of the following films.
  - The vast majority of lesions are **purely lytic, sharply defined/punched out**, with **Endosteal scalloping** when abutting the cortex.
- **CT**
  - Does **NOT** have a major role in the diagnosis of disseminated multiple myeloma; however, it may be useful for determining the extent of the extraosseous soft tissue component in patients with a large disease burden.
  - It may also better assess the risk of fracture in severely affected bones.
- **MRI**
  - MRI is generally **more sensitive** in detecting **multiple lesions** compared to the standard plain film skeletal survey.
  - Infiltration and replacement of bone marrow are exquisitely visualised, and newer scanners are able to perform whole body MRI scans for this purpose, shown to be superior to both CT and skeletal surveys.

- **Bone Scan**
  - o Bone scintigraphy appearance of patients with disseminated multiple myeloma is **variable** due to the potential lack of osteoblastic activity. Bone scans may also be **normal**. Therefore, bone scans usually do **NOT** contribute significant information to the workup of patients with suspected or established disseminated multiple myeloma.
- **PET Scan**
  - o PET-CT has had a growing role in the management of this disease, as it is effective in identifying the distribution of disease.
  - o **^{18}F-FDG uptake** by the myeloma lesions corresponds to areas of **bone lysis** seen on CT.

Ans: (b) Bone scan

Ref: *Radiology Review*

11. MUGA scan not useful in:

(a) Left ventricular ejection fraction
(b) Regional wall motion
(c) Regional wall perfusion
(d) Stroke volume

Explanation:

MUGA scan (multigated acquisition scan) is used to detect **ventricular function, ejection fraction, stroke volume or regional wall motion**

- **Myocardial Necrosis** is best demonstrated by **Tc99m Pyrophosphate**.
- Tc 99m pyrophosphate binds to the calcium released at the site of necrosis and gives the area of infarct as HOT uptake.
- **Thallium 201, Tc99m Tetrofosmin and Tc99m Pyrophosphate** are used for detecting **myocardial** perfusion and the area of infarct appears cold on **perfusion imaging**.

Ans: (c) Regional wall perfusion

Ref: *Radiology Review*

PSYCHIATRY

1. **Analeptics will:**

(a) Depress CNS (b) Stimulate CNS
(c) Causes seizures (d) Control seizures

Explanation:

ANALEPTICS

- Analeptic drugs are basically **CNS stimulants***.
- They also stimulate respiration by neural and other mechanisms.
- They are grouped based on their mechanism of action:
  - o **Serotonin receptor agonists** – *Buspirone*
  - o **AMPA agonists** – *Ampakines* (under trial)
  - o **Adenosine antagonists** – *Caffeine* (Methylxanthines)
  - o **Potassium channel blockers** – *Doxapram*
- **Uses:**
  - o Serotonin receptor agonists – **Depression***
  - o AMPA agonists – Used for research purposes
  - o Adenosine antagonists – **Bronchodilator** (Respiratory distress syndrome, Reactive airway disease)
  - o Potassium channel blockers – **Reversal of respiratory depression** *(Following anesthesia, drug overdose, neonatal apnea, respiratory failure etc.)*
- **Side Effects:**
  - o Excessive CNS stimulation → Irritability, anxiety, tremors, palpitations, seizures, insomnia, elevated pulse and BP.

Ans: (b) Stimulate CNS

Ref: *Kaplan and Sadock's Comprehensive Textbook of Psychiatry, 10th edition*

2. **Drug of choice for treating Attention Deficit Hyperactivity Disorder (ADHD) in a 6-year-old boy whose father has a history of substance abuse:**

(a) Methylphenidate (b) Atomoxetine
(c) Clonidine (d) Dexamphetamine

Ans: (b) Atomoxetine

Ref: *Stahl's Essential Psychopharmacology, 4th edition*

Explanation:

Treatment for ADHD

A. **Pharmacotherapy:** (Note: *Drugs reserved till 6 years of age*)
  - Three types of drugs used currently:

Stimulants (Amphetamines, Methylphenidate)

- They are **first-line** drugs
- They act by several mechanisms which ultimately end up in **enhancing monoamine actions**
- Most importantly **catecholamine** (epinephrine, norepinephrine) and **dopamine** are enhanced
- Complications: Seizures, Psychosis, Dependence
- *Hence contraindicated if a person is having/had/family history of these conditions*

Atomoxetine

- It is a **Norepinephrine reuptake inhibitor (NRI)**
- It *has no side effect profile like amphetamines.*

- Hence, useful when in conditions where stimulants are contraindicated.
- Contraindicated in **hypertension, arrhythmias, pheochromocytoma**
- It is useful in **adults** also.

Clonidine

- It improves attention by **increasing noradrenergic tone** in **locus coeruleus** and **prefrontal cortex** (binding to **postsynaptic α2A adrenergic receptors**)
- It controls hyperactivity by **suppressing sympathetic outflow**.

B. Psychotherapy

a. Behavior therapy (Positive reinforcement)
b. Neurofeedback

3. Least common conduct disorder seen in girls:

(a) Run away from home
(b) High risk sexual behavior
(c) Aggressive behavior involvement with law/antisocial
(d) Emotional bullying

Explanation:

- Behaviors which are disturbing to others are common in childhood.
- In this group, *the characteristic psychopathology is the behaviour(s) itself*.

Following three disorders included:

- Attention deficit hyperactive disorder
- Oppositional defiant disorder
- Conduct disorder

Attention deficit hyperactive disorder (ADHD) is characterized by:

- Poor attention, Hyperactivity and Impulsivity.

Oppositional Defiant Disorder (ODD)

- Features of **ADHD** may be present
- Plus, they **do *opposite*** of what being told and don't follow rules [*defiant*]
- Behavior mostly restricted in the **family** itself

Conduct Disorder (CD)

- Features of **ODD** may be present
- PLUS
  - **Cruelty to other children**/animals
  - **Aggression**
  - Emotional bullying
  - **Lying, stealing**
  - **School truancy**
  - Running away from home
  - Risk-taking behavior like sexual promiscuity
  - Speed driving
  - Engaging in dangerous sports/games
- Good number of CD children goes on to develop **Antisocial personality disorder (ASPD)** in adulthood.

Gender Differences of ODD/CD:

- **Boys** will present with more of **externalizing behavior**, like **aggression** to others, involvement with **law/police.**
- **Girls** will have more **internalizing problems**, like **suicide attempts**, **illegal relationships** etc.

Rx for ODD and CD (Juvenile delinquency):

- Behavior therapy (Contingency Management).

Ans: (c) Aggressive behavior involvement with law/antisocial

Ref: 1. Keenan K, Loeber R, Green S, Conduct Disorder in Girls: A Review of the Literature, Clin Child Fam Psychol Rev 1999, 2: Page 3-19
2. Zahn-Waxler C, Shirtcliff EA, Marceau K, Disorders of Childhood and Adolescence: Gender and Psychopathology, Annu Rev Clin Psychol, 2008, 4, Page 275-303

4. **Biological marker for antisocial behaviour in boys:**

(a) Low serum testosterone
(b) Low resting pulse rate
(c) Increased urinary dopamine levels
(d) Shortened REM latency

Explanation:

- A **biological marker** (or simply biomarker) is a *measurable indicator* of any biological state or condition. Biomarkers are useful to examine normal biological processes, pathological processes, or responses to any intervention.
- Human behavior is due to neuro-humoral mechanism (Neurological and Endocrine). Hence, chemicals (neurotransmitters, hormones), neurological responses, anatomical changes of brain can be used as biomarkers of behavior.

Antisocial Behavior

- **Antisocial behavior** is any behavior which is harmful to others. This may range from **lying** to **killing**. *The harm may be directed towards an individual or group of individuals or an institution or property*. A person or a group of people (gang) can indulge in anti-social behavior.
- It is seen in following disorders:
  - Its characteristic of **antisocial personality disorder (ASPD)**
  - **Disruptive behavior disorders** (ADHD, Oppositional defiant disorder, Conduct disorder). Note, some of them may go on to develop ASPD in future
  - Harm to others can occur in **delirium** (altered consciousness); **dementia** (memory impairment); **substance intoxication / withdrawal**; **mania/hypomania** (irritable mood)
- **Biomarkers** of **antisocial behavior** are divided into:
  - **Positive correlation**: Testosterone (well proven marker)
  - **Negative correlation**: Pulse rate (resting)
  - **Unclear**: Dopamine and Serotonin (and their metabolites level)
- Currently, **hyperdopaminergia and hyposerotonin** in brain are implicated with higher level of aggression and antisocial behavior. This is reflected in level of metabolites in CSF/urine of these neurotransmitters **(High HVA – for Dopamine; Low 5-HIAA–for Serotonin)**
- From a common sense point of view, antisocial behavior people have no/low empathy/sympathy; hence they sleep well even after crime (no shortening of REM latency) don't feel anxious/remorse (no sympathetic stimulation while doing crime/post crime – low pulse rate).

Ans: (b) Low resting pulse rate

Ref: 1. Valencia M, Arias JMC, Potential Biomarkers in Personality Disorders: Current State and Future Research, International Journal of Psychological Research 2016; 9(1): 98-112
2. Sjoberg, R.L., et al. A Non-additive Interaction of a Functional MAO-A VNTR and Testosterone Predicts Antisocial Behavior, Neuropsychopharmacology 2007; 33: 425-430
3. Todd A, et al. Low Resting Heart Rate and Antisocial Behavior: A Brief Review of Evidence and Preliminary Results from a New Test, Criminal Justice and Behavior 2009; 36(11): 1125-1140
4. Herbert C. Quay, Anne E. Hogan, Handbook of Disruptive Behavior Disorders, 1st edition, 1999

5. **According to Faulk classification, the husband battered wife syndrome is common in:**

(a) Dependent but suspicious husband
(b) Normal quiet husband
(c) Dependent active
(d) Dependent passive

Explanation:

- Violence between any two "individuals" who are related / or in a relationship denote.
  - **Abuse** (act of commission)
  - **Neglect** (act of omission).

- Types of **abuses / neglect:**
  - *Emotional* abuse / neglect
  - *Physical* abuse / neglect
  - *Sexual* abuse / neglect
- **Family** is the **unit of society. Marital (domestic) violence** is a **medico-legal** problem.
- **Battered person syndrome** is a condition where a **person** suffers **abuse** from **another person.**
- **Victims** - persons who are **dependent** on others **like wives, children and elderly.**
- **Perpetrators** - usually **males (spouse**), or **females (in case of children**).
- Typically **husband abuses wife (battered wife syndrome)** and **wife abuses children** (displacement - defense mechanism) - **battered baby syndrome.**
- Several studies were carried out to identify the characteristics of people who batter.
- **Faulk**, in 1974 published a paper classifying persons who abuse others.
- According to **Faulk**, there are **five types of men in a relationship:**
  - **Stable / affectionate**
  - **Dominating**
  - **Violent / bullying**
  - **Dependent passive**
  - **Dependent suspicious**
- **Battering** happens in all but **frequency and intensity varies**.
- **Least common** with men who are **stable and affectionate.**
- **Dominating** husband wants to **control wife.**
- **Bullying husband** uses violent methods even for trivial problems.
- **Dependent passive** man tries to **please wife** and **battering is less common**.
- **Dependent but suspicious** man is jealous hence **abuse wife more.**
- **Battered wife syndrome** logically comes under stress related disorders in ICD-10 (**Adjustment disorder, acute stress disorder, PTSD).**
- **Battered wife experiences**
  - **Depression**
  - **Fear** (not only with spouse but also with others)
  - Dislike her body, aversion towards sex
  - Belief that spouse is **omnipotent** (and she can't escape/others can't help).
- **Battered baby syndrome** is characterized by:
  - **Retinal bleed**
  - **Fractures**
  - **Soft tissue injuries**
  - **Subdural hematoma**
  - Cannot be explained by accidental trauma or other medical conditions.
- **Head injury** might be due to **violent shaking** *(syn. shaken baby syndrome/abusive head trauma).*
- **Head injury in BBS** result in **subdural hematoma, retinal bleeding even brain tissue damage (diffuse axonal injury) without other injuries.**
- **Long bone fractures** are multiple in **BBS** exhibit different healing stages (indicating chronic abuse), without corresponding external injury.
- **Domestic violence in India–Legal issues.**
- **Protection of Women from Domestic Violence Act, 2005** defines domestic violence and protects (women) victims.
  - It is a **civil law**, i.e., it **doesn't meant for *penalizing the perpetrator*** *(which is described in Section **498A** in The Indian Penal Code)*
  - **Patriarchal social structure and Dowry system** are believed to be causative dynamics behind violence against women in India.
- **Sexual Harassment of Women at Workplace** (Prevention, Prohibition and Redressal) Act came into force in **2013.**
  - **Sec. 354** of the Indian Penal Code describes **sexual harassment offence** and penalties shall be for a man committing such an offence.

Ans: (a) Dependent but suspicious husband

Ref: *Faulk M. (1974, July), Men Who Assault Their Wives, Medicine, Science and the Law, Page 180-183*

JIPMER–NOVEMBER 2017

ANATOMY

1. **Uncinate process of ethmoid attached anteriorly to:**

(a) Sphenoid
(b) Ethmoid
(c) Frontal
(d) Lacrimal bone

Explanation:

Uncinate Process

- Is a thin, hook like structure projecting downward and backward from the ***middle concha of ethmoid bone*** and joins with ethmoidal process of inferior nasal concha.
- Its posterosuperior margin is free, forming the ***hiatus semilunaris.***
- It is related anteriorly the descending process of ***lacrimal bone.***
- It is frequently removed during **sinus surgery.**

Parts of Ethmoid Bone

(a) ***Cribriform plate*** (crista galli)-horizontally aligned.
(b) ***Perpendicular plate.***
(c) ***Two lateral labrynth*** (superior and middle concha).
  - Agger nasi is a projection in the middle concha (contains anterior ethmoid air cells).

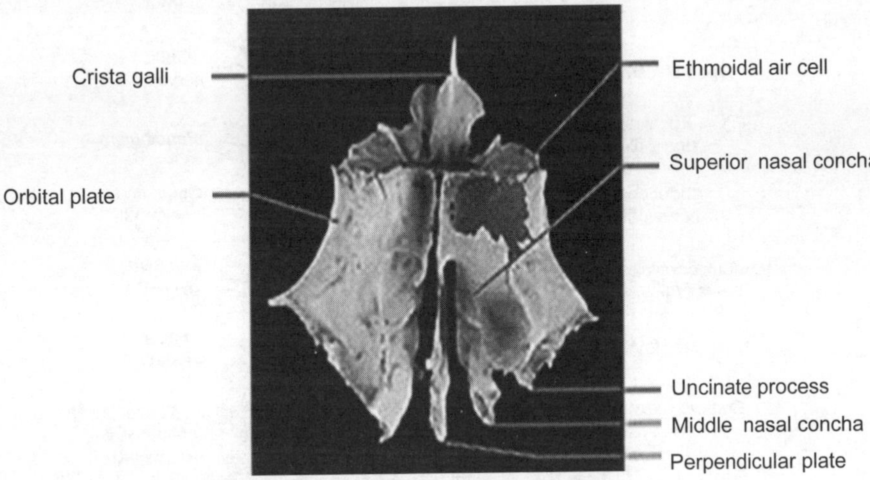

Ans: (d) Lacrimal bone

Ref: Gray's Anatomy, The Anatomical Basis of Clinical Practice, 41st edition, 2016, page 480 & 481

2. **Cranial nerve emerging between pyramidal and olive eminence is:**

(a) 6th CN
(b) 7th CN
(c) 11th CN
(d) 12th CN

Explanation:

- ***Pyramid:*** A prominent elongated ridge, which contains descending corticospinal axons, that lies immediately lateral to the ventral median fissure.
- ***Olive:*** Lateral to the pyramid and the ventrolateral sulcus is an oval prominence, which contains the inferior olivary nuclear complex.
- The lateral margin of the pyramid is indicated by a shallow ventrolateral sulcus. A linear series of rootlets forming the ***hypoglossal nerve*** emerge from this sulcus.

Exit of cranial nerve from the base of brain:

Cranial nerve	**Superficial origin at the base of brain**
1-Olfactory	Orbital gyri (inferior surface of frontal lobe)
2-Optic	Optic chiasma in front of infundibulum of pituitary gland
3-Oculomotor	Medial side of cerebral peduncle
4-Trochlear	Dorsal surface of midbrain below inferior colliculus [winds round the sides of cerebral peduncle and appear in the ventral surface of brain] **Note:** ***The only cranial nerve emerging from the dorsal surface of brain***
5-Trigeminal	Ventral surface of pons. Junction between pons and middle cerebellar peduncle
6-Abducent	Lower border of pons at its junction with pyramid
7-Facial	Lower border of pons between the olive and inferior cerebellar peduncle
8-Vestibulocochlear	Junction of pons and medulla behind and lateral to facial nerve
9-Glossopharyngeal	Medulla, upper part of posterolateral sulcus (lateral side of olive)
10-Vagus	Medulla, posterolateral sulcus below the 9th nerve (lateral side of olive)
11-Accessory	Medulla, posterolateral sulcus below the 10th nerve
12-Hypoglossal	Medulla, ventrolateral sulcus between pyramid and olive

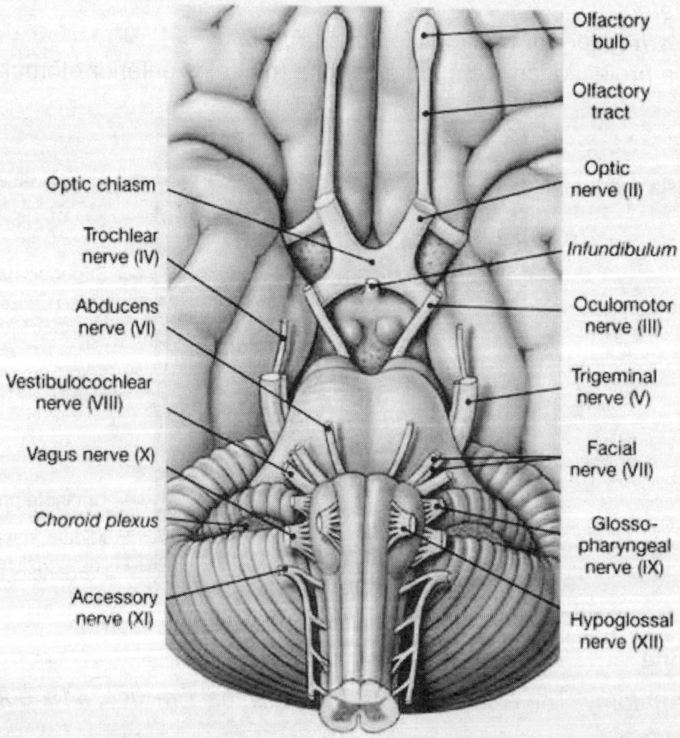

Ans: (d) 12th CN

Ref: Gray's Anatomy, The Anatomical Basis of Clinical Practice, 41st edition, 2016, page 311

3. **Primitive streak develops from:**

(a) Mesoderm
(b) Epiblast
(c) Hypoblast
(d) Neural plate

Explanation:

Primitive Streak

- Appears about ***15th day*** of development.
- Formed by active migration and invagination of ***pleuripotent ectodermal cells*** (***epiblast***) into the space between epiblast and hypoblast.
- ***Gastrulation****–The process of invagination of pleuripotent cells in between epiblast and hypoblast.
- **Primitive streak** acts as ***primary organizer*** – Induces the differentiation of notochord and intraembryonic mesoderm.
- **Primitive streak** from its cranial end gives origin to definitive ***notochord***–forerunner in the development of vertebral column.
- Notochordal cells persist as ***nucleus pulposus*** in the center of intervertebral disc.
- Primitive streak ***disappears at 26th day*** of development.
- If persist gives the development of ***sacrococcygeal teratoma.***

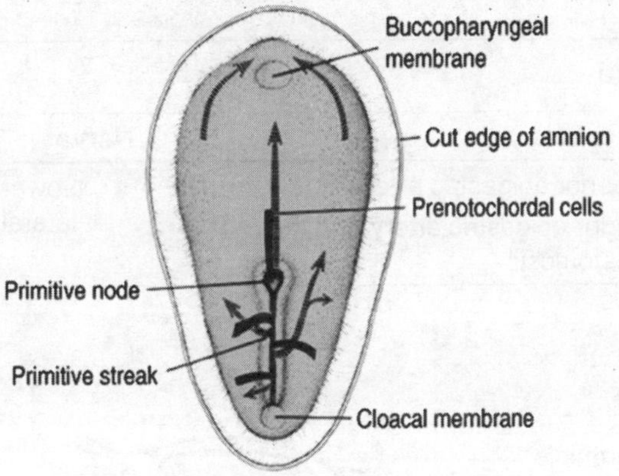

Ans: (b) Epiblast

Ref: Essentials of Human Embryology, A.K. Datta, 5th edition, 2005, page 38-42

4. **Trophoblast gives rise to all the following *except*:**

(a) Cytotrophoblast
(b) Syncytiotrophoblast
(c) Intra-embryonic mesoderm
(d) Extra-embryonic mesoderm

Explanation:

The outer cell mass of blastocoele developed into trophoblast.

Derivatives of Outer Cell Mass (Trophoblast)

(a) Cytotrophoblast.
(b) Syncytiotrophoblast.
(c) Placenta.
(d) Extra-embryonic mesoderm.

- **Intra-embryonic mesoderm or secondary mesoderm** – developed from primitive streak [cells from the sides of the primitive streak actively proliferate and migrate between ectodermal and endodermal layers of germ disc].

Ans: (c) Intra-embryonic mesoderm

Ref: Essentials of Human Embryology, A.K.Datta, 5th edition, 2005, page 34-42

5. **Rectus sheath is formed by:**

(a) External and internal oblique aponeurosis
(b) External, internal oblique and transverse abdominis aponeurosis
(c) Internal oblique and transverse abdominis aponeurosis
(d) Internal oblique, transverse abdominis aponeurosis and transversalis fascia

Explanation:

Formation of rectus sheath:

Region	Anterior wall	Posterior wall
I-Upper [above the costal margin]	External oblique aponeurosis	Deficit – Rectus muscle rests directly on 5,6,7th costal cartilage
II-Middle [from the costal margin to the level of anterior superior iliac spine]	External oblique and anterior lamina of internal oblique aponeurosis	Posterior lamina of internal oblique and transverse abdominis aponeurosis
III-Lower [below the region II]	External oblique, internal oblique and transverse abdominis aponeurosis	Deficit – Fascia transversalis alone
Note: Only in region II–Middle, internal oblique aponeurosis divides into an anterior and posterior lamina to enclose rectus abdominis muscle.		

Contents of Rectus sheath

Muscles	Blood vessels	Nerves
• Rectus abdominis • Pyramidalis	• Superior epigastric artery • Inferior epigastric artery and their anastomosis	• Lower 6th intercostal nerves (entering from lateral margin)

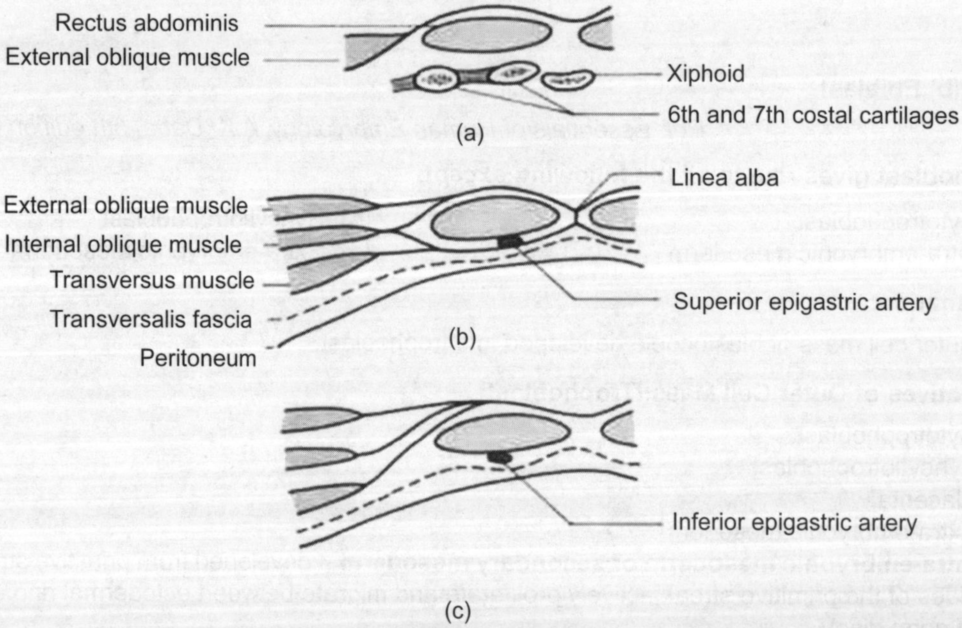

Ans: (b) External, internal oblique and transverse abdominis aponeurosis

Ref: Human Anatomy, Regional and Applied, BD Chaurasia's, Vol.2, 4th edition, 2006, page 205 & 206

6. **Which of the following structures is not derived from mesoderm?**

(a) Suprarenal medulla
(b) Renal cortex
(c) Cardiac musculature
(d) Skeletal musculature

Explanation:

Derivatives of Ectoderm, Mesoderm and Endoderm:

Ectoderm *(surface ectoderm and neuroectoderm)*	**Mesoderm**	**Endoderm**
• Central nervous system • Peripheral nervous system • Sensory epithelia of the eye, ear and nose • Epidermis and its appendages (hair and nails) • Mammary glands • Pituitary gland • Subcutaneous glands • Enamel of teeth • Neural crest cells, derived from neuroectoderm, give rise to the cells of the spinal, cranial (cranial nerves V, VII, IX and X), and autonomic ganglia • Ensheathing cells of the peripheral nervous system • Pigment cells of the dermis • Muscle • Connective tissues • Bone of pharyngeal arch origin • ***Suprarenal medulla*** • Meninges (coverings) of the brain and spinal cord	• Connective tissue • Cartilage • Bone • Striated muscles • Smooth muscles • Heart • Blood vessels • Lymphatic vessels • Kidneys • Ovaries • Testes • Genital ducts • Serous membranes lining the body cavities (pericardial, pleural and peritoneal) • Spleen • Cortex of suprarenal glands	• Epithelial lining of the gastrointestinal and respiratory tracts • Parenchyma of the tonsils • Thyroid and parathyroid glands • Thymus • Liver • Pancreas • Epithelial lining of the urinary bladder and most of the urethra • Epithelial lining of the tympanic cavity • Tympanic antrum • Pharyngotympanic (auditory) tube

Derivatives of Neural Crest Cells

• Connective tissue and bones of the face and the skull • Cranial nerve ganglia • C cells of the thyroid gland • Conotruncal septum in the heart • Odontoblasts • Dermis in the face and neck	• Dorsal root ganglia • Sympathetic ganglia • Parasympathetic ganglia of the G.I.T. • ***Adrenal medulla*** • Schwann cells • Leptomeninges • Melanocytes

Ans: (a) Suprarenal medulla

Ref: Langman's Medical Embryology, T.W. Sadler, 13th edition, 2016, page 112-114

7. **Blood supply of hippocampus:**

(a) Anterior choroidal artery
(b) Medial striate artery from middle cerebral artery
(c) Lateral striate artery from middle cerebral artery
(d) Anterior cerebral artery

Explanation:

Anterior Choroidal Artery

- ***Arises*** from **internal carotid artery.**
- Undergoes long subarachnoid course and enters the inferior horn of lateral ventricle where hippocampus is located.
- Supplies ***hippocampus*.***
- It also supplies:
  - o ***Optic tract, uncus, amygdala, globus pallidus.***
  - o ***Lateral geniculate body.***
  - o ***Posterior limb and retrolentiform part of internal capsule.***

Ans: (a) Anterior choroidal artery

Ref: Essentials of Neuroanatomy, A.K. Datta, 3rd edition, 2007, page 176

8. **All are true regarding trachea *except*:**

(a) C shaped cartilages
(b) Outer diameter is 20 mm
(c) More than 20 hyaline cartilages
(d) Isthmus of thyroid gland related at 2, 3, 4th tracheal rings

Explanation:

TRACHEA

- *Length of trachea is* ***10-11 cm.***
- ***Diameter: External transverse diameter*** is typically **2 cm in adult males and 1.5 cm in adult females.**
- Mean transverse diameter is greater than anteroposterior diameter up to the age of 6 years, after that **the two diameters are nearly equal.**
- ***Internal transverse diameter*** (lumen) is about ***12 mm.***
- In the first postnatal year, the tracheal diameter does not exceed 4 mm.
- The **second to fourth tracheal cartilages** are crossed by the **isthmus** of the thyroid gland.
- Trachea is lined by **respiratory epithelium,** i.e., **ciliated pseudostratified columnar epithelium with more number of goblet cells.**
- ***Extent:*** Trachea extends from the level of **C6 (Cricoid cartilage) to the upper border of T5** (Just below the sternal angle). At T5 it divides into right and left principal bronchi.
- ***Structure:*** Wall is made up of cartilage and fibromuscular membrane.
- **Tracheal rings** are varies from **16-20** in number. Consists of ***16–20 "C" shaped incomplete rings of hyaline cartilage*** and intervening fibroelastic tissue.
  - o ***Isthmus of thyroid gland*** related at ***2, 3, 4th tracheal rings.***

Ans: (c) More than 20 hyaline cartilages

Ref: Gray's Anatomy, The Anatomical Basis of Clinical Practice, 41st edition, 2016, page 965 & 966

Version – 2

True regarding trachea is:

(a) Consists of 12 incomplete rings of cartilage
(b) 15 cm long in the adult
(c) Lined by nonciliated pseudostratified columnar epithelium
(d) 2nd, 3rd and 4th tracheal rings are related with isthmus of thyroid.

Ans: (d) 2nd, 3rd and 4th tracheal rings are related with isthmus of thyroid

Ref: The Anatomical Basis of Clinical Practice, 39th edition, 2008, page1076

9. **Upper covering layer of cochlear duct is:**

(a) Tectorial membrane
(b) Basilar membrane
(c) Stria vascularis
(d) Vestibular membrane

Explanation:

Cochlear Duct (Scala Media)

- **Boundaries:** Bounded by the following structures.
  - o Medially by **vestibular or Reissner's membrane.**
  - o Laterally by **stria vascularis.**
  - o Below by the **tympanic lip of the osseous spiral lamina** in the medial part and **basilar membrane** in the lateral part.
- **Basilar membrane** is subdivided into a:
  - o Lateral part (**zona pectinata**).
  - o Medial part (**zona arcuata**) upon which rests the organ of Corti.
- Projecting free edge of osseous spiral lamina has 2 lips:
  - o **Tympanic lip** which gives attachment to basilar membrane.
  - o **Vestibular lip** which gives attachment to tectorial membrane. [**Note:** Vestibular membrane attached to somewhat away from the tip of vestibular lip.]
- **Tectorial membrane**
  - o Acellular protein rich fibrillated gelatinous structure.
  - o Attached to the **vestibular lip of osseous lamina.**
  - o Covers the stereocilia of the inner and outer hair cells.
- **Vestibular or Reissner's membrane** - separates the scala media from scala vestibule.
- **Basilar membrane** - separates the scala media from scala tympani.

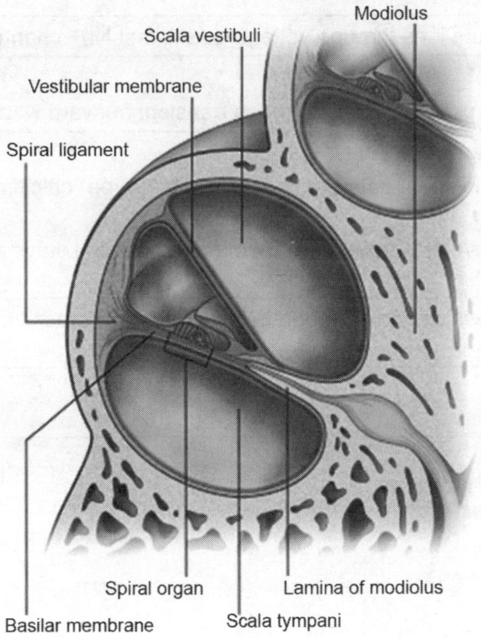

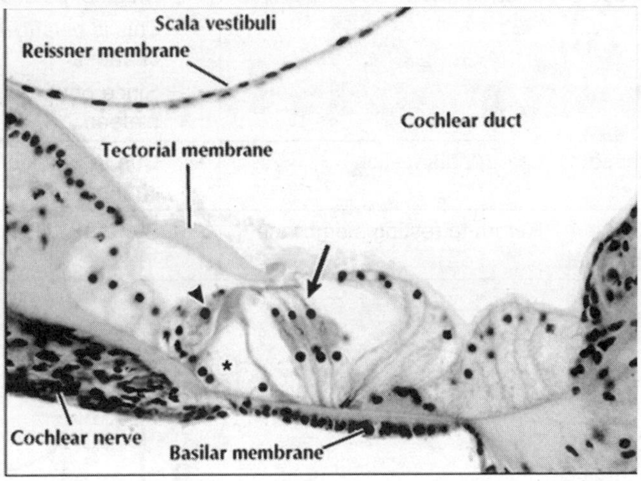

Ans: (a) Tectorial membrane

Ref: Essentials of Human Anatomy, Head and Neck, Vol.2, A.K. Datta, 3rd edition, 2003, page 353-355

PHYSIOLOGY

1. **Long acting calcium channel act in which part of action potential?**
   (a) 0 (b) 1 (c) 2 (d) 3

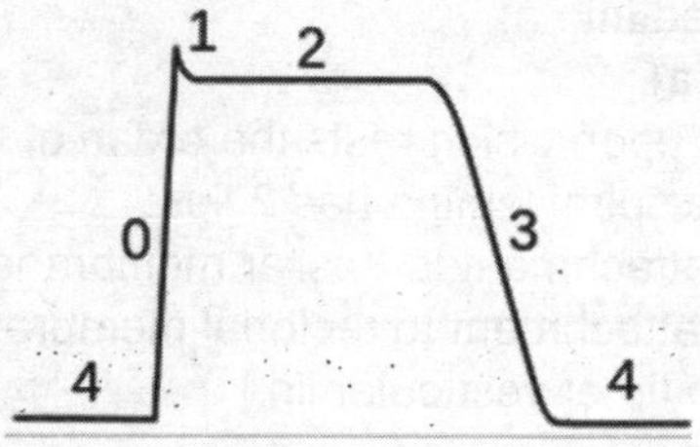

Explanation:

Ventricular Action Potential

- Ventricular action potential has five phases. They are:

Phases	Ions responsible
Phase 0 – Rapid depolarization	• Due to entry of sodium ions through voltage-gated, fast Na+ channels
Phase 1 – Initial repolarization	• Due to inactivation of fast Na+ channels • Also due to efflux of potassium ions through transient outward K^+ channels
Phase 2–Plateau phase	• Efflux of potassium ions continue • This is balanced by influx of **calcium ions** through (L-type) calcium channels • Since both are positively charged ions, membrane potential stays as plateau
Phase 3 – Late repolarization	• Due to Efflux of potassium ions through delayed rectifier potassium channels
Phase 4 – Return to resting membrane potential	• By Na K ATPase

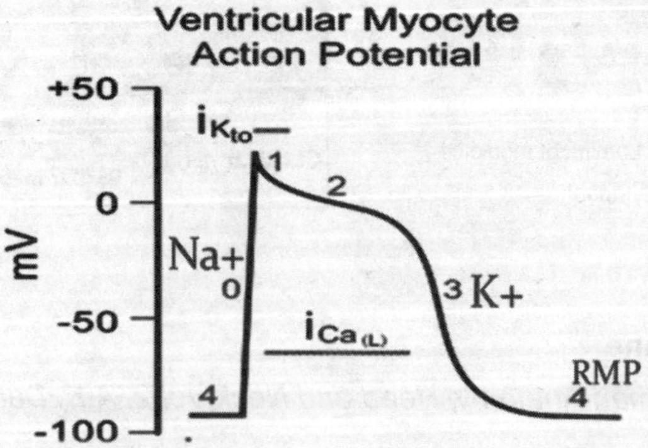

Ans: (c) 2

Ref: Ganong, 25th edition, page 521

2. **True regarding peripheral chemoreceptor:**
   (a) Sensitive to hypoxia (b) Sensitive to central PCO_2
   (c) Sensitive to pH (d) None of the above

Explanation:

Mechanism of Peripheral Chemoreceptor Stimulation

- Whenever there is **low PO_2 (hypoxia),** O_2-sensitive **K^+ channels** in **glomus cells** close.
- Accumulation of **K^+** inside the glomus cells leads to a state of **depolarization.**
- Such depolarization open calcium channels leading to **calcium influx.**
- Influx of calcium causes release of the neurotransmitter **dopamine** which stimulates the afferent nerve endings.
- Once stimulated, peripheral chemoreceptors produces:
  - o ***Hyperpnea.***
  - o ***Bronchoconstriction*.***
  - o ***Dilation of the upper airway.***
  - o ***Increased blood pressure*.***
  - o ***Tachycardia*.***

Ans : (a) Sensitive to hypoxia

Ref: *Ganong, 25th edition, page 521*

3. **Which factor is not freely circulating in blood?**

(a) Factor 9 (b) Factor 10 (c) Factor 12 (d) Factor 3

Explanation:

- Coagulation factor III is a cell surface glycoprotein. This factor enables cells to initiate the blood coagulation cascades, and it functions as the high-affinity receptor for the coagulation factor VII.
- **Clotting factors.**

Clotting factors		
Factor	**Name**	**Deficiency leads to**
I	Fibrinogen	Afbrinogenemia
II	Prothrombin	Hypoprothrombinemia (hemorrhagic tendency in liver disease)
III	Thromboplastin	**Only coagulation factor not found in the plasma***
IV	Calcium	
V	Proaccelerin, labile factor	Parahemophilia
VII	Proconvertin, stable factor	Hypoconvertinemia
VIII	Antihemophilic factor (AHF), antihemophilic factor A	Hemophilia A (classic hemophilia)
IX	Plasma thromboplastic component (PTC), Christmas factor, antihemophilic factor B	Hemophilia B (Christmas disease)
X	Stuart-Prower factor	Stuart-Prower factor deficiency
XI	Plasma thromboplastin antecedent (PTA), antihemophilic factor C	PTA deficiency
XII	Hageman factor, glass factor	Hageman trait
XIII	Fibrin-stabilizing factor, Laki-Lorand factor	Abnormal clot solubility

Ans: (d) Factor 3

Ref: *Ganong, 25th edition, page 575*

4. Actions of GLP are all *except*:

(a) Increases insulin release
(b) Decreases glucagon release
(c) Increases gastric emptying
(d) Reduces appetite

Explanation:

The Main Actions of GLP-1 are:

- ***Stimulate insulin secretion*** (i.e., to act as an incretin hormone).
- ***Inhibit glucagon secretion.***
  (Limits postprandial glucose excursions)
- ***Inhibits gastrointestinal motility*** and secretion.
  Thus, acts as an **"enterogastrone"** and a part of the **"ileal brake"** mechanism.
  (GLP-1 ***decreases gastrointestinal motility*** *via direct inhibitory effects on gastric/intestinal smooth muscle and also inhibits postprandial acid secretion).*
- GLP-1 also appears to be a physiological regulator of **appetite and food intake**.
- It **induces satiety**, **reduces food intake** hence leading to **reduced weight gain.**
- **Recent discovery:** (b) is able to **promote β-cell mass expansion.**

Hence, the correct option would be option (c).

The properties of GLP-1 described above, including glucose-dependent stimulation of insulin secretion and expansion of β-cell mass, coupled with the inhibition of glucagon secretion and food intake, suggest that it would greatly complement current β-cell therapies.

Also Note:

Synthesis of GLP:

- Formed in L cells of lower GIT.
- Secreted as **Preproglucagon**.
- Human **preproglucagon:** Found in **pancreatic A cells**, in **L cells** in the lower gastrointestinal tract and brain.
- It is the product of a single mRNA, but it is *processed differently in different tissues.*
- **Pancreatic A cells:** Processed to **glucagon, major proglucagon fragment (MPGF)** and residual **glicentin-related polypeptide (GRPP).**
- **Intestinal L cells:** Processed to **glicentin, glucagon-like polypeptides 1 and 2 (GLP-1** and **GLP-2)**, residual **glicentin-related polypeptide (GRPP)** and some **oxyntomodulin** is also formed.
- **Levels of GLP rise after food intake.** Principally sugars and fats release GLP.

Ans: (c) Increases gastric emptying

Ref: Ganong's Review of Medical Physiology, 25th edition, page 442/Physiol Rev. 2007; 87(4):1409-39/ Patrick E. et al. Diabetes 2002 Dec; 51(suppl 3): S434-S442

5. A 60-year-old patient, known case of hypertension for the past 25 years underwent renal artery Doppler which showed narrowing and turbulence in right renal artery. If radius of artery is reduced by one-third, resistance increases by _____.

(a) 3 times
(b) 9 times
(c) 25 times
(d) 81 times

Explanation:

Determinants of Resistance to Flow (Poiseuille's Equation)

- There are three primary factors that determine the **resistance to blood flow** within a single vessel:
  - ***Vessel diameter (or radius*).***
  - ***Vessel length*.***
  - ***Viscosity of the blood*.***
- Of these three factors, the most important quantitatively and physiologically is **vessel diameter.**
- **Vessel diameter** changes because of **contraction** and **relaxation** of the **vascular smooth muscle** in the wall of the blood vessel.

- Very small changes in vessel diameter lead to **large changes in resistance**.
- Vessel length does not change significantly and blood viscosity normally stays within a small range (except when hematocrit changes).
- **Vessel resistance** (R) is directly proportional to the **length (L)** of the **vessel** and the **viscosity** (η) of the blood, and **inversely proportional** to the radius to the **fourth power (r^4)**.

$$R \propto \frac{\eta L}{r^4 \mathrm{I}}$$

- Because changes in **diameter and radius** are directly proportional to each other (D = 2r; therefore D ∝ r), **diameter** can be substituted for **radius** in the following expression.
- Vessel having twice the **length** of another vessel (and each having the same radius) will have twice the resistance to flow.
- **Viscosity** of the blood increases 2-fold, the resistance to flow will increase 2-fold.
- An increase in radius will reduce resistance. Change in radius alters resistance to the fourth power of the change in radius.
- For example, a 2-fold increase in radius decreases resistance by 16-fold! Therefore, vessel resistance is exquisitely sensitive to changes in radius.
- Similarly reducing the radius by 1/3rd increases the resistance by $1/3^4$ = 1/81 = **81 times.**

Ans: (d) 81 times

Ref: *Ganong, 25th edition, page 573*

6. **When capillary and interstitial hydrostatic pressures are 3 mm of Hg and 0 mm of Hg and colloid oncotic pressure of capillaries and interstitum is 25 mm of Hg and 5 mm of Hg, what is the Net filtration pressure?**

(a) 17 mm Hg (b) 33 mm Hg (c) 23 mm Hg (d) 20 mm Hg

Explanation:

The rate of filtration at any point along a capillary depends on a balance of forces sometimes called the **Starling forces** which are:

- **Hydrostatic pressure gradient** (Difference between Capillary Hydrostatic pressure and Interstitial Hydrostatic pressure).
- **Osmotic pressure gradient** (Difference between Capillary Osmotic pressure and Interstitial Osmotic pressure).

Fluid movement across the capillary depends on **net filtration pressure, which is the difference between the hydrostatic pressure gradient and oncotic pressure gradient.**

Net Filtration Pressure = k [(Pc - Pi) - (πc - πi)]

k = capillary filtration coefficient
Pc = capillary hydrostatic pressure
Pi = interstitial hydrostatic pressure
πc = capillary colloid osmotic pressure
πi = interstitial colloid osmotic pressure

Replacing the values we get:
Net Filtration Pressure = (3 - 0) - (25 - 5)
= – 17 mm Hg.
The **minus sign** indicates that fluid movement is inward into the capillary.

So, the answer is 17 mm Hg

Ans: (a) 17 mm Hg

Ref: Ganong's, Review of Medical Physiology, 25th edition, page 578-579

7. **When the pulmonary arterial pCO_2 is constant and ventilation is increased three folds, alveolar pCO_2 will decrease by:**

(a) 66% (b) 33% (c) 25% (d) 55%

Explanation:

Relationship Between Alveolar Ventilation and Expired pCO_2

This is given by the Alveolar Ventilation Equation,

$$P_{A_{CO_2}} = 0.863 \cdot \frac{\dot{V}_{CO_2}}{\dot{V}_A}$$

- Where, $PACO_2$ is Alveolar PCO_2, VCO_2 is CO_2 produced in the body, V_A is alveolar ventilation.
- VCO_2 is CO_2 produced in body determines the pulmonary arterial CO_2.

In the question given:

- Pulmonary arterial CO_2 is constant, i.e., VCO_2 is constant, only alveolar ventilation is tripled.
- Replacing it,

$$PACO_2 = 0.863 \times \frac{V\,CO_2}{3\,VA}$$

- So, $PACO_2$ will be decreased by 1/3rd, i.e., 33%.

Alveolar ventilation equation states that, if **CO_2 production is constant**, the **alveolar PCO_2** is **inversely** related to **alveolar ventilation.**
Therefore, if ventilation is increased by **3 times** the **alveolar PCO_2** will be reduced to **1/3rd** of its former value.

Ans: (b) 33%

Ref: Walter F. Boron, Emile L. Boulpaep. Medical Physiology: A Cellular and Molecular Approach, updated 2nd edition, Chapter 31

8. **If the concentration of inhaled O_2 is doubled, the resultant effect will be:**

(a) Partial pressure of oxygen decreases
(b) Doubles the amount of oxygen dissolved in blood
(c) Increase in amount of oxygen bound with haemoglobin
(d) None of the above

Explanation:

- If the inspired partial pressure of oxygen is **doubled**, the amount of oxygen in solution **doubles** but does not double the amount of oxygen in the body because most of oxygen content is bound to **haemoglobin.**

Transport of Oxygen

- Oxygen is transported in blood in two forms. They are:
    - Oxygen in dissolved form **(3%)** = 0.003 × PaO_2.
    - Oxygen combined with hemoglobin **(97%)** = 1.4 × Hb in g/dL × % saturation.
- **Total oxygen content** in blood = Oxygen in Dissolved form + Oxygen Combined with hemoglobin.
- Therefore, **Total oxygen content in blood=** [0.003 × PaO_2] + [1.4 × Hb in g/dL × % saturation].

Oxygen Transport in Dissolved Form

- According to Henry's law, the amount of dissolved gas is proportional to its partial pressure.
- For **each mm Hg of PO_2**, there is **0.003 ml O_2/100 ml of blood.**
- We know that the normal arterial blood have **PO_2 of 100 mm Hg.** So, the amount of dissolved oxygen is 0.003 ml * 100 = 0.3 ml O_2/100 ml of blood.

Oxygen transported in dissolved form = 0.3 ml O_2/100 ml of blood

Oxygen Transport Combined with Hemoglobin

- Once the oxygen enters pulmonary capillaries from alveoli, much of it combines with the oxygen carrier protein in RBCs called Hemoglobin.

Calculation of PAO_2 (Arterial PO_2)

- $PAO_2 = (FiO_2 \times [Patm - PH_2O]) - (PaCO_2/R)$.
  – PAO_2 is alveolar O_2 pressure.
  – FiO_2 is fraction of inspired oxygen (room air ~0.20).
  – Patm is atmospheric pressure (~760 mm Hg at sea level).
  – PH_2O is vapor pressure of water (47 mm Hg at 37°C).
  – $PaCO_2$ is partial pressure of CO_2 (normally 40).
  – R is the respiratory quotient (typically ~0.8).
- $PAO_2 = 0.21 \times (760\text{-}47) - (40/0.8)$.
- PAO_2 =100 mm Hg.

Ans: (b) Doubles the amount of oxygen dissolved in blood

Ref: Diving and Oxygen, Peter Wilmshurst, BMJ, 1998 Oct 10; 317(7164): 996–999

9. **A patient presents with right to left shunt. Oxygen content in arterial and venous side are 18 and 14 ml/100 ml respectively. Oxygen content at pulmonary capillary is 20. What is the percentage shunting of cardiac output?**

(a) 23% (b) 33% (c) 43% (d) 53%

Explanation:

- The shunt as a fraction of cardiac output is given by the formula **(Cc.oxygen - Ca.oxygen)/(Cc.oxygen - Cv. oxygen).**
- **Here in this formula, Cc.oxygen denotes oxygen content in capillaries, Ca.oxygen denotes oxygen content in artery, Cv.oxygen denotes oxygen content in veins.**
- So, here in this question, oxygen content at pulmonary capillary is **20**, oxygen content in arterial and venous side are **18 and 14 ml / 100 ml.**
- The answer is **20-18/20-14 = 33%.**

Ventilation – Perfusion Ratio (V/Q Ratio) – Clinical Importance

- Imbalances in ventilation and perfusion commonly leads to ventilation perfusion mismatch that ultimately affects the gas exchange.

Ventilation – Perfusion Ratio (V/Q Ratio) = Zero (0)

- This means that ventilation (numerator) is zero. So, the ratio becomes zero.
- Physiological cause of non-uniform ventilation is:
  - Shunt blood perfused regions – Oxygenation of shunt blood doesn't occur because there is no ventilation.
- Pathological causes of non-uniform ventilation are:
  - Collapse of lung (emphysema).
  - Foreign body obstruction.
  - Bronchoconstriction due to asthma.
  - Compression of airways by tumor.
  - Pulmonary fibrosis.
  - Pneumothorax.

Ventilation – Perfusion Ratio (V/Q Ratio) = ∞ (Infinity)

- This means that the perfusion is nil (denominator). So, the ratio becomes infinity.
- Physiological cause of non-uniform perfusion is:
  - Dead spaces – No gas exchange happens.
- Pathological causes of non-uniform perfusion are:
  - Pulmonary embolism.
  - Compression of pulmonary vessels by high alveolar pressures.
  - Tumor occluding pulmonary vessels.

Ans: (b) 33%

Ref: West Respiratory Physiology, 9th edition, page184

10. Resting muscle length means?

(a) Length of actin and myosin before contraction.
(b) The length of the muscle at which the active tension is maximal.
(c) Relaxed length of the muscle.
(d) Length at which muscle has minimal tension.

Ans: (b) The length of the muscle at which the active tension is maximal

Ref: Ganong, 25th edition, page 101

Explanation:

Few important terms in length and tension of skeletal muscle
Passive tension: • It is primarily due to the elastic protein titin in muscle. Seen only in the unstimulated muscle. **Active tension:** • If the muscle is stimulated, Actin and myosin interact, muscle contracts and develops active tension. **Total tension:** • It is the sum of active tension and passive tension. **Resting length (Optimum length)** • The length of the muscle at which the active tension is maximal is usually called its **resting length**. All the muscles in body generates maximum tension at resting length. **Equilibrium length:** • Refers to the length of the relaxed muscle cut free from its bony attachments.

BIOCHEMISTRY

1. **Defect in alpha oxidation of fatty acid leads to:**

(a) Dicarboxylic aciduria
(b) Zellweger syndrome
(c) Jamaican Vomiting Sickness
(d) Refsum disease

Explanation:

Refsum Disease

- Neurologic disorder due to defect in ***alpha oxidation*** of fatty acid.
- Results in the accumulation of **branched chain fatty acid**, **phytanic acid**, which is found in dairy products, plants and ruminant fat.

Jamaican Vomiting Sickness

- Caused by eating the **unripe fruit** of the **akee tree**, which contains the toxin **hypoglycin.**
- This inactivates **medium- and short-chain acyl-CoA dehydrogenase**, inhibiting ***β-oxidation*** and causing **hypoglycemia**.

Dicarboxylic Aciduria

- Characterized by the excretion of **C6 - C10 ω-dicarboxylic acids** and by **nonketotic hypoglycemia.**
- Caused by a lack of mitochondrial **medium-chain acyl-CoA dehydrogenase.**

Zellweger (cerebrohepatorenal) syndrome

- Inherited absence of peroxisomes in all tissues.
- Accumulate **C26- C38 polyenoic acids** in **brain tissue.**
- The disease causes severe neurological symptoms, and most patients die in the first year of life.

Types of Fatty Acid Oxidation

A. ***Beta oxidation***
  - Major mechanism.
  - Occurs in mitochondrial matrix.
  - Oxidation occurs at beta carbon (refer below), 2-C units are released as acetyl CoA per cycle.

B. ***Alpha oxidation***
  - Predominantly occurs in **brain and liver.**
  - Suited for Branched chain fatty acid (e.g. Phytanic acid).
  - Beta oxidation cannot occur initially because of the presence of branched methyl groups, but it can proceed after decarboxylation.
  - Alpha oxidation (decarboxylation) followed by beta oxidation.

C. ***Omega oxidation***
  - Minor mechanism.
  - Gains importance during defect in beta oxidation.

D. ***Peroxisomal beta oxidation***
  - Mainly for long chain fatty acid oxidation.

Ans: (d) Refsum disease

Ref: Harper's Illustrated Biochemistry, 30th edition, page 231

2. **Which of the following is a peroxisomal disorder?**

(a) Zellweger syndrome
(b) Dicarboxylic aciduria
(c) Jamaican vomiting sickness
(d) Refsum disease

Explanation:

Zellweger (Cerebrohepatorenal) Syndrome

- Inherited absence of peroxisomes in all tissues.
- Peroxisomal system is active for oxidation of very long chain fatty acids accumulate C26-C38 polyenoic acids in brain tissue.
- Cause a generalized loss of peroxisomal function leading to multi organ involvement.
- The disease causes severe neurological symptoms, and most patients die in the first year of life.

Ans: (a) Zellweger syndrome

Ref: Harper's Illustrated Biochemistry, 30th edition, page 231

3. **All are true regarding xeroderma pigmentosa *except*:**

(a) Base excision repair defect
(b) Skin manifestations are seen usually within 2 years
(c) Usually patients die in 2nd or 3rd decade
(d) Metastasis of malignant tumors commonly occur in these patients

Explanation:

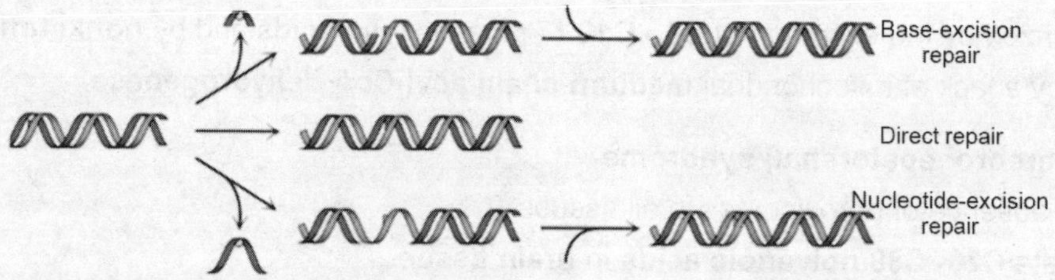

Repair Pathways: Different pathways are used to repair damaged regions in DNA.

- **Base excision repair**, the damaged base is removed and replaced.
- **Direct repair**, the damaged region is corrected in place.
- **Nucleotide excision repair**, a stretch of DNA around the site of damage is removed and replaced.

Human Diseases Due to Defective DNA Repair

Defective Nonhomologous End Joining Repair (NHEJ)
- Severe combined immunodeficiency disease (SCID)
- Radiation sensitive severe combined immunodeficiency disease (RS-SCID)

Defective Homologous Repair (HR)
- AT-like disorder (ATLD)
- Nijmegen breakage syndrome (NBS)
- Bloom syndrome (BS)
- Werner syndrome (WS)
- Rothmund-Thomson syndrome (RTS)
- Breast cancer suspectibility 1 and 2 (BRCA1, BRCA2)

Defective DNA Nucleotide Exicision Repair (NER)
- Xeroderma pigmentosum (XP)
- Cockayne syndrome (CS)
- Trichothiodystrophy (TTD)

Defective DNA Base Excision Repair (BER)
- MUTYH-associated polyposis (MAP)

Defective DNA Mismatch Repair (MMR)
- Hereditary nonpolyposis colorectal cancer (HNPCC)

Xeroderma Pigmentosum (XP)

- Rare human skin disease.
- Autosomal recessive.
- Patients are at increased risk for the development of cancers of the skin exposed to the ultraviolet (UV) light contained in sun rays.
- The basis of this disorder is **defective DNA repair**.
- **UV light** causes **cross-linking of pyrimidine residues**, preventing normal DNA replication.
- Such DNA damage is repaired by the **nucleotide excision repair** system.
- **Skin manifestations**
    - In infancy, severe changes in the skin become evident and worsen with time.
    - Dry skin → marked atrophy of the dermis.
    - Affected homozygote is extremely sensitive to sunlight or ultraviolet light.
    - Skin cancer usually develops at several sites. Many patients die before age 30 from metastases of these malignant skin tumors.
- **Eye manifestations**
    - Keratoses appear, the eyelids become scarred, and the cornea ulcerates.
- **Pathophysiology**
    - UV light induces cross-links between adjacent pyrimidines along one strand (same) of DNA, produces pyrimidine dimers, usually thymine – thymine bulky adducts, which normally are excised by the nucleotide excision repair mechanism. *XP can be produced by a defect in the excinuclease that hydrolyzes the DNA backbone near a pyrimidine dimer.*
    - In normal skin fibroblasts, half the pyrimidine dimers produced by ultraviolet radiation are excised in less than 24 hours. In contrast, almost no dimers are excised in this time interval in fibroblasts derived from XP patients.
    - Defects in DNA repair systems are expected to increase the overall frequency of mutations and, hence, the likelihood of a cancer-causing mutation.

Types of defects in DNA-repair systems and conditions associated

DNA repair mechanisms	Diseases associated
Mismatch repair	• Hereditary nonpolyposis colon cancer syndrome • Muir-Torre syndrome
Nucleotide excision repair	• Xeroderma pigmentosum • Cockayne's syndrome • Trichothiodystrophy
Base excision repair	• **Gross defects –** Not compatible with life • **Partial defects –** Colorectal cancer and lung cancers
Recombinational repair	• Ataxia telangiectasia (ATM gene, genome instability syndrome) • Bloom syndrome (RecQ DNA helicase; BLM gene) • Fanconi anemia (BRCA-2) • Werner syndrome (WRNp protein–RecQ DNA helicase)

Ans: (a) Base excision repair

Ref: Harper's Illustrated Biochemistry, 30th edition, page 390

Version-2

All true about Xeroderma pigmentosa *except*:

(a) Autosomal dominant
(b) Onset of squamous cell carcinoma by 2nd-3rd decade/Non-melanotic cancer by the age of 9 years
(c) Skin manifestations are seen usually within 2 years
(d) Nucleotide excision repair defect

*"Multiple oculo-cutaneous malignancies are a common manifestation on sun-exposed facial areas in patients with Xeroderma pigmentosum (XP) [1]. Commonly seen are the **basal cell carcinoma** and the **squamous cell carcinomas** which manifest in the **early first decade** in contrast to fifth and sixth decade in the general population."*

- Basal cell carcinoma (BCC) is the most common non-melanotic cancer, followed by squamous cell Ca.

Ans: (a) Autosomal dominant

Ref: Harper's Illustrated Biochemistry, 30th edition, page 390

4. **All are true about GIP (Glucose dependent insulinotropic Polypeptide) *except*:**

(a) GIP stimulates glucagon release
(b) GIP is inhibited by insulin
(c) GIP inhibits GLP-1
(d) GIP in T2DM worsens post prandial hyperglycemia

Explanation:

- GIP and GLP-1(glucagon like peptide -1) are **incretin** hormones (**enhance insulin secretion**), also affect glucagon secretion.
- Secreted by **enteroendocrine intestinal k cells** upon nutrient stimulation.
- GIP gene located on **chr 17q**, structurally related to secretin family. Binds to G protein coupled receptors
- GIP acts as **a bifunctional blood glucose stabilizing hormone, means it has effects on insulin and glucagon responses highly dependent on blood glucose levels.**

Other Options

Option (d)

- GIP has short lived insulinotropic effect in T2DM, it worsens postprandial hyperglycemia most likely through suppressive effect on GLP 1.

Option (b)

- Inhibition of GIP release by insulin and glucose stimulation.

Option (a) and (c)

- ***GIP enhances postprandial glucagon and GLP 1 suppresses it.***
- ***Both share common properties as incretins, but they also possess different biological characteristics.***
- *Sulfonylureas and incretins acts synergistically to stimulate insulin secretion, so combination drugs potentially cause hypoglycemia.*

GIP has **many additional actions** than insulinotropic activity like:

- Promote growth of pancreatic beta cell.
- Stimulate adipogenesis.
- Increase expression of anti-apoptotic Bcl-2 (resulting in reduced beta cell death).
- Inhibits gastric acid and pepsin release.
- Involves in number of c AMP dependent intracellular pathways.

Ans: (c) GIP inhibits GLP-1

Ref: (Review article by Christensen MB, dan Med J 2016) and for option (d) diabetes, 2009 (Exogenous GIP worsens post prandial hyperglycemia in T2DM) and for option (b) Inhibition of GIP release by insulin and glucose, diabetes, 1980

5. **Odd chain fatty acids can form glucose by which pathway?**

(a) By forming propionyl CoA
(b) By forming glycerol
(c) Acetyl CoA entering TCA cycle
(d) By lactic acid formation

Explanation:

- Fatty acids with an odd number of carbon atoms are oxidized by the pathway of β-oxidation, producing acetyl CoA (2C) until a three-carbon (propionyl-CoA) residue remains.
- End product of even chain FA oxidation – acetyl CoA (2C).

- End product of odd chain FA oxidation--acetyl CoA units **+ 1 propionyl CoA**(3C).
- Propionyl CoA is converted to succinyl-CoA (steps mentioned below), a constituent of the citric acid cycle, which after few steps, enters in to gluconeogenesis.

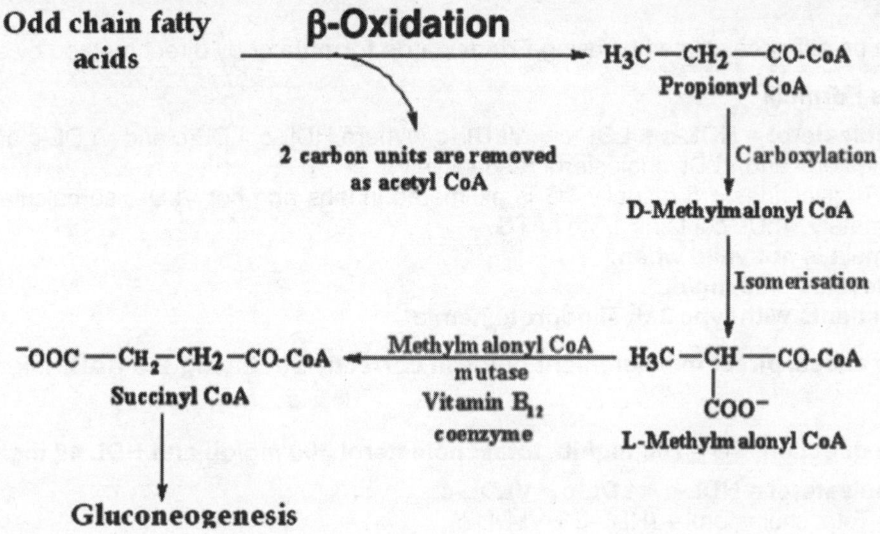

Only 2 enzymes in our body requires **vit B12** as cofactor.

- **Methyl malonyl CoA mutase (AKA methylmalonyl-CoA isomerase).**
- **Methionine synthase** (Synthesis of Methionine by methylation of homocysteine).
  - Hence, **the propionyl residue from an odd-chain fatty acid is the only part of a fatty acid that is glucogenic.**
  - **Even chain fatty acids cannot synthesize glucose, because PDH reaction is irreversible.**
  - Gluconeogenesis is glucose synthesized from **non-carbohydrate** sources like lactate, propionyl CoA and Glucogenic amino acids. **So glucose derived from glycogen break down (carbohydrate source) is NOT gluconeogenesis.**

Ans: (a) By forming Propionyl CoA

Ref: Harper's Illustrated Biochemistry, 30th edition, page 225,558; Styer Biochemistry, 7th edition, page 650

6. **Lipoprotein lipase is activated by:**

(a) Apo C1 (b) Apo C2 (c) Apo C3 (d) Apo A1

Explanation:

Lipoprotein Lipase (LPL)

- Located on the walls of blood capillaries, anchored to the endothelium by negatively charged proteoglycan chains of heparan sulfate.
- It is not active in adult liver.
- It is not normally found in blood. However, following injection of **heparin,** lipoprotein lipase is released from its heparan sulfate binding sites into the circulation.
  - **Apo C-II**–LPL activator.
  - **Apo A-II and apo C-III** are LPL inhibitors.
  - **Apo A-I - lecithin: cholesterol acyltransferase (LCAT)** activator.
- HDL concentrations vary reciprocally with plasma triacylglycerol concentrations and directly with the activity of lipoprotein lipase.

Ans: (b) Apo C2

Ref: Harper's Illustrated Biochemistry, 30th edition, page 257

7. **A patient's lipid profile is as follows, TG – 200 mg/dL, total cholesterol 300 mg/dL, and HDL 40 mg/dL. Calculate LDL level in this patient.**

(a) 40 mg/dL (b) 100 mg/dL (c) 220 mg/dL
(d) 260 mg/dL (e) 40 mg/dL

Explanation:

- **LDL** can be either calculated by using **Friedewalds formula** or by direct method by an auto analyser.

Friedewalds Formula

- **Total cholesterol = HDL-c + LDL-c + VLDL-c** (Where HDL-c, LDL-c and VLDL-c are HDL cholesterol, LDL cholesterol and VLDL cholesterol respectively).
- VLDL = Triglycerides ÷ 5 (usually TG is estimated in labs and not VLDL, so calculate VLDL from TG). Approximately, VLDL contains 1/5th of TG.
- This formula **is not valid when:**
  - **TG levels > 400 mg/dL*.**
  - **In patients with type 3 dyslipoproteinemia*.**
- **In those cases, direct measurement helps in correctly stratifying the CAD risk and goals of treatment.**

In the given question, TG – 200 mg/dL, total cholesterol 300 mg/dL and HDL 40 mg/dL.

- **Total cholesterol = HDL-c + LDL-c + VLDL-c.**
- **LDL-c** = Total cholesterol – (HDL-c + VLDL-c).
- VLDL-c = TG/5.
- LDL-c = Total cholesterol – (HDL-c + TG/5).
- So 300 = 40 + LDL-c + (200/5).
- LDL = 300 – (40+200/5).
- LDL = 300 – (40+40) = **220 mg/dL.**

Ans: (c) 220 mg/dL

Ref: Internet Source

8. **Bends in alpha helix structure are formed by which amino acid?**

(a) Glycine (b) Lysine (c) Methionine
(d) Glutamine (e) Alanine

Explanation:

Glycine Unique Features

- Except glycine, the a-carbon of every amino acid is chiral.
- Smallest amino acid, so accommodated in **peptide bends easily.**

Interior of Cytosolic Proteins Contains

- Hydrophobic AA (Ala, branched chain AA (V, Leu, IL) and aromatic AA (F, Tyr, Trp).

Helix Breakers

- **Valine, threonine and isoleucine**–Branches at the beta-carbon atom and tends to destabilize alpha helices because of steric clashes.
- **Serine, aspartate and asparagine** also tend to disrupt a helices because their side chains contain hydrogen-bond donors or acceptors in close proximity to the main chain, where they compete for main-chain NH and CO groups.
- **Proline** is a **helix breaker** because it lacks an NH group and because its ring structure prevents it from fitting in to the helix.

Important Points to Remember

- **Proteins** contain only **L–amino acids.**
- **Right handed alpha helix** are the most **common*.**

Ans: (a) Glycine

Ref: Styer Biochemistry, 7th edition, page 40

9. Keshan's cardiomyopathy due to deficiency of:

(a) Chromium (b) Selenium (c) Magnesium (d) Copper

Explanation:

Selenium

- Selenium is a trace element mineral.
- Cofactor for enzymes like:
  - Glutathione peroxidase.
  - Deiodinase.
  - Thioredoxin reductase.
- Selenium containing AA – **Selenocysteine (21st AA).**
- Toxicity occurs due to foods grown on soil containing high selenium levels, leads to **dilated endemic cardiomyopathy** or **Keshan's disease**, named after **Keshan county, China** where the disease was first discovered.

Ans: (b) Selenium

Ref: Bhagawan's Textbook of Biochemistry, 4th edition, page 893, Selenium Deficiency

10. Corneal vascularization is seen in deficiency of which vitamin?

(a) B1 (b) B2 (c) B3 (d) B4

Explanation:

- Riboflavin causes corneal vascularization and corneal opacity. It is also associated with night blindness in some communities.

Riboflavin (Vitamin B2)

- **Functions:** Oxidation reduction reaction, cellular respiration, carbohydrate, amino acid, fatty acid metabolism.
- **Requirement:** 0.5 – 1.5 mg.
- **Sources:** Milk, milk products, egg, liver, green leafy vegetables, wheat.
- **Deficiency:**
  - **Ariboflavinosis:** Photophobia, Cheilosis, Stomatitis, Glossitis.
  - **Neovascularisation of cornea*.**
  - Nasolabial dyssebacea.
- Urinary excretion of riboflavin < 30 mg/24 hours suggests low or deficient intakes.
- Erythrocyte gluthathione reductase (EGR) with and without added FAD >1.4.
- **Treatment**
  - 3-10 mg/day oral supplementation of Vitamin B2 riboflavin.

Ans: (b) B2

Ref: Harper's Biochemistry, 30th edition

11. Which of the following is a lipotropic factor?

(a) Sphingomyelin (b) Choline (c) Cardiolipin (d) Orotic acid

Explanation:

- Lipotropic factors are those whose deficiency causes fatty liver. These factors also aids in the recovery of fatty liver, but does not cure the condition.

Fatty Liver

- Imbalance in the rate of formation of TG and export causes fatty liver.
- Accumulation of triacylglycerides in the liver.
- Normally liver contains approximately 5% of fat, unlike adipose tissue, liver is not a storage organ for fat. So excess deposition causes fatty liver.

Factors Causing Fatty Liver

- **Raised levels of plasma free fatty acids** (due to increased mobilization of fat from adipose tissue or from the hydrolysis of lipoprotein triacylglycerol by lipoprotein lipase in extrahepatic tissues). E.g. DM, starvation, high fat diet.
- **Increased influx of FFA in to the liver**→ VLDL not able to cope up with the pace of influx and esterification of FFA→**accumulation of TG.**
  - Remember VLDL carries endogenous TG and chylomicrons carry exogenous/dietary TG.
- **Impairment in lipoprotein synthesis, protein deficiency, essential fatty acid and vitamin deficiencies** (e.g., linoleic acid, pyridoxine, and pantothenic acid).
- Alcoholism.
- Multiple metabolic disorders.
- Antibiotic puromycin, ethionine (α-amino-γ-mercaptobutyric acid), carbon tetrachloride, chloroform, phosphorus, lead and arsenic.

Lipotropic Factors

- Will not protect the organism against these agents, but appears to aid in recovery.
- **Common examples:**
  - **Choline*.**
  - **Methionine, serine, glycine.**
  - **Betaine, Inositol.**
  - **Folic acid, Vit B12.**

Ans: (b) Choline

Ref: Harper's Illustrated Biochemistry, 30th edition, page 261 and Satyanarayana, page 328

12. **Microsatellite is:**

(a) Extra-chromosomal DNA
(b) 2-4 nucleotides repeats
(c) Decrease in number of repeats leads to disease
(d) They occur only in centromere

Explanation:

- In human DNA, at least **30%** of the genome consists of repetitive sequences.
- Repetitive sequence DNA can be broadly classified as:
  - Moderately repetitive.
  - Highly repetitive.

	Highly repetitive	**Moderately repetitive (2 types)**
Sequence length	5 to 500 bp repeated many times in tandem	• Long interspersed repeat sequences **(LINEs)** **6 to 7 kbp** **20000-50000 copies/genome** • Short interspersed repeat sequences **(SINEs)** **70-300 bp.** **E.g. Alu family (10% of genome)** **>100,000 copies/genome**
Location	Clustered In centromeres and telomeres	Not clustered but are interspersed with unique sequences
Function	Transcriptionally inactive, some in structural role of chromosome.	

Microsatellite Repeat Sequences

- Repeat sequences exists as **both** dispersed and grouped tandem arrays.
- The sequences consist of **2 to 6 bp** repeated up to 50 times. Usually dinucleotide repeats of AC.
- Microsatellite number is a **heritable trait, heterozygous** (at a loci, number of repeats vary in both chromosome).
- PCR detects microsatellite polymorphism.
- Association of this polymorphism with disease provides the first clue in genetic basis of a disease.
- Trinucleotide sequences that increase in number (microsatellite instability) can cause disease.

Disease	Repeat sequence
CAG (remember as **hunt**er needs **cag**e)	Huntingtons chorea
CGG (remember as EGG is fragile)	Fragile X syn
CAG	SMA, Kennedys disease

Ans: 2-4 nucleotides repeats

Ref: Harper's Illustrated Biochemistry, 30th edition, page 378

13. Tomcat urine odor is seen in:

(a) Multiple carboxylase deficiency
(b) Phenylketonuria
(c) Hawkinuria
(d) Maple syrup diesase

Explanation:

Multiple Carboxylase Deficiency

- **Tom cat urine:** Multiple carboxylase deficiency (methyl malonyl CoA carboxylase, pyruvate carboxylase, propionyl CoA carboxylase).
- **Clinical features:**
  - Neurologic disorder resembling Werdnig Hoffmann's disease.
  - Ketoacidosis.
  - Failure to thrive.
  - Dermatitis (Generalized erythematous rash and skin exfoliation).
- **Treatment**
  - Leucine restriction.
  - **Biotin administration** (cofactor for carboxylases).

Defect in many metabolic pathways leads to accumulating substances, which gives different urine odour, thus providing a clue in diagnosis.

Disease	Sample	Odour
PKU	Urine and body	Mousy odour
DKA	Breath	Sweety or fruity
Maple syrup (MSUD)/branched chain ketonuria	Urine	Maple syrup/caramel/boiled Chinese herbal medicine
Oasthouse urine disease (methionine malabsorption)	Urine	Yeast/celery/malt/brewery
Tom cat urine-multiple carboxylase deficiency	Urine	Smells like cat urine
Isovaleric academia (sweat feet syn)	All body fluids	Sweaty feet/socks, ripe cheese

Ans: (a) Multiple carboxylase deficiency

Ref: Textbook of Pediatric Emergency Medicine, page 1566

14. Importance of pyruvate to lactate formation in anaerobic glycolysis is production of:

(a) FAD (b) NADH to NAD (c) ATP (d) NAD to NADH

Explanation:

- A cell can perform aerobic respiration through TCA cycle in mitochondria, in situations when there is no oxygen/mitochondria (RBC), it will perform anaerobic respiration.

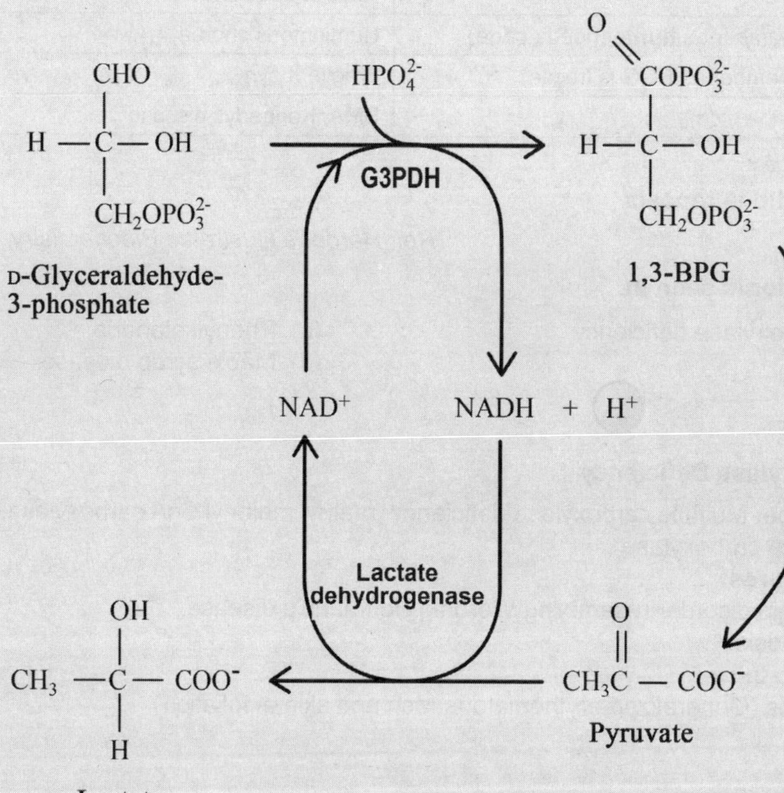

Lactic acid fermentation

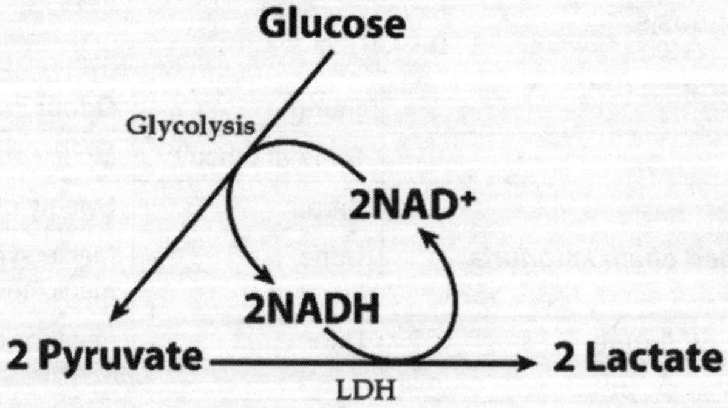

- NAD produced in the reaction catalyzed by LDH is used to maintain **glycolysis**. If NAD is deficient, Glycolysis will come to halt.

Ans: (b) NADH to NAD

Ref: Internet Source

PHARMACOLOGY

1. **Table sugar is not used in treating hypoglycaemia secondary to:**

(a) Acarbose (b) Metformin
(c) Glipizide (d) Insulin

Explanation:

For hypoglycemia treatment due to oral anti diabetic drugs, table sugar will not be useful if the patient has taken Alpha Glucosidase Inhibitors like **Acarbose**, miglitolol and voglibose.

Alpha Glucosidase Inhibitors

- **Acarbose, miglitolol and voglibose.**
- MOA: Inhibit α glucosidase in intestinal brush border.
- Because the above drugs competitively and reversibly inhibit α glucosidase.
- α glucosidase is required for breakdown of complex carbohydrate like sucrose, maltose.
- So if you give table sugar which contains sucrose, sucrose will not be broken down to glucose and will not be absorbed from GIT.
- So complex carbohydrate like sucrose, maltose are not cleaved, and glucose is not formed.
- **Acarbose** can decrease the absorption of **digoxin** and **miglitol** can decrease the absorption of **propranolol and ranitidine.**

Better to give glucose only in these situations.

Additional info:

Alpha Glucosidase Inhibitors

- Decrease post prandial glucose.
- Increase GLP in circulation.

ADRs:

Malabsorption, flatulence, diarrhea and abdominal bloating.

Other Options:

Metformin:

- Chances of hypoglycaemia are least with metformin. Even if there is hypoglycaemia that can be managed with table sugar, which will be broken down to glucose.

Glipizide:

- One of the major adverse effect of sulfonylureas is hypoglycaemia, so patient on Glipizide should be advised to carry sugar, chocolate or glucose tablets with them as an emergency treatment for hypoglycaemia.

Insulin:

- Once again major adverse effect of insulin is hypoglycemia. Best treatment for hypoglycemia is with IV dextrose.

Ans: (a) Acarbose

Ref: GG, 12th edition, page 1264

2. **DPP-IV inhibitor used in renal failure:**

(a) Linagliptin (b) Sitagliptin (c) Vildagliptin (d) Saxagliptin

Explanation:

- Patients with T2DM have dysfunction in **incretin hormones** (such as **glucagon-like peptide-1** or **GLP-1** and **glucose-dependent insulinotropic polypeptide or GIP**).
- By inhibiting the **dipeptidyl peptidase-4 (DPP-4)** enzyme, it is possible to slow the inactivation of GLP-1 and GIP, promoting blood glucose level decrease in a glucose-dependent manner.
- **Linagliptin** is a **dipeptidyl peptidase-4 inhibitor DPP IV inhibitor.**
- Linagliptin is approved by FDA and **EMA** for the **T2DM** treatment as an **anti-hyperglycemic** agent that can be used as **monotherapy** or in **combination** with other medications (metformin, sulphonylurea, pioglitazone, metformin plus sulphonylurea or insulin).

NOTE:

- Linagliptin is safe in renal failure, as it is eliminated majorly by biliary excretion and it also undergoes enterohepatic recycling.

Chemical and metabolic characteristics of DPP-4 inhibitors

Inhibitor	Chemical Structure	Metabolites	Route of Elimination
Linagliptin	Based on Xanthine	Negligible	Biliary(> 70% unchanged); <6% via kidney
Saxagliptin	Cyanopyrrolidine	Metabolized in the liver to active metabolite (via P450 3A4/5)	Renal (12-29% unchanged and 21-52% as metabolite)
Sitagliptin	Based on β-amino acid	Negligible	Renal (80% unchanged)
Vildagliptin	Cyanopyrrolidine	Hydrolyzed to inactive metabolite (P450 enzyme-independent)	Renal (22% unchanged and 55% as primary metabolite)
Alogliptin	Pyrimidine	Demethylated, acetylated	Renal

Ans: (a) Linagliptin

Ref: Hohl A, Ronsoni MF, Guedes EP, de Melo TG, Lauand F (2014), Linagliptin: DPP-4 Inhibition in the Treatment of Type 2, Diabetes Mellitus, J Diabetes Metab Disord Control 1(1): 00005, DOI: 10.15406/jdmdc,2014.01.00005

3. **All are true regarding insulin 'AFREZZA' *except*:**

(a) Inhalable insulin
(b) Bolus insulin not needed
(c) Given in multiple doses
(d) Used in combination with short acting insulin

Explanation:

AFREZZA

- Approved in 2014.
- For both **Type I and Type II diabetes.**
- Rapid acting **inhaled insulin**, administered at the beginning of each meal.
- Inhaled insulin formulation (2.5 μm) and technosphere technology.
- Available as single-use cartridges of **4 and 8 units.**

Remember:

- Not a substitute for long acting insulin.
- Must be **used in combination with long acting insulin** in Type I diabetes.
- Not recommended for treatment of **Diabetic Ketoacidosis** or in patient who **smoke.**
- Not be used in patients with **active lung cancer.**

How to Use

- AFREZZA should only be administered via oral inhalation using the AFREZZA Inhaler.
- AFREZZA is administered using a single inhalation per cartridge.
- Administer AFREZZA at the beginning of the meal.

Use Restricted in:

- During episodes of hypoglycemia.
- Asthma.
- Active lung cancer.
- Chronic obstructive pulmonary disease.
- Hypersensitivity to regular insulin.

Ans: (d) Used in combination with short acting insulin

Ref: Inhaled Insulin–current Direction of Insulin Research Journal of Clinical and Diagnostic Research, 2017 Apr, Vol 11(4): OE01-OE02

4. Anti-Graft rejection drug used in autologous transplantation is:

(a) Amphotericin B (b) Methotrexate (c) Cyclosporine (d) Tacrolimus

Explanation:

Tacrolimus:

- Preferred now for organ transplantations due to higher potency and easier monitoring of blood levels.
- Tacrolimus may be useful in patients whose rejection reaction is not suppressed by cyclosporine.
- It is particularly valuable in **liver transplantation** because its absorption is not dependent on bile.
- Being more potent, it is also suitable for suppressing acute rejection that has set in.

Sirolimus:

- Used in stem cell transplant as well.
- Not recommended for liver transplant.
- Sirolimus coated stents are being used to reduce the incidence of **coronary artery restenosis**, by inhibiting endothelial proliferation at the site.

Cyclosporine

- Most effective drug for prevention and treatment of graft rejection reaction.
- It is routinely used in renal, hepatic, cardiac, bone marrow and other transplantations.

Amphotericin B

- Antifungal drug.

Methotrexate:

- Folate antagonist.
- Potent immunosuppressant which markedly depresses cytokine production and cellular immunity.
- Has anti-inflammatory property.
- Used as a first line drug in many **autoimmune diseases** like rapidly progressing rheumatoid arthritis severe psoriasis, pemphigus, myasthenia gravis, uveitis, chronic active hepatitis.

Ans: (d) Tacrolimus

Ref: Goodman and Gillman, 13th edition

5. Which of the following is a Guanylate cyclase C agonist used in inflammatory bowel disease?

(a) Lubiprostine (b) Linaclotide (c) Tegaserod (d) Methyl naltrexone

Explanation:

Linaclotide

- Guanylate cyclase agonist.

- Activation of **GC-C** results in an increase in both intracellular and extracellular concentrations of cyclic guanosine monophosphate (cGMP).
- Elevation of intracellular cGMP stimulates secretion of **chloride** and **bicarbonate** into the **intestinal lumen**, mainly through activation of the cystic fibrosis transmembrane conductance regulator (**CFTR**) ion channel.
- Results in **increased intestinal fluid and accelerated transit.**

Indications:

- Treatment of **chronic constipation.**
- Treatment of **irritable bowel syndrome with constipation.**

NEW DRUG

Plecanatide (Jan. 2017)

- **Approved for the treatment of chronic idiopathic constipation in adults.**
- It is a guanylate cyclase-C (GC-C) agonist.
- Both plecanatide and its active metabolite bind to GC-C and act locally on the luminal surface of the intestinal epithelium.

Lubipristone

- Bicyclic fatty acid metabolite analogue of **prostaglandin E1** activates **type-2-chloride channels.**
- Used in treatment of:
  - o **Chronic constipation** in adults.
  - o **Irritable bowel syndrome** with **constipation (IBS-C)** in **adult women.**
- It promotes the secretion of a **chloride-rich fluid** and so improves **stool consistency** and promotes increased frequency by reflexly activating motility.
- The drug is **poorly bioavailable**, acting only in the lumen of the bowel.
- **Side effects:** Nausea, headache, diarrhea, allergic reactions and dyspnea.

Methylnaltrexone

- Peripheral Mu (μ) opioid antagonist.
- No analgesic effect.
- FDA approved for the treatment of **opioid-induced constipation** in patients receiving palliative care when laxative therapy is insufficient.

Alvimopan

- Peripheral mu (μ) opioid antagonist.
- Used in Opioid-induced constipation.

Ans: Linaclotide

Ref: GG, 12th edition, page 1334

6. **New drug for tardive dyskinesia:**

(a) Safinamide (b) Tetrabenazine (c) Valbenazine (d) Deutetrabenazine

Explanation:

Valbenazine:

- Vesicular monoamine transporter 2 (**VMAT2) inhibitor.**
- Specifically indicated for the **treatment of adults with tardive dyskinesia**.
- Supplied as a capsule for oral administration.

Tetrabenazine:

- Centrally-acting dopamine depletor.
- Selective and reversible.
- Used in **chorea associated with Huntington's disease.**

Deutetrabenazine: (Approved in April 2017)

- It is a vesicular monoamine transporter 2 **(VMAT2) inhibitor.**
- Specifically indicated for the treatment of **chorea associated with Huntington's disease**.
- Supplied as a tablet for oral administration.

Safinamide:

- **MAO B inhibitor.**
- Approved for treatment of **on off phenomena** seen with **levodopa** in parkinson's disease.

Ans: (c) Valbenazine

Ref: https://www.accessdata.fda.gov/drugsatfda_docs/label/2017/209241lbl.pdf

7. **Monoclonal antibody acting as enzyme is called as:**

(a) Granzyme
(b) Abzyme
(c) Lipozyme
(d) None of the above

Explanation:

Abzymes

- Abzymes are **antibodies with catalytic activity**.
- They combine the specificity and substrate turnover efficiency of the enzymes with the selective targeting of the antibodies.

Lipozyme

- An **enzyme** of the **hydrolase class** that catalyzes the reaction of **triacylglycerol** and **water** to yield **diacylglycerol** and a **fatty acid anion**.
- It is produced by glands on the **tongue** and by the **pancreas** and initiates the **digestion of dietary fats.**

Granzymes:

- **Serine proteases** that are released by **cytoplasmic granules** within **cytotoxic T cells** and **natural killer (NK) cells**.
- They induce **programmed cell death** in the target cell, thus eliminating cells that have become cancerous or are infected with viruses or bacteria.

Note:

- Natural Abzymes with proteolytic activity are called **Protabzymes*.**
- DNA hydrolyzing activity are called **DNA Abzymes*.**

Ans:(b) Abzyme

Ref: Biotechnology, Vol. XI, Abzymes–A Challenge for the Medical Biotechnology and Public Health - I. Getov, T. Argirova

8. **Which of the following does not penetrate intact skin?**

(a) Scopalamine
(b) Nitroglycerine
(c) Clonidine
(d) Dexmeditomidine

Explanation:

Simple way to answer this is to ask, whether these are available as Transdermal patch. **Scopolamine, Nitroglycerine and Clonidine** are available as Transdermal patch because they can penetrate intact skin.

Scopolamine is L-Hyoscine.

Hyoscine:

- Most effective drug for **motion sickness.**
- Valuable in highly susceptible individuals and for vigorous motions.
- Drug should be given **prophylactically** (0.2 mg oral), because administration after symptoms have set in is less effective; action lasts **4–6 hours.**
- A **transdermal preparation** applied behind the pinna **4 hours before journey** has been shown to **protect for 3 days.**

- Side effects with low oral doses and transdermal medication are few, but dry mouth and sedation can occur: driving is risky.
- Another anticholinergic used for motion sickness is **Dicyclomine.**

Nitroglycerine:

- Sublingual route is used when terminating angina or aborting an imminent one is the aim.
- Cutaneous application as ointment was found to produce haemodynamic effects for 4–6 hours.
- A transdermal patch in which the drug is incorporated into a polymer bonded to adhesive plaster has been developed which provides steady delivery for 24 hours.
- It starts working within **60 min** and has a **bioavailability** of 70–90%.
- However, development of tolerance and dependence may jeopardise its value.
- It is advised that the patch be taken off for 8 hours daily.
- A transmucosal dosage form which has to be stuck to the gums under the upper lip has also been produced—acts in 5 min and releases the drug for 4–6 hours.

Clonidine:

- Is a **partial agonist** with **high affinity** and **high intrinsic activity at α2 receptors**, especially **α2A subtype** in **brainstem.**
- Also activates **imidazoline receptors.**
- Activation of medullary imidazoline receptors also causes **decreased sympathetic outflow** and **fall in BP.**
- Transdermal delivery patch permits continuous administration of clonidine as an alternative to oral therapy. The drug is released at an approximately constant rate for a week; 3-4 days are required to reach steady-state concentrations in plasma. When the patch is removed, plasma concentrations remain stable for **~8 hours** and then decline gradually over a period of several days.

Dexmeditomidine:

- Acts by stimulation of **central α2 adrenergic receptors**.
- Known to cause **sedation and analgesia.**
- Used for **sedating critically ill/ventilated patients** in **intensive care units.**
- Also being used as an **adjunct to anaesthesia.**
- Analgesia and sedation are produced with little respiratory depression, amnesia or anaesthesia.
- Sympathetic response to stress and noxious stimulus is blunted.
- It is administered by **I.V. infusion.**

Ans: (d) Dexmeditomidine

Ref: KDT, 7th edition, page 384

9. Which drug has inverse agonist activity at benzodiazepine receptors?

(a) Flumazenil (b) Beta carboline (c) Naltrexone (d) Zopiclone

Explanation:

Inverse agonist activity at benzodiazepine receptors.

- **Beta carbolines.**

Flumazenil

- A selective competitive antagonist of **BZD receptors (Bz1).**
- Blocks action of **benzodiazepines, zaleplon and zolpidem** but not other sedative/hypnotics.
- Blocks **psychomotor**, **cognitive** and **memory** impairment of BZs.

Zopiclone

- **Agonist** at **BZD receptor.**

Naltrexone:

- Pure antagonist at **opioid receptor.**

Drugs affecting $GABA_A$-receptor gated chloride channel	
GABA	Endogenous agonist at $GABA_A$ receptor → promotes Cl^- influx
Muscimol	Agonist at $GABA_A$ site
Bicuculline	Competitive antagonist at $GABA_A$ receptor
Picrotoxin	Blocks Cl^- channel noncompetitively; acts on picrotoxin sensitive site
Barbiturates	Agonist at an allosteric site; prolong GABA action; and open Cl^- channel
Alcohol, Inhalational anaesthetics, Propofol	Open Cl^- channel directly; allosteric facilitation of GABA
Benzodiazepines	Agonist at an allosteric BZD site →facilitate GABA action
β-Carboline (DMCM)	Inverse agonist at BZD site → impede GABA action
Flumazenil	Competitive antagonist at BZD site

Ans: (b) Beta carboline

Ref: KDT, 7th edition, page 404

10. PCSK9 inhibitor drug:

(a) Reslizumab (b) Brodalumab (c) Alirocumab (d) Ixekizumab

Explanation:

- **Anti-PCSK-9 mab:** Inhibits proprotein convertase subtilisin/kexin type 9 (PCSK9).
- PCSK9 is a protein that targets **LDL receptors** for degradation and thereby reduces the liver's ability to remove **LDL-C.**

Alirocumab:

- Human monoclonal **IgG2.**
- Directed against human proprotein convertase subtilisin kexin 9(PCSK9).
- Binds to PCSK9 and inhibits circulating PCSK9 from binding to the low density lipoprotein (LDL) receptor (LDLR), preventing PCSK9-mediated LDLR degradation and permitting LDLR to recycle back to the liver cell surface.
- By inhibiting the binding of PCSK9 to LDLR, evolocumab increases the number of LDLRs available to clear LDL from the blood, thereby lowering LDL-C levels.
- **Use:**
  - o Homozygous familial hypercholesterolemia.
  - o Heterozygous familial hypercholesterolemia.

Brodalumab: (Feb. 2017)

- Approved for the treatment of moderate-to-severe **plaque psoriasis.**
- It is a human monoclonal immunoglobulin **G antibody [interleukin (IL)-17 receptor A].**

Ixekizumab:

- Humanized interleukin-17A antagonist.
- Treatment of adults with **moderate-to-severe plaque psoriasis** who are candidates for systemic therapy or phototherapy.

Reslizumab:

- An **interleukin-5 antagonist** monoclonal antibody **(IgG4 kappa).**
- Indicated for add-on maintenance treatment of patients with **severe asthma** aged 18 years and older, and with an eosinophilic phenotype.

Ans: Alirocumab

Ref: https://www.accessdata.fda.gov/drugsatfda_docs/label/2015/125522s000lbl.pdf

11. Lubiprostone is a:

(a) Chloride channel activator
(b) Chloride channel inhibitor
(c) Sodium channel activator
(d) Sodium channel inhibitor

Explanation:

Lubipristone

- Bicyclic fatty acid metabolite analogue of **prostaglandin E1** activates **type-2-chloride channels.**
- Used in treatment of:
    - o **Chronic constipation** in adults.
    - o **Irritable bowel syndrome** with **constipation (IBS-C)** in **adult women**.
- It promotes the secretion of a **chloride-rich fluid** and so improves **stool consistency** and promotes increased frequency by reflexly activating motility.
- The drug is **poorly bioavailable**, acting only in the lumen of the bowel.
- **Side effects:** Nausea, headache, diarrhea, allergic reactions and dyspnea.

Ans: Chloride channel activator

Ref: GG, 12th edition, page 1334

12. Newer monoclonal antibody approved for rheumatoid arthritis is:

(a) Durvalumab
(b) Pembrolizumab
(c) Nivolumab
(d) Sarilumab

Explanation:

Sarilumab:

- FDA Approved in May 2017.
- Monoclonal antibody against IL-6 receptor.
- Used in treatment of adults with **rheumatoid arthritis.**
- **200 mg** once every two weeks, administered as a **subcutaneous injection.**

Durvalumab:

- **MOA: Programmed death-ligand 1 (PD-L1)** blocking antibody.
- **Indications**: Locally advanced or metastatic **urothelial carcinoma** who:
    - o Have disease progression during or following platinum-containing chemotherapy.
    - o Have disease progression within 12 months of neoadjuvant or adjuvant treatment with platinum-containing chemotherapy.

Pembrolizumab and nivolumab

- Two humanized antibodies against **programmed cell death 1 (PD-1) receptor.**
- Approved for the treatment of **unresectable or metastatic melanoma** and for other cancers.

Ans: Sarilumab

Ref: https://www.accessdata.fda.gov/drugsatfda_docs/label/2017/761037s000lbl.pdf

13. Tetraethyl ammonium acts by blocking which of the following channels?

(a) Na+
(b) Cl-
(c) K+
(d) Ca

Explanation:

Tetraethylammonium

- **Ganglionic blocker** which blocks **voltage-gated K+ channels.**
- Tried previously for treatment of **Phantom Limb.**
- Marshall first described the "nicotine-paralyzing" action of Tetraethylammonium (TEA) on ganglia in 1913.

- TEA was largely overlooked until the effects of the ion on the cardiovascular system and autonomic ganglia were analyzed.
- It is of **historical importance** only.

Ans: (c) K+

Ref: GG, 12th edition, page 272

14. Denosumab is used in:

(a) Osteomalacia (b) Osteoarthritis (c) Osteoporosis (d) Osteosarcoma

Explanation:

Denosumab

- RANKL binds to its cognate receptor RANK on the surface of precursor and mature osteoclasts, and stimulates these cells to mature and resorb bone.
- **Osteoprotegerin (OPG),** which competes with RANK for binding to RANKL, is the physiological inhibitor of RANKL.
- **Denosumab** is a human monoclonal antibody that binds with high affinity to **RANKL**, mimicking the effect of OPG, and thereby reducing the binding of RANKL to RANK.
- Denosumab **blocks osteoclast formation** and **activation**. It increases **BMD** and **decreases bone turnover markers** when given subcutaneously once every 6 months.
- **Indications:**
  - o Prevention of skeletal-related events in patients with **bone metastases from solid tumors.**
  - o Treatment of adults and skeletally mature adolescents with **giant cell tumor of bone** that is unresectable or where surgical resection is likely to result in severe morbidity.

Ans: (c) Osteoporosis

Ref: GG,12th edition, page 1287

15. Dopamine agonist among the following is:

(a) Cabergoline (b) Seligiline (c) Entacapone (d) Amantadine

Explanation:

Dopamine agonists

Ergot-derived DAs	**Non-ergot DAs**
• Bromocriptine • Lisuride • Pergolide • **Cabergoline**	• Ropinirole and pramipexole (anti-oxidants) • Rotigotine • Apomorphine

Other Options:

- **Seligiline** is a **MAO-B inhibitor** used in treatment of parkinson's **disease.**
- **Entacapone** is a **peripheral COMT inhibitor**, used in treatment of **parkinson's disease**. Doesn't cross BBB.

Amantadine:

- Antiviral drug.
- Used for the **prophylaxis** and **treatment** of **influenza A.**
- Found to have **anti-parkinsonian** activity.

Ans: (a) Cabergoline

Ref: GG, 12th edition, page 358

16. All the following drugs are used in the treatment of metastatic breast cancer *except*:

(a) Ixabifilone (b) Abemaciclib (c) Ribociclib (d) Sunitinib

Explanation:

Ribociclib

- Is a **kinase inhibitor.**
- Specifically indicated in combination with an **aromatase inhibitor** as initial endocrine-based therapy for the treatment of **postmenopausal women** with **hormone receptor (HR)-positive**, **human epidermal growth factor receptor 2 (HER2)-negative advanced** or **metastatic breast cancer.**

Sunitinib

- Competitively inhibits the binding of ATP to the tyrosine kinase domain on the **VEGF receptor-2.**
- Also inhibits other protein tyrosine kinases (FLT3, PDGFR-α, PDGFR-β, RET, CSF-1R and c-KIT).
- **Indications:**
  - o Metastatic **renal-cell cancer.**
  - o Advanced **renal-cell carcinoma** and GIST that have developed resistance to imatinib as a consequence of c-KIT mutations.
- Causes **hand-foot syndrome.**

Ixabepilone:

- Belongs to **epothilones** group of drugs.
- Approved for **breast cancer** treatment.
- Used as monotherapy for **metastatic breast cancer.**
- **Mechanism of action:**
  - o They bind to β tubulin similar to taxanes.
  - o Trigger microtubule nucleation at multiple sites away from the centriole.
  - o This chaotic microtubule stabilization triggers cell-cycle arrest at the G2-M interface and apoptosis.
  - o Epothilones bind to a site distinct from that of taxanes.
  - o These are **cell cycle specific drugs.**
  - o **M phase specific.**

Abemaciclib:

- Is a kinase inhibitor.
- **Indications:**
  - o In combination with **fulvestrant** for the treatment of women with hormone **receptor (HR)-positive**, human epidermal growth factor receptor 2 (**HER2)-negative** advanced or **metastatic breast cancer** with disease progression following endocrine therapy.
  - o As **monotherapy** for the treatment of **adult patients with HR-positive, HER2-negative advanced or metastatic breast cancer** with disease progression following endocrine therapy and prior chemotherapy in the metastatic settings.

Ans: (d) Sunitinib

Ref: www.accessdata.fda.gov

17. Time dependent pharmacokinetics is seen in:

(a) Ofloxacin (b) Amikacin (c) Penicillin (d) Ciprofloxacin

Explanation:

Time-Dependent Killing Agents

- These drugs reach a ceiling at which higher concentrations do not result in increased effect. Instead, these agents are active against **bacteria** only when the drug concentration above the MIC. The duration above MIC (**T>MIC**) predicts clinical efficacy for **all β-lactams like penicillins, cephalosporins.**

- The longer the concentration of the β-lactam remains above the MIC for an infecting pathogen during the dosing interval, the greater the killing effect.
- *Examples:* **Cephalosporins, Penicillins, Macrolides, Clindamycin.**

Concentration-Dependent Killing

- The higher the drug concentration, the higher the rate and extent of bacterial killing.
- **Aminoglycosides** fit into the **Cmax/MIC** model of pharmacodynamics activity, and a particular peak serum concentration is often targeted to achieve optimal killing.
- ***Examples:*** **Amikacin, gentamicin, azithromycin, ketolides.**
- **Fluoroquinolones: Ciprofloxacin, ofloxacin.**
    - These are different class of antibacterial agents for which the **AUC/MIC** is a predictor of efficacy. For example, studies have found that an AUC/MIC ratio of >30 will maximize killing of S. pneumoniae by fluoroquinolones.

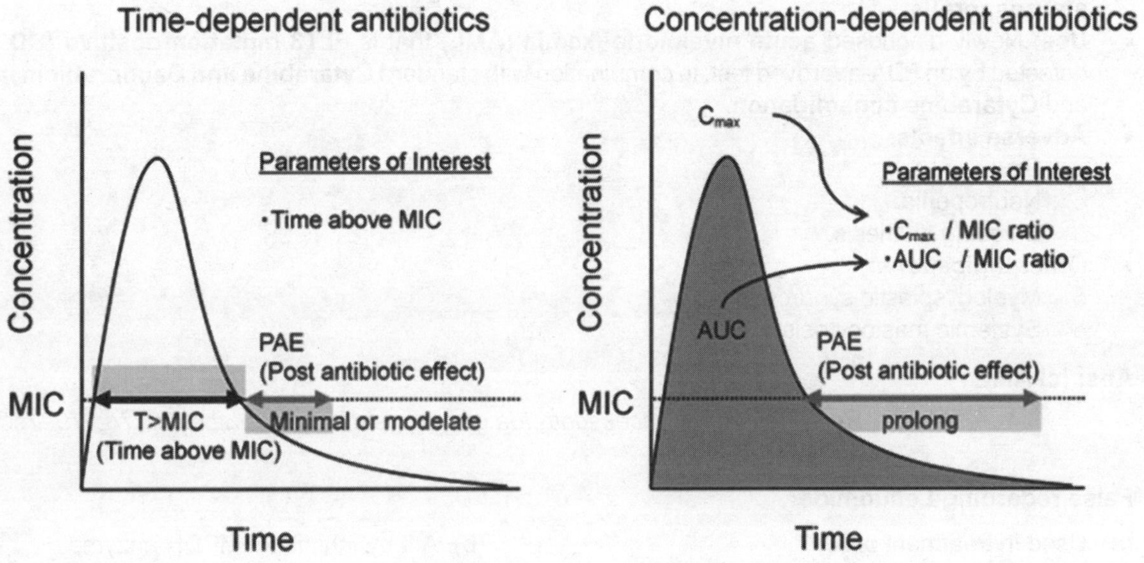

Ans: (c) Penicillin

Ref: Harrison, 19th edition, page 935

18. Tetrabenazine acts on:

(a) MAO B
(b) Vesicular monoamine transporter
(c) Dopamine
(d) COMT

Explanation:

Tetrabenazine

- It is a **vesicular monoamine transporter 2 (VMAT2) inhibitor.**
- Indicated for the treatment of **chorea** associated with **Huntington's disease**.
- Reversible high affinity inhibitor of monoamine uptake into granular vesicles of presynaptic neurons.
- Secondary depletion at low doses, as well as a weak D2 post synaptic receptor blocker in high doses.
- TBZ depletes all three monoamines, but particularly **dopamine.**

MAO-B INHIBITOR IS SELEGILINE

Dopamine receptor agonists

- **Ergot-derived Das**
    - Bromocriptine, lisuride, pergolide, **cabergoline.**
- **Non-ergot Das**
    - Ropinirole and pramipexole (anti-oxidants), rotigotine, apomorphine.

COMT Inhibitor

- Entacapone and tolcapone.

Ans: (b) Vesicular monoamine transporter

Ref: Diana Paleacu, Tetrabenazine in the Treatment of Huntington's Disease, Neuropsychiatry Dis Treat 2007 Oct; 3(5): 545–551

19. Midostaurin used in:

(a) CML (b) ALL (c) AML (d) CLL

Explanation:

Midostaurin

- **MOA:** Tyrosine kinase inhibitor.
- It is a semi-synthetic derivative of **staurosporine**, an alkaloid from the bacterium **Streptomyces staurosporeus.**
- **Use:** Newly diagnosed **acute myeloid leukemia (AML)** that is **FLT3 mutation positive (CD 135*)** as detected by an FDA-approved test, in combination with standard **Cytarabine and Daunorubicin induction** and **Cytarabine consolidation.**
- **Adverse effects:**
    - o Fever.
    - o Neutropenia.
    - o Bleeding diathesis.
- **Other indications:**
    - o Myelodysplastic syndrome*.
    - o Systemic mastocytosis*.

Ans: (c) AML

Ref: https://www.accessdata.fda.gov/drugsatfda_docs/label/2017/207997s000lbl.pdf

20. False regarding Lefluomide:

(a) Used in treatment of RA (b) Act by inhibiting IMPDH enzyme
(c) Inhibits proliferation of T and B cells (d) It is contraindicated in pregnancy

Explanation:

LEFLUOMIDE

- Immunomodulator that inhibits proliferation of stimulated lymphocytes in patients with active Rheumatoid arthritis.
- Arthritic symptoms are suppressed and radiological progression of disease is retarded.

MOA:

- Leflunomide is rapidly converted in the body to an active metabolite, which **inhibits dihydroorotate dehydrogenase** and **pyrimidine synthesis** in actively dividing cells.
- Antibody production by B-cells may be depressed.
- The active metabolite has a long t½ of 2–3 weeks.
- Inhibits proliferation of T and B cells.

Adverse effects

- Diarrhoea, headache, nausea, rashes, loss of hair, thrombocytopenia, leucopenia, increased chances of chest infection and raised hepatic transaminases.

Contraindications:

- It is not to be used in **children** and **pregnant/lactating women.**

NOTE:

- Leflunomide is an alternative to Methotrexate or can be added to it, but the combination is more hepatotoxic.
- Combination with sulfasalazine improves benefit.
- Leflunomide doesn't inhibit inosine monophosphate dehydrogenase (**IMPDH**).

Inosine Monophosphate Dehydrogenase (IMPDH)

- NAD-dependent enzyme that controls de novo synthesis of guanine nucleotides.
- Important target enzyme for anticancer drugs and also for antiviral, antiparasitic, and immunosuppressive chemotherapy.
- The field of IMPDH inhibitor research is highly important for providing potential therapeutics against a validated target for disease intervention.

Ans: (b) Act by inhibiting IMPDH enzyme

Ref: KDT, 7th edition, page 212

21. Cobicistat is used along with which of the following antiretroviral drug?

(a) Indinavir (b) Darunavir
(c) Ritonavir (d) Saquvinavir

Explanation:

Cobicistat

- Mechanism – Inhibitor of cytochrome **P450 (CYP) 3A enzymes.**
- Indicated as a pharmacokinetic enhancer (i.e., booster) of the HIV-1 protease inhibitors **atazanavir* and darunavir*** in adults.

Ritonavir

- Acts as pharmacokinetic booster by **inhibiting CYP3A4.**
- Used at lower dose for this purpose.
- Combinations of **darunavir, lopinavir, fosamprenavir and atazanavir** with ritonavir are approved for **once daily administration.**

Ans: (b) Darunavir

Ref:http://www.gilead.com/~/media/Files/pdfs/medicines/hiv/tybost/tybost_pi.pdf

22. Patient with DVT on therapeutic dose of Warfarin came with complaints of breathlessness and hypotension. True statement regarding this:

(a) Warfarin to be continued for 6 months (b) Maintain INR at 3.5 and continue
(c) Maintain INR at 2 and continue (d) Discontinue warfarin

Explanation:

INR Ranges When Treating with Warfarin

- 1.5–1.9
  - Higher rate of recurrent venous thromboembolism.
- <1.7
  - Increased risk of **cardioembolic stroke.**
- 2.0–3.0
  - Warfarin is administered in doses that produce above INR.
  - **This the recommended INR while treating with warfarin.**
  - This INR is effective as higher intensity treatment and produces less bleeding.
- 2.5–3.5
  - Allowed in special situations like in patients with mechanical heart valves, particularly those in the mitral position or older ball and cage valves in the aortic.
- >4.5
  - Increase in **bleeding.**

Note:

In a study, patients receiving long-term warfarin therapy for unprovoked venous thromboembolism demonstrated a higher rate of recurrent venous thromboembolism with a target INR of 1.5–1.9 compared with a target INR of 2.0–3.0.

So, in this case patient with DVT on therapeutic dose of Warfarin came with c/o breathlessness, hypotension. May be he has unprovoked venous thromboembolism and recurrent venous thromboembolism, so maintain INR at 2.0 to 3.0 and continue warfarin.

IMPORTANT:

Warfarin induced bleeding

- The INR should be maintained in the therapeutic range to minimize the risk of bleeding.
- In asymptomatic patients whose INR is between 3.5 and 10, warfarin should be withheld until the INR returns to the therapeutic range.
- If the INR is over 10, oral vitamin K should be administered, at a dose of 2.5–5 mg.
- Higher doses of oral vitamin K (5–10 mg) produce more rapid reversal of the INR but may render patients temporarily resistant to warfarin when the drug is restarted.
- Patients with serious bleeding need more aggressive treatment. These patients should be given 5–10 mg of vitamin K by slow IV infusion. Additional vitamin K should be given until the INR is in the normal range.
- Treatment with vitamin K should be supplemented with fresh-frozen plasma as a source of the vitamin K–dependent clotting proteins.
- Four factor prothrombin complex concentrates, which contain all four vitamin K–dependent clotting proteins, are the treatment of choice for:
    - Life-threatening bleeds.
    - Rapid restoration of the INR into the normal range in patients requiring urgent surgery or intervention.
    - Patients who cannot tolerate the volume load of fresh-frozen plasma.

Ans: (c) Maintain INR at 2 and continue

Ref: Harrison, 19th edition, page 755

23. All can cause serotonin increase *except:*

(a) MDMA (b) Amphetamine (c) Meperidine (d) LSD

Explanation:

- Amphetamines such as **methylene dioxy methamphetamine MDMA (Ecstasy),** which directly releases **serotonin** from **nerve terminals.**
- **Meperidine** also increases release of serotonin at nerve terminals.
- So these drugs should not combine with SSRIs to avoid serotonin syndrome.
- Symptoms of the **serotonin syndrome** include **hyperthermia, muscle rigidity, myoclonus, tremors, autonomic instability, confusion, irritability, and agitation**; this can progress toward **coma and death.**
- Treatment symptomatic with avoiding all the serotinergic drugs and administering **nonselective serotonin antagonists.**

LSD:

- Potent **serotonin 5-HT2 receptor agonist.**
- It doesn't increase serotonin release.

Ans: (d) LSD

Ref: GG, 12th edition, page 412

24. Which is not an osmotic laxative?

(a) Sorbitol (b) Magnesium
(c) Polyethylene glycol (d) Bisacodyl

Explanation:

Polyethylene Glycol

- **Osmotic purgative,** due to high molecular weight.

- **Used**
  - o Prior to surgery.
  - o Constipation.

Sorbitol

- **Lactulose** and **sorbitol** are both non-absorbable disaccharides, which pass unchanged into the colon where they are metabolized by bacteria into formic, acetic and lactic acids.
- The organic acids produced increase intraluminal fluid in the colon.

Magnesium

- Magnesium ions release **cholecystokinin** which augments **motility and secretion**, contributing to purgative action of magnesium salts.
- All inorganic salts used as osmotic (saline) purgatives have similar action—differ only in dose, palatability and risk of systemic toxicity.
- Magnesium salts are contraindicated in **renal insufficiency.**
- Sodium salts should not be given to patients of **CHF** and other sodium retaining states.

Bisacodyl

- **Stimulant laxative.**
- Available as 5 mg (infant) and 10 mg (adult) suppository.
- Irritates anal and rectal mucosa ⇛ reflex increase in motility ⇛ evacuation in 20-40 min.
- Can cause inflammation and mucosal damage.
- Bisacodyl activated by esterases in intestine so taken at bedtime.

Ans: (d) Bisacodyl

Ref: KDT, 7th edition, page 675

25. Warfarin induced skin necrosis is seen in:

(a) Protein C deficiency
(b) Sickle cell anemia
(c) Factor V leiden deficiency
(d) Antithrombin 3 deficiency

Explanation:

"Warfarin-induced skin necrosis is seen in patients with congenital or acquired deficiencies of protein C or protein S." Ref: Harrison

Warfarin Induced Skin Necrosis

- A rare complication of warfarin.
- **Skin necrosis** is seen **2–5 days** after initiation of therapy.
- **Well-demarcated erythematous lesions** form on the **thighs, buttocks, breasts or toes.**
- **Center of the lesion** becomes **progressively necrotic**.
- **Skin biopsies** from border of these lesions reveals **thrombi** in the microvasculature.
- Warfarin skin necrosis is seen with congenital or acquired deficiencies of **protein C or protein S.**
- Warfarin causes precipitous **fall in plasma levels of proteins C or S,** thereby eliminating this important anticoagulant pathway.
- The resultant **procoagulant** state triggers **thrombosis**.
- Treatment involves **discontinuation of warfarin** and **reversal with vitamin K**.
- An alternative anticoagulant, such as **heparin or LMWH**, should be given in patients with **thrombosis**.
- **Protein C concentrate** can be given to protein C–deficient patients to accelerate healing of the skin lesions; **fresh-frozen plasma** may be of value if protein C concentrate is unavailable and for those with protein S deficiency.
- Occasionally, **skin grafting** is necessary when there is **extensive skin loss**.
- Because of the potential for **skin necrosis**, patients with known **protein C or protein S deficiency** require overlapping treatment with a **parenteral anticoagulant** when initiating **warfarin therapy**.

Ans: (a) Protein C deficiency

Ref: Harrison's 19th edition, page 756 and K.D. Tripathi, Essentials of Medical Pharmacology, 6th edition

26. The risk of carbamazepine induced Stevens-Johnson syndrome is increased in the presence of which of the following genes?

(a) HLA-B 1507 (b) HLA-B 1502 (c) HLA-B 57 (d) HLA-B

Explanation:

Carbamazepine:

- Used in treatment of:
  - ***Partial seizures.***
  - ***Bipolar disorder.***
  - ***Trigeminal neuralgia.***
  - ***Chronic pain.***
- Associated with hypersensitivity reactions.
- The reactions may be simple **urticaria** to life-threatening cutaneous disorders, including **Stevens-Johnson syndrome (SJS) and toxic epidermal necrolysis (TEN).**
- These hypersensitivity reactions are associated with **HLA-B*1502** status of the individual.
- There is correlation between **HLA-B*1502** and **carbamazepine-SJS/TEN** in Han Chinese.
- So current guidelines is do genotyping Asian patients before starting the therapy.
- Important to suggest **HLA-B*1502 carriers** to avoid not only **carbamazepine** but also other structurally related anticonvulsants, such as **phenytoin, oxcarbamazepine and possibly lamotrigine.**

Ans: (b) HLA-B 1502

*Ref: Carbamazepine, HLA-B*1502 and Risk of Stevens-Johnson Syndrome and Toxic Epidermal Necrolysis: US FDA Recommendations*

27. Lenalidomide coadministration with which another drug increases the risk of thrombosis?

(a) Alcohol (b) Barbiturate (c) Glucocorticoids (d) Antibiotics

Explanation:

*"**Lenalidomide** may increase the risk of deep venous thrombosis and pulmonary embolus. Concurrent use of **corticosteroids** may further increase this risk." Ref: Lippincott's The Chemotherapy Source Book*

LENALIDOMIDE

- Anti-angiogenesis agent.
- **Mech of Action:**
  - Thalidomide analogue.
  - **Immunomodulatory agent** that **inhibits angiogenesis** in cells.
  - Exact mechanism is **not known.**
  - Believed to **inhibit** bone marrow secretion of **IL-6, VEFG and TNF alpha.**
- **Indications:**
  - **Transfusion dependent anemia** due to low or intermediate risk **MDS** associated with deletion **5q** cytogenetic abnormality.
  - **Multiple myeloma.**
- **Adverse Effects:**
  - **Myelosuppression.**
  - Diarrhea, mild rash.
  - **Teratogen.**
  - Increased risk of deep venous thrombosis (especially when given along with corticosteroids).

Ans: (c) Glucocorticoids

Ref: Lippincott's The Chemotherapy Source Book, Michael Clinton Perry, 4th edition, page 606

28. Which of the following drugs cause prolonged QT syndrome (Torsade de pointes) when given along with Ritonavir?

(a) Darunavir (b) Saquinavir (c) Amprenavir (d) Tipranavir

Explanation:

- Among the given options only **Darunavir** is used along with **Ritonavir**.

Ritonavir:

- Acts as pharmacokinetic booster by inhibiting **CYP3A4.**
- Used at lower dose for this purpose.
- Combinations of **darunavir, lopinavir, fosamprenavir, and atazanavir** with **ritonavir** are approved for once-daily administration.
- A **peptidomimetic HIV protease inhibitor.**
- Is active against both **HIV-1 and HIV-2.**
- Metabolized primarily by **CYP3A4** and to a lesser extent by **CYP2D6.**
- Induces its own metabolism.
- Ritonavir is used a **pharmacokinetic enhancer** by inhibiting **CYP 3A4 inhibitor** and it is used it low dose for this action.

QT prolongation (Torsade de pointes) is seen with:

Adverse Effects of Protease Inhibitors

Common side effects seen with all protease inhibitors include:

- **Nausea, vomiting.**
- **Diarrhea**, abdominal discomfort.
- Lipodystrophy.
- Hypercholesterolemia.
- Hypertriglyceridemia.

Specific ADR of Different Protease Inhibitors

- **Ritonavir**–Perioral paresthesia.
- **Fosamprenavir**–Skin eruption.
- **Atazanavir**–Cholelithiasis, cholecystitis.
- **Darunavir**–Rash, hepatotoxicity.
- **Indinavir**–Crystalluria, nephrolithiasis, hair loss, dry skin, insulin resistance.
- **Nelfinavir**–Chronic diarrhea.
- **Tipranavir**–Fatal hepatotoxicity, intracranial hemorrhage.
- **Atazanavir** is a **protease inhibitor** that does **not** cause **dyslipidemia** unlike **amprenavir**, **saquinavir**, **nelfinavir**.
- **Tipranavir** is one of the **HIV protease inhibitors** that has a high incidence of **raised cholesterol** and **triglycerides**.

Common Pharmacokinetic Drug Interactions Associated with Torsade de Pointes			
Inhibition of CYP 3A4		**Inhibition of CYP 2D6**	
Inhibitors	**Substrates**	**Inhibitors**	**Substrates**
Antifungals • Itraconazole • Ketoconazole • Posaconazole • Voriconazole **Macrolides** • Erythromycin • Clarithromycin • Azithromycin **Protease inhibitors** • Atazanavir • Darunavir/ritonavir • Fosamprenavir • Indinavir • Nelfinavir • Saquinavir • Tipranavir	Amiodarone Disopyramide Dofetilide Pimozide	**Neuropsychiatrics** • Bupropion • Duloxetine • Fluoxetine • Paroxetine **Antifungal** • Terbinafine	Flecainide Quinidine Thioridazine

Ans: (a) Darunavir

Ref: Li M, Drug-Induced QT Prolongation and Torsade de Pointes, P&T, 42(7):473-77

PATHOLOGY

1. Type of hereditary hemorrhagic telangiectasia commonly associated with ALK-1 mutation is:

(a) Type 1 (b) Type 2

(c) Type 3 (d) Type 4

Explanation:

Hereditary Hemorrhagic Telangiectasia (HHT or Osler-Weber-Rendu Syndrome)

- Inherited disorder characterized by malformations of various blood vessels (vascular dysplasia), potentially resulting in bleeding (hemorrhage).
- There are totally **6 types** till date.
- **Chronic nose bleeding** is usually the **first sign***.
- **Genetics.**

Type	Mutation
HHT 1	ENG gene
HHT 2	ALK 1 gene
HHT 3	Unidentified gene in Ch 5 (putative)
HHT 4	Ch 7p14

Ans: (b) Type 2

Ref: Genetic Home Reference

2. α1-antitrypsin deficiency chromosome is located at:

(a) 10 (b) 14

(c) 17 (d) 11

Explanation:

Alpha 1-Antitrypsin Deficiency:

α1-Antitrypsin deficiency is an autosomal recessive disorder of protein folding marked by very low levels of circulating α1-Antitrypsin (α1AT).

- α1AT deficiency leads to the development of **pulmonary emphysema**, because the activity of destructive proteases is not inhibited.
- It also causes **chronic liver disease** as a consequence of hepatocellular accumulation of the misfolded protein.
- **Cutaneous necrotizing panniculitis** also occurs in a minor subset of patients.
- The gene, located on **chromosome 14.**
- **The most common clinically significant mutation is PiZZ; homozygotes for the PiZZ protein have circulating α1AT levels that are only 10% of normal.**
- α1AT deficiency is characterized by the presence of round-to-oval **cytoplasmic globular inclusions in hepatocytes,** which on routine hematoxylin and eosin stains are acidophilic, but are strongly periodic acid-Schiff (PAS)-positive and diastase-resistant.

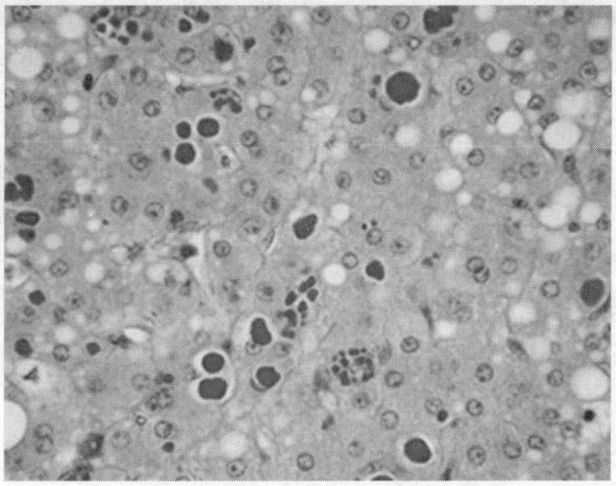

Fig: PAS positive globules in liver

Ans: (b) 14

Ref: Robbins Pathology, 9th edition, page 850

3. Bone marrow examination reveals leukoerythroblastic picture with dacryocytes. There was also positive history of dry tap during bone marrow aspiration. What is the probable diagnosis?

(a) Abundant fat cells laden bone marrow
(b) Primary myelofibrosis
(c) Fatty degeneration with erythroid cell hyperplasia with megakaryocytes
(d) Vitamin B12 deficiency

Explanation:

- **Leukoerythroblastic picture with dacryocytes (tear drop cells)** is a classical picture of **Myelofibrosis*.**

Myelofibrosis:

- **The hallmark of primary myelofibrosis is the development of obliterative marrow fibrosis.** The replacement of the marrow by fibrous tissue reduces bone marrow hematopoiesis, leading to cytopenias and extensive extramedullary hematopoiesis.
- **Mutations:**
  - o **Activating JAK2 mutations** are present in 50% to 60% of cases activating MPL mutations in an additional 1% to 5% of cases.
  - o A new mutation – **CALR (calreticulin)** mutation is seen in a rest.
- The chief pathologic feature is the extensive deposition of collagen in the marrow by non-neoplastic fibroblasts.

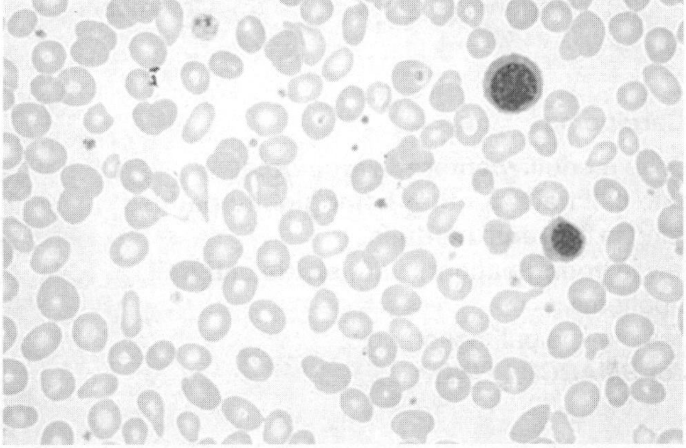

- Two nucleated erythroid precursors and several teardrop-shaped red cells (dacryocytes) are evident in the above peripheral blood smear.

Ans: (b) Primary myelofibrosis

Ref: Robbins Pathology, 9th edition, page 620-621

4. **Blister cells are seen in:**

(a) Thalassemia
(b) Chronic liver disease
(c) Sickle cell anemia
(d) G6PD disease

Explanation:

- **Blister and Bite cells** are seen in **G6PD deficiency***.

G6PD Deficiency:

- X linked recessive.
- Causes both **intra-vascular and Extravascular hemolysis.**
- Trigger factors – Infection, drugs, Fava beans.
- **Peripheral smear:**
  - o **Spherocytes***.
  - o **Reticulocytes***.
  - o **Heinz bodies* (denatured Globin).**
  - o **Bite cells*.**
- Confirmatory – **Enzyme analysis***.

Bite Cells

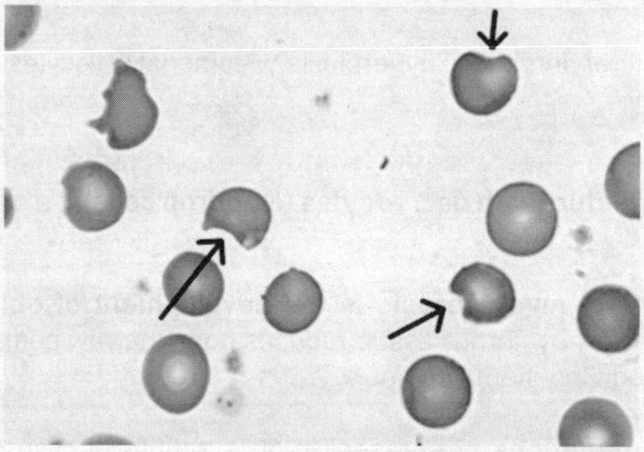

Ans: (d) G6PD disease

Ref: Robbins Pathology, 9th edition, page 634

5. **Sickle cell disease associated with which type of renal cell carcinoma?**

(a) Medullary (b) Papillary (c) Chromophobe (d) Colloid

Explanation:

Medullary Renal Cell Carcinoma

- Rare, highly aggressive **medulla centered carcinoma.**
- Associated with **sickle cell trait*** or **other hemoglobinopathies*.**
- Rare carcinoma arising in the **renal medulla.**
- Occurs predominately in **young patients with sickle cell trait.**
- Variety of histologic patterns.
- **Sickled erythrocytes** may be pathognomonic.
- Majority show **loss of *SMARCB1 / INI1**.**
- **Poor prognosis*.**

Ans: (a) Medullary

Ref: WHO, Urogential System, page 122

6. **Chromosomes involved in early onset Alzheimer's disease:**

(a) 1, 14, 21 (b) 1, 13, 22 (c) 3, 14, 20 (d) 3, 14, X

Explanation:

Genes Involved in Alzheimers Disease

- **Early onset Alzehimer's disease** involves three genes:
  - o **APP**–Ch 21.
  - o **PSEN1 (Presenilin 1)** – Ch 14.
  - o **PSEN 2 (Presenilin 2)** – Ch 1.

Genes causing autosomal dominant AD	• APP • PSEN1 • PSEN 2 All can cause early onset disease but PSEN2 is associated with a broad range of onset ages.
Susceptibitity genes	• Apolipoprotein E gene (APOE) – ε2 allele: associated with decreased risk – ε3 allele: neutral – ε4 allele: high-risk • SORL1

Ans: (a) 1,14,21

Ref: Genetic Home Reference

7. **Cell responsible for 'Graft versus host disease' (GVHD) is:**

(a) Donor T cell (b) Donor B cell

(c) Host T cell (d) Host B cell

Explanation:

Graft versus host disease occurs in any situation in which **immunologically competent cells** or their precursors are transplanted into **immunologically crippled patients** and the transferred cells recognize **alloantigens** in the host.

- It occurs most commonly in the setting of **allogenic one marrow transplantation.**
- The ***immunocompetent T cells*** present in the donor marrow recognize the ***recipient's HLA antigen*** as foreign ***antigen*** and reacts against them. Both **CD4$^+$** and **CD8$^+$T** cells recognize and attack host tissues.
- There are two types of GVHD – Acute and Chronic.

Characteristic Organs Affected in GVHD are:

- **Skin:** Epidermis and hair follicles are damaged.
- **Liver:** Small bile ducts show segmental disruption.
- **Intestines:** Destruction of the crypts and mucosal ulceration may be noted.

Ans: (a) Donor T cell

Ref: Robbins Pathology, 9th edition, page 236

8. **Loss of 'y' chromosome is associated with which of the following renal cell carcinoma?**

(a) Papillary (b) Chromophobe

(c) Clear cell (d) Collecting duct carcinoma

Explanation:

A direct question from Robbin's Pathologic Basis of Disease.

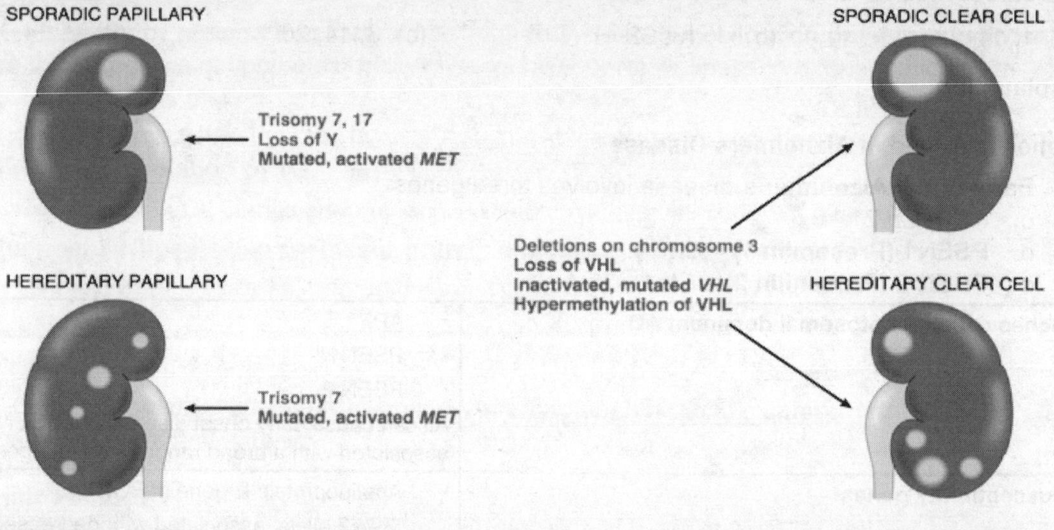

Ans: (a) Papillary

Ref: Robbins Pathology, 9th edition, page 954

9. All the following are criteria for diagnosing severe aplastic anemia *except*:

(a) BM cellularity <25% (b) Reticulocyte < 1%
(c) Platelet <20k (d) ANC <1500

Explanation:

Criteria for Aplastic Anemia (ASH)

Classification	Criteria
Severe	BM cellularity <25% (or <50% if <30% of BM is hematopoietic cells) AND ≥ 2 of the following: • Peripheral blood neutrophil count $<0.5 \times 10^9$/L • Peripheral blood platelet count $<20 \times 10^9$/L • Peripheral blood reticulocyte count $<20 \times 10^9$/L
Very severe	As above, but peripheral blood neutrophil count must be $<0.2 \times 10^9$/L
Non-severe	Hypocellular BM with peripheral blood values not meeting criteria for severe aplastic anemia

Ans: (d) ANC <1500

Ref: WHO, Hematopoietic System, page 221

10. Flow cytometry is used to:

(a) Antibody response T lymphocytes (b) Separate blood cells
(c) Distinguish between leukocytes (d) To get differential leukocyte count

Explanation:

Flow cytometers (FC or FCM) are automated instruments that quantitate properties of single cells, one cell at a time.

- They can measure **cell size**, **cell granularity**, the amounts of **cell components.**
- Simply measuring cell size and granularity is sufficient to distinguish the major categories of leukocytes in peripheral blood.
- This is the basis for clinical instruments that do **automated complete blood counts (CBC).**
- Adding **fluorescent probes** to the cells enables quantitation of **specific structures ("flow cytofluorometry").**

The most common use of flow cytofluorometry:

- To diagnose **leukemia and lymphoma.**
- To diagnoses various **RBC disorders** (PNH, Hereditary spherocytosis).
- Quantification of **CD4+ vs. CD8+** T lymphocytes in blood – in **HIV patients.**

Ans: (c) Distinguish between leukocytes

Ref: Robbins Pathology, 9th edition, page 334

11. TRAP positivity is seen with:

(a) CML (b) Hairy cell leukemia (c) CLL (d) Follicular lymphoma

Explanation:

Hairy Cell Leukemia

- Rare chronic leukemia that commonly presents with **massive splenomegaly**, with tumor cells containing **hair-like projections.**
- Also known as **leukemic reticuloendotheliosis*.**
- **Clinical:**
  - o Commonly presents with **massive splenomegaly** with **obliteration of white pulp** and involvement of red pulp, pancytopenia (50%), **marrow fibrosis, monocytopenia, infections in 1/3.**
  - o Bone marrow aspiration biopsies **unsuccessful** ("**dry tap**") in **30 - 50%** due to marrow fibrosis.
- **Peripheral Smear:**
  - o Tumor cells are larger than small lymphocytes, modest pale blue a granular cytoplasm with circumferential threadlike extensions seen with phase contrast microscope, round or indented/folded (oval) nuclei, no distinct nucleoli.
- **Bone Marrow:**
  - o Prominent cell borders ("**fried egg appearance**") with formalin fixation.
- **Stains:**
  - o ***TRAP.***
  - o ***B cell markers.***
  - o ***CD 11c, CD25, CD103.***
  - o ***Annexin A1.***

Ans: (b) Hairy cell leukemia

Ref: Robbins Pathology, 9th edition, page 603

12. Apoptotic genes regulating programmed cell death type 2, autophagy is:

(a) p53 (b) BAX (c) BCL-2 (d) None of the above

Explanation:

Autophagy:

- **Autophagy is a process in which a cell eats its own contents** *(Greek:* ***auto,*** *self;* ***phagy,*** *eating).*
- It involves the delivery of cytoplasmic materials to the lysosome for degradation.
- Autophagy is an adaptive response that is enhanced during nutrient deprivation, allowing the cell to cannibalize itself to survive.

Autophagy can be categorized into three types:

- ***Chaperone-mediated*** **autophagy** (direct translocation across the lysosomal membrane by chaperone proteins).
- ***Microautophagy*** (inward invagination of lysosomal membrane for delivery).
- ***Macroautophagy*** (hereafter referred to as *autophagy*), the major form of autophagy involving the sequestration and transportation of portions of cytosol in a double-membrane bound autophagic vacuole (autophagosome).

There are many genes and proteins involved in autophagy; BCL2 is one among the notable ones.

Ans: (c) BCL-2

Ref: Genetic Home Reference

13. Which of the following is HMB45 negative?

(a) Melanoma
(b) Angiomyolipoma
(c) Tendon clear cell sarcoma
(d) Juxtaglomerular tumor

Explanation:

HMB 45: Human Melanoma Black: **Positive staining is seen in:**

- Melanoma (85-90%, see exceptions under negative staining).
- Angiomyolipoma.
- Clear cell sarcoma of soft tissue.
- Clear cell "sugar" tumor.
- Epithelioid sarcoma (occasional).
- Kidney: t(6;11)(p21;q12) renal cell carcinoma.
- Lymphangioleiomyomatosis (also stains non-proliferative cells).
- Melanocytosis.
- PEComa.
- Pheochromocytoma.
- Pigmented neural tumors (some), including some nerve sheath tumors, some neurofibromas pigmented neuroectodermal tumor of infancy.
- Tuberous sclerosis complex components.

Ans: (d) Juxtaglomerular tumor

Ref: Dab Immunohistochemistry Basics, HMB45

14. Read the pedigree chart and identify the pattern of transmission:

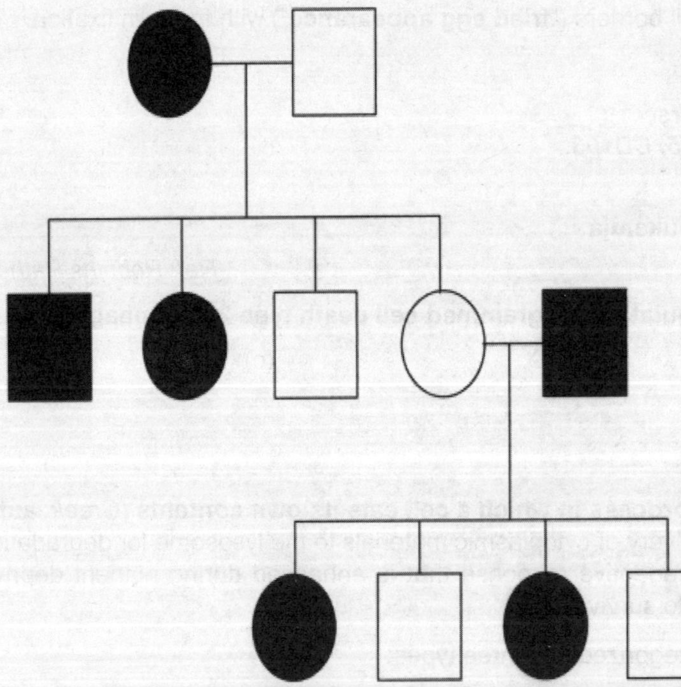

(a) Autosomal dominant
(b) Autosomal recessive
(c) X-linked dominant
(d) X-linked recessive

Explanation:

For two pedigree questions below (please follow this simple Flowchart).

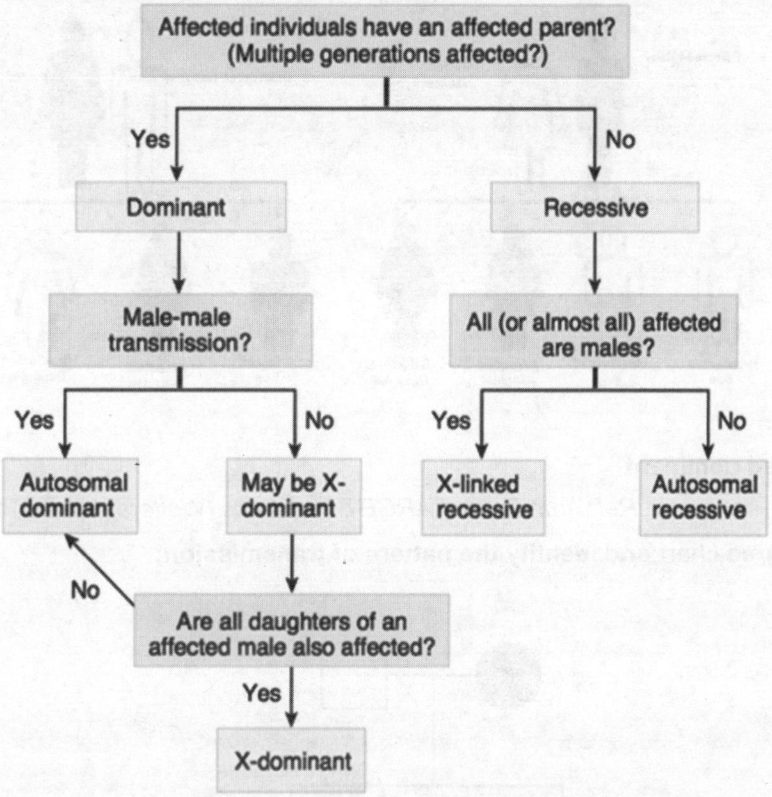

X-linked Dominant Inheritance

- **Daughters of affected male always inherit the disorder.**
- **More females are affected**, but have milder phenotype.
- **No male-to-male transmission.**
- **Both males and females are affected**; often **more females** than males are affected.
- **Does not skip generations**.
- **Affected sons** must have an **affected mother.**
- **Affected daughters** must have either **an affected mother or an affected father.**
- **Affected fathers** will **pass the trait** on to all their **daughters.**
- **Affected mothers** if **heterozygous** will pass the trait on to **1/2 of their sons and 1/2 of their daughters.**
- Affected males with normal mates have no affected sons and no normal daughters **(Criss cross inheritance*).**
- Some disorders may be **lethal in males.**

X-linked dominant diseases

- **Vitamin D resistant rickets** (X-linked hypophosphatemia)*
- **Incontinentia pigmenti***
- **Rett's syndrome***
- Goltz syndrome
- Fragile X syndrome
- Alport syndrome
- Aicardi syndrome
- Orofacial digital syndromes

X LINKED DOMINANT

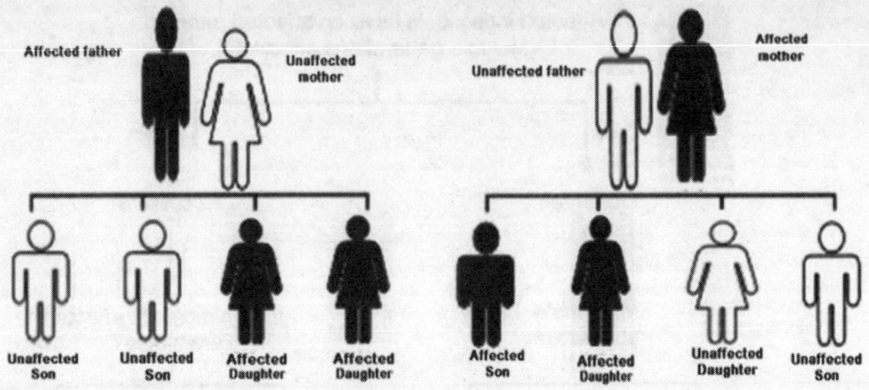

Ans: (c) X-linked dominant

Ref: Arun Babu, TARGET Pediatrics (Wolters Kluwer), 1st edition, page 126-127

15. Read the pedigree chart and identify the pattern of transmission:

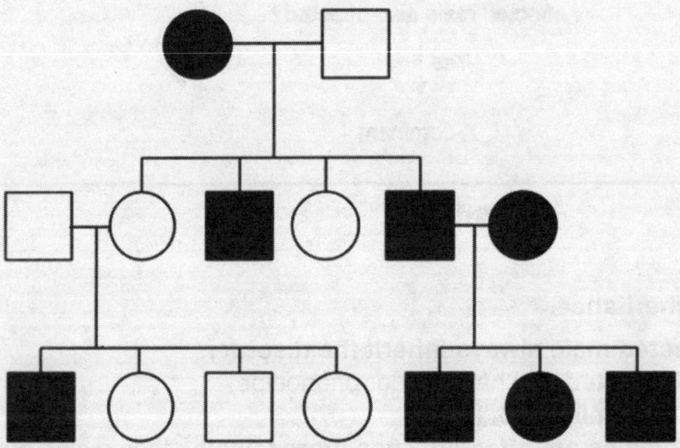

(a) Autosomal dominant
(b) Autosomal recessive
(c) X-linked dominant
(d) X-linked recessive

Explanation:

X-LINKED RECESSIVE INHERITANCE

- **Males are affected and female are carriers** and they transmit the disease.
- **No male to male transmission.**
- Female carriers have a 25% risk for having an affected son, a 25% risk for a carrier daughter, and a 50% chance of having a child that does not inherit the mutated X-linked gene.
- Females are **Carriers** only (Do not manifest the disease).
- Females transmit mutant genes to **50% sons.**
    - **Affected males have carrier daughters and unaffected sons** females are **Carriers** only (Do not manifest the disease).
    - Females transmit mutant genes to **50% sons.**
- A significant proportion of isolated cases are due to new mutations.

- Only rarely will a female manifest the signs of an X-linked disease; this is usually due to **atypical lionization,** a new mutation in the other X chromosome, a carrier with **Turner's syndrome**, **or X-autosome translocation.**

NEET PG Key

- **When females can rarely manifest X-linked recessive disease:**
  - o **Atypical lionization** (Selective inactivation of one copy of X chromosome).
  - o **New mutation** in the other X chromosome.
  - o Carrier with **Turner's syndrome.**
  - o **X-autosome translocation.**

X-LINKED RECESSIVE DISEASES

System	Disorder
Nervous	**Fragile X syndrome** **Colour blindness**
Immune	Agammaglobulinemia **Wiskott Aldrich syndrome**
Metabolic	Diabetes insipidus Lesch Nyan syndrome Hunter syndrome Fabry syndrome
Hematologic	**Hemophilia A & B** Chronic granulomatous disease G6PD deficiency
Musculoskeletal	Duchenne muscular dystrophy

X LINKED RECESSIVE

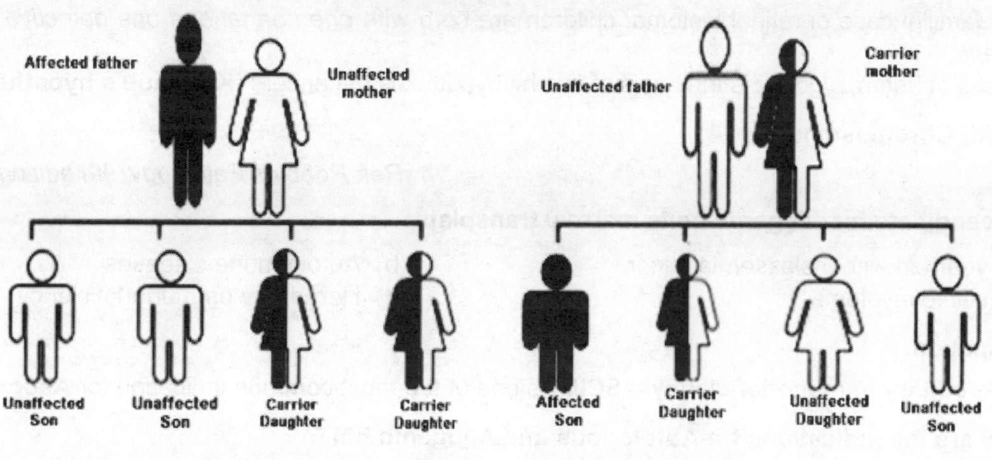

Ans: (d) X-linked recessive

Ref: Arun Babu, TARGET Pediatrics (Wolters Kluwer), 1st edition, page 126-127

16. Dohle like inclusions in neutrophils along with giant platelets is characteristic of:

(a) Bernard-Soulier syndrome
(b) Chediak-Higashi syndrome
(c) May Hegglin anomaly
(d) Pelger-Huet anomaly

Explanation:

May Hegglin anomaly (MHA), also known as **Döhle leukocyte inclusions** with **giant platelets** and **macrothrombocytopenia** with **leukocyte inclusions**, is a rare genetic disorder of the blood platelets that causes them to be abnormally large.

Bernard-Soulier syndrome (BSS), also called **hemorrhagiparous thrombocytic dystrophy**, is a rare **autosomal recessive** coagulopathy (bleeding **disorder**) that causes a deficiency of **glycoprotein Ib (GpIb),** the receptor for von Willebrand factor.

Chédiak-Higashi syndrome is a rare autosomal recessive **disorder** that arises from a mutation of a **lysosomal trafficking regulator protein**, which leads to a decrease in phagocytosis. The decrease in phagocytosis results in recurrent pyogenic infections, albinism and peripheral neuropathy.

Characteristic feature is giant inclusions in WBC in peripheral smear.

Pelger-Huet anomaly (PHA) has **unusual shape** (**bilobed**, **peanut or dumbbell-shaped** instead of the normal trilobed shape) and unusual structure (coarse and lumpy).

Ans: (c) May Hegglin anomaly

Ref: Robbins, Pathologic Basis of Disease, 8th edition

17. All are true regarding retinoblastoma *except*:

(a) They play major role in cell cycle regulation/Tumour suppression
(b) Require deletion of 2 Rb genes (two hit)
(c) Autosomal dominant
(d) Chromosome 13p14

Explanation:

The location of **RB is 13q14. Not 13p14.**

Retinoblastoma:

RB gene is a **tumor suppressor gene**.

- RB – Is an **autosomal dominant** condition.
- In the active or hypophosphorylated state, it is present in the non-multiplying cells.
- The RB inactivation results in cell multiplication by activation of the transcription factor E2F.
- Retinoblastoma is a prime example of a tumor, which is associated with loss of heterozygosity. This term is mostly used in the context of oncogenesis.
- Retinoblastoma develops when both the normal alleles of the Rb gene are inactivated or altered.
- In familial case of retinoblastoma, children are born with *one normal and one defective copy of the Rb gene.*
- Loss of heterozygosity is the basis of two hit hypothesis of cancers (**Knudson's hypothesis**).

Ans: (d) Chromosome 13p14

Ref: Robbins Pathology, 9th edition, page 292-294

18. Best candidate for allogenic bone marrow transplant:

(a) 6-year-old with thalassemia minor
(b) Autoimmune diseases
(c) Multiple myeloma
(d) Hereditary ommunodeficiency

Explanation:

- **Hereditary immunodeficiency** – **SCID**, is one of the most common indication for **Allogenic BMT.**

Below are the indications for Autologous and Allogenic BMT

	Autologous Transplantation*	**Allogenic Transplantation†**
Malignancies	Multiple myeloma	Acute myeloid leukemia
	Non-Hodgkin lymphoma	Acute lymphoblastic leukemia
	Hodgkin disease	Chronic myeloid leukemia
	Acute myeloid leukemia	Myelodysplastic syndromes
	Neuroblastoma	Myeloproliferative neoplasms
	Ovarian cancer	Non-Hodgkin lymphoma
	Germ-cell tumors	Hodgkin disease
		Multiple myeloma
		Juvenile chronic myeloid leukemia

Contd.

Non-malignant disorders	Autoimmune disease Amyloidosis	Aplastic anemia Paroxysmal nocturnal hemoglobinuria Fanconi's anemia Diamond-Blackfan anemia Thalassemia major Sickle cell anemia Severe combined immunodeficiency Wiskott-Aldrich syndrome Inborn errors of metabolism Congenital neutropenia syndromes

* More than 30,000 autologous transplantations are performed annually worldwide, two-thirds for multiple myeloma or non-Hodgkin lymphoma.

† More than 24,000 allogeneic transplantations are performed annually worldwide, more than half for acute leukemias.

Ans: (d) Hereditary immunodeficiency

Ref: Wintrobe, Hematology, 13th edition

19. Carbohydrate tumor marker for breast cancer:

(a) CA 15-3 (b) CA 125 (c) CA 34 (d) CA 19-9

Explanation:

Carbohydrate Tumor Markers:

- Carbohydrate-rich tumor markers are specific antigens either found on the surface of tumor cells or may also be secreted as products by the tumor cells.
- The carbohydrate tumor markers are further classified as high-molecular weight mucins and blood group antigen-related markers.
- In current nomenclature, the carbohydrate antigens are abbreviated "CA" and are also referred to more generally as "cancer antigens", followed by their number of discovery, such as 125, 549 and so on.

Few important tumor markers below:

CA-125	Ovarian cancer
CA-19-9	Colon cancer, pancreatic cancer
CA-15-3	Breast cancer
p53, APC, RAS mutations in stool and serum	Colon cancer
p53 and RAS mutations in stool and serum	Pancreatic cancer
p53 and RAS mutations in sputum and serum	Lung cancer
p53 mutations in urine	Bladder cancer

Ans: (a) CA 15-3

Ref: WHO, Breast and Female Genital Tract

20. Which of the following markers increases the risk of recurrent carcinoma breast?

(a) Ca 125 (b) Ca 19-9 (c) Ca 27-29 (d) PSA

Explanation:

Breast Carcinoma Recurrence:

ASCO recommends that the following tests and imaging tests are not used to watch for a recurrence when a person has no signs or symptoms that the breast cancer has returned:

- Tumor marker tests for **CEA, CA 15-3 and CA 27-29.**
- CT scan.
- PET scan.
- Bone scan.

Ans: (c) Ca 27-29

Ref: ASCO Guidelines

21. **Marker of bone formation / Osteoclast markers are all *except*:**

(a) Pyridinoline
(b) TRAP
(c) C telopeptide
(d) Procollagen 1 C propeptide

Explanation:

Biochemical Markers of Bone Formation

- Bone specific alkaline phosphatase.
- Procollagen type 1C and 1N propeptide.
- Osteocalcin.
- Alkaline phosphatase (not very specific).

Ans: (d) Procollagen 1 C propeptide

Ref: Robbins Pathology, 9th edition, page 1180

22. **Marker of bone resorption / Osteoclast marker is:**

(a) Alkaline phosphatase
(b) Procollagen 1 N propeptide
(c) C – telopeptide
(d) Osteocalcin

Explanation:

Biochemical Markers of Bone Resorption

- Amino and carboxy terminal crosslinking telopeptide of bone collagen.
- Pyridinoline.
- Free lysyl-pyridinoline.
- Tartarate-resistant acid phosphatase (TRAP).
- Hydroxyproline (not very specific).

Ans: (c) C-telopeptide

Ref: Robbins Pathology, 9th edition, page 1180

23. **All are markers of Wilms' tumor *except*:**

(a) Desmin
(b) Vimentin
(c) TTF 1
(d) Cytokeratin

Explanation:

Wilms' Tumour

- Grossly, Wilms' tumor tends to present as a large, solitary, well-circumscribed mass and on cut section, the tumor is soft, homogeneous, and tan to grey with occasional foci of hemorrhage, cyst formation and necrosis.
- **Microscopically,** Wilms' tumors are characterized by the *classic triphasic combination of blastemal, stromal, and epithelial cell types* observed in the vast majority of lesions
- ***Anaplasia:*** Marker of **unfavorable histology**; associated with poor treatment response; defined as hyperchromatic, pleomorphic nuclei that are 3× larger than adjacent cells and have abnormal mitotic figures.
- **Immunohistochemisty: Positive for:**
    - Epithelium:WT1, Keratin, EMA, Cd57.
    - Blastemal: WT1, Desmin, Vimentin.
    - Stromal: weak WT1.

ALSO NOTE:

TTF-1 Positive Tumours

- **Lung carcinoma:** Small cell (90%), adenocarcinoma (75%); large cell (40%); squamous cell (5%).
- **Thyroid:** Hyperplastic and neoplastic thyroid tissue, but less common / lower levels in undifferentiated thyroid carcinomas.

- **Other tumors:**
  - Small cell carcinomas of lung and various sites.
  - Colorectal carcinomas to lung may be positive.
  - Small cell carcinoma of bladder.

Ans: (c) TTF-1

Ref: Robbin's Pathology, 9th edition, page 479

24. Exocrine pancreatic insufficiency, marrow failure with neutropenia is characteristic of:

(a) Fanconi syndrome
(b) Diamond Blackfan syndrome
(c) Shwachman-Diamond syndrome
(d) Dyskeratosis congenita

Explanation:

Below is the list of inherited bone marrow failure syndromes:

Syndrome	Inheritance patterns and genes	Characteristic haematological neoplasms	Risk of myeloid neoplasm	Other phenotypic findings	Diagnostic testing
Fanconi anaemia	AR: FANCA XLR: FANCB, FANCC, BRCA2 (FANCD1), FANCD2, FANCE,FANCF, FANCG, FANCI, BRIPI (FANCJ), FANCL, FANCM, PALB2 (FANCN), RAD51C, SLX4 (BTBD12)	MDS, AML	MDS: 7% AML 9%	Bone marrow failure, low birth weight, short stature, radial anomalies, congenital heart disease, microphthalmia, ear anomalies, deafness, renal malformafons, hypogonadism, cafe-au-lait spots, solid tumours	Screening: chromosomal breakage analysis Gene sequencing for relevant mutations
Severe congenital neutropenia	AD: ELANE, CSF3R, GFI1 AR: HAX1, G6PC3 XLR: WAS	MDS, AML	21-40%	HAX1: neurodevelopmental G5PC3 cardiac and other	Gene sequencing for relevant mutations
Shwachman-Diamond syndrome	AR: SBDS	MDS, AML, ALL	5-24%	Preceding isolated neutropenia, pancreatic insufficiency, short stature, skeletal abnormalities including metaphyseal dysostosis	Gene sequencing for SBDS mutations
Diamond-Blackfan anaemia	AD: RPS19, RPS17, RPS24, RPL35A, RPL5, RPL11, RPS7, RPS26, RPS10 XLR: GATA1	MDS, AML, ALL	5%	Small stature, congenital anomalies (e.g. craniofacial, cardiac, skeletal, genitourinary)	Screening: elevated erythrocyte adenosine deaminase and haemoglobin F Gene sequencing for relevant mutations
Telomere biology disorders including dyskeratosis congenita and syndromes due to TERC or TERT mutation	XLR: DKC1 AD: TERT, TERC, TINF2, RTEL1 AR: NOP10, NHP2, WRAP53, RTEL1, TERT, CTC1	MDS, AML	2-30%	Nail dystrophy, abnormal skin and pigmentation, oral leukoplakia, pulmonary fibrosis, hepatic fibrosis, squamous cell carcinoma	Telomere length measurement by flow-FISH If abnormal, gene sequencing for relevant mutations

Ans: (c) Shwachman-Diamond syndrome

Ref: WHO, Hematolymphoid Malignancy, 2017, page 127

25. Blueberry muffin is seen in all *except:*

(a) Rhabdomyosarcoma
(b) Nephroblastoma
(c) Neuroblastoma
(d) Syphilis

Explanation:

Blueberry Muffin Syndrome

- Descriptive term used when an infant is born with multiple blue/purple marks or nodules in the skin.
- These are due to the presence of clusters of blood-producing cells in the **skin** (extramedullary erythropoiesis), or bleeding into the **skin** (purpura) or spreading cancer (metastases).

Causes of Blueberry Muffin Babies:

Tumours such as:

- Congenital leukaemia cutis.
- Langherhans cell histiocytosis.
- Neuroblastoma.
- Congenital rhabdomyosarcoma.

Blood disorders such as:

- Haemolytic disease of the newborn – Rhesus or ABO incompatibility.
- Hereditary spherocytosis.
- Twin-twin transfusion syndrome.

Congenital infections such as:

- Rubella.
- Toxoplasmosis.
- Cytomegalovirus.
- Herpes simplex.
- Coxsackie virus.
- Parvovirus.
- Epstein-Barr virus.
- Syphilis.

Ans: (b) Nephroblastoma

Ref: Robbins Pathology, 9th edition, page 475

26. **Myd88 L265p mutation is seen in:**

(a) Multiple myeloma
(b) Waldenstrom's macroglobulinemia
(c) ALL
(d) Chronic myeloid leukemia

Explanation:

Waldenstrom Macroglobulinemia

- Indolent neoplasm.
- Also known as **lymphoplasmacytic lymphoma.**
- Involves **bone marrow** (100%), **liver, spleen, lymph nodes** (15 - 20%).
- Rare sites of involvement **lung and testis** (PGIMER exam options).
- **IgM secretion.**
- **MYD88 mutation** – virtually in all cases.
- Associated with **cold agglutinin AIHA** and **Hyperviscosity syndrome** in 15%.

Ans: (b) Waldenstrom's macroglobulinemia

Ref: Robbins 9th edition, page 538

27. **An 18-year-old patient's hemogram shows Hb 12 g%, RBC count of 6 million, decreased MCV (56), decreased MCH (29) and RDW of 14. What is the most probable diagnosis?**

(a) Iron deficient stores
(b) Sideroblastic anemia
(c) Beta thalassemia trait
(d) Normal lab parameters

Explanation:

This is a pretty straightforward question. Same topic of RDW was asked in the AIIMS exam also.

Data:

- Decreased MCV, MCH, Normal RDW and Hb-12 (without age and gender we will consider Hb-15 to be the ideal) its reduced.
- So it's a microcytic hypochromic anemia with normal RDW.

Red Cell Distribution Width

This is a beautiful concept. We will learn it with the help of a simple fictional example. Examples are always trustworthy. If we arrange RBC's on the basis of their **anisocytosis**. We will get a distribution range - That is RDW.

(1) **Iron Deficiency Anemia** – IDA is an ongoing state. Some days you dates milk shake or a piece of meat– That day your iron requirement will be met with so the RBC produced on the particular day will be looking normal (just for example) and the day preceding and later is going to be iron deficient. Resultant will be a population of microcytic and normal sized RBC's - A bigger range of cells - Wider RDW (holds good for any nutritional deficiency so megaloblasti also has I elevated RDW).

(2) In **thalassemia**, which is a genetic defect. How much ever you are going to eat. All the RBC's from the marrow are going to be small --> all are microcytic (gathered over a common point) - the range of RDW will be normal (though it's microcytic). Hope this will clear doubt with RDW.

Normal Value

- RDW-SD 39-46 fL.
- RDW-CV 11.6-14.6% in adult.

Condition with Increased RDW

- Iron deficiency anaemia.
- Folate/Vit B12 deficiency anaemia.

Now we will see the question again, it's more evident the answer is thalassemia.

Ans: (c) Beta thalassemia trait

Ref: Robbins Pathology, 9th edition

28. False about familial polyposis colon cancer syndrome:

(a) Autosomal recessive transmission
(b) Associated with fibroma and osteomas
(c) Associated with brain tumors
(d) 100% chance of colon carcinomas

Explanation:

"Colorectal adenocarcinoma develops in 100% of untreated FAP patients, often before age 30." Ref: Robbins

FAMILIAL ADENOMATOUS POLYPOSIS (FAP)

- ***Autosomal dominant*** disorder.
- Patients develop numerous ***colorectal adenomas*** as ***teenagers***.
- It is caused by mutations of the adenomatous polyposis coli, or **APC gene.**
- Some FAP patients without APC loss have mutations of the **base-excision repair gene *MUTYH*.**
- ***At least 100 polyps*** are necessary for a diagnosis of classic FAP, and as many as several thousand may be present.
- These growths are morphologically indistinguishable from ***sporadic adenomas***.
- ***Colorectal adenocarcinoma*** develops in ***100%*** of ***untreated FAP patients*** before age ***30***.
- ***Prophylactic colectomy*** is the standard therapy for individuals carrying APC mutations.
- Colectomy prevents colorectal cancer, but patients remain at risk for neoplasia at other sites.
- **Adenomas** may develop elsewhere in the **GI tract**, particularly adjacent to the **ampulla of Vater and in the stomach.**
- FAP is associated with a variety of **extra-intestinal manifestations** including:
  - Congenital hypertrophy of the retinal pigment epithelium.
  - Gardner syndrome; and
  - Turcot syndrome.

- **Gardner syndrome**
  - Osteomas of mandible, skull and long bones.
  - Epidermal cysts.
  - Desmoid tumors.
  - Thyroid tumors.
  - Dental abnormalities (Unerupted and supernumerary teeth).
- **Turcot syndrome**
  It is rare and characterized by:
  - Intestinal adenomas.
  - Tumors of the central nervous system.
  - **Two third** patients have **APC gene mutation** and develop **medulloblastomas**.
  - The remaining **one third** have mutations genes involved in DNA repair and develop **glioblastomas**.

HEREDITARY NON-POLYPOSIS COLORECTAL CANCER (Lynch syndrome) HNPCC

- Familial clustering of cancers at several sites including the ***colorectum, endometrium, stomach, ovary, ureters, brain, small bowel, hepatobiliary tract and skin.***
- Colon cancers occur at ***younger ages*** than sporadic colon cancers and are often located in the right colon
- HNPCC is caused by inherited mutations in genes that encode proteins responsible for the ***detection, excision, and repair of errors*** that occur during ***DNA replication.***
- There are at least five such **mismatch repair genes**, but the majority of HNPCC cases involve **MSH2** and **MLH1**.
- Defects in mismatch repair lead to the ***accumulation of mutations*** at rates up to **1000 times higher than normal**, mostly in regions containing ***short repeating DNA sequences*** referred to as **microsatellite DNA**.
- The human genome contains approximately ***50,000 to 100,000 microsatellites***, which are prone to undergo expansion during DNA replication and represent the most frequent sites of mutations in HNPCC.
- The basic pathogenesis is due to ***mismatch repair deficiency*** and the resulting ***microsatellite instability***

Common Patterns of Sporadic and Familial Colorectal Neoplasia

Etiology	Molecular Defect	Target Gene(s)	Transmission	Side	Histology
Familial adenomatous polyposis (70% of FAP)	APC/WNT pathway	*APC*	Autosomal dominant	None	• Tubular • Villous • Typical adenocarcinoma
Familial adenomatous polyposis (<10% of FAP)	DNA mismatch repair	*MUTYH*	None, recessive	None	• Sessile serrated adenoma • Mucinous adenocarcinoma
Hereditary nonpolyposis colorectal cancer	DNA mismatch repair	*MSH2, MLH1*	Autosomal	Right side	• Sessile serrated adenoma • Mucinous adenocarcinoma
Sporadic colon cancer (80%)	APC/WNT pathway	*APC*	None	Left side	• Tubular • Villous • Typical adenocarcinoma
Sporadic colon cancer (10% to 15%)	DNA mismatch repair	*MSH2, MLH1*	None	Right side	• Sessile serrated adenoma • Mucinous adenocarcinoma

Ans: (a) Autosomal recessive transmission

Ref: Robbins Pathologic Basis of Disease, 8th edition

29. Good prognostic factor in ALL:

(a) Age > 10
(b) Hyperdiploidy
(c) MLL gene rearrangements
(d) t(1:19)

Explanation:

Common Chromosomal Abnormalities in the Acute Leukemias of Childhood

Disease	Subtype	Chromosomal Abnormality	Influence on Prognosis
ALL	Pre-B	Trisomy 4 and 10	Favorable
		t(12;21)	
	Pre-B	t(4;11)	Unfavorable
	Pre-B	t(9;22)	Unfavorable
	B-cell	t(8;14)	None
	General	Hyperdiploidy	Favorable
	General	Hypodiploidy	Unfavorable

Prognosis

Most children with ALL can now be expected to have long-term survival, with the survival rate >80% at 5 years from diagnosis.

Important Prognostic Factors

- Choice of appropriate risk-directed therapy.
- Type of treatment chosen.
- Type of ALL.
- Stage of disease.
- Age of the patient.
- Rate of response to initial therapy (favorable if the patient responds in <1 month).

Poor Prognostic Indicators

- Age <1 year or >10 years at diagnosis.
- Leukocyte count of >100,000/μL at diagnosis; or a
- Slow response to initial therapy.
- Hypodiploidy.
- Philadelphia chromosome.
- MLL gene rearrangements.
- Translocations [t(1:19) or t(4;11)].

Favorable Prognostic Indicators

- Rapid response to therapy.
- Hyperdiploidy.
- Trisomy of specific chromosomes.
- Rearrangements of TEL/AML1 genes.

Ans: (b) Hyperdiploidy

Ref: Robbins Pathologic Basis of Disease, 8th edition and Nelson, Textbook of Pediatrics

30. MHC gene is located in:

(a) Chromosome 12
(b) Chromosome 6
(c) Chromosome 7
(d) Chromosome 8

Explanation:

- **MHC gene is located in short arm of chromosome 6.**

Major Histocompatibility Complex

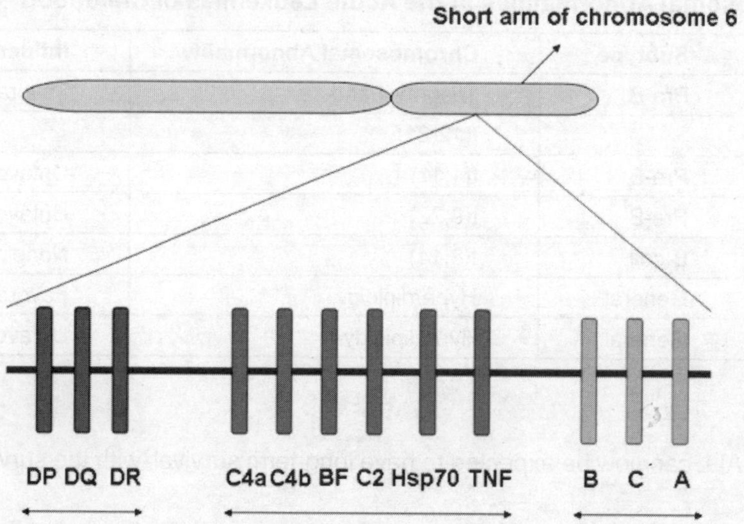

MHC Restriction

- T cells recognise only immunogens that are bound to major histocompatibility complex (MHC).
- There are 2 types of MHC proteins:
  - Class I: Expressed virtually by all somatic cells. Present substances to $CD8^+$ T cells.
  - Class II: Expressed only by activated macrophages, dendritic cells and B cells. Present antigen to $CD4^+$ T cells.
- **HLA class I antigens (A, B and C)** are found on the surface of virtually **all nucleated cells**. They are the principal antigens involved in **graft rejection** and **cell mediated cytolysis**. Class I molecules may function as **components of hormone receptors.**
- **HLA class II antigens** are more restricted in distribution, being found only on **antigen presenting cells** of the immune system such as **macrophages**, **dendritic** cells, **B cells** and **activated T cells.**
- T cells normally do not possess MHC II, **only activated T cells** may express **MHC II** molecules.

MHC Class I	MHC Class II
Found on virtually every cell in the body (except RBCs)	Found on B-cells, macrophages and other antigen presenting cells
Presents "endogenous" antigens, such as viral fragments or tumor proteins	Presents "exogenous" antigens, such as digested fragments of foreign cells
Presents antigen to cytotoxic T cells	Presents antigen to helper T cells

Ans: (b) Chromosome 6

Ref: Robbins Pathologic Basis of Disease, 9th edition

31. **Clinical features of 22q11 mutation syndrome (Catch22/ Velocardiofacial syndrome/Digeorge syndrome):**

(a) Hypercalcemia
(b) Conotruncal abnormalities
(c) Thymic hyperplasia
(d) Dysmorphogenesis of the 1st and 2nd pharyngeal pouches

Explanation:

Chromosome 22q11.2 Deletion Syndromes

- Cayler cardiofacial syndrome.
- Conotruncal anomaly face syndrome.
- DiGeorge syndrome.
- Shprintzen syndrome.
- Velocardiofacial syndrome.

THYMIC HYPOPLASIA (DIGEORGE SYNDROME)

- Results from dysmorphogenesis of the **3rd and 4th pharyngeal pouches.**
- **Hypoplasia or aplasia** of the **thymus and parathyroid glands**.
- Anomalies of the great vessels (**right-sided aortic arch).**
- **Esophageal atresia.**
- **Bifid uvula.**
- Congenital heart disease (**conotruncal**, atrial and ventricular septal defects).
- **Facial features: Short philtrum of the upper lip**, hypertelorism, an antimongoloid slant to the eyes, mandibular hypoplasia, and low-set, often notched ears.
- Cases often present with **hypocalcemic seizures** during the neonatal period.

Genetics and Pathogenesis

- Occurs in both males and females.
- Microdeletions of specific DNA sequences from chromosome 22q11.2.
- A **T-box transcription** family member, **TBX1 gene** mutation is found in majority cases.
- Excess of 22q11.2 deletions of maternal origin.
- **Conotruncal heart defects** and **22q deletions** are observed in **DiGeorge** syndrome, **velocardiofacial** syndrome, and **conotruncal** anomaly face syndrome.
- The **CATCH 22 syndrome** (cardiac, abnormal facies, thymic hypoplasia, cleft palate, hypocalcemia) includes the broad clinical spectrum of conditions with 22q11.2 deletions.

Ans: (b) Conotruncal abnormalities

Ref: Nelson, 20th edition, page 1019

32. **Lymphoid malignancy arising from thymic cells are:**

(a) Hairy cell leukemia
(b) Burkitt lymphoma
(c) Pre-B cell ALL
(d) Pre-T cell ALL

Explanation:

Summary of Major Types of Lymphoid Leukemias and Non-Hodgkin Lymphomas

Diagnosis	Cell of Origin	Genotype	Salient Clinical Features
NEOPLASMS OF IMMATURE B AND T CELLS			
B-cell acute lymphoblastic leukemia/lymphoma	Bone marrow precursor B cell	Diverse chromosomal translocations; t(12;21) involving *CBFα* and *ETV6* present in 25%	Predominantly children; symptoms relating to marrow replacement and pancytopenia; aggressive
T-cell acute lymphoblastic leukemia/lymphoma	Precursor T cell (often of **thymic origin**)	Diverse chromosomal translocations, *NOTCH1* mutations (50% to 70%)	Predominantly adolescent males; **thymic** masses and variable bone marrow involvement; aggressive
NEOPLASMS OF MATURE B CELLS			
Burkitt lymphoma	Germinal-center B cell	Translocations involving **c-*MYC*** and Ig loci, usually **t(8;14)**; subset **EBV-associated**	Adolescents or young adults with extranodal masses; uncommonly presents as "leukemia"; aggressive

Contd.

Contd.

Diffuse large B-cell lymphoma	Germinal-center or post-germinal-center B cell	Diverse chromosomal rearrangements, most often of ***BCL6* (30%), *BCL2* (10%), or c-*MYC* (5%)**	All ages, but most common in adults; often appears as a rapidly growing mass; 30% extranodal; aggressive
Extranodal marginal zone lymphoma	Memory B cell	**t(11;18), t(1;14),** and t(14;18) creating *MALT1-IAP2*, *BCL10-IgH*, and *MALT1-IgH* fusion genes, respectively	Arises at **extranodal sites** in adults with chronic inflammatory diseases; may remain localized; indolent
Follicular lymphoma	Germinal-center B cell	t(14;18) creating *BCL2-IgH* fusion gene	Older adults with generalized lymphadenopathy and marrow involvement; indolent
Hairy cell leukemia	Memory B cell	No specific chromosomal abnormality	Older males with pancytopenia and splenomegaly; indolent
Mantle cell lymphoma	Naive B cell	**t(11;14)** creating *CyclinD1-IgH* fusion gene	Older males with disseminated disease; moderately aggressive
Multiple myeloma/solitary plasmacytoma	Post-germinal-center bone marrow homing plasma cell	Diverse rearrangements involving IgH; 13q deletions	Myeloma: Older adults with lytic bone lesions, pathologic fractures, hypercalcemia, and renal failure; moderately aggressive Plasmacytoma: Isolated plasma cell masses in bone or soft tissue; indolent
Small lymphocytic lymphoma/chronic lymphocytic leukemia	Naive B cell or memory B cell	**Trisomy 12**, deletions of **11q, 13q and 17p**	Older adults with bone marrow, lymph node, spleen, and liver disease; autoimmune hemolysis and thrombocytopenia in a minority; indolent
NEOPLASMS OF MATURE T CELLS OR NK CELLS			
Adult T-cell leukemia/ lymphoma	Helper T cell	HTLV-1 provirus present in tumor cells	Adults with cutaneous lesions, marrow involvement, and hypercalcemia; occurs mainly in Japan, West Africa, and the Caribbean; aggressive
Peripheral T-cell lymphoma, unspecified	Helper or cytotoxic T cell	No specific chromosomal abnormality	Mainly older adults; usually presents with lymphadenopathy; aggressive
Anaplastic large-cell lymphoma	Cytotoxic T cell	Rearrangements of ALK	Children and young adults, usually with lymph node and soft-tissue disease; aggressive
Extranodal NK/T-cell lymphoma	NK cell (common) or cytotoxic T cell (rare)	EBV-associated; no specific chromosomal abnormality	Adults with destructive extranodal masses, most commonly sinonasal; aggressive
Mycosis fungoides/ Sézary syndrome	Helper T cell	No specific chromosomal abnormality	Adult patients with cutaneous patches, plaques, nodules, or generalized erythema; indolent
Large granular lymphocytic leukemia	Two types: Cytotoxic T cell and NK cell	No specific chromosomal abnormality	Adult patients with splenomegaly, neutropenia, and anemia, sometimes, acco mpanied by autoimmune disease

Ans: (d) Pre-T cell ALL

Ref: Robbins Pathologic Basis of Disease, 9th edition

33. Schistocytes in peripheral are seen in all *except*:

(a) MAHA
(b) Sickle cell anemia
(c) DIC
(d) HUS

Keratocytes/Schistocytes

- **Keratocytes *("horn cells, helmet cells*")** and **schistocytes** ("***fragmented cells***") are damaged red blood cells.
- Such damage characteristic occurs from ***fibrin deposits.***
  - DIC.
  - Microangiopathic hemolytic anemia.
  - Thrombotic thrombocytopenic purpura (TTP).
  - Prosthetic heart valves.
  - Severe valvular stenosis.
  - Malignant hypertension.
  - March hemoglobinuria.
- However, keratocytes and schistocytes also occur in:
  - Normal newborns.
  - Bleeding peptic ulcer.
  - Aplastic anemia.
  - Pyruvate kinase deficiency.
  - Vasculitis.
  - Glomerulonephritis.
  - Renal graft rejection.
  - Severe burns.
  - Iron deficiency.
  - Thalassemia.
  - Myelofibrosis with myeloid metaplasia.
  - Hypersplenism.
  - Post-splenectomy.
- Clinical correlation is recommended, with the appropriate diagnostic studies.
- These cells are pathologic and should never be ignored.

Ans: (b) Sickle cell anemia

Ref: Robbins Pathologic Basis of Disease, 8th edition

34. Feature of autosomal dominant disorder:

(a) Present early in life
(b) Complete penetrance common
(c) New germ cell mutations in old fathers
(d) Male to male transmission not possible

Explanation:

Autosomal Dominant Inheritance Pattern

- **Successive** or **multiple generations** of family are affected.
- One **faulty copy of gene** (i.e., mutant allele) in **any autosome** and one copy of normal allele.
- Disease **phenotype** is seen in all such individuals.
- Patients having disease have **50% chance** of passing on the disease to the **next generation.**
- Both **males** and **females** are affected equally.
- Both **males and females** can **transmit** the condition to progeny.
- There is atleast one instance of **Male to male transmission.**
- Disease **manifests in heterozygous state**, so at least one parent of an index case is usually affected.
- When an affected person marries an unaffected one, every child has one chance in two of having the disease.
- Clinical features can be modified by variations in **penetrance** and **expressivity**.
- Some individuals inherit the mutant gene but are phenotypically normal. This is referred to as **incomplete penetrance**.

- Penetrance is expressed in mathematical terms. Thus, 50% penetrance indicates that 50% of those who carry the gene express the trait.
- In practice, penetrance risk is **less than 10%.**
- If a trait is seen in all individuals carrying the mutant gene but is expressed differently among individuals, the phenomenon is called variable **expressivity**. For example, manifestations of neurofibromatosis type 1 range from brownish spots on the skin to multiple skin tumors and skeletal deformities.
- In many conditions the **age at onset is delayed**.
- Symptoms and signs may not appear until adulthood (as in Huntington disease).
- Many autosomal dominant diseases (e.g., achondroplasia) have been shown to be associated with **increasing paternal age.**
- **Paternal age** is an important determinant in **new germ cell mutation**, causing both **autosomal dominant** and **X-linked recessive illnesses.**

Two Types of Mutations Seen in AD

- **Loss-of-function mutations**
  - **Most common.**
  - Affect regulatory proteins; and
  - Also affects subunits of multimeric proteins.
- **Gain-of-function mutations**
  - Less common.
  - Normal proteins with toxic properties.
  - Increase a normal activity (e.g, Activating mutation of erythropoetin receptor – Polycythemia).

Common Autosomal Dominant Disorders

System	Disorder
Nervous	Huntington disease
	Neurofibromatosis
	Myotonic dystrophy
	Tuberous sclerosis
Urinary	Polycystic kidney disease
Gastrointestinal	Familial polyposis coli
Hematopoietic	Hereditary spherocytosis von Willebrand disease
Skeletal	Marfan syndrome
	Ehlers-Danlos syndrome
	Osteogenesis imperfecta
	Achondroplasia
Metabolic	Familial hypercholesterolemia
	Acute intermittent porphyria

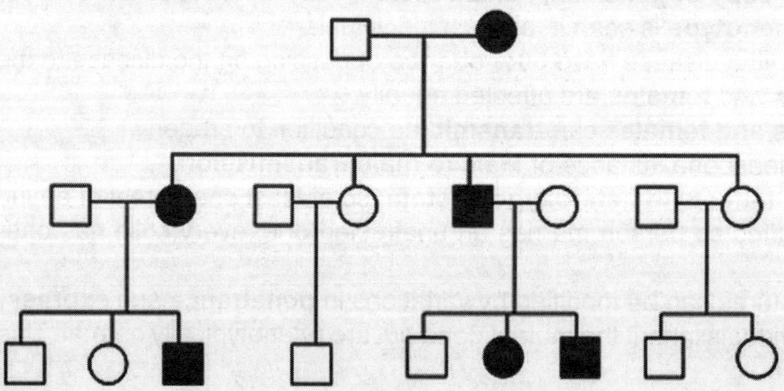

PEDIGREE OF AUTOSOMAL DOMINANT TRANSMISSION

Also Note:

Autosomal Recessive Inheritance

- Both copies of genes are mutated.
- It occurs when **both parents are carriers** of the defective gene.
- Having one **normal allele** and **one defective allele** in **each parent.**
- Each parent passes on their defective gene to the next progeny causing disease.
- There is **25% chance of transmission** when both parents are carriers.

Ans: (c) New germ cell mutations in old fathers

Ref: Robbins Pathologic Basis of Disease, 8th edition, page 140-141

MICROBIOLOGY

1. **All of the following have operculated eggs *except*:**
   (a) Clonorchis sinensis
   (b) Diphyllobothrium latum
   (c) Hymenolepis dimunita
   (d) Fasciola hepatica

Explanation:

Parasites with Operculated Eggs:

- Fasciola hepatica.
- Fasciolopsis buski.
- Paragonimus westermani.
- Opisthorchis felineus.
- Fasciola gigantica.
- Clonorchis sinensis.
- Opisthorchis viverrini.
- Diphyllobothrium latum.

Ans: (c) Hymenolepis dimunita

Ref: Paniker's Textbook of Parasitology, 6th edition, page 127,129,156

2. **All the following spread by auto infection *except*:**
   (a) Taenia solium
   (b) Strongyloides stercoralis
   (c) Hymenolepis nana
   (d) Ascaris lumbricoides

Explanation:

Parasite Causing Autoinfection:

- Taenia solium.
- Enterobius vermicularis.
- Capillaria philippinensis.
- Hymenolepis nana.
- Strongyloides stercoralis.
- Cryptosporidium parvum.

Ans: (d) Ascaris lumbricoides

Ref: Paniker's Textbook of Parasitology, 6th edition, page 149-151

3. **A Sabin Feldman test is used for the diagnosis of:**
   (a) Toxoplasma
   (b) Cryptococcus
   (c) Cyclospora
   (d) Ankylostoma

Explanation:

The Diagnostic Test of Importance in Parasitology:

Entero or string test	Giardia lamblia
Montenegro and Napier's aldehyde test	Leishmania donovani
Casoni's test	Echinococcus granulosum
Frenkel's and Sabin Feldman dye test	Toxoplasma gondii
Fairley's test	Schistosoma haematobium

Ans: (a) Toxoplasma

Ref: Paniker's Textbook of Parasitology, 6th edition, page 96-103

4. Which of the following is true regarding transmission of Toxoplasma?

(a) Vertical
(b) Ingestion of uncooked cyst
(c) Organ transplantation
(d) All of the above

Explanation:

- ***Toxoplasma gondii*** is an obligate intracellular Apicomplexan parasite.
- Definitive host: Cat (Felidae).
- Intermediate/accidental host: Other animals.
- 3 Stages:
  - Tachyzoites in Pseudocyst.
  - Bradyzoites in Tissue cyst.
  - Sporozoites in Oocyst (excreted in cat feces).

Modes of Infection in Human:

- Ingestion of oocysts.
- Consumption of raw/undercooked meat.
- Handling of infected meat.
- Transplacental.
- Organ transplantation and blood transfusion.
- Accidental inoculation of tachyzoites.

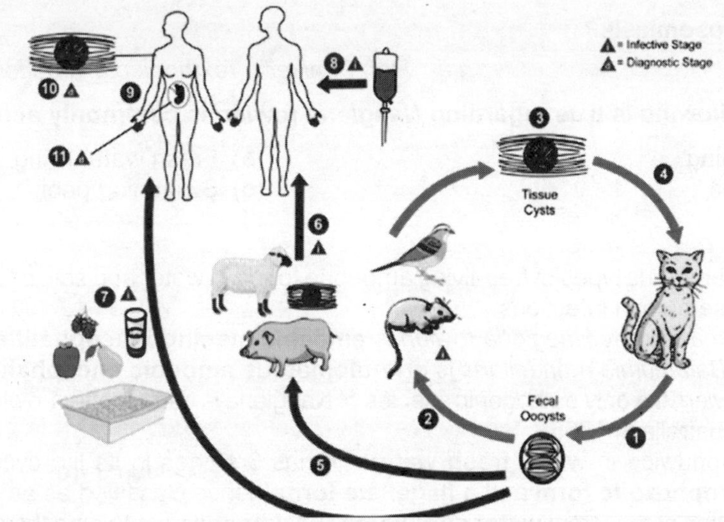

Ans: (d) All of the above

Ref: Paniker's Textbook of Parasitology, 6th edition, page 96-103

5. **A HIV positive individual having diarrheal episodes stool examination reveals an oocyst of size 8-10 Micron, what could be the diagnosis?**

(a) Cyclospora (b) Cryptococcus
(c) Cryptosporidium parvum (d) Isospora

Explanation:

Cryptosporidium Parvum:

- **Cryptosporidia** were first observed in the gastric mucosal crypts of laboratory mice by Tyzzer in 1907. Its importance as a pathogen causing diarrhea in animals was recognized in 1971 and the first case of human infection reported in 1976.
- Cryptosporidium has assumed great importance as a frequent cause of **intractable diarrhea in AIDS patients.**
- Natural infection with ***C. parvum*** is present in many species of birds such as chicken, turkey, and of animals including cattle, sheep, goats and cats.
- The oocysts of Cryptosporidium in stool samples are **modified acid fast (cold Ziehl-Neelsen) stain positive**, measuring about **6-10 µm.**

Ans: (c) Cryptosporidium parvum

Ref: Paniker's Textbook of Parasitology, 6th edition, page 105,106

6. **Winter bottom sign is seen in:**

(a) Toxoplasmosis (b) Trypanosomiasis (c) Cryptosporidiosis (d) Leishmaniasis

Explanation:

African Sleeping Sickness:

- This infection is caused by ***Trypanosoma brucei gambiense*** is endemic in West and Central Africa.
- The vector for this disease is **tsetse flies (*Glossinia palpalis*)**. The incubation period is about 1 to 2 weeks.
- The illness is chronic and can persist for many years. There is an initial period of Parasitemia, following which they are localized predominantly in the lymph nodes.
- The important clinical features are intermittent fever, chill, and headache at this stage and hepatosplenomegaly with lymphadenopathy particularly in the posterior cervical region **(Winterbottom sign).**
- With the invasion of CNS, this occurs after several months, the **sleeping sickness stage** starts. This is marked by increasing headache, mental dullness, apathy and sleepiness. The patient falls into profound coma followed by death from asthenia.

Ans: (b) Trypanosomiasis

Ref: Paniker's Textbook of Parasitology, 6th edition, page 45-48

7. **Which of the following is true regarding *Naegleria fowleri* is commonly acquired by?**

(a) Salt water living (b) Fresh water living
(c) Sulfur springs (d) Swimming pool

Explanation:

- Among the numerous types of free-living amoebae found in water and soil, a few are potentially pathogenic and can cause human infections.
- The disease caused by *Naegleria fowleri* is **amoebic meningoencephalitis (PAM)** and *Acanthamoeba culbertsoni, Balamuthia mandrillaris* is **granulomatous amoebic encephalitis (GAE)** respectively.
- *Naegleria fowleri*, the only pathogenic species of Naegleria is named after Fowler who, with Carter described it first from Australia in 1965.
- It is found worldwide in **warm fresh waters**. It has 3 stages in its life cycle–a **dormat cyst form**, an **amoeboid trophozoite form** and **a flagellate form** (hence classified as an amoeboflagellate).
- Human infection comes from **water containing the amoebae** containing the amoebae and usually follows swimming or diving in ponds.

Ans: (b) Fresh water living

Ref: Paniker's Textbook of Parasitology, 6th edition, page 31-35

8. In Toxoplasmosis the oocyst seen in______ and pseudocyst is seen in_____ respectively.

(a) Tissue, faeces (b) Human, cats (c) Cats, human (d) Feces, tissue

Explanation:

Human ingesting either **tissue cysts or oocysts**→→ rupture of cyst wall and release of organisms→→ invade the small intestinal epithelium→→ via mesenteric lymph nodes→→ disseminates throughout the body and multiplies intracellularly.

Pseudocyst (tachyzoites)	Tissue cyst (bradyzoites)
Placenta, liver, L.N, spleen, skeletal muscles, lungs, heart, retina and choroid.	Brain and skeletal muscles.

Ans: (c) Cats, human (cat faeces and human tissue)

Ref: Paniker's Textbook of Parasitology, 6th edition, page 96-103

9. Whole cell pertussis vaccine used to prevent infection can protect against:

(a) Mild form of Bordetella pertussis
(b) Bordetella parapertussis
(c) Severe Bordetella pertussis
(d) Chronic carriers of Bordetella pertussis

Explanation:

Pattern in Pre-Vaccination Era

- Limited data on the distribution of pertussis in unvaccinated (pre-vaccine) populations indicate that infection was ubiquitous, with most individuals infected in childhood, of whom an appreciable proportion, > 50 %, exhibited classical disease.
- Approximately 80% cases occurred in children under 5 years in some parts of the USA, and less than 3% cases in persons aged 15 years or above (Fales 1928).
- Case fatality rates were also high, in particular in infancy. Similar patterns were observed in other countries, including in Africa (e.g., Senegal, Kenya and South Africa) and South Asia (India).

Patterns in Post-Vaccination Era

- The introduction of effective infant vaccination with high coverage was accompanied by a steep decline in the number of pertussis cases and deaths in children worldwide. Pertussis surveillance remains difficult and in need of strengthening.
- A shift toward pertussis in older age groups (adolescents and young adults) has been reported in recent years in some high income countries, in particular those which now use acellular pertussis vaccines.
- The age shifts may, in part, be explained by an increasing awareness and recognition of less typical disease manifestations in older subjects, as well as more sensitive laboratory testing. It has also been suggested that waning of vaccine-derived immunity, combined with lower naturally-acquired immunity and boosting (as a result of lower community transmission) may play a role in increased susceptibility in adolescents and adults.
- Several high income countries which introduced aP vaccines experienced resurgence of pertussis in recent years, including relatively large numbers of cases in adolescents and adults. The reasons for these resurgences are not yet clear.

Ans: (a) Mild form of Bordetella pertussis

Ref: Ananthanarayan and Paniker's Microbiology, 10th edition, page 343 and www.who.int/immunization/sage/.../2_wP_summary_WG_23Mar2015_submitted.pdf

10. Ingested RBCs (Erythrophagy) seen in:

(a) Naegleria fowleri
(b) Entamoeba histolytica
(c) Entamoeba coli
(d) Acanthamoeba

Explanation:

Entamoeba Histolytica:

- ***E. histolytica*** occurs in three forms–**the trophozoite, precystic and cystic stages**. The trophozoite or the vegetative form is the growing or feeding stage of the parasite.
- It is irregular in shape and varies in size from about **12 to 60 μm**. It is **large and actively motile in freshly passed dysenteric stools**, while in convalescents and carriers, it is much smaller.
- The **protoplasm** is differentiated into a thin outer layer of clear, transparent, refractive ectoplasm and an inner finely granular endoplasm having a ground glass appearance.
- **Typical amoeboid motility** is due to the pseudopodia, which is crawling or gliding movement and not a free swimming one.
- The **endoplasm** contains the nucleus, food vacuoles and granules. The nucleus is not clearly seen in the living trophozoite, but can be distinctly demonstrated in preparations stained with **iron-haematoxylin or Gomorri's trichrome stains**.
- The **karyosome** is anchored to the inner surface of the nuclear membrane by fine radiating fibrils called the lining network giving a **cartwheel appearance**.
- The trophozoites from acute dysenteric stools often contain **phagocytosed erythrocytes**. This feature is diagnostic as phagocytosed red cells **are not found in any other commensal intestinal amoebae**.

Ans: (b) Entamoeba histolytica

Ref: Paniker's Textbook of Parasitology, 6th edition, page 14-20

11. Ziemans dots are seen in:

(a) Plasmodium malariae (b) Plasmodium vivax
(c) Plasmodium falciparum (d) Plasmodium knowelsi

Explanation:

Plasmodium species	**Dots/stipplings**
Plasmodium falciparum	**Maurer's clefts**; Basophilic stippling
Plasmodium ovale	**Schuffner's dots and James dots**
Plasmodium vivax	**Schuffner's dots**
Plasmodium malariae	**Ziemann's dots**

Ans: (a) Plasmodium malariae

Ref: Paniker's Textbook of Parasitology, 6th edition, page 65-70

FORENSIC MEDICINE

1. **A 32-year-old woman presents to ER with history of ingestion of crushed plant seed (Picture). She was treated with stomach wash and activated charcoal. She is at risk of developing which of the following electrolyte disturbance?**

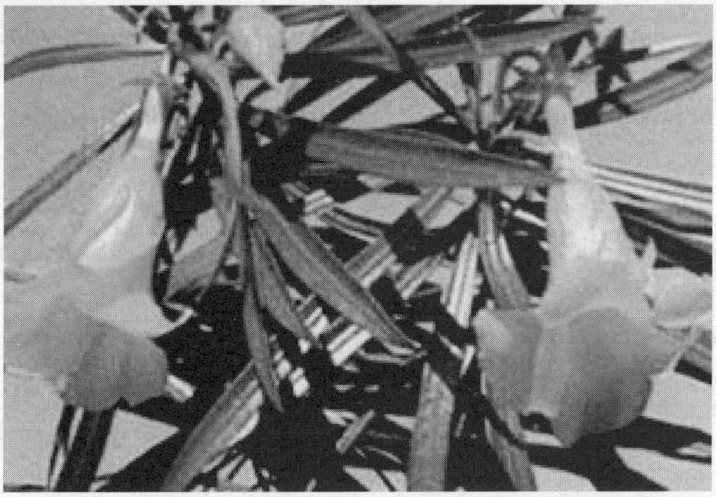

(a) Hypocalcemia (b) Hypercalcemia (c) Hypokalemia (d) Hyperkalemia

Explanation:

- Picture shows yellow oleander plant (Cerebra thevetia).

Yellow Oleander Poisoning (Cerebera thevetia)

- All parts – poisonous.
- Active principles–Glycosides – Thevetin + thevotoxin = cardiac poison and cerberin = acts like strychnine.
- Fatal Dose: Seeds – 8-10; root – 15-20 gm.
- **Sign and Symptoms**
  - o Most common– **Bradycardia** with AV block, hypotension, lethargy, dizziness and GI distress.
  - o Others–Convulsions, electrolyte disturbances (especially **hyperkalemia**), hypertension and coma.
- **Treatment**
  - o **Sodium molar lactate** transfusion with **glucose** and 1 mg **atropine**, 2 cc **adrenaline** and 2 mg **noradrenaline.**

Ans: (d) Hyperkalemia

Ref: VV Pillay, Modern Medical Toxicology, 4th edition, page 344

2. **Minimum duration within which a consumer should initiate dispute case?**

(a) 1 year (b) 6 months (c) 2 years (d) 5 years

Explanation:

Consumer Protection Act (CPA), 1986

Hospitals covered	Hospitals exempted
• Charging fees for consultation or treatment • Charging a token fees like for registration • Treating poor for free but charging fees to rich	• Offering free treatments

Power of Consumer Courts (Quasi Judiciary)

- District level – upto 20 lakh.
- State level – 20 lakh - 1 crore.
- National level – > 1 crore.

Limitation Period

- Case need to be filed within 2 years.

Ans: (c) 2 years

Ref: Consumer Protection Act (CPA), 1986 http://ncdrc.nic.in

3. Maximum number of times a woman can become pregnant for surrogacy is:

(a) 1 (b) 2 (c) 3 (d) 4

Explanation:

According to Section 3.10.8 of ICMR Guidelines "No woman may act as a surrogate more than thrice in her lifetime."

ICMR Guidelines (2005) on Assisted Reproductive Technology Procedures

- Surrogacy arrangement will continue to be governed by contract amongst parties. But such an arrangement should not be for commercial purposes.
- A surrogacy arrangement should provide for financial support for surrogate child in the event of death of the commissioning couple or individual before delivery of the child, or divorce between the intended parents and subsequent willingness of none to take delivery of the child.
- A surrogacy contract should necessarily take care of life insurance cover for surrogate mother.
- One of the intended parents should be a donor as well, because the bond of love and affection with a child primarily emanates from biological relationship.
- Legislation itself should recognize a surrogate child to be the legitimate child of the commissioning parent without there being any need for adoption or even declaration of guardian.
- The birth certificate of the surrogate child should contain the name of the commissioning parent only.
- Right to privacy of donor as well as surrogate mother should be protected.
- Sex-selective surrogacy should be prohibited.
- Cases of abortions should be governed by the Medical Termination of Pregnancy Act 1971 only.

Features of Surrogacy (Regulation) Bill, 2016, introduced by Union Government, are as following:

- As per the draft bill, commercial surrogacy is banned. Any payment to a woman opting to be a surrogate mother is prohibited.
- Surrogacy for singles, foreigners and persons of Indian origin is also banned as per the new proposed bill.
- Only a blood relative aged 25 to 35 years can become a surrogate.
- The woman opting to become a surrogate mother should be married and with a child of her own.
- The draft Bill also bans egg donation.
- In other words, surrogacy will be allowed only in an altruistic form and there will be no monetary benefits for the surrogate mother.
- This proposed bill is yet to be passed as of January 2018.

Ans: (c) 3

Ref: ICMR National Guidelines for ART Clinics in India, page 69

4. Gastric lavage is allowed in which corrosive poisoning?

(a) Paint thinner ingestion (b) Lysol ingestion
(c) Crude toilet disinfectant ingestion (d) Battery acid ingestion

Explanation:

- Paint thinner usually contains kerosene and other petroleum distillates.
- Lysol is a carbolic acid (phenol) derivative.

- Crude toilet disinfect contains hydrochloric acid.
- Battery acid is nothing but sulphuric acid.

Gastric lavage

Indications	Contraindications	
	Absolute	**Relative**
Ingested poisons (within 3 hours)	Corrosives **except** *carbolic* acid* and *Oxalic* acid*	• Convulsants and unconscious • Coma • Foreign body ingestion • Petroleum distillates • Esophageal varices

Tube:

- Ewald or Boas tube – 1.5 mt in length, 1 cm in diameter with marking at 50 cm.
- Lavacuator (ideal tube).

Lavage Fluid:

(i) Warm water (most commonly used) (ii) Saline (0.9% or 0.45%).

Ans: (b) Lysol ingestion

Ref: VV Pillay, Modern Medical Toxicology, 4th edition, page 20

5. **Enzyme that can be traced in semen sample of 8 - 10 weeks is:**

(a) Acid phosphatase test
(b) ALP test
(c) LDH
(d) CPK enzyme

Explanation:

SEMINAL STAIN EXAMINATION

a. **Invisible stains**
   - On UV light - fluoresces (bluish white on a dark background).

   False positives
   - Other body fluids, e.g., blood, pus, saliva etc.
   - Also fabric whiteners.

b. **Florence test – For Choline (seminal vesicle)**
   - Stain extract + Florence solution (potassium iodide, iodine and water) = dark-brown rhomboid crystals of choline per iodide (larger than haemin crystals).
   - A negative reaction is proof that stain is not seminal.

c. **Barberio's test – For Spermin (Prostatic secretion)**
   - Stain extract + aqueous or alcoholic soln. of picric acid = yellow, long needle shaped crystals (of spermin picrate).

d. **Acid phosphatase test – Highest concentration in seminal fluid**
   - 20 to 400 times more than any other body fluid.
   - Undiluted semen – 300-360 Bodanksy units.
   - 100 B units/ml – indicative of semen.
   - Test is conclusive in the absence of demonstrable sperms or in azoospermia.

e. **CPK enzyme**
   - Spermatozoa contain a high concentration of CPK, which is more than double than found in any other body fluid.
   - Normal conc. – 385 to 1400 units/ml.

- 400 units/ml – conclusive of seminal stain.
- **Can Be Detected Even In 6 Months Old Stain.**

f. **Aluminium molybdate test**
- Detects phosphorus.

g. **P30 – PSA prostate specific antigen**
- A glycoprotein derived from prostatic epithelial cells.
- Found in – semen, male urine and blood (only for male).
- Detected in old and dried stains too.
- Reliable indicator of semen.

h. **Monoclonal antibody mouse anti-human semen-5 (MHS-5)**
- Secreted by seminal vesicle epithelium.
- Only found in semen.
- Highly reliable for semen.

i. **LDH isoenzyme of spermatozoa (LDH C4)**
- Detected on electrophoresis.
- Absolute proof of semen.

j. **Demonstration of spermatozoa**

In living

- Motile sperms seen 12 hours after ejaculation into vagina.
- Complete sperm are seen upto 26 hours (2-3 days).
- Then separate into head and tail – identifiable, upto 120 hours.

In the dead

- Seen in vagina up to 1 or 2 weeks.
- Up to a fortnight in uterine cavity.

k. **Species identification**
- Precipitin test.
- LDH isoenzyme pattern.
- Y bodies on human spermatozoa heads.

Absolute Proof of Semen

- One unbroken spermatozoa.
- LDH isoenzymes detection.

Ans: (d) CPK enzyme

Ref: Essentials of Forensic Medicine and Toxicology by Narayan Reddy, 34th edition

6. **A 20 years old boy presents with alleged history of ingesting rat killer poison. He is also having spontaneous bleeding tendencies following that. What is the initial management?**

(a) Liver transplantation
(b) N acetyl cysteine
(c) Vitamin K
(d) Platelet/FFP transfusion

Explanation:

- Rodenticides very commonly involved in human poisoning include phosphorus, zinc and aluminium phosphide, long acting anticoagulants (especially bromadiolone) etc.
- The spontaneous bleeding manifestations exhibited by the patient is likely due to poisoning with anticoagulants.
- **Vitamin K1** is the antidote in such cases.
- **Mode of action:** Oral anticoagulants are vitamin K antagonists, administration of vitamin K1 sets right the anomaly.
- **Dose:** 50-100 mg, 3 to 4 times a day orally for 1 to 2 days.

Ans: (c) Vitamin K

Ref: VV Pillay, Modern Medical Toxicology, 4th edition, page 335

PSM

1. **If a woman experiences 2.5 accidental pregnancies after using a contraceptive method, Pearl index:**

(a) 0.1 per 100 woman years

(b) 100 per 1000 woman years

(c) 10 accidental pregnancies per 1000 woman years using contraceptives

(d) 10 accidental pregnancies per 100 woman years using contraceptives

Explanation

Pearl index = (Total accidental pregnancies/total months of exposure) × 1200

= [2.5/(25×12)]×1200

= 10 per 100 woman years

25 years is considered as the average fertile period for a woman for calculation.

Contraceptive Effectiveness

Assessed by measuring the number of unplanned pregnancies that occur during a specified period of exposure and use of contraceptive method. Two methods are used:

1. Pearl index.
2. Life table analysis.

The numerator "total accidental pregnancies" includes all unwanted pregnancies irrespective of the outcome, i.e.,

- Livebirth.
- Abortion.
- Stillbirth; or
- Still not terminated.

Disadvantages

- A minimum of 600 months of exposure is necessary for obtaining a valid "failure rate" value.
- Life table analysis:
  - o Calculates failure rate per month of use.
  - o More precise than Pearl Index.

Ans: (d) 10 accidental pregnancies per 100 women years using contraceptives

Ref: Park, 24th edition, page 544; Principles and Practice of Community Medicine by Dr Asma Rahim, 2nd edition, page 439

Version -2

Contraceptive failure 10/100 women years means:

(a) 0.1 accidental pregnancy per 100 woman year using contraceptives

(b) 100 accidental pregnancy per 1000 woman year using contraceptives

(c) 10 accidental pregnancy per 1000 woman year using contraceptives

(d) 10 accidental pregnancy per 100 woman year using contraceptives

Explanation:

Named after **Raymond Pearl**

$$\textbf{Pearl Index (Failure Rate)} = \frac{\textbf{Total number of accidental pregnancies}}{\textbf{Total woman months of exposure}} \times 1200$$

- A **Pearl Index** of **10 per HWY** means that **10 out of 100 woman** will become pregnant if they are using that particular method of contraception in one year.
- To interpret effectiveness of a contraceptive method a **minimum of 600 months** of exposure is usually considered as **necessary**.

Other methods of evaluation are:

- Method failure.
- User failure.
- Life table analysis.

Pearl Index of various contraceptives used are:

- **Calendar Method** - 9 / 100 HWY (9%)
- **BBT Method** - 1 - 2 / 100 HWY (1-2%)
- **Cervical Mucus Method** - 3 / 100 HWY (3%)
- **Symptothermal Method** - 2 / 100 HWY (2%)
- **Foam Tablets** - 0.5%
- **Condoms** - 12%
- **Condoms correctly used** - 3%
- **IUCD** - 1-2%
- **OCP** - 0.1%

Ans: (d) 10 accidental pregnancy per 100 woman year using contraceptives

Ref: AH Suryakantha, Community Medicine with Recent Advances, 3rd edition, page 651

2. **A study is planned to check stool occult blood positivity using hemoccult test among a group of participants aged 50-75 years. The test is repeated if result is positive. No repeating if the test is negative. What is the effect on sensitivity and specificity?**

(a) Sensitivity increases specificity decreases
(b) Sensitivity decreases specificity increases
(c) Sensitivity unchanged specificity increases
(d) Sensitivity increases specificity unchanged

Explanation:

- When two sequential tests are used and those who test positive by the first test are brought in for the second test, there is a net loss in sensitivity, but a net gain in specificity.

Summary of tests in series and parallel

Characteristic	**Tests in series**	**Tests in parallel**
Procedure	A population is subjected to one screening test. We retest those who tested positive on the first test.	Multiple tests are used simultaneously at the same time.
Net sensitivity	Decrease	Increase
Net specificity	Increase	Decrease
Positive predictive value	Increase	Decrease
Negative predictive value	Decrease	Increase

Ans: (b) Sensitivity decreases specificity increases

Ref: Leon Gordis, Epidemiology, 5th edition, page 100 and page 115 Question 8

Version - 2

A study is planned to check stool occult blood positivity using Hemoccult test among a group of participants aged 50 – 75 years. The test is repeated if result is positive. No repeating if the test is negative. What is the effect of this on sensitivity and specificity?

(a) ↑ specificity ↓ sensitivity
(b) ↓specificity ↑ sensitivity
(c) ↑specificity ↑ sensitivity
(d) No effect

Explanation:

- The **sequential/serial testing**–Two sequential tests are used and those who **test positive by the first test** are brought in for the second test. When we retest those who tested positive on the first test, there is a **loss in net sensitivity and a gain in net specificity**.
- The **simultaneous testing,** because an individual who tests positive on any one or multiple tests is considered positive, there is a **gain in net sensitivity and net loss in specificity**.

Basic measures used in evaluation of a diagnostic test are:

a. Sensitivity and specificity.
b. Predictive values – positive predictive value and negative predictive value.

Sensitivity	Ability of the test to identify **true positives** (TP)
Specificity	Ability of the test to identify **true negatives** (TN)
Positive predictive value	Probability that a patient with positive test result truly has the disease
Negative predictive value	Probability that a patient with negative test result truly does not have the disease

Ans: (a) ↑ specificity ↓ sensitivity

Ref: Leon Gordis, Epidemiology, 5th edition, page 99

3. **True about single exposure, common vector outbreak:**

(a) Explosive onset
(b) Secondary waves occur
(c) Cases occur in varying incubation periods
(d) Depends on herd immunity

Explanation:

Point Source Epidemic

- Here simultaneous brief exposure to the disease agent takes place. The resultant cases occur within one incubation period.

Features (as shown in Figure)

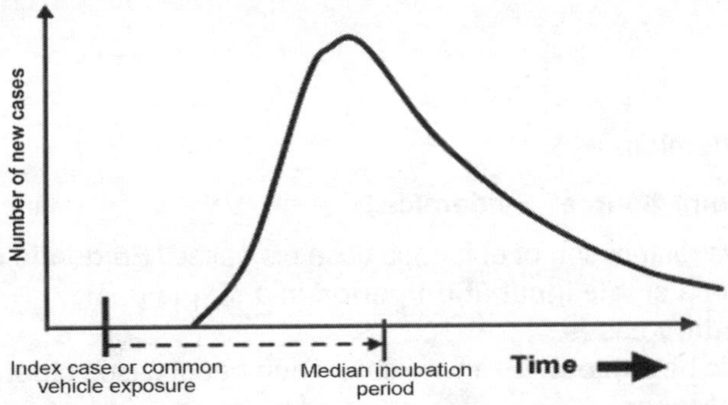

- Epidemic curve rises and falls rapidly.
- There are no secondary waves.
- Epidemic tends to be explosive.

- Clustering of cases within a narrow interval of time.
- All cases occur within one incubation period.

Examples:

- Bhopal Gas Tragedy–1984.
- Chernobyl explosion–1986.
- Minamata disease–due to methyl mercury poisoning.

Continuous Exposure Epidemic

- Sharp rise in number of cases and fall in number of cases interrupted by "secondary waves/peaks", e.g. Contaminated well in a village, prostitute in STD outbreak.

Propagated Epidemics

- Gradual rise and gradual fall over a long time.
- The rate of spread depends upon:
  - Herd immunity.
  - Contact.
  - Secondary attack rate.

  E.g. Hepatitis A and polio epidemics.

Ans: (a) Explosive onset

Ref: Park, 24th edition, page 69; Leon Gordis, Epidemiology, 5th edition, page 29; Principles and Practice of Community Medicine by Dr Asma Rahim, 2nd edition, page 107

Version - 2

True About Single Exposure, Common Vector Outbreak

(a) All cases does not occur within one incubation period
(b) Frequent secondary cases
(c) Explosive
(d) Secondary wave present

Explanation:

Types of Epidemics

Three major types of epidemics may be distinguished.

A. **Common - Source epidemics**
   (a) Single exposure or "point source" epidemics.
   (b) Continuous or multiple exposure epidemics.
B. **Propagated epidemics**
   (a) Person-to-person
   (b) Arthropod vector
   (c) Animal reservoir
C. **Slow (modern) epidemics.**

Single Exposure or "Point Source" Epidemics

- The graph of the time distribution of epidemic cases is called "**Epidemic curve**".
- All cases occur within a **single incubation period** in a **single peak.**
- There are **no secondary cases**.
- The epidemic tends to be **explosive** with maximum number of cases **clustered** around **one point of time**.
- Epidemic will be **explosive**.

  The common source epidemics are frequently but not always due to exposure to an infectious agent, e.g.
- **Bhopal gas tragedy** (air pollution).
- **Minamata** disease in Japan (contaminated food chain).

- **Chernobyl** tragedy (radiation pollution).

Ans: (c) Explosive

Ref: Park's Preventive and Social Medicine, 23rd edition, page 64

4. **Case act as its own control in which of the following study?**

(a) Cross over study
(b) Retrospective study
(c) Prospective study
(d) Case control study

Explanation:

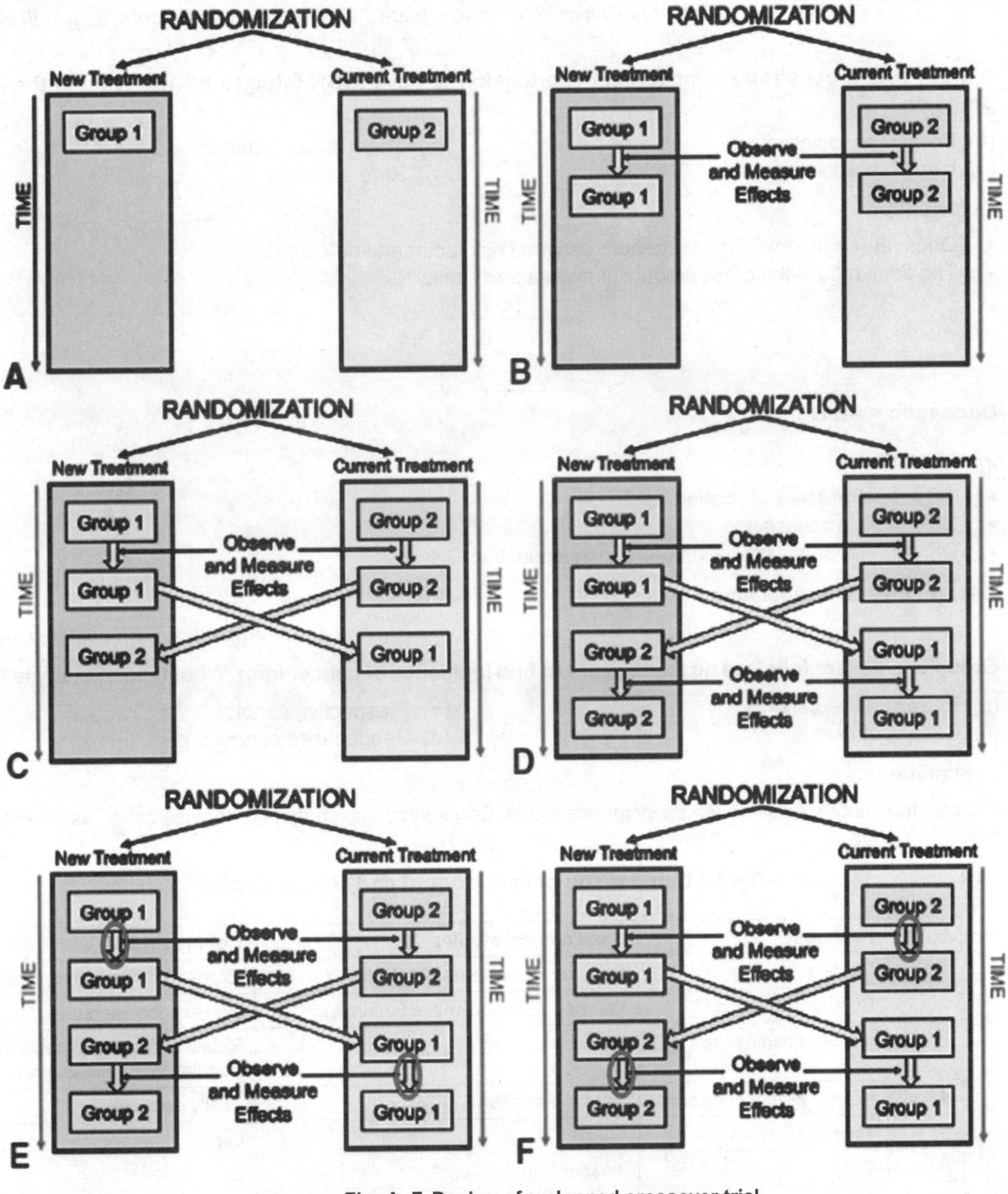

Fig: A–F, Design of a planned crossover trial

There are two types of cross over in clinical trials

Planned cross over	Unplanned cross over
Patients are randomized to therapy A and therapy B and after being observed for a certain period of time on one therapy, they are switched for another therapy.	Patients during the study may change over to other treatment.
Cases themselves act as controls.	Cases wont be taken as controls as randomization is affected.

Ans: (a) Cross over study

Ref: Park, 24th edition, page 88; Principles and Practice of Community Medicine by Dr Asma Rahim, 2nd edition, page 116; Leon Gordis, Epidemiology, 5th edition

5. **A study found odds ratio of maternal hypertension to have IUGR fetus to be 1:5. What is the interpretation?**

(a) Positive association
(b) Common association
(c) Inverse association
(d) Rare outcome

Explanation:

- Odds ratio is the measure of strength between risk factor and outcome.
- The odds ratio is the cross product of entries as in table.

A	B
C	D

Odds ratio = AD/BC

Interpretation

- OR > 1 – Positive association.
- OR = 1 – No association.
- OR < 1 – Inverse association (here in this question OR= 0.2).

Ans: (c) Inverse association

Ref: Park, 24th edition, page 78

6. **Group of smokers followed up for 10 years to find incidence of cancer lung. What type of study is this?**

(a) Retrospective cohort
(b) Prospective cohort
(c) Case control study
(d) Randomized control trials

Explanation:

Cohort study is otherwise called as incidence study. Cross sectional study is otherwise called as prevalence study.

Table: Comparison of case control and cohort studies

S.No.	Features	Case control studies	Cohort studies
1	Study group	Persons with disease (outcome)	Exposed persons (risk factor)
2	Comparison group	Persons without disease (controls)	Non exposed persons
3	Measurements of risk	Odds ratio	Relative risk, attributable risk, Population attributable risk
4	Natural history of disease	Hard to establish	Easily establish
5	Time of study	Short	Long
6	Cost	Inexpensive	Expensive
7	Sample size needed	Small	Large

Contd.

8	Best when	Disease is rare	Exposure is rare
9	Bias	Selection bias (occur during selection of cases and controls)	Hawthorne bias

Ans: (b) Prospective cohort study

Ref: Park, 24th edition, page 80; Leon Gordis, Epidemiology, 5th edition

7. Variation of sample mean from population mean is:

(a) Standard error of the mean
(b) Standard error of proportion
(c) Standard error of difference between two means
(d) Standard error of difference between two proportions

Explanation:

Concept of Standard Error:

- Suppose I want to measure haemoglobin levels of adolescent girls of entire India. Ideally I have to travel entire India from Kashmir to Tamilnadu. It is not possible. I am in Pondicherry. I measure Haemoglobin levels of adolescent girls of Pondicherry and calculate sample mean and standard deviation. From this I calculate standard error (SE) = sd/√n, then I calculate 95% confidence interval = mean ± 2 SE.
- Standard error of mean = SD/√N.
- Standard error of mean is inversely related to sample size. Hence larger the sample size, the mean will be precise.
- Standard error of sample proportions = p= √pq/n.
- Standard error between two means= $SD_1/\sqrt{n_1}+SD_2/\sqrt{n_2}$
- Standard error of difference between two proportions = $\sqrt{p_1q_1/n1 \pm p_2q_2/n_2}$

Ans: (a) Standard error of the mean

Ref: Park, 24th edition, page 887

8. What is true regarding increasing sample size *except*?

(a) Decreases power of the study
(b) Standard error of mean decreases
(c) Confidence interval widens
(d) Decreases alpha error

Explanation:

- **Sample size:** No. of subjects/patients in study. Represented by symbol "n".
- Calculated by formula $4pq/d^2$ where p=prevalence q=100-p.
- d-precision
- More sample size increases the power of study thereby reducing alpha error.
- **Option (b):** Standard error= SD/√n.
- Hence increasing sample size will reduce the standard error, i.e., make more precise.
- **Option (c):** Increasing sample size narrows the confidence interval.

Ans: (a) Decreases power of the study

Ref: Leon Gordis, Epidemiology, 5th edition, page 155; Principles and Practice of Community Medicine, page 624

9. A city with 800 deaths per year. Mortuary, body stored for average duration of 8 days with 80% occupancy in a year. What number of mortuary beds needed?

(a) 22 (b) 17 (c) 7 (d) 34

Explanation:

- 80% of total number on body days per year = 800 × 8= 6400.

- 100% = (6400÷80) × 100 = 8000.
- Number of mortuary beds needed = 8000/365 = 21.92=22.

Ans: (a) 22

Ref: Textbook of Forensic Medicine and Toxicology – Krishan Vij and Internet

10. Loss of inter-personal communication is managed by:

(a) Group counselling (b) Individual counselling
(c) Check telecommunications (d) Improving language

Explanation:

There are many channels of health communication.

They are:

(a) Inter-personal communication.
(b) Mass media.
(c) Traditional or folk media:
   - Interpersonal communication is the most common method of communication.
   - Otherwise called as face to face communication.
   - Most persuasive and effective than other communication.
   - When the message relayed via mass media gets diffused in community, it is picked up by inter-personal and informal networks.
   - By improving the telecommunications via media, we can improve face to face communication.

Ans: (c) Check telecommunications

Ref: Park, 24th edition, page 881

ENT

1. **Politzer bag maneuver used to test:**

(a) Eustachian tube (b) Larynx (c) Esophagus (d) Nasal cavity

Explanation:

- Politzer bag is used for testing the eustachian tube.
- The bag can also be used to ventilate the middle ear.
- Other eustachian tube function tests are:
    - Valsalva test.
    - Eustachian tube catheterization.
    - Toynbee's test.
    - Tympanometry as a part of impedance audiometry.
    - Radiological test using radiopaque dye, saccharine or methylene blue test can be done only when there is a perforation in the tympanic membrane.
    - Sonotubometry in which a tone is presented to the ear and the recording taken from a microphone in the external auditory canal.

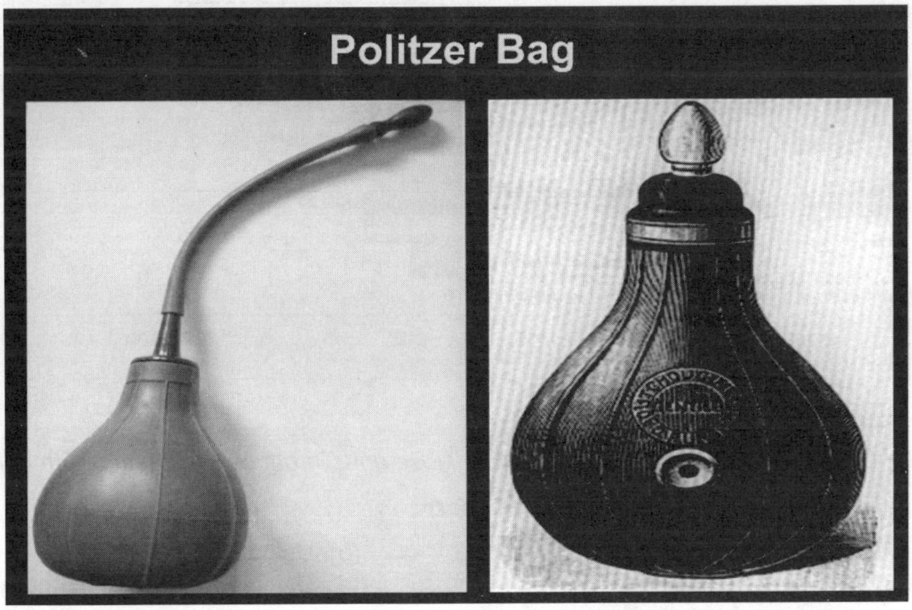

Ans: (a) Eustachian tube

Ref: Diseases of the Ear, Nose and Throat by PL Dhingra, 6th edition, 2010, page 59

2. **Patient presents with severe hearing loss. For the amount of decibel loss he has, which of the following sound can be heard by him?**

(a) Rustling of leaves (b) Start of car engine at 10 feet
(c) Sound of Niagara falls (d) Noisy environment night street

Explanation:

- **Severe hearing loss** means that the patients hearing loss is in the range of **71-91dB.**
- In such hearing loss only the sound of Niagara falls **[> 90 dB]** will be heard.
- **Other options:**
    - o The **sound of rustling of leaves** is 15 dB.
    - o **Car engine** at 10 feet is 70 dB.
    - o **Noisy environment night street** is 80 dB.
- The Levels of hearing loss are:
    - o **Mild:** 26-40 dB.
    - o **Moderate:** 41-55 dB.
    - o **Moderately severe:** 56-70 dB.
    - o **Severe:** 71-91 dB.
    - o **Profound:** More than 91 dB.
    - o Total.

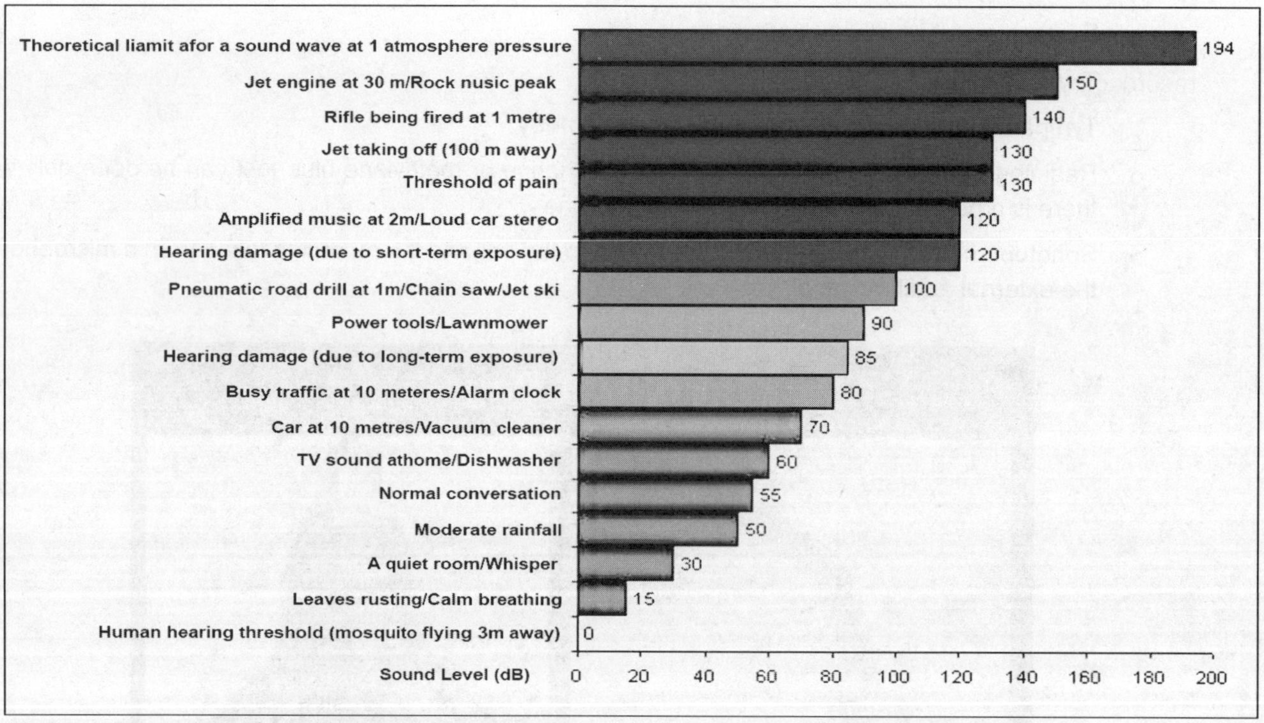

Ans: (c) Sound of Niagara falls

Ref: Diseases of the Ear, Nose and Throat by PL Dhingra, 6th edition, 2010, page 38

3. **False regarding hearing assessment in newborn:**

(a) Done for all normal babies to assess hearing (b) Using BERA
(c) Using OAE (d) Using pure tone audiometry

Explanation:

- The assessment of newborn hearing is now **universal**, which means that all neonates should be screened for hearing loss.
- In **pure tone audiometry** a tone is presented to the ear and the patient responds by raising his hand. It's a **subjective test** and depends on the patient's ability to understand and response to the sound and therefore cannot be used in **mentally challenged, uncooperative individuals, neonates and infants.**
- The screening can be done using either of the 2 tests which are:

A. **OAE–Otoacoustic emissions,** which are low intensity sounds produced by outer hair cells of the cochlea and can be detected by using microphones placed in the external auditory canal.

- Sedation does not affect OAE.
- Types are:
  - **Spontaneous OAE** – healthy individuals with hearing loss < 30 dB.
  - **Evoked OAE** – elicited by a sound stimulus and are of the following type:
    - Transient evoked OAE (TEOAE) – evoked by clicks.
    - Distortion product OAE (DPOAE) – two tones are simultaneously presented to the cochlea to produce distortion products.

Uses

- Screening test of hearing in neonates.
- Differentiate between a cochlear and retro cochlear lesion.

OAE may be absent in:

- 50% of normal population.
- Lesions of the cochlea.
- Middle ear disorders.
- Hearing loss > 30 dB.

B. **BERA – Brainstem evoked response audiometry,** in which brainstem responses to auditory stimulus are recorded using electrodes placed on the scalp.

- Also called BAER or BAEP or ABR (auditory brainstem response).
- Tests the integrity of central auditory pathway.
- Non invasive test.
- Normally 7 waves are seen in the first 10 milliseconds.
- I, III and V waves are most important.
- Absolute latency, inter wave latency and the amplitude of the waves is measured.
- Site for generation of waves are:
  - Wave I – distal CN VIII.
  - Wave II – proximal CN VIII.
  - Wave III – cochlear nucleus.
  - Wave IV – superior olivary complex.
  - Wave V – lateral lemniscus.
  - Wave VI and VII – inferior colliculus.

Uses

- Screening for hearing in infants.
- Threshold estimation in infants.
- To diagnose retro cochlear pathology and brainstem lesions.
- Monitor VIII N in surgery of acoustic neuroma.

Also Note

- **Pure tone audiometry** (PTA) is **subjective test.**
- **Impedance audiometry, OAE and BERA** are **objective tests.**

Ans: (d) Pure tone audiometry

Ref: Diseases of the Ear, Nose and Throat by PL Dhingra, 6th edition, 2010, page 26-28 and 118

4. **Abductor of vocal cord:**

(a) Cricothyroid
(b) Cricoarytenoid
(c) Posterior cricoarytenoid
(d) Lateral cricoarytenoid

Explanation:

- **Only muscle** which **abducts** the vocal cord is **Posterior cricoarytenoid** which is supplied by the **recurrent laryngeal nerve.**
- Muscles of the larynx are divided into **intrinsic** and **extrinsic** groups.

Intrinsic muscles of the larynx

Those acting on the vocal cord	**Abductors**	Posterior cricoarytenoid
	Adductors	Lateral cricoarytenoid Interarytenoid Thyroarytenoid
	Tensors	**External** – Cricothyroid **Internal** – Vocalis
Those acting on the laryngeal inlet	**Opening the inlet**	Thyroepiglottis (part of thyroarytenoid)
	Closing the inlet	Interarytenoid (oblique part) Aryepiglottic (posterior oblique part of interarytenoid)

Extrinsic muscles of the larynx

Elevators	Primary	**Stylopharyngeus** **Salpingopharyngeus** **Palatopharyngeus** **Thyrohyoid**
	Secondary	**Mylohyoid** **Stylohyoid** **Digastric** **Geniohyoid**
Depressors	**Sternohyoid** **Sternothyroid** **Omohyoid**	

- All the **intrinsic muscles** of the larynx are supplied by **recurrent laryngeal** nerve except **cricothyroid** which is supplied by the **external laryngeal branch of superior laryngeal nerve.**

Ans. (c) Posterior cricoarytenoid

Ref: Diseases of the Ear, Nose and Throat by PL Dhingra, 6th edition, 2014, page 283

5. **Young's operation done in:**

(a) Rhinophyma
(b) Atrophic rhinitis
(c) Rhinitis sicca
(d) Hypertrophic rhinitis

Explantation:

Young's Operation

- It is done as a treatment of ***atrophic rhinitis.***
- It involves ***closure of the nasal cavity*** affected with atrophic rhinitis by creating ***mucocutaneous flaps.***
- These flaps are sutured together in two layers: first the mucosal layer, then the skin layer.
- The ***nasal cavity*** is kept ***closed for a period of 9 months.***
- Re-examination is done after 9 months – if the crusts have disappeared, a revision surgery is performed and the nasal cavity is reopened.
- The theory behind this procedure is that the closed nasal cavity has time to heal.

Ans: (b) Atrophic rhinitis

Ref: Diseases of the Ear, Nose and Throat by PL Dhingra, 5th edition, 2010, page 170

OPHTHALMOLOGY

1. **The following features are seen in high myopia *except*:**

(a) Tilted optic disc
(b) Anterior staphyloma
(c) Vitreous syneresis
(d) Macular chorioretinal atrophy

Explanation:

- Pathological myopia is associated with abnormal increase in axial length of the eyeball especially the posterior segment leading to weakening of the posterior segment resulting in **Posterior Staphyloma**.
- Anterior staphyloma occurs due to sloughing of the total cornea in corneal ulcer.
- Myopia and astigmatism is strongly associated with tilted optic disc.

PATHOLOGICAL MYOPIA

- A rapidly progressive refractive error resulting in high myopia (>-6 D) and is usually associated with degenerative changes in the eye.

Etiopathogenesis: Genetic factors and general growth process→abnormal increased growth in retina → the sclera due to its distensibility stretches along with the retina. But the choroid being more vascular undergoes degeneration because of stretching, which in turn causes retinal degeneration.

Ocular Features:

- Increased axial length, prominent eyeballs.
- **Anterior segment:** Large cornea, anterior chamber is deep, pupils are slightly large and react sluggishly to light.
- **Posterior segment:**

Vitreous: Vitreous liquefaction (syneresis), opacities and posterior vitreous detachment.

Retina:

- **Optic disc:** Large pale myopic disc with temporal myopic crescent and nasal supertraction crescent. Tilted optic disc can also occur.
- **Macula:** Foster - Fuch's spots (subretinal neovascularization and choroidal hemorrhage) and chorio retinal atrophic patches.
- Peripheral retinal degenerations like Lattice, Cystoid, etc. will lead to retinal hole/tear and then retinal detachment.
- Posterior staphyloma due to ectasia of the sclera.

Ans: (b) Anterior staphyloma

Ref: A.K. Khurana's Comprehensive Ophthalmology, 6th edition, page 135, 39-40; Kanski Clinical Ophthalmology, 8th edition, page 796

2. **Pathology in keratomalacia:**

(a) Accumulation of desquamated debris
(b) Absence of mucus
(c) Breakdown of collagen fibers in corneal stroma
(d) Infection with corynebacterium xerosis

Explanation:

Keratomalacia

Sterile Corneal ulcer secondary to vitamin A deficiency.

Xerophthalmia

- Spectrum of ocular disease ranging from night blindness to corneal melting caused by vitamin A deficiency.
- Nutritional blindness.
- VIitamin A is essential for the synthesis of retinal photo pigments and conjunctival glycoproteins.
- Vitamin A deficiency is a systemic disease affecting cells and organs throughout the body

Causes: Malnutrition, malabsorption, chronic alcoholics, diseases which precipitate malnutrition like measles, malaria, diarrhoea, acute illness in children.

Classification	Ocular Signs
XN	Night blindness
X1A	Conjunctival xerosis
X1B	Bitot's spots
X2	Corneal xerosis
X3A	Corneal ulceration-keratomalacia involving one-third or less of the cornea
X3B	Corneal ulceration-keratomalacia involving one-half or more of the cornea
XS	Corneal scar
XF	Xerophthalmic fundus

XN: Night Blindness

- EARLIEST SYMPTOM; responds rapidly to vitamin A therapy [within 24-48 hours]

X1 A and X1 B: Conjunctival Involvement

- The conjunctival epithelium undergoes KERATANISING METAPLASIA, i.e., the normal columnar epithelium is transformed into stratified squamous epithelium. Goblet cells will be lost (mucin secretion is reduced) and keratinization occurs.
- Conjunctival xerosis–dryness of the conjunctiva usually starts at the temporal side.
- Keratin + saprophytic bacilli [CORYNEBACTERIUM XEROSIS] accumulate on the xerotic surface→ FOAMY APPEARANCE == BITOT'S SPOT.
- Begin to resolve within 2-5 days and disappear by 2 weeks of treatment.
- In chronic cases, the spots will not disappear.

X2:Corneal Xerosis

- Lustreless dry appearance, in the inferior limbus.
- Responds within 2-5 days, disappear within 2 weeks of treatment.

X3A and X3B: Keratomalacia

- COLLIQUATIVE NECROSIS/LIQUAFACTIVE NECROSIS→**sterile** corneal melting due to collagen breakdown without any signs of inflammation.
- Round or oval punched out ulcers involving the inferonasal quadrant.
- Perforation→adherent leucoma, anterior staphyloma, phthisis bulbi.

XS: Corneal Scarring

- Nebula, macula, leucoma.

XF: Xerophthalmic Fundus/Uyemura's Fundus

- Small yellowish white lesions in the peripheral retina.

Treatment:

- Medical emergency especially in malnourished infants.
- **Vitamin A dosage:**
  2 lakh I.U. – Orally or 1 lakh I.U. – I.M.
  3 doses are given = Day 1, Day 2 and within 1-4 Weeks.
- Children between 6-11 Months: Half the Dose.
- Children < 6 Months: Quarter the Dose.

Ocular Lesions:

Lubricants, broad spectrum antibiotics and cycloplegic.

Ans: (c) Breakdown of collagen fibers in corneal stroma

Ref: Kanski Clinical Ophthalmology, 8th edition, page 212

3. Congenital glaucoma is associated with all *except*:

(a) Shallow anterior chamber
(b) Large cornea
(c) Watering of the eyes, photophobia and blepharospasm
(d) Haab's striae

Explanation:

Primary congenital glaucoma is caused by impaired aqueous outflow due to maldevelopment of the anterior chamber angle (trabeculodysgenesis) resulting in high IOP. It is not associated with any other ocular or systemic abnormalities.

Depending upon the age of onset, congenital glaucomas are termed as:

- True congenital glaucoma (40%) in which IOP is elevated during intrauterine life.
- Infantile glaucoma (55%) which manifests prior to age 3.
- Juvenile glaucoma, the least common, in which IOP rises between 3 and 16 years of age.

Prevalence: 1 in 10,000; boys are commonly affected.

Sporadic: 90%; autosomal recessive – 10%.

Buphthalmos: When the IOP increases before the age of 3, due to elasticity of cornea and sclera, the eyeball enlarges. It is termed as Buphthalmos (bull like eyes). After 3 years of age, the fibrous coat loses its elasticity and so the eyeball will not enlarge in size if the IOP rises. Because of the same reason, the optic disc cupping is reversible in case of congenital glaucoma once IOP is reduced.

Symptoms:

- **Classic triad:** Lacrimation, photophobia and blepharospasm.

Signs:

- **Cornea:**
  - Corneal edema (cloudy cornea).
  - Corneal enlargement (>13 mm in diameter).
    - Horizontal diameter at birth is 10 mm and by the age of 2 years , it reaches the adult size of about 11.7 mm.
- **Haab's striae:** Descemet's membrane break → seen in peripheral cornea and concentric to the limbus.
- **Sclera:** Due to enlargement of eyeball, it will become thin and appears blue due to the underlying uveal tissue.
- **Anterior Chamber:** Deep.
- **IRIS:** Iridodonesis and atrophic patches.
- **Lens:** Flat due to stretching of zonules and subluxate backward.
- Axial myopia due to increase in axial length.

P.S: Both pathological myopia and buphthalmos have similar anatomical findings.

Differential diagnosis:

Cloudy cornea	Large cornea	Lacrimation
Mnemonic: STUMPED • Sclerocornea • Trauma (forceps injury–Descemets rupture will be vertical) • Ulcer (Interstitial keratitis) • Mucoploysaccharidosis • Peter's anomaly • Endothelial dystrophy • Dermoid	• Megalo cornea • High myopia • Buphthalmos	• Congenital glaucoma • Congenital nasolacrimal duct obstruction • Conjunctivitis • Corneal abrasion/ulcer • Foreign body • Epithelial dystrophy → recurrent corneal erosions • Aberrant eyelashes • Entropion

Ans: (a) Shallow anterior chamber

Ref: A.K. Khurana's Comprehensive Ophthalmology, 6th edition, page 225-228; Kanski, Clinical Ophthalmology, 8th edition, page 385-388

MEDICINE

1. An asymptomatic patient on regular health checkup has platelet counts of 8,00,000. Next line of management is:

(a) Follow up and observe

(b) Bone marrow biopsy

(c) Plasmapheresis

(d) Phelobotomy + Packed cell transfusion

Explanation:

An elevated platelet count in an asymptomatic patient without cardiovascular risk factors requires no therapy.

When the platelet count rises above 1 × 10^6/μL, a substantial quantity of high-molecular-weight von Willebrand multimers are removed from the circulation and destroyed by the enlarged platelet mass, resulting in an acquired form of von Willebrand's disease.

THROMBOCYTOSIS

- Thrombocytosis, also called thrombocythemia, is generally defined as a platelet count greater than a defined upper limit of normal that may vary between **350,000/μl to 600,000/μl,** depending on the laboratory or medical reference. The most common cut off for normal is **<450,000/μl.**
- Elevated platelet counts are often an incidental or unexpected finding on a complete blood count (CBC) conducted to evaluate an unrelated condition.
- For those individuals found to have thrombocytosis without associated bleeding or thrombosis, the first challenge is to find the cause.
- The causes of thrombocytosis are separated into two categories:

  A. **Autonomous (primary) thrombocytosis**

  - Occurs as a result of myeloproliferative disorders, myelodysplastic disorders, or rarely as a result of a hereditary condition.

  B. **Reactive (secondary) thrombocytosis** is:

  - Most often a normal physiologic response to coexistent inflammatory condition (e.g., infection, chronic inflammatory condition).

Management of essential thrombocytosis by risk factors

Risk category	**Risk factors**	**Management**
Low	Age <60 and no prior cardiovascular event	Nil. Follow-up and observe
Intermediate	Generic cardiovascular risk factors	Low dose aspirin (no consensus)
High	Age >60 and/or prior cardiovascular events	Myelosuppression + Low dose aspirin

Ans: (a) Follow-up and observe

Ref: Harrison's Principles of Internal Medicine, 19th edition, page 678

2. **'Pie in the sky' visual field defect seen in lesions of:**

(a) Optic tract (b) Temporal cortex (c) Optic chiasma (d) Occipital cortex

Explanation:

- If an infarct occurs at the middle cerebral artery **Superior Division** - it will affect the upper portion of the optic radiations in the **parietal** lobe and will give a contralateral **Inferior Quadrantopsia** ("pie on the floor" visual defect).
- If an infarct occurs at the middle cerebral artery **Inferior Division** - will affect the lower portion of the optic radiations in the **temporal** lobe and will give a contralateral **Superior Quadrantopsia** ("pie on the sky" visual defect).

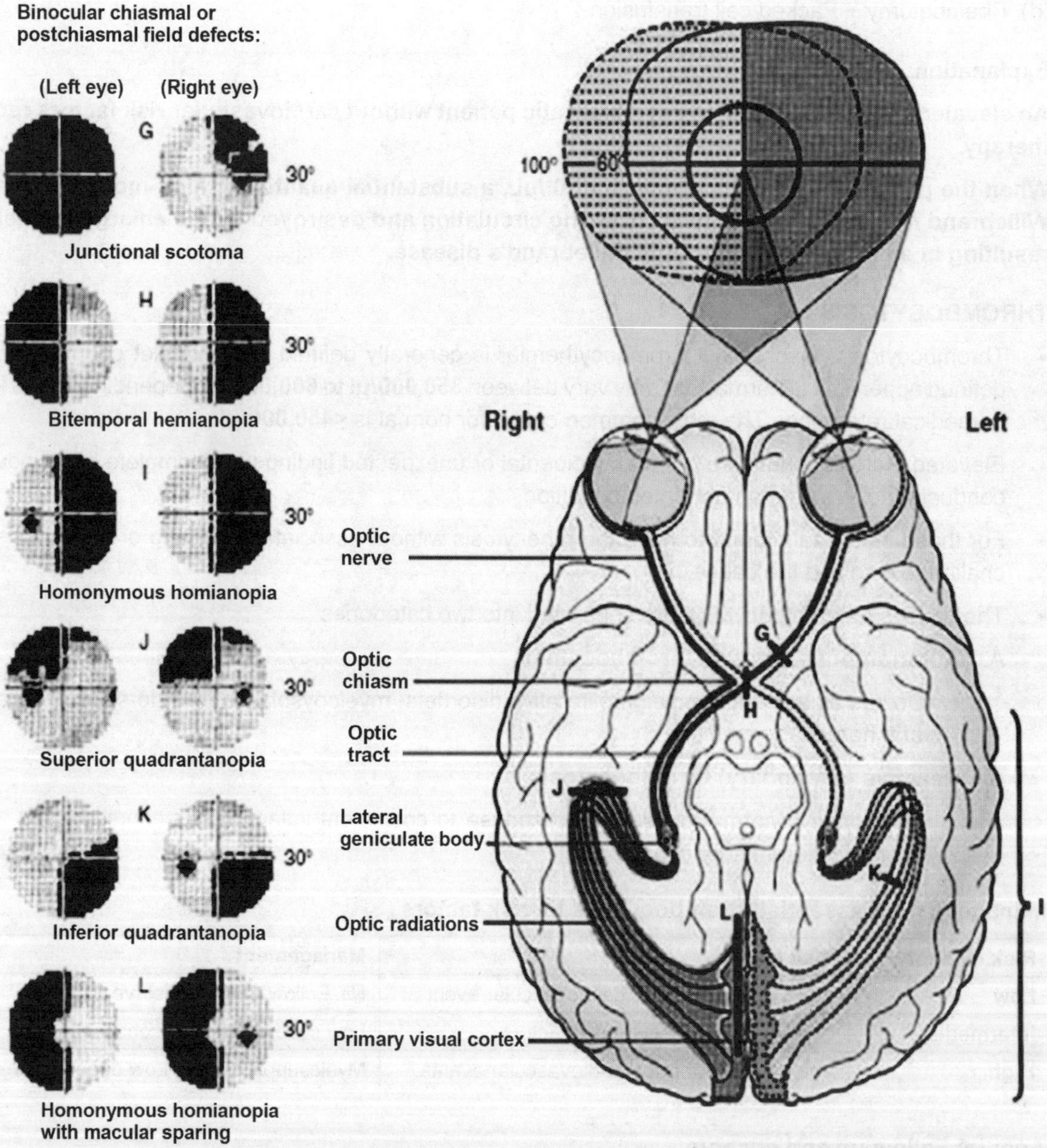

Ans: (b) Temporal cortex

Ref: Harrison's Principles of Internal Medicine, 19th edition, page198

3. **A tall male presents with absent pubic, axillary hair, infantile genitalia, high LH, FSH levels and XY karyotype. What is the most probable diagnosis?**

(a) Vanishing testis syndrome
(b) Noonan syndrome
(c) Adrenal hyperplasia
(d) Klinefelter syndrome

Explanation:

Classic form of Klinefelter syndrome (47,XXY)–due to meiotic non-disjunction of the sex chromosomes. Mosaic forms of Klinefelter syndrome (46,XY/47,XXY)–due to chromosomal mitotic non-disjunction within the zygote.

Causes of hypergonadotrophic hypogonadism in males:

- Klinefelter's syndrome.
- Noonan's syndrome.
- Cryptorchidism.
- Testicular agenesis/atrophy.

Klinefelter syndrome

- Syndrome of male hypogonadism.
- Most common cause of hypogonadism and infertility in males.
- Most common sex chromosomal aneuploidy in males.
- Occurs when there are **two or more X chromosomes** and **one or more Y chromosomes.**
- **Increased maternal age** predisposes to **meiotic nondisjunction** of X chromosomes.
- **Clinical features**
  - o **Low IQ.**
  - o **Tall stature.**
  - o **Poor muscle tone.**
  - o **Reduced secondary sexual characteristics.**
  - o **Gynaecomastia.**
  - o **Small testes/infertility.**
- **Diagnosis**
  - o Low testosterone levels.
  - o High FSH, LH levels.

Ans: (d) Klinefelter syndrome

Ref: Harrison's Principles of Internal Medicine, 19th edition, page 2350

4. **An HIV positive male with yellow white patches on fundoscopy. Best management is:**

(a) INH + Rifampicin and PYZ
(b) Ganciclovir + steroid
(c) Sulfadoxine plus pyramethamine
(d) Amphotericin

Explanation:

Ophthalmologic Diseases in HIV:

- Most common abnormal finding is **cotton wool spots*** due to **retinal ischemia** and **microvascular disease.**
- **CMV retinitis:**
  - o Common in patients with CD 4 count<100.
  - o Painless progressive loss of vision.
  - o Characteristic retinal appearance is **perivascular hemorrhage** and **exudate**.
  - o Oral valganciclovir, IV gancyclovir, IV foscarnet.
  - o Combination with gancyclovir and foscarnet more effective.
- **Varicella zoster:**
  - o Acute retinal necrosis syndrome.
  - o Progressive outer retinal necrosis.

- **P. jiroveci:**
  - o Widespread peripheral pale grey lesions.
  - o Bilateral slightly elevated yellow white plaques in the choroid.
- **Toxoplasmosis:** Choriotetinitis in association with congenital toxoplasmosis.
- **Kaposi's sarcoma:** Involves eyelid and conjunctiva.
- **Syphilis:** Uveitis.

Ans: (c) Sulfadoxine plus pyramethamine

Ref: Harrison's Principles of Internal Medicine, 19th edition, page 1267

5. An HIV patient on ART presents with seizures, unilateral facial nerve palsy. CT scan shows ring enhancement lesion. Best treatment is:

(a) Acyclovir
(b) Amphotericin B
(c) INH, Rifampicin and Ethambutol
(d) Sulphadiazine and pyrimethamine

Explanation:

Cause of seizures in HIV patient:

- HIV encephalopathy: 7-50%.
- Cerebral toxoplasmosis: 15-40%.
- Cryptococcal meningitis: 8%.
- Primary CNS lymphoma: 15-30%.
- Progressive multifocal leukencephalopathy: 20%.
- CNS tuberculosis.

Cause for ring enhancing lesson in HIV infected patients:

- Toxoplasmosis.
- Primary CNS lymphoma.
- Tuberculosis.
- Fungal abscess.
- Bacterial abscess.

'Eccentric target sign' **on MRI – Toxoplasmosis*:**

- Standard therapy for toxoplasmosis in HIV patients consists of **pyrimethamine**, **sulfadiazine**, and **folinic acid** in combination. **Trimethoprim-sulfamethoxazole** (TMP-SMZ) can be used as an **alternative regimen.**

Ans: (d) Sulphadiazine and pyrimethamine

Ref: Harrison's Principles of Internal Medicine, 19th edition, page 1265,1266

6. Prophylactic antifungal drug used in HIV patients:

(a) Itraconazole
(b) Posaconazole
(c) Terconazole
(d) Voriconazole

Explanation:

Prophylactic Antifungal for Opportunistic Infections in HIV Patients

- **Fluconazole 400 mg daily:**
  - o For **Coccidiodes immitis** when **CD4 count <250.**
  - o For **Cryptococcus neoformans** when **CD4 count <100.**
- **Itraconazole 200 mg daily:**
  - o For **Histoplasma capsulatum** when **CD4 count <150.**
  - o For **Penicillium marneffi CD4 count <100.**

Ans: (a) Itraconazole

Ref: Harrison's Principles of Internal Medicine, 19th edition, page 1252

7. **A new drug approved for treatment of 'off phenomenon' in Parkinsonism:**

(a) Safinamide
(b) Evenamide
(c) Lacosamide
(d) Ziconotide

Explanation:

- **Safinamide is** orally active, selective, reversible **monoamine oxidase-B inhibitor** with both **dopaminergic** and **non-dopaminergic** (glutamatergic).
- Used as an **add-on treatment** for **Parkinson's disease** during **"off" episodes.**

Contraindicated in liver disease, albinism, retinitis pigmentosa, diabetic neuropathy and uveitis.

Ans: (a) Safinamide

Ref:https://www.medscape.com/viewarticle/877524

8. **True statement regarding migraine in pregnancy is:**

(a) Ketorolac is preferred
(b) NSAIDs are first line drugs
(c) Improved symptoms with pregnancy
(d) Sumatriptan preferred over chlorpromazine

Explanation:

Treatment of Acute Migraine

NSAIDs	Naproxen, Ibuprofen,Tolfenamic acid Diclofenac, Acetominophen
5-HT1 Receptor Agonists	**Oral**: Ergotamine, Naratriptan, Rizatriptan, Sumatriptan, Frovatriptan, Almotriptan, Eletriptan, Zolmitriptan **Nasal:** Sumatriptan, Zolmitriptan **Parenteral:** Dihydroergotamine, Sumatriptan
Dopamine Receptor Antagonists	**Oral:** Metoclopramide, Prochlorperazine **Parenteral:** Chlorpromazine, Metoclopramide, Prochlorperazine
Others	**Nasal:** Butorphanol **Parenteral:**Opioids

Migraine during Pregnancy

- Improvement in 'migraine without aura'.
- Worsening of 'migraine with aura'.
- **Ergot derivatives** are **contraindicated** due to possibility of uterine hypertonicity and vascular disruption leading on to miscarriage.
- Safety of **Triptans during pregnancy is not fully confirmed.** Can be used only if other drugs are not effective.
- **Treatment**
  - o First line: NSAIDs and paracetamol.
  - o Triptans are avoided.
- **Prophylaxis: Magnesium, Metoprolol.**

Ans: (b) NSAIDs are first line drugs

Ref: Harrison's Principles of Internal Medicine, 19th edition, page 2592

9. **Slow saccadic movement present in all *except*:**

(a) Alzheimer's disease
(b) Huntington's chorea
(c) Progressive supranuclear palsy
(d) Spinocerebellar ataxia

Explanation:

Causes of Slow Saccades

- Drug ingestion (very common).
- Drowsiness or fatigue (common).
- **Basal ganglia syndromes**
    - **Huntington's chorea** (global saccadic paresis, accompanied by chorea).
    - **Progressive Supranuclear Palsy** (PSP) -- (vertical slow first).
    - **Wilson's disease** (extremely rare, accompanied by tremor, eye abnormalities).
- **Cerebellar syndromes**
    - **Ataxia telangiectasia.**
    - Joseph's disease (SCA-3).
    - Spinocerebellar ataxia.
- **Peripheral oculomotor weakness (cranial nerve palsies, myopathy)**
    - 6th and 3rd nerve palsies (common) (link to sixth nerve).
    - Miller Fisher syndrome (rare, saccadic slowing plus areflexia and ataxia).
    - Progressive external ophthalmoplegia (PEO).
    - Mitochondrial myopathy.
    - Thyroid disorders (common, mainly vertical).
    - Lambert-Eaton myasthenic syndrome.
    - Myasthenia gravis.
- **White matter diseases**
    - Adrenoleukodystrophy*.
    - Internuclear ophthalmoplegia.
    - PPRF (parapontine reticular formation lesions) such as due to MS (multiple sclerosis) or brainstem stroke.
- **Miscellaneous disorders**
    - **Parkinsonism*.**
    - Niemann-Pick disease (extremely rare).
    - Wernicke's ophthalmoplegia (extremely rare).
    - Following cardiac surgery (global saccadic paresis).
    - Kennedy's disease (SMA-4, extremely rare).
- **Others**
    - Sleep.
    - Intoxication.
    - Elderly.

Ans: (a) Alzheimer's disease

Ref: Harrison's Principles of Internal Medicine, 19th edition, page 2606

10. True statement regarding glycemic control in ICU patient:

(a) Monitoring of blood insulin levels far better than sugar levels in SICU patients
(b) Maintenance of normoglycemia in medical ICU is of no use
(c) Target glucose range of 140–180 mg/dL (7.8–10.0 mmol/L) is recommended
(d) Stringent goals, such as 110–140 mg/dL required for all patients

Explanation:

- **Insulin therapy** should be initiated for treatment of **persistent hyperglycemia** starting at a threshold **180 mg/dL** (10.0 mmol/L).
- Target glucose range of **140–180 mg/dL** (7.8–10.0 mmol/L) is recommended for the majority of critically ill patients and non-critically ill patients.

- Stringent goals, such as **110–140 mg/dL** (6.1–7.8 mmol/L), may be appropriate for selected patients, if this can be achieved without significant hypoglycemia.

Ans: (c) Target glucose range of 140–180 mg/dL (7.8–10.0 mmol/L) is recommended

Ref: Standards of Medical Care in Diabetes—2018, January 2018, Volume 41, Supplement 1, Diabetes Care 2018;41(Suppl. 1):S3 | https://doi.org/10.2337/dc18-SPPC01

11. Prophylactic antifungal used in autologous stem cell transplant recipient is:

(a) Lipoic amphotericin B
(b) Fluconazole
(c) Itraconazole
(d) Posaconazole

Explanation:

Infection Prophylaxis in Stem Cell Transplant Recipients

Organism	**Agent**	**Approach**
Bacterial	Levofloxacin	750 mg PO or IV daily
Fungal	Fluconazole	400 mg PO qd to day 75
Pneumocystis carinii	Trimethoprim sulfamethoxazole	1 double-strength tablet PO bid 2 days/week until day 180 or off immunosuppression
Herpes simplex	Acyclovir	800 mg PO bid to day 30
Varicella-zoster	Acyclovir	800 mg PO bid to day 365
Cytomegalovirus	Ganciclovir	5 mg/kg IV bid for 7 days, then 5 (mg/kg)/d 5 days/week to day 100

Ans: (b) Fluconazole

Ref: Harrison's Principles of Internal Medicine, 19th edition, Chapter 139e-4

12. A 50 years male, chronic alcoholic with MMS score of 20/30 presents with tremors, proximal weakness and has cerebral lesions in MRI. What is the next investigation?

(a) CSF AFB
(b) CSF oligoclonal bands
(c) CSF protein
(d) CSF culture and gram stain

Explanation:

Investigations for Multiple Sclerosis:

- **MRI:**
  - Lesions are frequently oriented perpendicular to the ventricular surface, corresponding to the pathologic pattern of perivenous demyelination **(Dawson's fingers).**
- **CSF:**
  - **Lymphocytic pleocytosis** in acute phase and **Oligoclonal bands** of **IgG** between attacks.
- **Disease modifying drugs in multiple sclerosis:**
  - Interferon β1a.
  - Glatiramer acetate.
  - Natalizumab.
  - Fingolimod.
  - Mitoxantrone.
  - Cladribine.

Ans: (b) CSF oligoclonal bands

Ref: Harrison's Principles of Internal Medicine, 19th edition, page 2663

13. Flu like symptoms followed by radiographic evidence of consolidation in lung in a non-smoker is due to:

(a) Klebsiella (b) Staph aureus
(c) Streptococcus (d) Pseudomonas

Explanation:

S. aureus pneumonia commonly complicates influenza infection.

Factor	Possible Pathogen(s)
Alcoholism	*Streptococcus pneumoniae*, oral anaerobes, *Klebsiella pneumoniae*, *Acinetobacter* spp., *Mycobacterium tuberculosis*
COPD and/or smoking	*Haemophilus influenzae*, *Pseudomonas aeruginosa*, *Legionella* spp., *S. pneumoniae*, *Moraxella catarrhalis*, *Chlamydia pneumoniae*
Structural lung disease (e.g., bronchiectasis)	*P. aeruginosa*, *Burkholderia cepacia*, *Staphylococcus aureus*
Dementia, stroke, decreased level of consciousness	Oral anaerobes, gram-negative enteric bacteria
Local influenza activity	Influenza virus, *S. pneumoniae*, *S. aureus*
Exposure to bats or birds	*H. capsulatum*
Exposure to birds	*Chlamydia psittaci*

Ans: (b) Staph aureus

Ref: Harrison's Principles of Internal Medicine, 19th edition, page 805

14. Essential tremor does not exist in:

(a) Hand (b) Head (c) Lips (d) Voice

Explanation:

- Essential tremors involve head in ~30%, voice in ~20%, face/jaw in ~10%, lower limbs in ~10%.

Tremors

Tremor consists of alternating contractions of agonist and antagonist muscles in an oscillating, rhythmic manner.

It can be:

- **Rest tremor–Parkinsonism.**
- **Postural tremor– Essential tremor*.**
- **Kinetic tremor–Cerebellar tremor.**

Enhanced physiologic tremor (EPT) in association with anxiety, fatigue, a metabolic disturbance (e.g., hyperthyroidism, electrolyte abnormalities), drugs (e.g., valproate, lithium), or toxins (e.g., alcohol).

ESSENTIAL TREMOR

- Inherited condition characterized by kinetic tremor in the absence of other neurological signs.
- **Onset:** Childhood or late adulthood.
- **Etiology:** Unknown.
- **Clinical features:**
  - **Tremor:** Kinetic, postural tremor and during action (Writing, drinking).
  - More than 50% cases have intention component.
  - **Progression**: Slowly progressive; Unilateral to bilateral.
  - **Location:** Arm, head, voice, tongue, leg and trunk.
- **Treatment of Essential Tremor:**
  - **Beta blockers (Propanolol) and Primidone–standard drug therapies for ET.**
  - **Gabapentin and topiramate in selected cases.**

- **Botulinum toxin injections helpful for limb or voice tremor.**
- **Surgical therapies targeting the VIM nucleus of the thalamus for severe and drug-resistant cases.**

Ans: (c) Lips

Ref: Harrison's Principles of Internal Medicine, 19th edition, page 2618

15. A patient presents with polyuria and elevated prolactin levels. There is family history of father died due to renal stones. He has Ca2+ of 12 g% and PTH levels of 260 IU/L. Most likely diagnosis is:

(a) MEN 1 (b) PGA 1
(c) MEN 2 (d) Autoimmune polyendocrinopathy

Explanation:

Hyperprolactinemia with hyperparathyroidism (leading to renal stones in the family / polyuria) indicates MEN 1 syndrome as a likely answer.
Pituitary and pancreatic tumours are characteristic features of MEN 1 and do not occur in MEN 2 and hence ruled out (option (b) ruled out).
Hypothyroidism / Addison's are again characteristic features of PGA's and hence since both are not seen options (b) and (d) can be ruled out.

The characteristic features of MEN 1 are:

Parathyroid Hyperplasia>> Adenoma – Hyperparathyroidism is the most common presenting feature in > 80% patients.

Pituitary adenomas:

- **Anterior pituitary adenomas occur in MEN-1.**
- **Most common tumour is Prolactinoma > GH secreting pituitary adenoma.**
- **Pancreatic Neuroendocrine Tumours–Most common is the gastrinoma.**
- **Skin lesions–Most common is angiofibroma.**
- **Carcinoids of Foregut, Midgut and Thymus (approximately 10% of patients).**

MEN 1	MEN 2A	MEN 2B
Parathyroid adenoma Enteropancreatic tumour Foregut carcinoid Anterior pituitary tumour	Medullary thyroid cancer Pheochromocytoma Parathyroid tumours Cutaneous lichen amyloidosis	Medullary thyroid cancer Pheochromocytoma Marfanoid habitus Mucosal neuromas

Ans: (a) MEN 1

Ref: Oxford Handbook of Endocrinology, 3rd edition, page 587

16. All are true regarding familial adenomatous polyposis *except*:

(a) Associated endocrine involvement can be present
(b) More > 100 polyps in the colon
(c) Autosomal recessive
(d) Multiple duodenal polyps

Explanation:

FAMILIAL ADENOMATOUS POLYPOSIS (FAP)

Autosomal Dominant Disorder

Patients develop numerous *colorectal adenomas* as *teenagers*.

It is caused by mutations of the adenomatous polyposis coli, or APC gene (5q21).
Some FAP patients without APC loss have mutations of the *base-excision repair gene* ***MUTYH***.

- *At least 100 polyps* are necessary for a diagnosis of classic FAP, and as many as several thousand may be present.

- These growths are morphologically indistinguishable from *sporadic adenomas*.
- Colorectal adenocarcinoma develops in 100% of untreated FAP patients before age 30.
- *Prophylactic colectomy* is the standard therapy for individuals carrying APC mutations.
- Colectomy prevents colorectal cancer, but patients remain at risk for neoplasia at other sites.
- Adenomas may develop elsewhere in the GI tract, particularly adjacent to the ampulla of Vater and in the stomach.
- FAP is associated with a variety of extra-intestinal manifestations including:
  - Congenital hypertrophy of the retinal pigment epithelium.
  - Gardner syndrome; and
  - Turcot syndrome.

Gardner Syndrome

- Osteomas of mandible, skull, and long bones.
- Epidermal cysts.
- Desmoid tumors.
- Thyroid tumors.
- Dental abnormalities (Unerupted and supernumerary teeth).

Turcot Syndrome

- Intestinal adenomas.
- Tumors of the central nervous system.
- Two third patients have APC gene mutation and develop medulloblastomas.
- The remaining one third have mutations genes involved in DNA repair and develop glioblastomas.

Associated Tumours

- **Colorectal** cancer **under the age of 25 years.**
- **Papillary carcinoma of the thyroid.**
- Cancer of the **ampulla of Vater.**
- **Hepatoblastomas.**
- Primary brain tumours (**Turcot's syndrome**).
- **Osteomas** of the jaw.
- **CHRPE** (congenital hypertrophy of the retinal pigment epithelium).
- **Gardner's syndrome** can cause the development of cutaneous pathology, such as multiple epidermoid cysts and lipomata.

Clinical Features and Pathological Outlines

- Patients may develop gastric fundic gland polyps, gastric or small bowel flat adenomas, and gastric/duodenal carcinomas.
- Duodenal adenomas are very common.
- Extracolonic manifestations of classical FAP are less common in attenuated FAP.
- Classically reserved for patients with fewer than **100 colonic adenomatous** polyps.
- Polyps are usually more **proximal** (i.e., right sided) than in classic FAP.
- **Rectum** often **spared.**
- Polyps are flat, slightly raised, or plaque-like.
- May have minute central depression or umbilication.
- Adenomatous polyps are microscopically similar to sporadic-type adenomas.
- Extra-colorectal polyps and cancers are important primarily for surveillance purposes.

STRATEGIES FOR PREVENTION

Clinical Testing of APC Gene

- **Flexible proctosigmoidoscopy** at age **10-12 years**; repeat every **1-2 years** until age **35**; after age 35 repeat **every 3 years.**
- **Upper GI endoscopy** every **1-3 years** starting when polyps first identified.
- **Prophylactic panprotocolectomy.**

Here are the estimated cancer risks associated with classic FAP.

Cancers	Incidence
Colorectal cancer	Almost 100% if not treated
Desmoid tumor	10% to 20%
Small bowel (intestines)	4% to 12%
Pancreatic cancer	2%
Papillary thyroid cancer	2%
Hepatoblastoma (a type of liver cancer)	1.5%
Brain or central nervous system tumor	Less than 1%
Stomach cancer	0.5%
Bile duct cancer	Small, but increased
Adrenal gland cancer	Small, but increased

Ans: (c) Autosomal recessive

Ref: Bailey and Love, Short Practice of Surgery, 5th edition, chapter 7, page 94-95, 1149

17. A man is found comatose in his room, having taken an unknown number of sleeping pills. An arterial blood sample yields the following values: pH – 7.10, HCO_3- 12 meq/liter, $PaCO_2$ 66 mm Hg. This patient's acid-base status is most accurately described as:

(a) Uncompensated metabolic acidosis
(b) Uncompensated respiratory acidosis
(c) Simultaneous respiratory and metabolic acidosis
(d) Respiratory acidosis with partial renal compensation

Explanation:

Approach to Acid Base Disturbances

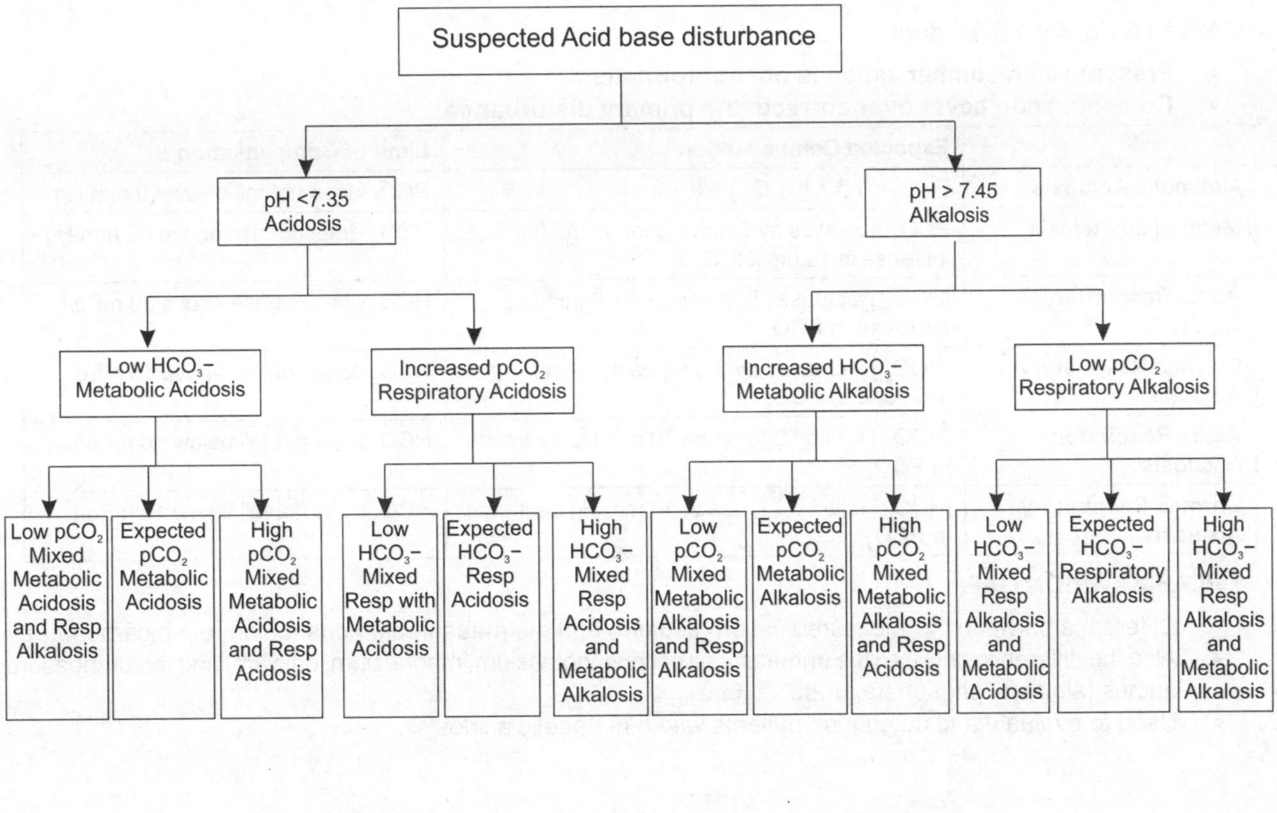

Normal levels of blood pH, pCO_2 and HCO_3

Blood levels criteria	Venous	Arterial
pH	7.35-7.40	7.38-7.45
pCO_2	45-50 torr	35-45 torr
HCO_3	24-25 mEq/L	23-27 mEq/L

Normal ABG Values

H^+ (35–45 nmol/L) < 35 = alkalaemia, > 45 = acidaemia
pH (7.35–7.45) < 7.35 = acidaemia, > 7.45 = alkalaemia
PO_2 (> 10.6 kPa or > 80 mm Hg in arterial blood on room air)
PCO_2 (4.7–6.0 kPa or 35–45 mm Hg in arterial blood)
SpO_2 (> 96% on room air)
HCO_3 (22–28 mmol/L)
BE (-2 to +2)
Lactate (0.4–1.5 mmol/L)

Stepwise approach for acid base disorders

pH < 7.35 = acidosis; pH > 7.45 = alkalosis
Primary change in HCO_3 → metabolic • If the change in HCO_3 is in keeping with the pH (i.e., acidosis + decreased HCO_3) the problem is metabolic • If the change in HCO_3 is opposite with the pH (i.e., acidosis + increased HCO_3) the problem is compensatory metabolic
Primary change in CO_2 → respiratory • If the change in **CO_2** is in keeping with the pH (i.e., acidosis + increased **CO_2**) the problem is respiratory • If the change in **CO_2** is opposite with the pH (i.e., acidosis + decreased **CO_2**) the problem is compensatory respiratory

Mixed Acid Base Disorders

- **Present when compensation is not appropriate.**
- **Compensation never over-corrects the primary disturbance.**

	Expected Compensation	**Limit of Compensation**
Metabolic Acidosis	$PCO_2 = 1.5 \times [HCO_3^-] + 8 \pm 2$	PCO_2 does not fall below 10 mm Hg
Metabolic Alkalosis	PCO_2 increases by 7 mm Hg for each 10 mEq/L increase in serum $[HCO_3^-]$	PCO_2 does not rise above 55 mm Hg
Acute Respiratory Acidosis	$[HCO_3^-]$ increases by 1 for each 10 mm Hg **increase in PCO_2**	HCO_3 does not rise above 30 mEq/L
Chronic Respiratory Acidosis	$[HCO_3^-]$ increases by 3.5 for each 10 mm Hg **increase in PCO_2**	HCO_3 does not rise above 45 mEq/L
Acute Respiratory Alkalosis	$[HCO_3^-]$ falls by 2 for each 10 mm Hg decrease **in PCO_2**	HCO_3 does not fall below 18 mEq/L
Chronic Respiratory Alkalosis	$[HCO_3^-]$ falls by 4 for each 10 mm Hg decrease **in PCO_2**	HCO_3 does not fall below 12 mEq/L

PLASMA ANION GAP

- Difference between the measured cation (sodium) and the measured anions (chloride + bicarbonate).
- Also the difference between the unmeasured cations (potassium, magnesium, calcium) and the unmeasured anions (albumin, phosphate, urate, sulfate).
- Used to evaluate and categorise patients with a metabolic acidosis.

- Metabolic acidosis is divided into subcategories:
  - o Increased anion gap acidosis.
  - o Normal anion gap acidosis.
- Normal anion gap is **4-11**.
- Formula: Anion Gap = **$[Na^+] - [Cl^-] - [HCO_3^-]$**.
- Increased anion gap metabolic acidosis occurs when there is an increase in unmeasured anions.
- Normal anion gap metabolic acidosis occurs when there is a decrease in the bicarbonate concentration without an increase in the unmeasured anions.
- Approximately 11 mEq of the anion gap is normally secondary to albumin.
- A 1 g/dL decrease in the albumin concentration decreases the anion gap by roughly 2.5 mEq/L. Increase in unmeasured cations, such as calcium, potassium, and magnesium, decreases the anion gap.

Ans: (c) Simultaneous respiratory and metabolic acidosis

Ref: TARGET Pediatrics (Wolters Kluwer) by Arun Babu, 1st edition, page 100

18. False regarding restrictive lung disease:

(a) FEV 1/FVC decreased
(b) FVC decreased
(c) TLC decreased
(d) FeV1 increased

Explanation:

How to Interpret Spirometry

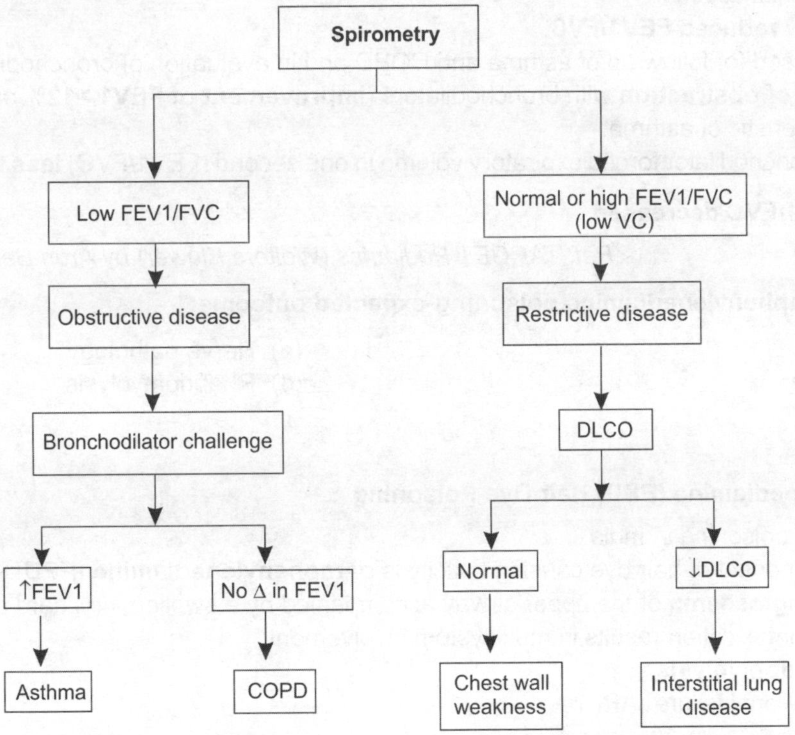

Spirometry	COPD	Restrictive lung diseases
FEV1	Low ++	Low+
VC	Low+	Low ++
FEV1/FVC	Low	Normal/high
RV	High	Low
FRC	High	Low

- **TLC**: Volume of air in the lungs following maximal inspiration **(N= 5-6 L).**

- **FVC:** Maximum amount of air exhaled following maximal inspiration **(N= 4.8 L).**
- **VT:** Volume of air entering and leaving lungs during normal respiration **(N= 500 ml).**
- **RV:** Volume of air remaining in the lungs after maximal expiratory effort **(N= 1.2 L).**
- **FRC:** Volume of air within the lungs at the end of normal respiration **(N= 2.5-3 L).**
- **FEV:** Volume of air exhaled in a given time during a forced vital capacity effort.
- **FEV1/FVC:** Proportion of a person's vital capacity that they are able to expire in the first second of expiration **(N= 80%).**

Restrictive Lung Disease:

- **FVC is reduced** because of reduction in intrathoracic air volume.
- **Normal or Increased FEV1/FVC.**
- *Examples are:*
  - ***Interstitial lung disease.***
  - ***Neuromuscular disorders.***
  - Mechanical compression like ***obesity, kyphoscoliosis, pneumothorax***.
- **TLC and RV** are reduced in all except in **neuromuscular disorders.**

Obstructive Lung Disease

- Two major types:
  - COPD.
  - Bronchial asthma.
- Both show **reduced FEV1/FVC**.
- **FEV1** is used for follow up of asthma and COPD and in evaluation of bronchodilator response.
- **Reversal of obstruction** with bronchodilators (**Improvement of FEV1 >12**% and minimum **of >200 ml**) is characteristic of asthma.
- A post-bronchodilator forced expiratory volume in one second (FEV1/FVC) **less than 0.7** confirms COPD.

Ans: (a) FEV1/FVC decreased

Ref: TARGET Pediatrics (Wolters Kluwer) by Arun Babu, 1st edition, page 378

19. Hair dye paraphenylenediamine poisoning-expected outcome:

(a) Blindness
(b) Nerve pathology
(c) Dermatitis
(d) Rhabdomyolysis

Explanation:

Paraphenylenediamine (PPD) Hair Dye Poisoning

- Emerging poisoning in India.
- Main component of hair dye causing toxicity is **paraphenylenediamine (PPD).**
- Severe **angioedema** of the upper airway accompanied by a swollen, dry, hard and protruding tongue.
- Systemic intoxication results in multisystem involvement:
  - **Rhabdomyolysis***.
  - Acute renal failure (ARF)*.
- **Management**
  - No specific antidote for PPD.
  - Treatment is mainly supportive.

JIPMER has reported a case of suicidal hair dye ingestion that presented with **cervicofascial edema, rhabdomyolysis** and **ARF**. Patient improved with dialysis and symptomatic management. This (Ref) case report was published in 2012. This yet again proves that JIPMER asks questions from its own publications. It is worth reading the abstract of all research articles published from JIPMER in the last 5 years (approximately around 75–100 articles per year). You can search 'JIPMER' from www.pubmed.com

Ans: (d) Rhabdomyolysis

Ref: Toxicol Int. 2012 Jan;19(1):77-78

20. In Vitamin A deficiency, respiratory tract infection due to:

(a) Keratinization of upper epithelial cells
(b) Lack of antibody production
(c) Dysfunction of epithelial layer
(d) Defective chemotaxis

Explanation:

- The most obvious function of vitamin A deficiency is maintenance of **epithelial functions**.
- Characteristic epithelial changes in vitamin A deficiency:
  - **Proliferation of basal cells.**
  - **Hyperkeratosis.**
  - Formation of **stratified cornified squamous epithelium**.
- **Squamous metaplasia** of the **renal pelvis, ureters, vaginal epithelium**, and the **pancreatic and salivary ducts** can lead to increased infections in these areas.
- In the **urinary bladder**, loss of **epithelial integrity** can result in **pyuria** and hematuria.
- Epithelial changes in the **skin** are manifested as **dry, scaly, hyperkeratotic patches,** commonly on the **arms, legs, shoulders and buttocks**.
- The combination of **defective epithelial barriers** to infection, **low immune response**, and **lowered response** to **inflammatory stress**, all because of insufficient vitamin A, can cause **poor growth** and infections in children.

Vitamin A (Retinol)

Source	GYO (green, yellow, orange) vegetables and fruits, milk and its products, egg yolk, fish, fish liver oil
RDA	1500 IU (500 mcg)
Functions	**Retinal**–Vision **Retinoid acid**–nuclear transcription factor, regulates genes (multiple function in immunity, cell growth integrity of skin and mucous membrane)
Clinical implications	**Xerophthalmia, Night blindness**, Hydrocephalus, Increased bacterial binding to mucous membrane
Investigations	Staining of eye with 1% Rose Bengal, Low Serum Retinol, **Dark Adaptometry**

WHO Vitamin A deficiency staging

X1A **X1B**	Xerosis conjunctiva Bitot spots
X2	Xerosis cornea
X3A **X3B**	Corneal ulceration Keratomalacia
XN	Night blindness
XS	Corneal scarring
XF	Fundoscopic changes

Ans: (c) Dysfunction of epithelial layer

Ref: Nelson's Textbook of Pediatrics, 20th edition, page 319

21. Flatbush diabetes is associated with:

(a) Type 1 DM
(b) Type 2 DM
(c) Diabetes insipidus
(d) Bronze diabetes

Explanation:

Flatbush Diabetes

- Described in African American **young adults** residing in an area named Flatbush in New York city, USA. Now increasingly seen in **Africa** as well.
- Variant of Type 1 diabetes but without any markers of autoimmunity.

- Also known as **atypical diabetes**, **type 1B diabetes**, **idiopathic type 1 diabetes** and **ketosis-prone type 2 diabetes**.
- These **young adult** patients presented with **diabetic ketoacidosis** but required **insulin** only for a **short period**. They were maintaining **euglycemia** for long period after tapering and stopping insulin.
- Exact mechanism of this condition is not known. Proposed mechanisms include:
  - Severe oxidative stress.
  - Glucotoxicity mediated beta cell dysfunction.
  - Insulin resistance.
- Most cases present with sudden onset of **very high blood glucose and ketosis (DKA).**
- Most of these patients were **overweight/obese***.
- Strong **family history*** of diabetes present (90%).
- No evidence of autoimmunity against islet cells.
- Beta cell function relatively preserved.
- Patients may relapse with DKA*.

Ans: (a) Type 1 DM

Ref: Bhansali A, et al. Clinical Rounds in Endocrinology: Volume II – Pediatric Endocrinology, page 423

22. ANCA negative vasculitis among the following is:

(a) Wegener's granulomatosis
(b) Churg-Strauss syndrome
(c) Polyarteritis nodosa
(d) Microscopic polyangiitis

Explanation:

Anti Neutrophilic Cytoplasmic Antibodies (ANCA)

It consists of two types:

- **Cytoplasmic c- ANCA Antibody**–Directed against Proteinase 3 antigen*.
- **Perinuclear p- ANCA Antibody**–Directed against myeloperoxidase antigen*.

ANCA Positive Vasculitis

- **Wegener granulomatosis** – c-ANCA.
- **Microscopic polyangiitiis** – p-ANCA.
- **Churg-Strauss syndrome** – Both c-ANCA and p-ANCA.

c-ANCA is seen in	p-ANCA is seen in
Wegener's granulomatosis*	Churg-Strauss syndrome
Microscopic polyangiitis (Rare)	Microscopic polyangiitis
Churg-Strauss syndrome (Rare)	Systemic lupus erythematosus
	Rheumatoid arthritis
	Crohn's disease

Ans: (c) Polyarteritis nodosa

Ref: Harrison's Principles of Internal Medicine, 19th edition

SURGERY

1. **All are true regarding circumcision *except*:**

(a) Hemorrhage due to bleeding from frenular artery
(b) Increase sexual drive
(c) Avoid correction of congenital anomaly
(d) Reduces sexually transmitted infections

Explanation:

Indications:

- Cultural or religious reasons.
- Phimosis.
- Paraphimosis.
- Balanoposthitis.
- STDs.

Medical Benefits

- Reduced urinary infections in infancy.
- Reduced incidence of STDs.
- Marked reduction in incidence of penile cancer.

Complications:

- Bleeding from **frenular artery** (which needs compression and if not controlled, requires reexploration in theatre).
- Infections.
- Meatal stenosis in infants (due to ammoniacal dermatitis in wet diapers).
- Uretherocutaneous fistulas.
- Removal of too much or too little skin.

Circumcision is not done in patients with hypospadias as prepucial skin can be used in surgical repair.

Ans: (b) Increase sexual drive

Ref: Glenn's Urologic Surgery, 7th edition, page 778

2. **A patient is diagnosed with pituitary tumour, prolactinoma encircling the carotid artery. What is the best line of management?**

(a) Wait and watch
(b) Transsphenoidal surgical resection
(c) Radiotherapy
(d) Combination
(e) Chemotherapy with somatostatin analogues

Explanation:

- Most of the tumors in sellar region are **benign pituitary adenomas**, but also include **craniopharyngiomas, meningiomas, aneurysm and rathke cleft cyst.**

- **Pituitary microadenomas** are **less than 1 cm** in size and **macroadenomas** are more than 1 cm.
- **Microadenomas** present with **endocrine effects**, whereas macroadenomas present with **visual field defects.**
- Majority of the adenomas are **prolactinomas** (30%), 20% are **non-functioning**, 15% **secrete GH** and 10% **secrete ACTH.**
- Baseline assessment of serum prolactin, FSH and LH, TFT and Fasting serum GH and cortisol is necessary.
- **Prolactinomas** are initially managed with dopamine agonists like **bromocriptine** and **cabergoline**.
- Compression of the chiasm with evidence of **visual compromise**, encasement of nearby **cavernous** sinus or **carotid arteries** are the indications of **surgical intervention.**
- **Surgical resection** is usually performed through **transsphenoidal approach** using a microscope or endoscope inserted through nose.
- Postoperative complications include **CSF leak, pituitary insufficiency and SIADH.**

Ans: (b) Transsphenoidal surgical resection

Ref: Bailey and Love, 27th edition, page 665-666

3. A patient undergoes surgery in pelvic region. Which vein is most likely to result in thrombosis?

(a) Iliac vein
(b) Femoral vein
(c) Calf vein
(d) IVC

Explanation:

- Venous Thromboembolism is dictated by **Virchow's Triad which is Stasis, Hypercoagulability and Endothelial Injury.**
- Causes for Venous Thromboembolism are:

Stasis	**Hypercoagulability**	**Endothelial Injury**
Advanced age Hospitalization Immobilization Long air haul travel Obesity Spinal cord injury	Factor V leiden Protein C, S deficiency Prothrombin gene mutation Antithrombin deficiency APLS Homocysteinemia Hyperfibrinogenemia Activated Protein C resistance Factor 7, 8, 9, 11 elevation Pregnancy Malignancy Nephrotic syndrome HRT and OCP use Puerperium	Major surgery IV cannulation Varicose veins Trauma

- **Most common presentation of a DVT is pain and swelling** usually in the calf, on one side. But bilateral presentation is seen in 30% of individuals.
- Physical signs include mild pitting oedema of the ankle, dilated surface veins, stiff calf and tenderness over the course of veins.
- Leg pain occur in 50% of patients with DVT but it is not specific. Tenderness occurs in 75% of patients and Pulmonary embolism in 10% of patients with confirmed DVT.
- **Homan's sign** – Dorsiflexion of the ankle causes pain in the calf.
- **Moses sign** – Squeezing of the calf muscles causes pain in the calf.
- Both these are suggestive of DVT, but negative test does not rule out DVT. Moses sign is contraindicated as it may dislodge thrombus and cause pulmonary embolism.
- Complications of DVT include **Phlegmasia alba dolens, Phlegmasia cerulean dolens, Post thrombotic Syndrome and Pulmonary Embolism.**
- Scores used to predict the risk of acquiring DVT include **Roger's score and Caprini score**.

Ans: (c) Calf vein

Ref: Schwartz Principles of Surgery, 10th edition, page 918-920

4. **Barium meal characteristic feature of malignant gastric ulcer is:**

(a) Hampton line
(b) Carmen meniscus sign
(c) Ulcer cap
(d) Ulcer crater

Explanation:

Radiological Features of Benign Gastric Ulcer:

- The primary sign is a collection of barium on the dependent wall.
- Benign ulcers are usually round, oval or linear in shape with a ring shadow may be seen if the ulcer is located on a non-dependent surface (as barium coats the edge of the ulcer crater).
- Presence of normal area gastricae extending to the ulcer crater is a good sign of a benign lesion.
- A benign ulcer will project beyond the stomach lumen.
- ***Hampton's line****:* A thin lucent line crossing the ulcer base (representing preserved gastric mucosa with undermining of the more vulnerable submucosa).
- ***Ulcer collar****:* More commonly there is a thicker smooth rim of lucency at the ulcer base.
- ***Ulcer mound****:* With increasing oedema a symmetrical gently sloping mass can be seen.

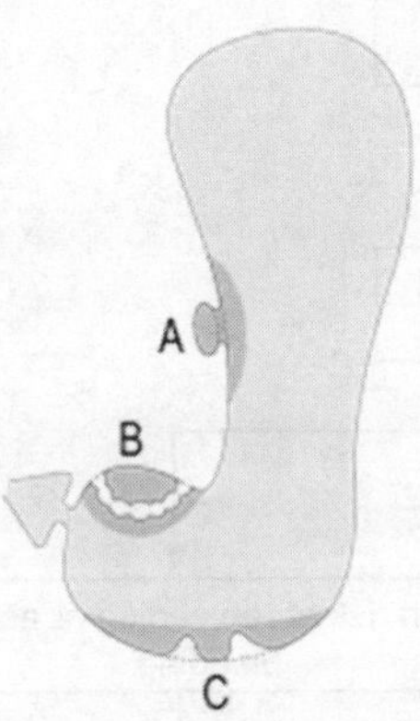

Graphical description of three types of gastric ulcer (the shading represents barium): A = benign, projecting, lesser curvature ulcer with collar (broken lines = Hampton's line) ► B = malignant, intraluminal ulcer with irregular nodular tumour rim which traps a lenticular barium collection that is convex relative to the gastric lumen (Carman meniscus sign) ► C = non-projecting benign greater curvature ulcer.[†]

Features Suspicious for Malignancy:

- Location within the fundus or proximal ½ of the greater curvature.
- Incomplete healing.
- Irregularity of the radiating folds.
- A residual mass.
- Loss of the mucosal pattern.
- **Carmen meniscus sign** is characterised by Lentiform shaped appearance of inner margin also looking convex in malignant ulcer as shown below.

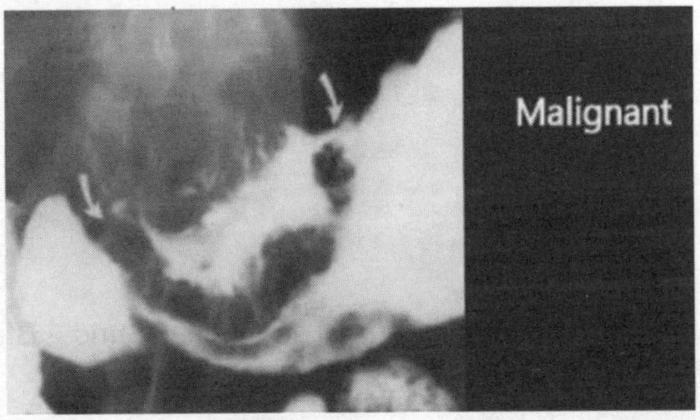

Ans: (b) Carmen meniscus sign

Ref: Grainger Allisons Radiology, page 254-255

5. Treatment of choice in bleeding gastric ulcer:

(a) TV and drainage (b) Antrectomy
(c) Distal gastrectomy (d) Under running of ulcer

Explanation:

- Patients with bleeding gastric ulcers presents in the emergency setting as **Hematemesis** or in the mild chronic setting as **Melena**.
- Most of the bleeding stops spontaneously and requires no intervention. However, persistent bleeding is associated with mortality.
- In the emergency setting, patient treatment algorithm is as follows:

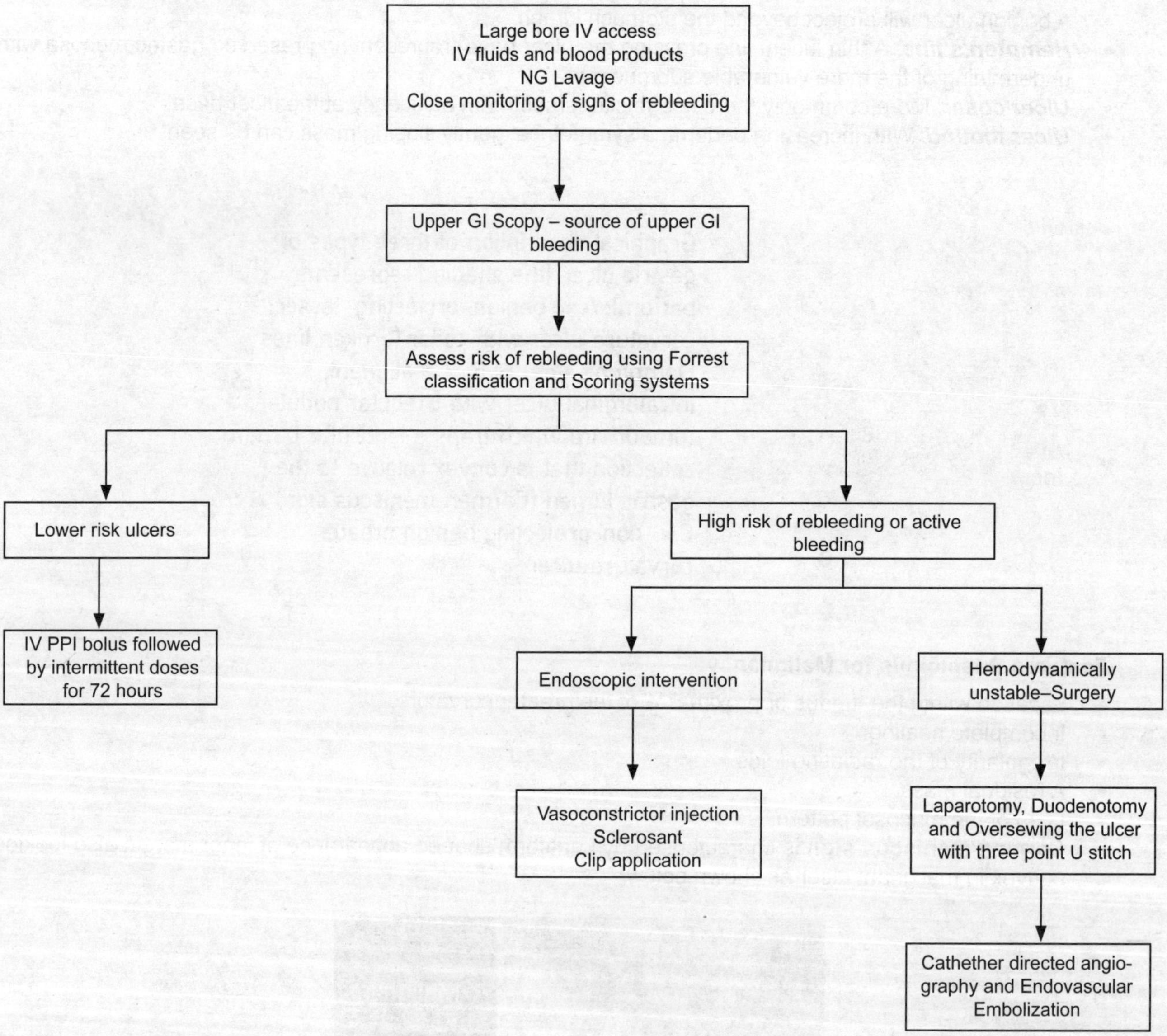

- **Rebleeding risk** is assessed by commonly used scoring systems – **Blatchford and Rockall Prediction scores.**

Ans: (d) Under running of ulcer

Ref: Sabiston's Textbook of Surgery, 20th edition, page 1202–1204

6. **Familial adenomatous polyposis is characterised by all *except*:**
   (a) Autosomal recessive transmission
   (b) More than 100 polyps in colorectal area
   (c) Polyps seen in duodenum
   (d) Extra intestinal manifestations are present

Explanation:

Hereditary cancers	Family history, Young age at onset Presence of other specific tumors and defects FAP and HNPCC
Sporadic cancers	Absence of family history, older age 60 – 80 years Isolated lesions in colon or rectum Specific mutation is present in all cells of affected individuals
Familial cancers	Genetic polymorphisms, Gene modifiers and defects in TyK Lifetime risk increases for members in families in which index case is young and relative is close

FAMILIAL ADENOMATOUS POLYPOSIS – HEREDITARY CANCER SYNDROME

APC gene 5q21	Mutation leads to Increased beta catenin levels and Wnt signal activation Earliest phenotype is Aberrant crypt formation Germline, somatic mutations seen and polymorphism	
CLASSIC FAP	**ATTENUATED FAP**	**GARDNERS SYNDROME**
More than 100 adenomatous polyps in colorectum Manifest by late second or early third decade Germline APC truncation mutations from codon 1250 – 1464 Autosomal dominant	Mutations close to the 5' end of the gene Far less than 100 polyps Tendency to spare the rectum	Profuse colonic polyps, Mesenteric desmoids Skull and Mandible osteomas Periampullary cancers

- Extraintestinal Manifestations of FAP – **CHRPE, PTC, Medulloblastoma, Gastric fundic polyps.**
- **The average age at discovery of a new patient with FAP is 29 years.**

Ans: (a) Autosomal recessive transmission

Ref: Sabiston Textbook of Surgery, 20th edition, page 1366-1369

7. **Hereditary pancreatitis is characterised by all *except*:**
   (a) 80% penetrance
   (b) 30% leads to chronic pancreatitis
   (c) Autosomal recessive inheritance
   (d) Pancreatic cancer risk is high

Explanation:

Hereditary Pancreatitis (PRSS1 and SPINK1 gene mutation)

- Mutations in the cationic trypsinogen gene (**PRSS1**) are responsible for 80% of the cases of hereditary pancreatitis and lead to **increased trypsin activity** and **chronic inflammation** in the pancreas.
- The **SPINK1 gene** codes for a **serine protease inhibitor** that inhibits active protein and mutations in this gene have been associated with hereditary pancreatitis.
- Individuals with hereditary pancreatitis have a greater than 50-fold increase in their risk for development of **pancreatic cancer** compared with unaffected individuals has long been noted that individuals with familial pancreatitis.
- **Autosomal Dominant** inheritance pattern.

- Disease penetrance is **80%.**
- Pancreatitis starts in **early childhood** and progresses to **chronic pancreatitis.**
- **Pancreatic cancer risk** is **50-60 times higher** than general people.

Ans: (c) Autosomal recessive inheritance

Ref: Sabiston, Textbook of surgery, 20th edition, page 1542

8. Early complication of TIPS procedure:

(a) Shunt stenosis and blockage
(b) Capsular haemorrhage
(c) Metabolic encephalopathy
(d) Recurrent variceal bleed

Explanation:

Portal Hypertension

- Defined when portal venous pressure is more than **5 mm of Hg.**
- Due to **prehepatic, hepatic and posthepatic conditions** causing **Portal hypertension,** patients present with **variceal bleeding.**
- Treatment of **acute variceal** bleed includes airway, breathing and circulation, cross matching and blood transfusion.
- **Initial Endoscopy** should be done **within first 24 hours** and the treatment options are:
  - ***Endoscopic Band ligation.***
  - ***Sclerotherapy.***
- **Endoscopic Band ligation** is considered **more effective** and associated with less **complications.**
- When both these are not available or failure is seen, **Balloon tamponade** using **Sengstaken-Blakemore tube** is done for **48 hours.**
- **Medical management** of **variceal bleed** includes **Octreotide** and then **vasopressin** in severe **bleeding.**
- **Endoscopic band ligation and Octreotide** is the combination therapy that is considered **more effective.**
- **TIPSS** (**Transjugular Intrahepatic Porto Systemic Shunts**) – Percutaneous invasive procedure where a stent which passes through the Right hepatic vein and connects Right portal branch thereby shunting both. Done in patients with resistant Ascites, End stage liver disease needing liver transplant as a standby procedure.

Complication of TIPS can be divided into:

- **Intra op complication**: Capsular hemorrhage.
- **Early Complication**: Hepatic Encephalopathy (34%).
- **Late Complication**: Recurrent Variceal bleed (19%).
- **Delayed Complication**: (6 months–1 year) Shunt stenosis due to neo intimal hyperplasia > shunt thrombosis. Shunt stenosis can be dilated by balloon. Total occlusion is seen in 15%.

Ans: (c) Metabolic encephalopathy

Ref: Sabiston Textbook of Surgery, 20th edition, page 1439-1440

9. Treatment of choice for simple cyst of liver:

(a) Percutaneous drainage
(b) Cysto enterostomy
(c) Deroofing
(d) Aspiration

Explanation:

Hepatic Cysts

- Mostly recognized as an **incidental finding during laparotomy,** during **autopsy** or on **imaging studies.**
- These are more **common in increasing age,** i.e., **> 40 years** of age and **higher female** incidence.
- Most are **asymptomatic.**
- Symptoms usually occur owing to **large size of the cyst** causing **compression effects.**
- **Symptoms:**
  - Early satiety.
  - Nausea and vomiting.

- o Abdominal mass.
- o Hepatomegaly.

- **Ultrasound** is the **preferred initial evaluation**, in which cysts appear as **anechoic masses** with **smooth margins** and **thin walls**.
- **CT** is needed for **precise localization** and **spatial relationships**, which are crucial to surgical planning.
- **Simple cysts** are **nonenhancing lesions** of **water density (0 to 10 HU),** whereas internal septations, papillary mural projections, wall irregularity and intracystic debris are **inconsistent** with simple cyst.
- On **MRI**, simple hepatic cysts appear as **low signal intensity** relative to liver parenchyma in **T1 weighted images** and **high signal intensity** in **T2 weighted images**, which **do not enhance** with **gadolinium contrast**.
- Treatment depends on symptoms.
- **Cysts** tend to be **asymptomatic** in **80 – 85%** long term, hence **non-operative treatment** is appropriate in **such situations.**
- **Symptomatic cysts** require **intervention** either in the form of:
  - o **Percutaneous aspiration;** or
  - o **Laparoscopic fenestration/deroofing.**
- **Percutaneous aspiration alone** has a **100% recurrence** rate; hence aspiration along with **sclerosant injection** or **ethanol ablation** is being tried although it has recurrence rates more than surgical approaches.
- **Surgical approach** can be either:
  - o **Open; or**
  - o **Laparoscopic.**
- **Laparoscopic** is quite challenging in inaccessible sites like **Segments VI, VII and IV A**, in such situations **open approach** is preferred.
- In either approaches, **excision of cyst wall to within 2 cm of the liver tissue** is needed allowing the **cyst to drain into the peritoneal cavity**.
- In case of **biliary communication**, the communication sites are **suture ligated** within the cavity or **Roux en Y cystojejunostomy** performed to allow biliary drainage.

Ans: (c) Deroofing

Ref: Shackelford's Surgery of the Alimentary Tract, 7th edition, page 1453-1456

10. Best method to visualise the proximal bile duct is by:

(a) Percutaneous transhepatic cholangiogram (b) EUS
(c) ERCP (d) Transabdominal USG

Explanation:

Percutaneous Transhepatic Cholangiography:

- It is a technique of cannulating the liver bile ducts directly using **Chiba or Okuda needle** and bile duct is cannulated.
- Stent can be placed and can help in drainage of bile also in strictures and malignancy.
- Proximal duct visualisation is done easily by passing water-soluble contrast.
- Multiple images can be taken which demonstrate areas of strictures or obstruction.
- Also enables placement of catheter to provide external biliary drainage or insertion of indwelling stents.
- **PTC** is usually preferred to **ERCP**, when a malignant stricture is at the level of confluence of right and left hepatic ducts or higher in a jaundiced patient.

Ans: (a) Percutaneous transhepatic cholangiogram

Ref: Bailey and Love, 27th edition, page 1193-94

11. Order of correction of Hypospadias:

(a) Straightening of penis–Balanoplasty–Urethroplasty
(b) Urethroplasty–Balanoplasty–Straightening
(c) Straightening–Urethroplasty–Balanoplasty
(d) Balanoplasty–Urethroplasty–Straightening

Explanation:

Hypospadias

- **Hypospadias** is a congenital condition associated with urethral meatus opening on the underside of penis or perineum, ventral chordee and dorsal hooded prepuce.
- It is the most common congenital abnormality of urethra.
- Depending on the site of opening, it is named distal and proximal hypospadias, with proximal hypospadias being more severe anomaly and associated with poor outcome even after repair.
- Best time for correction of hypospadias is within 12-18 months of age by paediatric urologist.
- Order of correction involves:
  - **Orthoplasty or chordee correction** (by Nesbitt).
  - **Urethroplasty**–The neourethra may be created by tubularization of the native urethral plate, especially if there is a deep glanular groove. Local tissue flaps employed for urethral reconstruction must be thin, non-hair-bearing, and easy to handle. They are often derived from distal penile shaft skin or prepuce.
  - And finally **Meatoplasty or Glanuloplasty.**
- **Hence, circumcision is not done in patients with hypospadias as prepucial skin can be used in surgical repair.**

Ans: (c) Straightening–Urethroplasty–Balanoplasty

Ref: *Operative Textbook of Paediatric Surgery, 7th edition, page 874-880*

12. **Identify the image given below:**

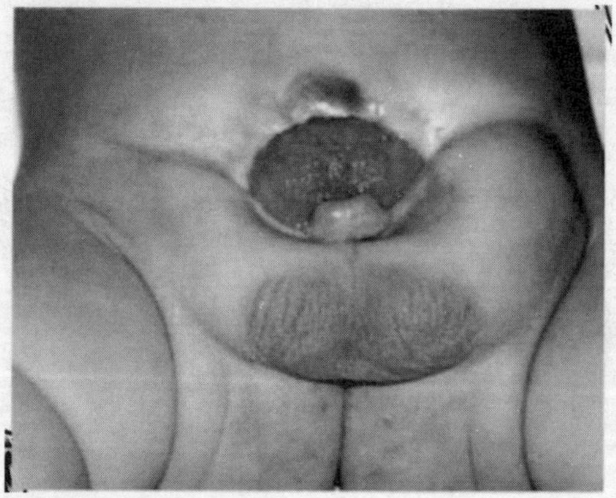

(a) Raspberry tumor (b) Ectopia vesica
(c) Exomphalos major (d) Umbilical hernia

Explanation:

Ectopia Vesicae or Bladder Exstrophy

- **Ectopia vesicae** is associated with complete **ventral defect of the urogenital sinus** with associated defect in the lower anterior abdominal wall.
- Pubic bones are widely separated.
- Urine spurts from lower abdominal wall.
- Posterior wall of bladder is seen.
- Associated with bilateral inguinal hernias.
- **Epispadias** is always associated.
- Treatment includes **bladder closure with sacral osteotomy** within 1 year of age and **antiureteral reflux procedure** with **bladder neck reconstruction.**
- Finally repair of **epispadias.**
- Complications include **stricture, hyperchloremic acidosis** and 20 fold increased risk of **Adenocarcinoma bladder.**

Ans: (b) Ectopia vesica

Ref: Bailey and Love, 27th edition, page 1424-25

13. A 35-year-old male came to hospital with dysuria and pus cells on examination. Urine culture came negative (sterile pyuria). After few hours patient deteriorated suddenly and died due to renal failure. Gross autopsy pictures of kidney shown. Family history renal disease present. What is the diagnosis?

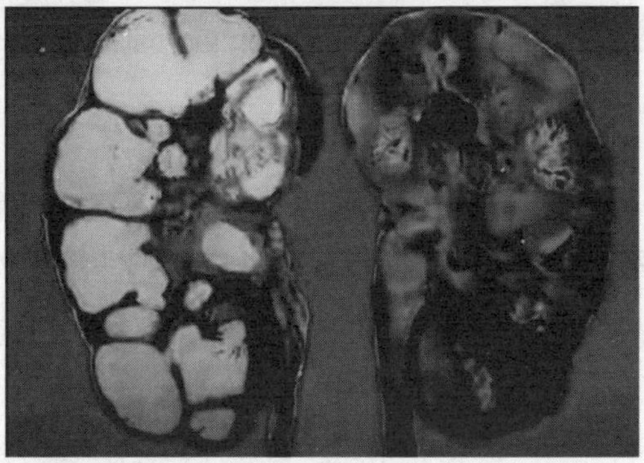

(a) Renal cell cancer
(b) Renal tuberculosis
(c) Cystic renal disease
(d) Metastasis

Explanation:

- **Most common site of genitourinary tuberculosis is – Kidney.**
- Genitourinary tuberculosis is always secondary to pulmonary infection, though in many cases has healed or is quiescent.
- Infection occurs via the **hematogenous route**.
- **Most sensitive modality to detect early TB–IVP (Blunting of Calyx).**

Advanced Changes in Kidney and Ureter:

- **Calcification.**
- **Cavities.**
- **Fibrosis leading to obstruction.**
- Fibrotic strictures of the pelvis or ureters lead to hydronephrosis.
- Strictures of the calyceal neck leads to hydrocalyces (or hydrocalicosis).

Bladder Changes:

- Bladder wall may appear thickened and trabeculated and bladder may be small, contracted (**thimble bladder****).
- In later stages VUR may develop.

Investigations for TB Renal Tract:

- Sterile pyuria is the rule in renal TB.
- The tubercle bacilli can be identified on AFB staining of 24 hours urine specimen or the first morning urine collected on 3 successive days. AFB staining is positive in about 60% of cases.

Recent Advance:

- **Computed tomography:** Shows advanced changes in Renal TB well but is less sensitive in early stages as it cannot be detailed calyceal anatomy.
- For early changes IVP is best. IVP is replaced by CT urography recently to detect the earliest changes in TB.

Sterile pyuria and the image – Both points to renal tuberculosis (Stage of Putty kidney).

Renal Tuberculosis:

- Most patients present with local symptoms such as frequent voiding; dysuria; pyuria; back, flank, or abdominal pain; and microscopic or macroscopic hematuria.
- Systemic symptoms of fever, weight loss, and anorexia are less common.

- Hematuria and **culture-negative pyuria** may be seen at urine analysis.

Urine analysis of sediment from a 24-hour specimen for acid-fast bacilli (AFB) is positive in 80-90% of cases of TB.

Putty Kidney:

- A **putty kidney** refers to a pattern of renal calcification associated with renal tuberculosis conventionally described on plain radiography.
- Calcification characteristically is very homogeneous and ground glass-like, representing calcified caseous tissue.

Ans: (b) Renal tuberculosis

Ref: Bailey and Love, 27th edition, page 1405

14. According to Weigert Meyer rule of duplication of ureter, the lower pole ureter in urinary bladder is:

(a) Lateral and cephalad to the upper pole ureter
(b) Lateral and caudal to the upper pole ureter
(c) Medial and cephlad to the upper pole ureter
(d) Medial and caudal to the upper pole ureter

Explanation:

Weigert-Meyer Rule:

- This rule applies in **Congenital Complete Duplication of Ureter.**
- In Complete Duplication of Ureter, where the **upper** and **lower** collecting duct systems are **separate** and drains **separately** through way of **two ureter.**
- The Rule states that "the **ureter which drains the upper collecting system will enter the bladder inferior and medial to the ureter draining the lower collecting system**".
- The **upper ureter** is considered **ECTOPIC** and the **lower ureter** is considered **ORTHOTOPIC**.
- **Ectopic ureters** are more prone for **Obstruction.**
- **Orthotopic ureters** are more prone for **Reflux** due to **perpendicular entry** into bladder musculature rather than **oblique entry**.

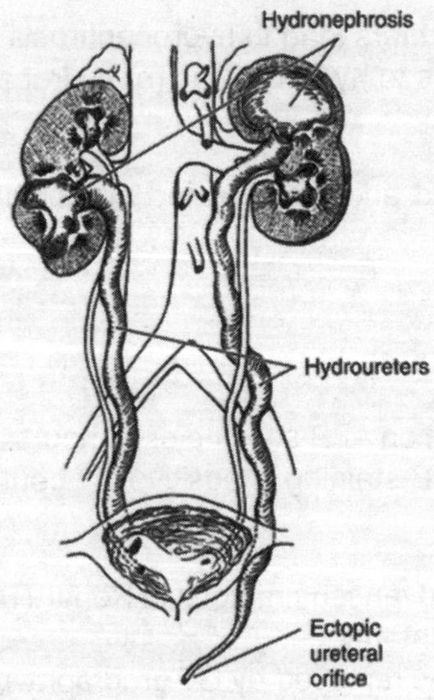

Ans: (a) Lateral and cephalad to the upper pole ureter

Ref: Campbell's Textbook of Urology, 11th edition, page 974-975

15. Sickle cell anaemia is associated with which type of RCC:

(a) Medullary (b) Papillary
(c) Chromophobe (d) Colloid

Explanation:

- **Renal medullary carcinoma** is a subtype of **RCC** that occurs almost exclusively in patients with the **sickle cell trait.**
- Arise from the **calyceal epithelium** near the **renal papillae** but is often highly infiltrative.
- The site of origin (renal papillae) and association with sickle cell trait suggest that a relatively hypoxic environment may contribute to tumorigenesis.
- Diagnosed in young **African-Americans**, often in the third decade of life.
- Mostly locally advanced and metastatic at the time of diagnosis.
- Most patients do not respond to therapy and succumb to their disease in a few to several months.
- Mean survival was only 15 weeks.
- Shares many histologic features with collecting duct carcinoma.

Most common type–**Clear cell RCC***
Most common type seen in Dialysis associated cystic disease–**Papillary RCC***
Most common type seen in sickle cell trait–**Medullary RCC***
Best prognosis–**Chromophobe RCC***

Ans: (a) Medullary

Ref: Campbell Urology, 11th edition, page 1333

16. **In lumbar sympathectomy, which root value is spared?**

(a) L1
(b) L2
(c) L3
(d) L4

Explanation:

LUMBAR SYMPATHECTOMY

Principles

- Increase blood flow (by vasodilatation).
- Nutritive value for small ulcers.
- Reduces ischemic rest pain.
- No effect on collateral circulation.

Indications

- Rest pain*.
- Ulcers*.
- Superficial gangrene*.
- Not useful for intermittent claudication**.
- Contraindicated if ABPI > 0.3 and in diabetics**.

(Diabetics have autonomic neuropathy already, so, there will not be any benefit on sympathectomy)

Ganglia Removed

- In unilateral cases L1,L2,L3 and L4 ganglionectomy advised.
- In bilateral cases L1 must be preserved at least on one side (to avoid retrograde ejaculation).

Structures Mistaken for Sympathetic Trunk:

- Lymphatic chain.
- Genitofemoral nerve.
- Psoas sheath.
- Psoas minor.

Ans: (a) L1

Ref: Sabiston, Textbook of Surgery, 20th edition, page 1764-66

17. **Klippel Trenanauy syndrome associated with all *except*:**

(a) Port wine stain
(b) Varicose veins
(c) Limb lengthening
(d) Fused vertebra

Explanation:

Venous Malformation

- Present at birth, but becomes obvious later as bluish compressible swellings.
- VM often develop thrombi and later phleboliths and are typically painful.
- Blood contained in extensive VM exhibits a localized intravascular coagulopathy.

SLOW-FLOW SYNDROMES

Klippel-Trenaunay Syndrome

Capillary lymphaticovenous malformation is often sporadic.

- Large or small capillary malformations (Portwine stain) over the extremity and buttock.
- Lymphedema involving the limb leading to limb hypertrophy.
- Lateral varicosities.
- All patients should be treated conservatively with compression hosiery, and LMWH is needed when they undergo surgery as they have increased of VTE.

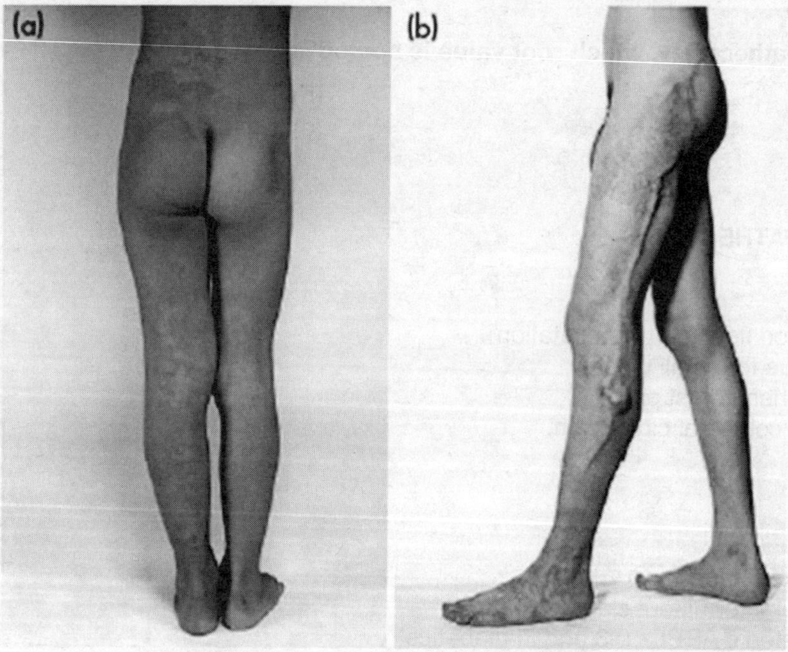

Ans: (d) Fused vertebra

Ref: *Bailey and Love, 27th edition, page 991*

18. **Oliver's sign is seen in:**

(a) Ascending aortic aneurysm
(b) Arch of aorta aneurysm
(c) Descending aortic aneurysm
(d) Aortic dissection

Explanation:

Oliver's Sign:

- It is an abnormal **downward movement of the trachea** during **systole** that can indicate a **dilation or aneurysm of the aortic arch***.

- Elicited by gently grasping the cricoid cartilage and applying upward pressure while the patient stands with his or her chin extended upward. Due to the anatomic position of the aortic arch, which overrides the left main bronchus, a downward tug of the trachea may be felt if an aneurysm is present. Also called as **Tracheal Tug sign.**
- Another sign that is associated with abnormal pulsation of the trachea in patients with a dilation or aneurysm of the aortic arch called **Cardarelli's sign.**
- It can be felt by a physician pressing on the thyroid cartilage and displacing it to the patient's left. This increases contact between the left bronchus and the aorta, allowing systolic pulsations from the aorta to be felt at the surface if an aneurysm is present.

Ans: (b) Arch of aorta aneurysm

Ref: Rutherford Vascular Surgery, 8th edition, page 2090

19. A biopsy from a mass in front of the neck revealed parafollicular cells. How do you follow up?

(a) Calcitonin (b) T4
(c) Thyroxine (d) Thyroglobulin

Explanation:

MEDULLARY THYROID CARCINOMA

- Tumors arise from parafollicular C cells from neural crest and not from thyroid cells, hence not dependent on TSH and do not take up radioactive iodine.
- May be familial in 25% or sporadic (mostly).
- Familial may be MEN associated and non-MEN associated.
- Seen in 50 – 60 years, mostly in superior poles. 1.5 :1 females.
- Secrete Calcitonin, CEA, CGRP, PG E2, F2 alpha, Histaminidases, Serotonin.
- 10 years survival rate is 45 – 80%, worst with MEN2B – 35% at 10 years.
- **Histology:** Characterisitic cell balls with amyloid stroma.

Features:

- Thyroid swelling.
- Rising calcitonin.
- Diarrhoea in 30% of individuals.
- Cushing's syndrome in 2 – 4% due to ectopic secretion of ACTH.
- Rising CEA levels.
- Lymph nodal spread is very common, 50 – 60%.
- Blood spread also common.

Treatment:

- Genetic screening – suspecting familial cases.
- Added by Serum calcitonin – Basal and stimulated by calcium or pentagastrin.
- Pheochromocytoma to be ruled out, before planning on surgery by 24 hours urine for catecholamines/ metanephrines.
- **Plan:** Total Thyroidectomy with Bilateral Prophylactic central neck dissection for all.
- Palpable / Image detected cervical nodes with Calcitonin >400 pg/ml -- Ipsilateral or Bilateral Selective (Posterolateral) Neck Dissection (LEVELS 2A,3,4,5).

Targeted Therapies:

Multikinase Inhibitors	Sorafenib, Sunitinib, Lenvatinib, Cabozanitinib
VEGFR inhibitors	Axitinib, Pazopanib
EGFR inhibitor	Vandetanib (only USFDA approved drug for advanced and progressive MTC
Anti CEA monoclonal antibody	Labetuzumab

Follow up:

- Serum calcitonin – best marker for recurrence.
- Replacement doses of thyroxine given. There is no role for TSH suppression or Radioactive iodine ablation in this.
- HRCT of neck/chest/liver or isotope scans like DMSA/I123 MIBG in cases of raised calcitonin or CEA levels.

Ans: (a) Calcitonin

Ref: Sabiston, Textbook of Surgery, 20th edition, page 909-910

20. False about the swelling is:

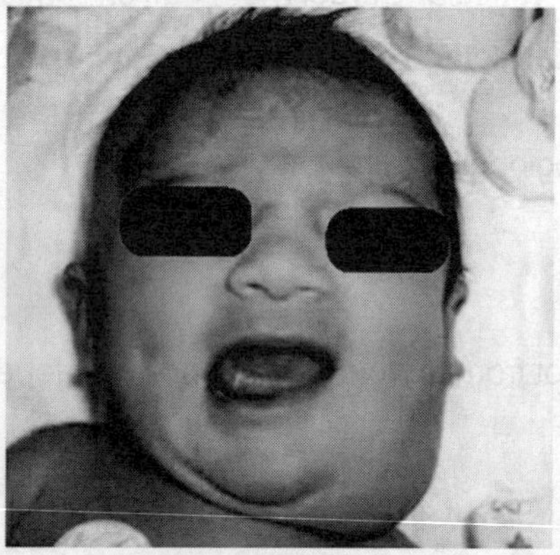

(a) Most common location is posterior fossa
(b) Filled with blood
(c) Filled with lymph
(d) Associated with Turner's syndrome

Explanation:

CYSTIC HYGROMA

- New terminology for cystic hygroma is **Cavernous Lymphangioma.**
- It is formed during embryological development of lymphatic system, when any of the jugular lymph sacs gets sequestered to develop into a lymphatic cyst.
- Most common site is **posterior triangle of neck***, followed by **axilla, retroperitoneum, cheek, mediastinum and groin.**
- It presents at **birth** with a huge cyst in the neck leading to obstructed labour.
- It is very large, smooth, cystic, fluctuant, brilliant **transilluminant** swelling which is not reducible.
- It is filled with **clear lymph** with **lining epithelium.**
- It attains **very large size**, to cause respiratory insufficiency and stridor.
- It is **multiloculated**, can get infected often, or can cause lymph ooze.
- Treatment is difficult surgically, as it involves several anatomical planes and cannot be excised completely.
- **Sclerosant injection** with **OKT32** or **Picibanil** is gained popularity.

Ans: (b) Filled with blood

Ref: Bailey and Love, 27th edition, page 754-755

21. A child with moderate to severe head injury is admitted in PICU. First line treatment are all *except*:

(a) IV mannitol
(b) Hypothermia
(c) Analgesia and sedation
(d) Controlled mechanical ventilation

Explanation:

Brain Trauma Foundation Recommendations for Traumatic Brain Injury:

Goals to Prevent Secondary Brain Injury
Maintain cerebral perfusion pressure at least 60 mm Hg
Keep intracranial pressure below 20 mm Hg
Maintain mean arterial pressure above 90 mm Hg
Never allow $PaCO_2$ less than 25 mm Hg

Measures (To do)	Avoided (Not recommended)
Keep **HOB elevated to 20–30'** or reverse trendelenberg position	Hypotonic fluids to be avoided
Intubation and optimal ventilation with PaO_2 >11kPa; pCO_2 = 4.5-5 kPa	**Steroids avoided or contraindicated**
Monitor ICP with ICP bolt monitor or **External ventricular drain** (advantage of therapeutic drainage of CSF)	Hyperventilation not in first 24 hours due to risk of hypocapnia induced cerebral vasoconstriction
Mannitol as temporizing measure (100 ml of 20% mannitol as bolus)	Pyrexia should be avoided
Sedation and paralysis with barbiturates	
Finally **Decompressive Craniectomy** if all measures fail	

- Check pituitary function, monitor for electrolyte imbalance and start on enteral nutrition within 72 hours of injury.
- **Infection prophylaxis** needed in severe traumatic brain injury or in patients with external ventricular drain.
- **Seizure prophylaxis** to be started to prevent early post traumatic fits (within 7 days). Risk factors are ICH, depressed skull fractures and dural tears.

Although mannitol is commonly used in the management of elevated ICP in adult and paediatric traumatic brain injury, the evidence supporting its use in paediatric patients is inconclusive and did not meet the standards for inclusion in the 2012 guidelines.

Ans: (a) IV mannitol

Ref: Bailey and Love, 26th edition, page 336-337; Sabiston, Textbook of Surgery, 20th edition, page 1919

OBSTETRICS AND GYNECOLOGY

1. **Stage IIB cervical carcinoma. Best line of management:**

(a) Type 3 hysterectomy (b) Chemotherapy

(c) Radiation therapy (d) Chemoradiation

Explanation:

Stage 0 (carcinoma in situ)

Treatment options for squamous cell carcinoma in situ include:

- Cryosurgery.
- Laser surgery.
- Loop electrosurgical excision procedure (LEEP/LLETZ).
- Cold knife conization.
- Simple hysterectomy.

Treatment options for adenocarcinoma in situ include:

- Hysterectomy.
- Cone biopsy.

Stage IA1

Treatment options for women who want to maintain fertility:

- Cone biopsy or a radical trachelectomy.
- Radical hysterectomy along with removal of the pelvic lymph nodes in case of lymphovascular invasion.

Treatment options for women who don't want to maintain fertility:

- A simple (total) hysterectomy.

Stage IA2

Treatment options for women who want to maintain fertility:

- Radical trachelectomy with pelvic lymph node dissection.

Treatment options for women who don't want to maintain fertility:

- Radical hysterectomy with removal of pelvic lymph nodes and sampling of the para-aortic lymph nodes.
- External beam radiation therapy (EBRT) to the pelvis plus brachytherapy.

Stages IB and IIA

The main treatment options are surgery, radiation, or radiation given with chemo (concurrent chemoradiation).

Stages IB1

- Type III hysterectomy with PLND. Most patients require post op. adjuvant chemo/radiotherapy.
- Radical trachelectomy can be done if lesion is less than 2 cms.
- Concurrent chemoradiation.

Stages IB2 and IIA

Treatment options:

- Chemoradiation: This is usually the standard treatment. The chemo may be cisplatin or cisplatin plus fluorouracil. The radiation therapy includes both external beam radiation and brachytherapy.
- Radical hysterectomy with pelvic lymph node dissection and para-aortic lymph node sampling followed by post operative adjuvant chemoradiation therapy.

Stages IIB, III and IVA

Treatment options:

Chemoradiation: The chemo may be cisplatin or cisplatin plus fluorouracil. The radiation therapy includes both external beam radiation and brachytherapy.

Stage IVB

Stage IVB cervical cancer is not usually considered curable. Treatment options include radiation therapy and/or chemotherapy. Most standard chemo regimens include a platinum drug (cisplatin or carboplatin) along with another drug such as paclitaxel (Taxol), gemcitabine (Gemzar), or topotecan. The targeted drug **bevacizumab (Avastin)** may be added to chemo.

Ans: (d) Chemoradiation

Ref: DC Dutta, Textbook of Gynecology, 7th edition, page 287

2. **A pregnant lady with gonorrhea with white discharge. Treatment of choice is:**

(a) Ceftriaxone single dose IM + Metronidazole for 14 days
(b) Ceftriaxone plus azithromycin single dose
(c) Ceftriaxone plus Doxycycline 100 mg for 7 days + Metronidazole for 14 days
(d) Ceftriaxone single dose IM

Explanation:

- Pregnant women infected with *N. gonorrhoeae* should be treated with dual therapy consisting of **ceftriaxone 250 mg in a single IM dose and azithromycin 1 g orally as a single dose.**
- As dual therapy, ceftriaxone and azithromycin should be administered together on the same day, preferably simultaneously and under direct observation. Ceftriaxone in a single injection of 250 mg provides sustained, high bactericidal levels in the blood.

Ans: (b) Ceftriaxone plus azithromycin single dose

Ref: https://www.cdc.gov/std/tg2015/gonorrhea.htm#preg

3. **Labour is said to be prolonged when combined first and second stage of labour crosses:**

(a) 12 hours (b) 18 hours (c) 24 hours (d) 36 hours

Explanation:

Prolonged Labour

- Labour is said to be prolonged when the combined duration of first and second stage is **more than 18 hours.**
- **Causes:**
  - Abnormal uterine action.
  - Malposition.
  - Malpresentation.
  - Macrosomia.
  - Fetal malformation.
  - Contracted pelvis.
  - Cephalopelvic disproportion.

- **Prolonged latent phase**–in primi more than 20 hours and in multi more than 14 hours.
- **Prolonged active phase**–this is the most common. Cervical dilatation less than 1.2 cm/hour in nullipara and less than 1.5 cm/hour in multipara.
- **Secondary arrest of dilatation**–there is arrest in cervical dilatation for atleast 2 hours.
- **Arrest of descent**–there is arrest of descent of fetal head for atleast one hour.

First stage of labor:

- Two phases of **cervical dilatation** are defined:
  - ***Latent phase.***
  - ***Active phase.***
- The ***latent phase*** corresponds to the **preparatory division**, and the ***active phase***, to the **dilatational division.**
- **Friedman** subdivided the **active phase** into the:
  - **Acceleration phase.**
  - **Phase of maximum slope.**
  - **Deceleration phase.**
- **Latent Phase**
  - The onset of latent labor, as defined by **Friedman** (1972), is the point at which the **mother perceives regular contractions**. The latent phase for most women ends at between **3 and 5 cm of dilatation**.
- **Prolonged Latent Phase**
  - Friedman and Sachtleben (1963) defined this by a **latent phase exceeding 20 hours in the nullipara and 14 hours in the multipara.**
- **Active Labor**
  - Cervical dilatation of **3 to 5 cm or more**, in the presence of **uterine contractions**, can be taken to reliably represent the threshold for active labor.
- **Protraction** as a ***slow rate*** **of cervical dilatation** or **descent.**
  - For **nulliparas** was **less than 1.2 cm dilatation per hour** or **less than 1 cm descent per hour.**
  - For **multiparas**, protraction was defined as **less than 1.5 cm dilatation per hour** or **less than 2 cm descent per hour.**

Second Stage of Labor

- This stage begins when **cervical dilatation is complete** and **ends with fetal delivery.**
- The **median duration** it is highly variable but is approximately:
  - **50 minutes for nulliparas.**
  - **20 minutes for multiparas.**
- The **mean length of first- and second-stage labor** was approximately:
  - **9 hours in nulliparous women** without regional analgesia, and that the **95th percentile** upper limit was **18.5 hours.**
  - Corresponding times for **multiparous women** were a mean of **6 hours** with a 95th percentile maximum of **13.5 hours.**

Ans: (b) 18 hours

Ref: Williams' Obstetrics, 24th edition

4. **An obese woman with type 2 diabetes and hypertension is diagnosed with endometriod type of endometrial carcinoma. Most probable gene defect expected in this condition is:**

(a) PTEN (b) p53 (c) MSH2 (d) BRCA 2

Explanation:

- The **most frequently altered gene in estrogen-dependent endometrioid endometrial carcinoma is PTEN.**
- In contrast, **p53 mutations or Her2/neu overexpression are more frequent in non-endometrioid tumors.**
- K-ras mutations are detected in approximately 15–30% of endometrioid carcinomas.
- A beta-catenin mutation was detected in about 20% of endometrioid carcinomas.

- **Lynch syndrome,** which is an autosomal dominant inherited disorder of cancer susceptibility and is characterized by a MSH2/MSH6 protein complex deficiency, is associated with the development of **non-endometrioid carcinomas.**

Also Know:

The genetic mutations most commonly associated with **endometrioid adenocarcinoma** are in the genes:

- **PTEN**, a tumor suppressor gene*.
- **PIK3CA**, a kinase.
- **KRAS**, a GTPase that functions in signal transduction.
- **CTNNB1,** involved in adhesion and cell signaling. The CTNNB1 (beta-catenin) gene is most commonly mutated in the squamous subtype of endometrioid adenocarcinoma.

PROGNOSTIC VARIABLES IN ENDOMETRIAL CA

- **Age:**
  - Younger women with endometrial cancer have better prognosis than older women.
- **Histologic Type:**
  - Nonendometrioid histologic subtypes account for about 10% of endometrial cancers and carry an increased risk for recurrence and spread.
- **Histologic grade.**
- **Tumour size:**
  - Significant prognostic factor for **lymph node metastasis** and survival in patients with endometrial CA.
- **Hormone receptor status:**
  - **Estrogen** and **progesterone** receptor levels are prognostic indicators.
  - Patients whose tumours are positive for one or both receptors have **longer survival times.**
  - Progesterone receptors levels appear to be stronger predictors of survival.
- **DNA ploidy and proliferative Index:**
  - The proportion of nondiploid tumours increases with **stage, lack of tumour differentiation, and depth of myometrial invasion.**
- **Myometrial invasion:**
  - Increasing depth of invasion is associated with increasing likelihood of extrauterine spread and recurrence.
- **Lymph-vascular space invasion.**
- **Isthmus and cervix extension:**
  - Involvement of isthmus and cervix is associated with increased risk for extrauterine disease, lymph node metastasis and recurrence.
- **Peritoneal cytology:**
  - Seems to have adverse effect on survival only if the endometrial cancer has spread to adnexa, peritoneum, or lymph nodes and not if the disease is otherwise confined to uterus.
- **Lymph node metastases.**
- **Intraperitoneal metastases.**
- **Molecular aberration.**
  - Inactivation of **PTEN tumor suppressor** gene is one of the earliest aberrations observed and most common genetic defect in **Type 1 cancer**.
  - Most frequent genetic alteration is **TP53 mutation** found in **Type 2 endometrial cancer**.

Ans: (a) PTEN gene

Ref: https://www.hindawi.com/journals/ogi/2010/984013/genetics of endometrial carcinoma

5. In a patient with history of pelvic inflammatory disease (PID), correct advice regarding pregnancy:

(a) Infertility and ectopic pregnancy are common
(b) Less chance for spontaneous conception
(c) No complications
(d) Increased abortions

Explanation:

Complications of Pelvic Inflammatory Disease

- **PID is the most common cause of ectopic pregnancy**. One episode leads to 12% chance of ectopic, the incidence rising steadily with each further episode. Chlamydial infection which is usually subclinical, is more likely to lead to ectopic pregnancy. Pelvic TB is yet another cause. Agglutination of tubal mucosal folds and formation of blind pockets, reduced ciliation and impaired tubal peristalsis leads to ovum entrapment and implantation in the tube.
- **Infertility** rate is 12%, after two episodes increases to 25% and after three raises to 50%. It is due to tubal damage and tubo-ovarian mass.
- Chronic pelvic pain.
- Hydrosalpinx.
- Pyosalpinx.

Ans: (a) Infertility and ectopic pregnancy are common

Ref: Sheila Balakrishnan, Textbook of Obstetrics, 2nd edition, page 156

6. Most reliable criteria for gestational age estimation in 1st trimester ultrasound is:

(a) CRL
(b) Femur length
(c) BPD
(d) Abdominal circumference

Explanation:

First trimester scan is also called **Dating scan.**

- Crown rump length [CRL] is measured from the top of the head to the bottom of the buttocks excluding limbs.
- **CRL between 9 and 11 weeks is the most accurate method of dating.**
- Error is about **+/-5 days.**
- **CRL in cm +6.5** gives a rough estimate of gestational age in weeks.
- Useful prior to amniocentesis and chorionic villous sampling and in diagnosis of fetal growth restriction.

Ans: (a) CRL

Ref: Textbook of Obstetrics by Sheila Balakrishnan, 2nd edition, page 476

7. Cordocentesis is done in which period of pregnancy?

(a) 11-14 weeks (b) 18-20 weeks (c) 22-26 weeks (d) 28-32 weeks

Explanation:

Cordocentesis:

- **Percutaneous cord blood sampling** with a fine needle under ultrasound guidance.
- **Common site is the umbilical vein at the placental cord insertion.**
- **Indications**–Assessment and treatment of Rh and platelet isoimmunisation, rapid karyotyping, hemoglobinopathies, genetic disorders, fetal infection, intravascular transfusion.
- Fetal loss 1-2%.
- **Highly accurate.**
- It is an invasive procedure for prenatal diagnosis.

	Chorion Villus Sampling	Amniocentesis	Cordocentesis
Time	• **Transcervical–10-12 weeks** • **Transabdominal–10 weeks to term**	**14-16 weeks** (early **12-14 weeks**)	**18-20 weeks**
Materials for study	Trophoblast cells	Fetal fibroblasts Fluid for biochemical study	Fetal white blood cells (others–infection and biochemical study)
Karyotype Result	Direct preparation–**24-48 hours** Culture–**10-14 days**	Culture **3-4 weeks**	**Culture: 24-48 hours**
Fetal Loss	**0.5-1%**	**0.5%**	**1-2%**
Accuracy	Accurate, may need amniocentesis for confirmation	Highly accurate	Highly accurate
Termination of pregnancy when indicated	Ist trimester–safe	2nd trimester–risky	2nd trimester–risky
Maternal effects following termination of pregnancy	Very little	More traumatic: Physically and psychologically	Same as amniocentesis

Ans: (b) 18-20 weeks

Ref: Textbook of Obstetrics by Sheila Balakrishnan, 2nd edition, page 503

8. Most important feature to diagnose fetal aneuploidy:

(a) Absent nasal bone
(b) Nuchal translucency
(c) Increase in frontomaxillary angle
(d) Reversal of ductus venosus flow

Explanation:

Ultrasound Markers of Fetal Aneuploidy:

- **Nuchal translucency is the single most powerful tool.** More than **3 mm** needs evaluation.
- Absence of nasal bone.
- Absence or reversal of flow in the ductus venosus on Doppler.
- Tricuspid regurgitation.
- Increase in frontomaxillary angle more than 85 deg.

Ans: (b) Nuchal translucency

Ref: Current Progress in Obstetrics and Gynecology, John Stud, Volume 1, page 17

9. True about 'capacitation' of sperm:

(a) Takes about 6-8 hours
(b) Acrosomal reaction occurs
(c) Zona pellucida reaction occurs
(d) Capacitation takes place in testis

Explanation:

- Capacitation is the physiochemical change in the **sperm by which it becomes hypermotile and is able to bind and fertilize a secondary oocyte.**
- **Capacitation takes place in the female genital tract and takes about 2-6 hours.**
- The changes involve cyclic AMP dependent phosphorylation with increase in intracellular pH.
- **Activation of acrosomal membranes** causes release of hyaluronidase, hydrolytic enzymes, proacrosin, acrosin, that help the sperm to digest the zona pellucida and enter the oocyte.
- **Acrosomal reaction is fusion of sperm plasma membrane and outer acrosomal membrane.**
- The sperm with acrosomal membrane bind with the zona protein.
- Acrosome sperm penetrate the zona pellucida fuse with the oocyte plasma membrane.
- The sperm head swells and the fused membrane vesiculates.

- Gamete fusion occurs.
- After 3-6 hours of insemination, one polar and two pronuclear bodies are visible and they migrate to the center of the oocyte.

Ans: (b) Acrosomal reaction occurs

Ref: Dutta Textbook of Obstetrics, 8th edition, page 22

10. Which layer of placenta disappears at the end of pregnancy?

(a) Decidua parietalis
(b) Decidua capsularis
(c) Decidua basalis
(d) Chorion frondosum

Explanation:

- The decidua is the endometrium of the pregnant uterus.
- Three layers of deciduas are:
  1. **Decidua basalis or serotina**–the portion of decidua in contact with the base of the blastocyst.
  2. **Decidua capsularis or reflexa**–the thin superficial compact layer covering the blastocyst.
  3. **Decidua vera or parietalis**–the rest of the decidua lining the uterine cavity.
- As the implanted embryo bulges towards the uterine cavity, the space between the decidua capsularis and the deciduas vera called the decidual space is gradually narrowed down and **by 4th month, it is completely obliterated** by the fusion of the decidua capsularis with the decidua vera.
- **The decidua basalis** however retains its characteristic appearance till term and **becomes the maternal portion of placenta**.

Ans: (c) Decidua basalis

Ref: DC Dutta, Textbook of Obstetrics, 8th edition, page 28

11. Pregnant patient comes at 34 weeks gestation with leaking. What examination will confirm leaking?

(a) Speculum examination
(b) USG
(c) Non stress test
(d) Amnisure

Explanation:

Premature Rupture of Membranes (PROM):

- Spontaneous rupture of membranes anytime **beyond 28th week but before the onset of labour is called prelabour rupture of the membranes**.
- When it occurs **before 37 completed weeks** it is called **preterm PROM (PPROM).**

Causes:

- **Polyhydramnios.**
- **Cervical incompetence.**
- **Multiple pregnancy.**
- **Chorioamnionitis.**
- **Low BMI.**

Confirmation of diagnosis:

- **Speculum examination–most confirmatory.**
- Vaginal pool for pH–6-6.2, **ferning pattern, orange blue discoloration of exfoliated cells.**
- Amnisure radioimmunoassay.
- Ultrasound.

Investigations

- Complete blood count, C reactive protein, urine routine and culture.
- High vaginal swab for Group B streptococcus.
- Vaginal pool for estimation of phosphatidyl glycerol and L:S ratio.
- USG for fetal biophysical profile, cardiotocography.

Complications:

Obstetric	Neonatal
• Chorioamniotis • Cord prolapse • Dry labour • Placental abruption	• Neonatal sepsis • RDS • IVH • NEC

Ans: (a) Speculum examination

Ref: DC Textbook of Obstetrics, 8th edition, page 369

Version – 2

A 34 weeks pregnant with complaints of leaking vaginal discharge. What examination will confirm premature rupture of membranes in this patient?

(a) Digital examination (b) USG exam (c) Speculum exam (d) Urine exam

Explanation:

>>The question is about the **'confirmatory test'** for PROM.

Preterm Premature Rupture of Membranes

This term defines spontaneous rupture of the fetal membranes before 37 completed weeks and before labour onset.

Diagnosis of Ruptured Membranes:

- **Sterile speculum** examination–ruptured membranes are diagnosed if amniotic fluid pools in the posterior fornix or clear fluid flows from cervical canal.
- **Litmus test**–PH of vaginal secretions normally ranges from **4.5 to 5.5** whereas that of amniotic fluid is usually **7.0 to 7.5**. Therefore red litmus paper turns **blue.**
- **Microscopic ferning.**
- **Nitrazine test**–yellow nitrazine paper turns blue.
- **Arborization or ferning of vaginal fluid**–Amniotic fluid crystallizes to form **fern like pattern** due to relative concentrations of sodium chloride, proteins and carbohydrates.
- **Detection of alpha fetoprotein** in vaginal vault has been used to identify amniotic fluid.
- **0.1% Nile blue sulfate test** (orange coloured cells seen).
- **USG** will show **oligohydramnios**
  - **False positive tests** results may occur with **coexistent blood, semen, or bacterial vaginosis** where results may occur due to scant fluid.

Ans: (c) Speculum exam

Ref: Williams' Textbook of Obstetrics

12. **An 11-year-old girl is raped by her uncle. Lateral wall smear which shows maturation index 0/100/0 (Basal, Intermediate and Superficial). Correct interpretation:**

(a) Abortion done (b) Pregnant
(c) Uses contraception (d) Premenstrual phase

Explanation:

Cytohormonal Study of Vagina:

- **The lateral wall of the upper third of the vagina which is most sensitive to hormonal influence** is lightly scraped with a wooden spatula. The material so collected is to be fixed and stained.
- **The exfoliated vaginal epithelial cells normally include parabasal, intermediate and superficial cells.**
  - The parabasal cells are small, round and **basophilic.**
  - The intermediate cells are transparent and **basophilic.**
  - The superficial cells are large, thin **acidophilic** with pyknotic nuclei.
- **The estrogen produces superficial cell maturation.**

- **Progesterone, pill, pregnancy androgen and corticosteroids, will produce intermediate cell maturation.**
- Whereas **lack of any hormone will produce parabasal cell predominance.**
- **The maturation index** relates to the relative percentage of parabasal, intermediate and superficial cells per 100 cells counted. It is expressed in three numbers; **the left one parabasal percentage, the intermediate in the center, and on the right the percentage of superficial cells.**

Age	MI	Inference
At birth	0/95/5	Maternal hormones
Childhood	80/20/0	Minimal hormones
Preovulatory	0/40/60	Estrogen ++
Mild secretory	0/70/30	Estrogen + progesterone+
During pregnancy	0/95/5	Predominantly progesterone+corticosteroid
Postpartum	100/0/0	Minimal hormonal stimulation
Postmenopausal	0/100/0 100/0/0	No estrogen

Ans: (b) Pregnant

Ref: DC Dutta, Textbook of Gynecology, 7th edition, page 92

13. Amiodarone belongs to which category of drugs in pregnancy?

(a) Category A (b) Category B (c) Category C (d) Category D

Explanation:

FDA Pregnancy Categories

Category A	**Adequate and well-controlled studies** have failed to demonstrate a risk to the fetus in the first trimester of pregnancy (and there is no evidence of risk in later trimesters).
Category B	**Animal reproduction** studies have **failed to demonstrate a risk to the fetus** and there are **no adequate and well-controlled studies** in pregnant women.
Category C	**Animal reproduction** studies have **shown an adverse effect on the fetus** and there are no adequate and well-controlled studies in humans, but potential benefits may warrant use of the drug in pregnant women despite potential risks.
Category D	There is **positive evidence of human fetal risk** based on **adverse reaction data** from investigational or marketing experience or studies in humans, but potential benefits may warrant use of the drug in pregnant women despite potential risks.
Category X	Studies in animals or humans have demonstrated **fetal abnormalities** and/or there is **positive evidence of human fetal risk** based on adverse reaction data from investigational or marketing experience, and the risks involved in use of the drug in pregnant women clearly outweigh potential benefits.

Drugs	Category
Acetaminophen	B
Phenacetin	B
Aspirin	C
Doxylamine	B
Meclizine	B
Cyclizine	B
Dimenhydrinate	B

Contd.

Penicillin, Ampicillin, Amoxycillin	B
Cloxacillin, Cephalosporins	B
Erythromycin	B
Gentamycin	C
Amikacin	C/D
Streptomycin	D
Sulphonamides	B/D
Tetracyclines	D
Metronidazole	B
Piperazine	B
Mebendazole	B
Antimalarials	C
Antifungals	C
Anti TB drugs	B and C
Ethambutol	B
INH	C
Rifampicin	C
Pyrazinamide	C
Vitamins B,C,D,E, folic acid	A
Thyroxin	A
Androgens	X
Estrogens	X
Progestogens–Hydroxyprogesterone	D
Medroxyprogersterone	D
Norethindrone	X
Bronchodilators	X
Norgestrel	C

Drug	Teratogenic Effect
Vitamin A and its derivatives including isotretinein, accutane and etretinate	Significant risk of spontaneous abortion and risk of many significant anomalies
ACE inhibitors	May cause kidney damage in the fetus when used in II and III trimester, decrease in the amount of amniotic fluid and deformities of face, limbs and lungs
Anticoagulants–warfarin	Use during I trimester produces defects like nasal hypoplasia and a depressed nasal bridge; termed as fetal warfarin syndrome. Use during II and III trimesters is associated with increased risk of fetal malformations
Heparin	Safe but if taken for long time osteoporosis and decrease in number of platelets in pregnant women occurs
Estrogen and androgens	Genital tract malformations
Thyroid preparations	
Methimazole	Overactive and enlarged thyroid gland
Carbimazole	Overactive and enlarged thyroid gland
Radioactive iodine	Underactive Thyroid gland in fetus
Propylthiouracil	Safe

Contd.

Anticonvulsants	
Carbamazepine	Risk of birth defects
Phenytoin, Phenobarbitone	Bleeding problem in the newborn which can be prevented if pregnant woman takes Vitamin K by mouth every day for a month before delivery or if the newborn baby is given an injection of Vitamin K soon after birth. Risk of birth defects
Trimethadione	Increased risk of miscarriage
Sodium valproate	Increased risk of birth defects in fetus; including a cleft palate and abnormalities of the heart, face, skull, hands or abdominal organs
Antidepressants–Lithium	Birth defects (mainly of the heart), lethargy, decreased muscle tone, underactivity of Thyroid gland **and nephrogenic diabetes insipidus** in the newborn. **Ebstein's anomaly** (tricuspid valve malformation) has been reported in a number of fetuses exposed to this drug
Aspirin and other Salicylates	Premature closing of ductus arteriosus, jaundice and bleeding problems in the woman during and after delivery and in the newborn
Antibiotics–Tetracycline	Slowed bone growth, permanent yellowing of the teeth and increased susceptibility to cavities in the body
Chloramphenicol	Gray Baby syndrome
Ciprofloxacin	Possibility of joint abnormalities (seen in animals)
Kanamycin and Streptomycin	Risk of ototoxicity
Sulfonamides	Jaundice and brain damage in newborn
Antineoplastic agents	
Oral hypoglycemic drugs	A very low level of sugar in the blood of newborn. Inadequate control of diabetes in the pregnant woman

Class III **anti arrhythmic** agents (such as **sotalol, amiodarone) are very effective drugs in patients with ventricular tachyarrhythmias**. During pregnancy, both drugs are of limited value: sotalol appears to be relatively safe, although there is a 3–5% risk of developing polymorphic or torsade de pointes **tachycardia**. Animal studies have revealed evidence of fetotoxicity. In humans, congenital goiter/hypothyroidism, hyperthyroidism, and neonatal bradycardia have been reported. US FDA pregnancy **category D**, but potential benefits may warrant use of the drug in pregnant women despite potential risks.

Ans: (d) Category D

Ref: FDA, Pregnancy Categories

ORTHOPEDICS

1. **Lisfranc's fracture dislocation involves:**

(a) Lunate (b) Scaphoid
(c) Trans metatarsal (d) Capitate

Explanation:

Lisfranc's Fracture Dislocation

- The **Lisfranc joint** consists of the **tarsometatarsal joint complex**, which includes the **three cuneiforms, cuboid and their articulations** with the **five metatarsal bones**.
- Dislocations of the Lisfranc joint are the **most common** dislocations of the **foot***.
- **Mechanism of injury:** These injuries usually result from high-energy injuries like:
  - o **Forced hyperflexion** in road traffic accidents **(Figure 1).**
  - o **Fall from height**.
- On X-ray, there is **increased space** between the **medial cuneiform** and the **second metatarsal** (due to rupture of Lisfranc ligament that runs between these points) called as **Fleck sign***.
- For treating the dislocation has to be **reduced** accurately either by **closed or open** means and has to be fixed with **K wires or screws**.

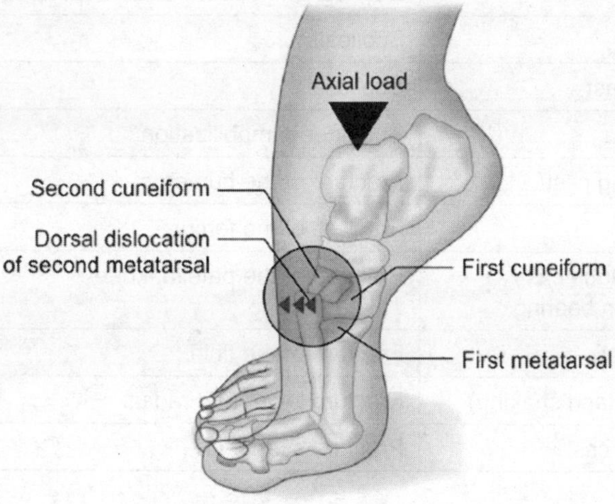

Fig. 1: Forced hyperflexion injury causing Lisfranc dislocation

Ans: (c) Trans Metatarsal

Ref: Fundamentals of Orthopedics, 2nd edition, Mohindra and Jain, Jaypee Publishers, page 160

2. **Tube cast is used for which of the following bones?**

(a) Knee (b) Ankle (c) Shoulder (d) Elbow

Explanation:

- **Tube (Cylinder) cast** (Figure) is applied for **undisplaced patellar fractures*** seen in injury around the **knee joint***.

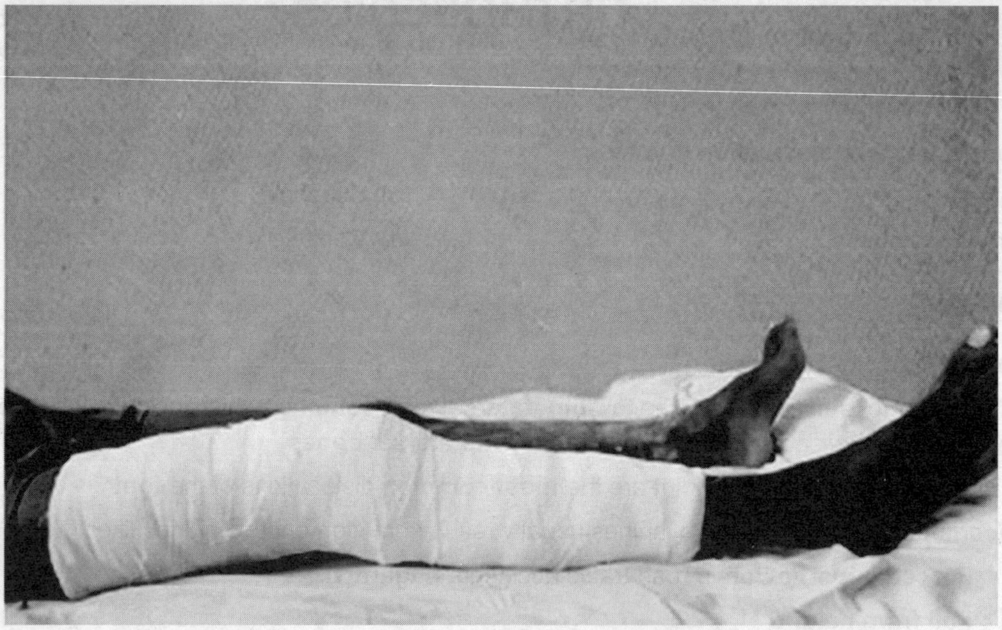

Fig. 2: Tube/Cylindrical cast applied for an undisplaced fracture of patella

Plaster Casts and Uses

Name of cast	**Uses**
Minerva cast	Cervical and upper thoracic spine disease
Risser's cast	Scoliosis
Turn-buckle cast	Scoliosis
Shoulder spica	Shoulder immobilization
U-Slab/hanging cast	Fracture of the humerus
Hip spica	Fracture of the femur
Cylinder cast/tube cast/ Patellar tendon bearing	Fracture of the patella, knee
Cast (PTB cast)	Fracture of the tibia
Colle's cast (Hand shaking)	Fracture lower end radius
Glass holding cast	Fracture scaphoid

Ans: (a) Knee

Ref: Fundamentals of Orthopedics, 2nd edition, Mohindra and Jain, Jaypee Publishers, page 148

3. **Kohler's disease is due to osteonecrosis of:**

(a) Calcaneum
(b) Tarsal bone
(c) Talus
(d) Humerus-Capitulum

Explanation:

- **Kohler's disease** is osteochondritis of **Navicula (a tarsal bone)**.
- In osteochondritis there occurs degeneration of osteochondral part of joint possibly due to a vascular etiology. However, exact etiology is unknown and the condition is categorized as under based on possible causative mechanisms.

Types of Osteochondritis

A. **Crushing type**
   - ***Freiberg's disease***: Metatarsal heads.
   - ***Kohler's disease***: Navicula **(Figure).**
   - ***Kienbock's disease***: Lunate.
   - ***Panner's disease***: Capitulum.
   - ***Scheuermann's disease***: Ring epiphysis of vertebrae.
   - ***Calve's disease***: Central bony nucleus of vertebrae.
   - ***Thiemann's disease***: Phalangeal epiphysis.

B. **Traction/pulling type**
   - **Osgood-Schlatter's disease:** *Tibial tuberosity.*
   - **Severe's disease:** *Calcaneal epiphysis.*
   - **Johansson-Larson syndrome:** *Patellar ligament (at its lower pole patellar attachment).*
   - **Iselin's disease:** *Base of fifth metatarsal.*
   - **Adam's disease:** *Medial epicondyle of humerus.*

C. **Splitting type**
   - Osteochondritis dissecans.

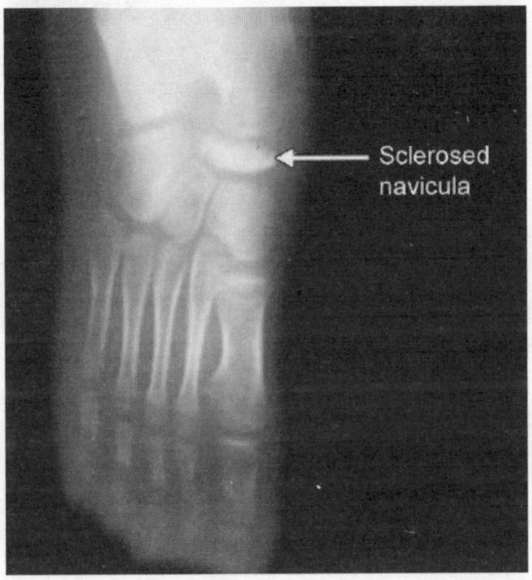

Fig. 3: Kohler's disease (Navicular osteochondritis)

Ans: (b) Tarsal bone

Ref: Fundamentals of Orthopedics, 2nd edition, Mohindra and Jain, Jaypee Publishers, page 44

PEDIATRICS

1. **A child presented with dog bite on neck and presented to hospital after 12 hours. He was sent for X-ray. What is your diagnosis?**

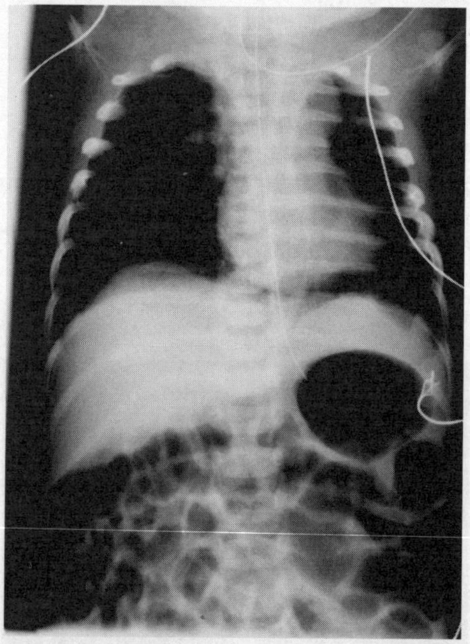

(a) Subcutaneous emphysema
(b) Pneumothorax
(c) Pneumoperitoneum
(d) Hydropneumothorax

Explanation:

Pneumothorax:

- Primary or secondary and can be spontaneous, traumatic, iatrogenic, or catamenial.
- **Primary spontaneous:** Without trauma or underlying lung disease with or without exertion (Valsalva) occurs Ehlers-Danlos disease and Marfan syndrome.
- **Secondary spontaneous** as a complication of an underlying lung disorder but without trauma, e.g., pneumonia, empyema, pulmonary abscess, gangrene, infarct, rupture of a cyst or an emphysematous bleb (in asthma), foreign bodies in the lung, cystic, lymphoma or other malignancies, and in graft vs host disease with bronchiolitis obliterans.
- Traumatic pneumothorax–External chest or abdominal blunt or penetrating trauma, ecstasy methylene dioxy meth amphetamine) abuse has been associated with pneumothorax.
- **Iatrogenic pneumothorax**–Tracheotomy, subclavian line placement, thoracentesis, transbronchial biopsy, acupuncture treatment.
- **Catamenial** pneumothorax–associated with menses, results from passage of intra-abdominal air through diaphragmatic defects.
- Pneumothorax with a serous effusion (hydropneumothorax) or a purulent effusion (pyopneumothorax).
- Bilateral pneumothorax–Lung transplantation and with *Mycoplasma pneumoniae* infection and tuberculosis.

- Air enters the pleural space -> the lung collapses.
- Hypoxemia - due to alveolar hypoventilation, ventilation-perfusion mismatch, and intrapulmonary shunt.
- **Simple pneumothorax** - intrapleural pressure = atmospheric pressure (lung collapses up to 30%).
- **Tension pneumothorax** - increasing positive pressure in the pleural space -> shift of mediastinal structures toward the contralateral side -> decreased venous return -> decreased cardiac output.
- Abrupt onset of chest pain, dyspnea, and cyanosis with respiratory distress, retractions, and markedly decreased breath sounds over the involved lung.
- The larynx, trachea, and heart may be shifted toward the unaffected side.
- Diagnosis by radiographic examination–Expiratory views accentuate the contrast between lung markings and the clear area of the pneumothorax.

Evidence of Tension

- Shift of mediastinal structures away from the side of air leak.
- Evidence of circulatory compromise; or
- On hearing a "hiss" of rapid exit of air under tension with the insertion of the thoracostomy tube.

Treatment

- Tension pneumothorax–Emergently require drainage by **needle thoracostomy**.
- Small or even moderate-sized pneumothorax in an otherwise normal child–resolve within about 1 week. 100% oxygen may hasten resolution in asthma children.
- >5% collapse or if the pneumothorax is recurrent or under tension, chest tube drainage is necessary.

Ans: (b) Pneumothorax

Ref: Nelson, Textbook of Pediatrics, 20th edition

2. **A 6-year-old boy with lymphoreticular malignancy has come for a cycle of chemotherapy. Which of the following investigations need to be done for next 4 hours to diagnose tumour lysis syndrome?**

(a) Urea, Creatinine, Chloride, Ca2+ and K+
(b) Urea, Creatinine, Phosphate, Ca2+ and K+
(c) Urea, Creatinine, Magnesium, Ca2+ and K+
(d) Urea, Creatinine, sodium and phosphate

Explanation:

Tumour Lysis Syndrome (TLS):

- Oncologic emergency triggered by the rapid release of intracellular material from lysing malignant cells.
- **AKI / acute *uric acid nephropathy*** (rapid accumulation of uric acid derived from the breakdown of nucleic acids) is central to the development of TLS.
- Renal failure then limits the clearance of **potassium, phosphorus**, and **uric acid** leading to ***hyperkalemia, hyperphosphatemia*, and secondary *hypocalcemia*** (phosphate chelation with calcium).
- **Hypocalcemia** of TLS may persist even after phosphate levels normalize, presumably because of **acute deficiencies of 1,25-vitamin D.**

Diagnosis by Cairo-Bishop Criteria

Cairo-Bishop criteria		
Laboratory TLS	**≥ 2 among**	**Clinical TLS**
Uric acid	≥ 476 umol/L	Laboratory TLS
Potassium	≥ 6 mmol/L	
Phosphorus	≥ 2.1 mmol/L (children) ≥ 1.5 mmol/L (adults)	And ≥1 among
Calcium	≤ 1.75 mmol/L	• Acute kidney injury • Seizure • Arrhythmia • Sudden death
Laboratory alterations should be measured within the same 24 hours and must occur within 3 days before and 7 days after therapy. TLS = tumour lysis syndrome		

Cancers Associated with TLS

- High - large-volume, highly metabolic malignancies such as B-cell ALL and Burkitt's lymphoma.
- Low risk - slow-growing hematologic malignancies (such as multiple myeloma).

Prevention

- Methods to increase GFR and urine output are appropriate regardless of risk category.
- Prophylactic use of recombinant urate oxidase before chemotherapy.

Management

Volume Expansion and Diuretics

- Augmenting potassium, phosphate and uric acid excretion.
- A robust urine flow rate will decrease the calcium-phosphate product in the renal tubules.
- Decreasing the risk of crystal formation and micro-obstruction.

Allopurinol

- Structural isomer of hypoxanthine.
- It is metabolized by xanthine oxidase to oxypurinol (inhibits the conversion of xanthine to uric acid).
- Treatment can elevate serum and urine xanthine levels.
- Allopurinol hypersensitivity syndrome—a constellation of rash, acute hepatitis and eosinophilia.
- Febuxostat is a novel xanthine oxidase inhibitor that does not have the hypersensitivity profile of allopurinol.

Urinary Alkalinization

- The solubility of uric acid is highly pH dependent.
- At a typical acidic urine pH of 5.0, the solubility of uric acid is 15 mg/dL vs 200 mg/dL at a pH of 7.0.
- A neutral urine pH may be achievable via the administration of bicarbonate with or without a carbonic anhydrase inhibitor.

Rasburicase

- Approved by the U.S. Food and Drug Administration in 2002 in children.
- It is an aspergillus-derived recombinant urate oxidase and catalyzes the conversion of uric acid to allantoin, carbon dioxide, and hydrogen peroxide.
- The latter can lead to devastating methemoglobinemia and hemolytic anemia in individuals with glucose-6-phosphate dehydrogenase deficiency.

Ans: (b) Urea, Creatinine, Phosphate, Ca2+ and K+

Ref: https://www.ncbi.nlm.nih.gov/pmc/articles/PMC4411564/

3. **Phocomelia:**

(a) Failure of calcification of cartilage
(b) Failure of membranous ossification
(c) Failure of development of flat bones
(d) Failure of development of long bones

Explanation:

Phocomelia Syndrome (PS)

- Rare birth defect that causes severe birth defects, especially of the **upper limbs**.
- The bones of the arms may be extremely **shortened** and **even absent.** The **fingers** of the hands may be **fused**.
- **Risk factors:**
  - Maternal **thalidomide therapy.**
  - **Genetic inheritance.**
  - **Roberts syndrome.**
- An extreme case results in the **absence of the upper bones of both the arms** and **legs** so that the hands and feet appear attached directly to the body. This is called **tetraphocomelia***.
- Other associated anomalies:
  - Encephalocele.
  - Hydrocephalus.
  - Bicornuate uterus.

- o Short neck.
- o Thrombocytopenia.
- o Renal and cardiac anomalies.

Ans: (d) Failure of development of long bones

Ref: Nelson, 20th edition

4. **A child with retarded growth came with triangular face, micrognathia, Tripod skull and fifth finger clinodactyly:**

(a) Russell-Silver syndrome
(b) Beckwith-Wiedemann syndrome
(c) Angelman syndrome
(d) Prader-Willi syndrome

Explanation:

Russell-Silver Syndrome

- Most cases occur sporadically, chromosome **11p15**, **maternal disomy** of **chromosome 7.**
- **Clinical features:**
  - o Intrauterine growth restriction and low birth weight.
  - o Poor appetite and feeding difficulties.
  - o Hypoglycemia, **short stature.**
  - o Scoliosis, Curving of the pinky finger (***clinodactyly***).
  - o **Characteristic facial features:** Prominent forehead; small, **triangular-shaped face**; a small jaw; a narrow chin; and down-turned corners of the mouth.
  - o Arms and legs of different lengths (body asymmetry).
  - o Delayed bone age.
  - o Head circumference is normal but may look bigger relative to small body size.
- **Possible risks include:**
  - o Metabolic syndrome.
  - o Uterine and vaginal dysgenesis (in females with 11p15-related RSS).
  - o Gonadal hypofunction or testicular cancer in males.
  - o Low muscle mass or low bone mineral density.
  - o Myoclonus dystonia (in people with chromosome 7-related RSS).

Syndromes with digit anamolies:

Digit anomaly	Physical feature	Syndrome associated
Clinodactyly	Medial or lateral curvature of digit (finger or toe), usually fifth or fourth finger, but can occur in any finger even thumb. Developmental arrest of the growth plate or Abnormal growth plate around the side of the bone – "bracketed epiphysis" typically occur in the middle pharynx and worsens with age.	• Down syndrome • Noonan syndrome • Edwards syndrome • TAR syndrome • Focal dermal hypoplasia (Goltz syndrome) • ***Russell-Silver syndrome*** • XXXX OR XXXXX females • Klinefelter syndrome • Turner syndrome • Carpenter syndrome • Cornelia de Lange syndrome
Syndactyly	Incomplete separation of the fingers. It most commonly occurs between the 3rd and 4th fingers and between the 2nd and 3rd toes	• Apert syndrome • Carpenter syndrome • de Lange syndrome • Holt-Oram syndrome • Orofaciodigital syndrome • Polysyndactyly • Trisomy 21 • Fetal hydantoin syndrome • Laurence-Moon-Biedl syndrome • Fanconi panctyopenia • Trisomy 13 • Trisomy 18

Contd.

Postaxial polydactyly	Extra finger or toe present on the lateral side of the hand or foot	• Carpenter syndrome • Ellis-van Creveld syndrome • Meckel-Gruber syndrome • Polysyndactyly • Trisomy 13 • Orofaciodigital syndrome • Rubinstein-Taybi syndrome
Preaxial polydactyly	Extra finger or toe present on the medial side of the hand or foot	
Brachydactyly	Having short digits	• Robinow syndrome • Albright Hereditary Osteodystrophy
Camptodactyly	Congenital deformity characterized by a flexed posture in the proximal interphalangeal joint. It is generally found in the little finger	• Antley-Bixler syndrome

Features of other syndromes:

Syndrome	**Beckwith-Wiedemann syndrome**	**Angelman syndrome**	**Prader-Willi syndrome**
Features	• Macrosomia • Macroglossia • Abdominal wall defects - omphalocele or umbilical hernia • Neonatal hypoglycemia • Hyperinsulinism • Hemihyperplasia/hemihypertrophy • Grooves in the ear lobes • Risk for Wilms tumor and hepatoblastoma • Intraorbital hypoplasia • Capillary nevus flammeus • Mandibular prognathism • Renal medullary dysplasia • Nephrocalcinosis	• Developmental delays • Learning disabilities • Ataxia • Hypotonia of the trunk • Hypertonia of the arms and legs • Unprovoked • Prolonged laughter and smiling • Prominent chin • Deep-set eyes • An abnormally wide mouth (marcostomia) with a protruding tongue • Widely-spaced teeth and an abnormally flat back of the head (brachycephaly) • Gastroesophageal reflux disorder	• Lethargy • Infantile hypotonia • Feeding difficulties • Disproportionately long • Narrow head (dolichocephaly) growth hormone deficiency • Short stature • Small genitals • An excessive appetite and obesity • Low normal intelligence with learning disabilities

Ans: (a) Russell-Silver syndrome

Ref: Nelson, Textbook of Pediatrics, 20th edition, page 2859

5. **Basic pathophysiology in Potter syndrome:**

(a) Maternal diabetes (b) Pulmonary hypoplasia
(c) Bilateral renal agenesis (d) Oligohydramnios

Explanation:

Potter Syndrome

- Oligohydramnios is the cause of the deformities observed in **Potter syndrome.**
- **Oligohydramnios** can be due to:
    - o **Bilateral renal agenesis / hypoplasia.**
    - o **Urinary tract obstruction.**
    - o **Polycystic kidneys.**
    - o **PROM.**
    - o **Uteroplacental insufficiency.**
- **Typical physical appearance** (**wide separated eyes** with **epicanthic folds, parrot beak nose, low set ears**, **redundant skin** and receding chin and **club foot**).

- **Pulmonary hypoplasia** resulting from **oligohydramnios.**
- **Compression** of the **neonate** in utero.
- Incidence–1 in 3,000 births.
- **Male predominance** (due to higher rate of **Eagle-Barrett (prune belly) syndrome** and **obstructive uropathy** secondary to **posterior urethral valves** in **males**).
- **Death** due to **pulmonary hypoplasia***.
- Potter syndrome / Potter sequence and oligohydramnios sequence are used interchangeably.

Ans: (d) Oligohydramnios

Ref: Nelson, Textbook of Pediatrics, 20th edition, page 833

6. Proximal muscle weakness atrophy in a child with PEM due to which electrolyte disturbance:

(a) Hypokalemia (b) Hypomagnesemia
(c) Hypophosphatemia (d) Hypocalcemia

Explanation:

Hypokalemia: • Heart and skeletal muscle (muscle weakness and cramps) are especially vulnerable to hypokalemia • Paralysis is a possible complication, generally only at levels <2.5 mEq/L (starts with the legs, followed by the arms) • Slows gastrointestinal motility (constipation levels <2.5 mEq/L) • Impairs bladder function, potentially leading to urinary retention • Causes polyuria and polydipsia	**Hypocalcemia:** • Muscular pain and cramps are early manifestations; they progress to numbness, stiffness, and tingling of the hands and feet positive Chvostek or Trousseau sign or laryngeal and carpopedal spasms. • Convulsions with or without loss of consciousness teeth erupt late and irregularly. Enamel formation is irregular, and the teeth may be unusually soft.
Hypophosphatemia: • Hypophosphatemia is a serum phosphate concentration **< 2.5 mg/dL (0.81 mmol/L)** • **Hemolysis** and **dysfunction of white blood cells**. • **Proximal muscle weakness and atrophy** • **Rhabdomyolysis** • **Cardiac dysfunction** • **Neurologic symptoms**, such as tremor, paresthesia, ataxia, seizures, delirium and coma	**Hypomagnesaemia:** • Magnesium levels **<0.7 mg/dL** • Causes **secondary hypocalcemia** by impairing the release of PTH by the parathyroid gland and through blunting the tissue response to PTH • Dominant manifestations of Hypomagnesaemia are due to **hypocalcemia**: **tetany**, **positive Chvostek and Trousseau signs** and **seizures**

Ans: (c) Hypophosphatemia

Ref: Nelson, Textbook of Pediatrics, 20th edition, page 833

7. An orthopedician adducts the flexed hip and gently pushes the thigh posteriorly in an effort to dislocate the femoral head of a neonate. What is this maneuver called?

(a) *Galeazzi sign* (b) Ortoloni test
(c) Telescopic sign (d) Barlow test

Explanation:

Developmental Dysplasia of the Hip (DDH)

- Ranges from simple acetabular **dysplasia**, acetabular dysplasia plus **subluxation** to **dislocation** of the hip joint.
- **Two major groups:**
  - **Typical** (otherwise normal individuals without defined syndromes or genetic conditions); and
  - **Teratologic** (with identifiable causes) – small, shallow acetabulum and a stiff hip joint at birth.
- 1–1.5 of 1000 live births, multifactorial etiology, involving both genetic and intrauterine environmental factors.
- Marked geographic and racial variation (Positive family history 12–33% of affected patients).

- Common – **female patients**, **left hip** (maternal hormones such as relaxin, which increases ligamentous laxity) and delivered by **cesarean section.**
- High rate of association in **tighter intrauterine space (oligohydramnios**, **large birth weight**, and **first pregnancy)** which supports the "**crowding phenomenon**" theory.

Untreated typical DDH have changes may include (hypertrophy of the lateral cartilage of the acetabulum (**neolimbus formation**), hypertrophy of the ligamentum teres, capsular laxity, **hourglass constriction of the hip capsule** and hypertrophy of the transverse acetabular ligament, and excess femoral anteversion).

Clinical Findings:

Characters	Barlow test	Ortolani test
Introduction	Provocative maneuver / assesses the potential for dislocation of a nondisplaced hip	Nonforced maneuver / reverse of Barlow test–attempt to reduce a dislocated hip
Method	Adducts the flexed hip and gently pushes the thigh posteriorly in an effort to dislocate the femoral head	Grasps the child's thigh between the thumb and index finger and, with the 4th and 5th fingers, lifts the greater trochanter while simultaneously abducting the hip
Positive test	The hip will be felt to slide out of the acetabulum and while relaxing the proximal push, the hip can be felt to slip back into the acetabulum	The femoral head will slip into the socket with a delicate "clunk" that is palpable but usually not audible

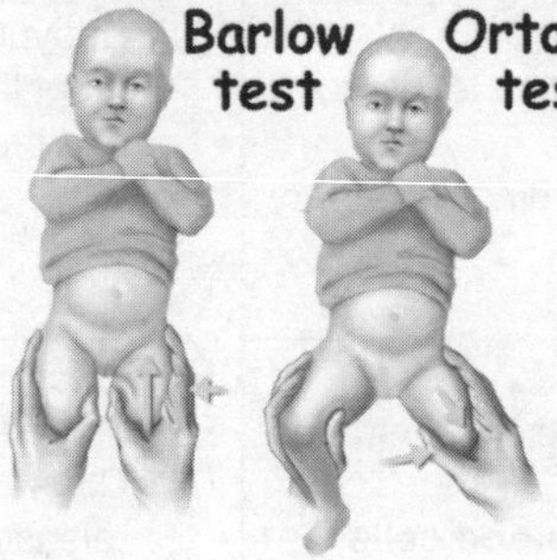

- **Hip click** - high-pitched sensation (or sound) felt at the very end of abduction during testing for DDH with Barlow and Ortolani maneuvers (originate in the ligamentum teres or occasionally in the fascia lata or psoas tendon and do not indicate a significant hip abnormality).
- **Hip clunk** - which is felt as the hip goes in and out of joint (signifies hip abnormality).
- **Infant (1 to 3 months of age)** - hip is no longer reducible, ***limited hip abduction*** **(**most reliable sign of a dislocated hip**)**, apparent shortening of the thigh, proximal location of the greater trochanter, asymmetry of the gluteal or thigh folds and pistoning of the hip.

Galeazzi sign (Shortening of the thigh): Placing both hips in 90 degrees of flexion and comparing the height of the knees, looking for asymmetry.
Klisic test Places the 3rd finger over the greater trochanter and the index finger of the same hand on the anterior superior iliac spine. • Normal hip - an imaginary line drawn between the two fingers points to the umbilicus. • Dislocated hip - the trochanter is elevated, and the line projects halfway between the umbilicus and the pubis.

Walking child–Limp (toe-walk on the affected side), a waddling gait, leg-length discrepancy, positive trendelenburg sign and excessive lordosis.

Ultrasonographic Findings:

- In < 6 mo of age - acetabulum and proximal femur are cartilaginous and not visible on plain radiographs and are best visualized with ultrasonography.
  - Dynamic assessment about the stability of the hip joint.
  - Monitor acetabular development, particularly of infants in Pavlik harness treatment.

Radiographic Findings:

> 6 mo of age. Anteroposterior view of the pelvis – use of several classic lines drawn on it			
Line	**Type**	**Landmarks**	**Interpretation**
Hilgenreiner line	Horizontal line	Drawn through the top of both triradiate cartilages (the clear area in the depth of the acetabulum).	• Perpendicular to the Hilgenreiner line • Ossific nucleus of the femoral head should be located in the medial lower quadrant of the intersection of these two lines
Perkins line	Vertical line	Through the most lateral ossified margin of the roof of the acetabulum	
Shenton line	Curved line	Drawn from the medial aspect of the femoral neck to the lower border of the superior pubic ramus	• Line is a continuous contour – normal • Two separate arcs / "broken" – in DDH
Acetabular index	Angle	Formed between the Hilgenreiner line and a line drawn from the depth of the acetabular socket to the most lateral ossified margin of the roof of the acetabulum (angle measures the development of the osseous roof of the acetabulum)	• Newborn, the acetabular index can be up to 40 degrees • By 4 months in the normal infant, it should be no more than 30 degrees
In older child			
Center-edge angle	Angle	Formed at the juncture of the Perkins line and a line connecting the lateral margin of the acetabulum to the center of the femoral head	• 6–13 years old, an angle >19 degrees – normal • > 14 years and older, an angle >25 degrees – normal

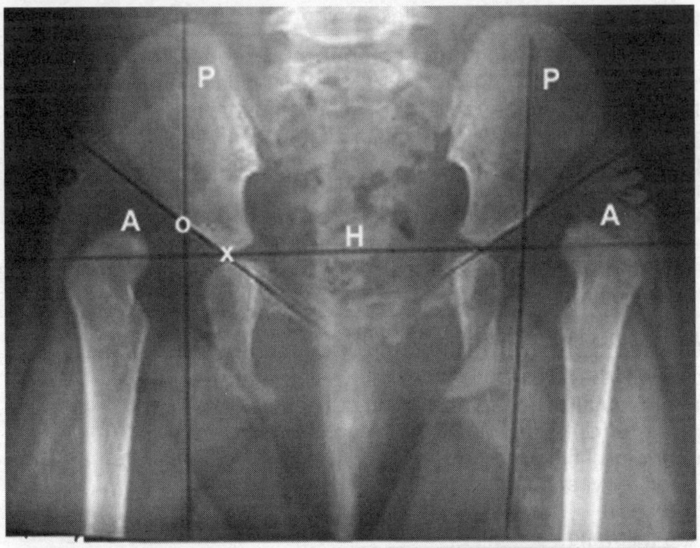

H - Hilgenreiner's Line
P - Perkins Line
A - Acetabular Index
x - triradiate cartilage
o - lateral border of acetabulum

Treatment Goals: Obtain and maintain a concentric reduction of the femoral head within the acetabulum.

Age	Treatment
< 6 months of age	• Triple diapers or abduction diapers no role. • Pavlik harness - In normal newborns with all degrees of hip dysplasia. • Other braces - von Rosen splint, Frejka pillow. • 1 and 6 mo of age - Pavlik harness (full-time basis for 6 weeks), hip instability resolves in 95% of cases. • 6 months of age, the failure rate for the Pavlik harness is >50% (increasingly active and crawling child).
6 months to 2 years	• *Closed reductions* under general anesthesia. And casting in human position of moderate flexion and abduction for 12 weeks. • The replaced by an abduction orthotic device for 2 months (until acetabular development is normal). • Failure to obtain a stable hip needs *open reduction.*
Older than 2 years of age	• **Open reduction** is usually necessary.
Sequlae: *Avascular necrosis of the Capital Femoral epiphysis (< 6 months of age),* redislocation, residual subluxation and acetabular dysplasia.	

Ans: (d) Barlow test

Ref: Nelson, Textbook of Pediatrics, 20th edition, page 3274

8. **Criteria for diagnosing SIRS all seen *except*:**

(a) Temp > 38.5 °C or < 36 °C
(b) RR > SD above normal for age
(c) Children <1 year old persistent bradycardia over 0.5 hour
(d) >50% immature neutrophils

Explanation:

Systemic Inflammatory Response Syndrome (SIRS)

- It's an inflammatory cascade that is initiated by the host in response to infection, occurs when the host defense system does not adequately recognize or clear the infection.

Infection	Suspected or proven infection or a clinical syndrome associated with high probability of infection
Systemic Inflammatory Response Syndrome (SIRS)	**2 out of 4 criteria, 1 of which must be abnormal temperature or abnormal leukocyte count** 1. **Core temperature** >38.5°C or <36°C (rectal, bladder, oral, or central catheter) 2. **Tachycardia**: Mean heart rate >2 SD above normal for age in absence of external stimuli, chronic drugs or painful stimuli; OR unexplained persistent elevation over 0.5–4 hr; OR in children <1 year old persistent bradycardia over 0.5 hr (mean heart rate <10th percentile for age in absence of vagal stimuli, β blocker drugs, or congenital heart disease) 3. **Respiratory rate** >2 SD above normal for age or acute need for mechanical ventilation not related to neuromuscular disease or general anesthesia 4. **Leukocyte count** elevated or depressed for age (not secondary to chemotherapy) or >10% immature neutrophils
Sepsis	SIRS plus a suspected or proven infection
Severe Sepsis	**Sepsis** plus 1 of the following: 1. **Cardiovascular organ dysfunction** defined as: Despite >40 mL/kg of isotonic intravenous fluid in 1 hr **Hypotension** <5th percentile for age, systolic blood pressure <2 SD below normal for age OR Need for **vasoactive drug** to maintain blood pressure OR 2 of the following: **Unexplained metabolic acidosis**: Base deficit >5 mEq/L **Increased arterial lactate** >2 times upper limit of normal **Oliguria**: Urine output <0.5 mL/kg/hr **Prolonged capillary refill** 5 sec **Core to peripheral temperature gap** >3°C 2. **Acute respiratory distress syndrome (ARDS)** as defined by the presence of a PaO_2/FiO_2 ratio ≤300 mm Hg, bilateral infiltrates on chest radiograph and no evidence of left heart failure OR **Sepsis** plus 2 or more organ dysfunctions (respiratory, renal, neurologic, hematologic or hepatic)

Contd.

Septic Shock	Sepsis plus cardiovascular organ dysfunction as defined above
Multiple Organ Dysfunction Syndrome (MODS)	Presence of altered organ function such that homeostasis cannot be maintained without medical intervention

Ans: (d) >50% immature neutrophils

Ref: Nelson, Textbook of Pediatrics, 20th edition, page 522

9. **Febrile seizure persisting continuously beyond ___ should be treated with midazolam nasal spray.**

(a) 3 minutes (b) 5 minutes (c) 8 minutes (d) 10 minutes

Explanation:

Febrile Seizures:

1. Between the age of 6 and 60 months with a temperature of 38°C (100.4°F) or higher.
2. That are not the result of central nervous system infection or any metabolic imbalance.
3. And that occur in the absence of a history of prior afebrile seizures.

Simple febrile seizure – Primary generalized, usually tonic–clonic, attack associated with fever, lasting for a maximum of 15 min, and not recurrent within a 24-hour period. Do not have an increased risk of mortality.

Complex febrile seizure – Prolonged (>15 min), is focal, and/or reoccurs within 24 hours, fold long-term increase in mortality.

Febrile status epilepticus is a febrile seizure lasting longer than 30 minutes.

Simple febrile seizure plus for those with recurrent febrile seizures within 24 hours.

Recurrence:

- 30% of those experiencing a first episode.
- 50% after 2 or more episodes; and
- 50% of infants younger than 1 year old at febrile seizure onset.
- 2-7% of children who experience febrile seizures proceed to develop epilepsy later in life.

Risk factor for recurrence

Major	Minor
• Age <1 year • Duration of fever <24 hours • Fever 38-39°C (100.4-102.2°F)	• Family history of febrile seizures • Family history of epilepsy • Complex febrile seizure • Daycare • Male gender • Lower serum sodium at time of presentation

Dravet syndrome* is the most severe of the phenotypic spectrum of febrile seizure-associated epilepsies.

Indication for Lumbar Puncture:

- All infants younger than 6 months of age who present with fever and seizure.
- Option in a child 6-12 months of age whose *Haemophilus influenzae* type B and *Streptococcus pneumonia* immunization.
- Status is unknown.

Indication for Electro Encephalogram (EEG):

- Do not predict the future recurrence of febrile seizures or epilepsy even if the result is abnormal.
- Performed within 2 weeks of a febrile seizure often have nonspecific slowing, usually posteriorly.
- Children with febrile status epilepticus.
- CT or MRI is not recommended in evaluating the child after a first simple febrile seizure.
- Child is neurologically abnormal, usually have unilateral swelling of their hippocampus acutely on MRI.

Treatment:

- Seizure lasts for longer than 5 min, acute treatment with diazepam, lorazepam, or midazolam is needed.
- Parents are very anxious concerning their child's seizures, intermittent oral diazepam (0.33 mg/kg every 8 hours during fever) / clonazepam (0.1 mg/kg/day).
- Antipyretics can decrease the discomfort of the child but do not reduce the risk of having a recurrent febrile seizure.
- Future epilepsy does not change with or without antiepileptic therapy.
- Iron deficiency is associated with an increased risk of febrile seizures.

Ans: (b) 5 minutes

Ref: Nelson, Textbook of Pediatrics, 20th edition, page 2829

10. Baby with fused eyes and single nasal chamber, undeveloped callosum. What is diagnosis?

(a) Holoprosencephaly (b) Schizencephaly (c) Plagiocephaly (d) Brachycephaly

Explanation:

Holoprosencephaly

Disorder of neuronal migration with defective cleavage of the prosencephalon (the forebrain of the embryo fails to develop into two hemispheres) and inadequate induction of the forebrain structures.
Cause - Mutations in the "sonic hedgehog" gene at 7q, maternal diabetes.

Three groups:

(1) Alobar–Severe facial anomalies, including lack of a nose and the eyes merged to a single median structure, e.g., cyclopia.
(2) **Semilobar**–Intermediate form.
(3) Lobar–Least severe form

Middle interhemispheric fusion (MIHF variant) or **syntelencephaly** - involves a segmental area of non-cleavage of the posterior frontal and parietal lobes.
Facial abnormalities - Cyclopia (**fused eyes and single nasal chamber**), cebocephaly, single central incisor tooth, premaxillary agenesis and anosmia.
A prenatal diagnosis - ultrasonography after the 10th week of gestation for more severe types.

Other disorder of neural migration:

Disorder	Pathology	Clinical features
LISSENCEPHALY/ AGYRIA	• Absence of cerebral convolutions, poorly formed sylvian fissure, giving the appearance of a 3–4 months fetal brain • Associated with enlarged lateral ventricles and heterotopias in the white matter	Presents with failure to thrive, microcephaly, marked developmental delay, and a severe seizure disorder. hypoplasia of the optic nerve and microphthalmia associated with **Miller-Dieker Syndrome (MDS)** • Gene LIS-1 (lissencephaly 1) that maps to chromosome region *17p13.3* is deleted • Prominent forehead, bitemporal hollowing, anteverted nostrils, a prominent upper lip, and micrognathia • CT and MRI scans typically show a smooth brain with an absence of sulci
SCHIZENCEPHALY	Presence of unilateral or bilateral clefts within the cerebral hemispheres	• Mental retardation, refractory seizures and microcephaly • Unilateral schizencephaly is a frequent cause of congenital hemiparesis • With spastic quadriparesis when the clefts are bilateral • CT scan is diagnostic and clearly demonstrates the size and extent of the cleft

Contd.

PORENCEPHALY	Presence of cysts - in sylvian fissure and typically communicate with the subarachnoid space, the ventricular system, or both, associated with microcephaly, abnormal patterns of adjacent gyri, and encephalocele	Mental retardation, spastic hemi- or quadriparesis, optic atrophy and seizures. **Pseudoporencephalic cysts** • Perinatal or postnatal period and result from abnormalities (infarction, hemorrhage) of arterial or venous circulation • Cysts extend to be unilateral • They do not communicate with a fluid-filled cavity; and • They are not associated with abnormalities of cell migration or CNS malformations • Present with hemiparesis and focal seizures in the 1st year of life

Ans: (a) Holoprosencephaly

Ref: Nelson, Textbook of Pediatrics, 20th edition, page 2640

11. **All are true regarding Hib vaccine *except*:**

(a) Protects against non capsulated H. influenza disease
(b) Catch up vaccination before 5 years
(c) Can be given in less than 6 months
(d) Given 2 weeks before splenectomy

Explanation:

Hemophilus Influenzae Type B (Hib) Conjugate Vaccines

- Capsulated H. influenzae has six serotypes of which type B - important invasive pathogen causing diseases such as meningitis, bacteremia, pneumonia, cellulitis, osteomyelitis, septic arthritis and epiglottitis.
- Natural protective immunity is acquired by the age of 3-4 years.
- No protection against - Non capsulated Hib disease - bronchitis, otitis media, sinusitis and some pneumonia.
- Vaccines should be stored at 2 to 8°C and the recommended dose is 0.5 ml intramuscularly.
- 90-100% efficacy against culture proven invasive Hib disease for 1 year after vaccination.

Age at initiation	**No. of doses**	**General measures**
Below 6 months	Three doses when initiated	Interval between two doses should be at least 4 weeks
Between 6 and 12 months	2 doses and 1 dose between 12 and 15 months, with a booster at 18 months	Catch up vaccination - 5 years of age
More than 15 months	Single dose	

- All individuals with functional/anatomic hyposplenia irrespective of age.

Vaccines recommended for functional/anatomical hypo or asplenia:

2 weeks prior to splenectomy

1. Hemophilus influenzae type B (hib) conjugate vaccines.
2. Meningococcal vaccines.
3. Pneumococcal vaccine.

Ans: (a) Protects against non capsulated H. influenza disease

Ref: Indian Academy of Pediatrics Guide Book on Immunisation, 2013–14

12. **Which of the following is true regarding whole cell pertussis vaccine?**

(a) Maternal antibody provides protection against pertussis
(b) Effectiveness against pertussis is more than diphtheria / tetanus
(c) Progressive neurological deficit is an absolute contraindication
(d) Not recommended for children more than 7 years of age

Explanation:

DTwP VACCINE

- **Triple antigen - tetanus** and **diphtheria** toxoids as well as **killed whole cell pertussis bacilli** adsorbed on insoluble **aluminium salts** which act as adjuvants.
- Diphtheria toxoid varies from 20 to 30 Lf and that of tetanus toxoid varies from 5 to 25 Lf per dose.
- Stored at **2 to 8°C,** never be frozen, and if frozen accidentally, should be discarded 0.5 ml intramuscularly.
- **No maternal antibody** for **protection** against **pertussis.**
- Three **primary doses** at **6, 10 and 14 weeks** and **2 boosters** at **15-18 months** and **5 years**.
- Effectiveness against **diphtheria/tetanus** of **three doses** of the vaccine exceeds **95%.**
- Vaccine against **pertussis** is lower and as per data from international trials ranges from 70-90%.
- **Adverse effects (pertussis component**)
    - o Fever more than 40.5°C.
    - o Persistent crying.
    - o Hypotonic hyporesponsive episodes.
    - o Seizures.
    - o Encephalopathy.
- No association with sudden infant death syndrome (SIDS), autism, chronic neurologic damage, infantile spasms, learning disorders and Reye's syndrome.
- **Absolute contraindications:**
    - o History of **anaphylaxis;** or
    - o Development of **encephalopathy within 7 days** following previous DTwP vaccination.
- **Relative contraindication:**
    - o Progressive/evolving neurological illnesses.
- **Precautions but not contraindications:**
    - o Persistent inconsolable crying of more than 3 hours duration.
    - o Hyperpyrexia (fever > 40.50 C)/HHE within 48 hours of DTwP administration; and
    - o Seizures with or without fever within 72 hours of administration of DTwP.
- **Not recommended** in children **above 7 years.**

Ans: (d) Not recommended for children more than 7 years of age

Ref: Indian Academy of Pediatrics Guide Book on Immunisation, 2013 - 14

13. Which of the following is false regarding neonatal resuscitation?

(a) T-tube delivers free flow oxygen
(b) Self-inflating bag needs reservoir
(c) Self-inflating bag can deliver free flow oxygen
(d) Flow inflating bag delivers free flow oxygen

Explanation:

The three types of equipment available for providing PPV in the newborn are:

(i) The Self inflating bag

Self inflating bag	
Avantages	• Will always refill after being squeezed, even without compressed gas source • Pressure limiting valve reduces risk of over-inflation
Disadvantages	• Will inflate even if there is no seal between mask and patient's face • Requires oxygen reservoir to provide high oxygen concentration • Cannot deliver free flow oxygen reliably with self inflating bag • Cannot be used to deliver continuous positive airway pressure (CPAP); can only deliver CPAP if postive end-expiratory pressure (PEEP) valve and pressurized gas is used.

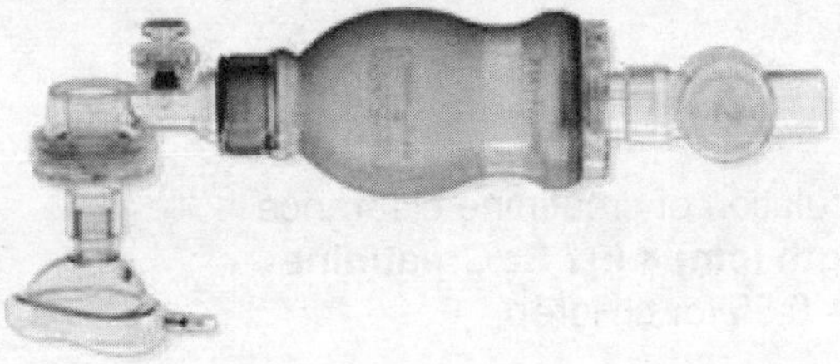

(ii) The Flow inflating bag (Anesthesia bag)

Flow inflating bag	
Advantages	• Can deliver free flow oxygen upto 100% depending on source • Easy to determine when there is a seal on the patient's face
Disadvantages	• Needs compressed gas source to work • Requires a tight seal between the mask and the patient's face to remain inflated • Usually does not have a safety pop-off valve; requires a pressure gauze to monitor pressure being delivered

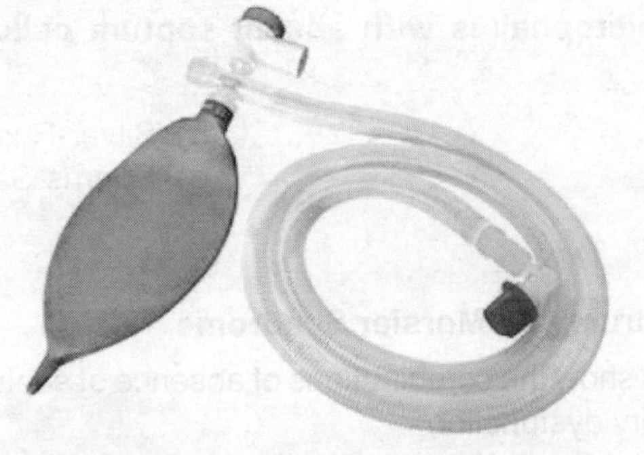

(iii) The T-piece resuscitator

T-piece resuscitator	
Advantages	• Consistent delivery of PIP and PEEP • Can be used to provide free flow oxgen reliably–21-100% (with blender) • Provider does not get tired from ventilation
Disadvantages	• Needs compressed gas with a blender • Requires pressures to be set prior to use • Changing inflation pressure during resuscitation is more difficult • Risks of prolonged inspiratory time

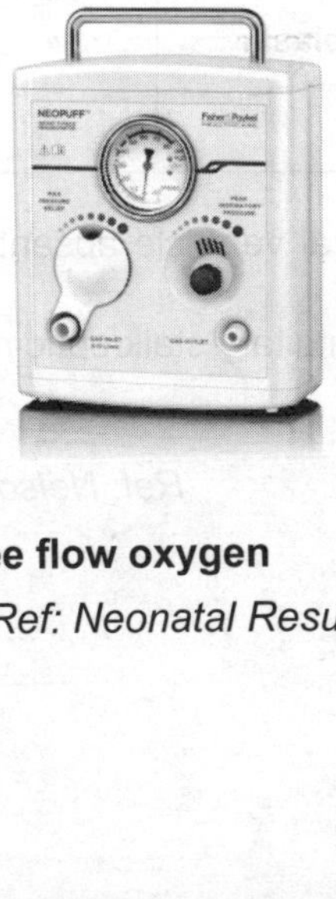

Ans: (c) Self-inflating bag can deliver free flow oxygen

Ref: Neonatal Resuscitation Protocol – India, 1st edition, page 35

14. Schwartz formula for creatinine clearance calculation. (Values) Urea – 49. Creat 2, length 85 cm and weight of 11 kg:

(a) 90 (b) 23 (c) 2.3 (d) 9

Explanation:

Schwartz equation: For calculation of creatinine clearance

CrCl (ml/min/1.73m^2) = [length (cm) × k] / Sr Creatinine

k = 0.45 for infants, k = 0.55 for children

In the above scenario

Crcl (Schwartz formula) = [85 × 0.55]/ 2

= 23.4 ml/min/1.73m^2

Other formulas to measure the creatinine clearance:

Cockcroft-Gault formula:

$$\text{Men} = \frac{(140 - \text{age}) \times \text{ideal weight}}{0.814 \times [\text{serum creatinine}]}$$

In women = 0.85 × creatinine clearance in men.

Ans: (b) 23

Ref: Nelson, Textbook of Pediatrics, 20th edition, page 2492

15. Hypoglycemia, jaundice, microphallus with absent septum pellucidum is characteristic of which syndrome?

(a) De Morsier syndrome (b) Silver-Russell syndrome
(c) Kallmann syndrome (d) Kearns-Sayre syndrome

Explanation:

Septo-optic Dysplasia Spectrum / De Morsier Syndrome

- Loss-of-function mutations show the combinations of absence of septum pellucidum, optic nerve hypoplasia and hypothalamo – pituitary dysfunction.
- *HESX1*, *OTX2*, and *SOX2* – Gene abnormalities and valproate / cocaine toxicity in utero.
- Hypoplasia of the optic nerve, abnormal formation of structures along the midline of the brain, and pituitary hypoplasia, agenesis of the septum pellucidum, partial or complete agenesis of the corpus callosum, malformation of the fornix, with a large chiasmatic cistern are seen.
- Nystagmus, visual impairment in infancy, anterior and/or posterior pituitary hormone deficiencies (Neonatal hypoglycemia, jaundice and microphallus) and seizures were the presenting features.
- Clinical presentation depends on presence or absence of schizencephaly.

With schizencephaly	Without schizencephaly
• Less severe visual impairment • Polymicrogyria, cortical dysplasia can be present • Referred to as **septo-optic dysplasia plus**	• Severe visual impairment • Hypothalamic-pituitary dysfunction common • Small ectopic posterior pituitary seen • Olfactory bulbs may be absent (Kallmann syndrome)

- CT brain – suggests enlarged lateral ventricle absent septum pellucidum, small optic apparatus, small bony optic foramen.
- MRI brain – suggests hypoplastic pituitary stalk/optic nerve.

Ans: (a) De Morsier syndrome

Ref: Nelson, Textbook of Pediatrics, 20th edition, page 2710

16. Formula to calculate intelligence quotient (IQ):

(a) Chronological age/Mental age × 100
(b) Mental age - Chronological Age × 100
(c) Mental age/Chronological age × 100
(d) Mental age + Chronological Age × 100

Explanation:

IQ = Mental Age / Chronological Age × 100

Distribution of intelligence in normal population

Classification of Types	I.Q. (Inteligence Quotient)
1. Near genius or genius	140 and above
2. Very superior	130-139
3. Superior	120-129
4. Above average	110-119
5. Normal or average	90-109
6. Below average	80-89
7. Dull or borderline	70-79
8. Feebleminded, moron	50-69
9. Imbecile	25-49
10. Idiot	0-24

Ans: (c) Mental age/Chronological Age × 100

Ref: Parks Textbook of Preventive and Social Medicine, 24th edition

17. An 8 days old neonate presents with hypoglycemia (Glucose – 17 mg%) and jaundice is diagnosed to have metabolic disorder. Most likely diagnosis:

(a) Hypothyroidism
(b) Galactosemia
(c) Glycogen storage disease
(d) Fatty acid oxidation defect

Explanation:

Galactosemia

- Due to deficiency of **galactose-1-phosphate uridyltransferase (GALT).**
- Newborn develop symptoms after ingestion of **lactose** (glucose-galactose disaccharide) through a standard formula or breast milk.
- **Clinical features**
  - Vomiting, diarrhea, feeding difficulties.
  - ***Hypoglycemia.***
  - ***Jaundice***, hepatosplenomegaly, liver dysfunction.
  - Renal tubulopathy.
  - Lethargy, irritability, seizures.
  - **Oil drop cataract.**
  - Increased risk of ***Escherichia coli* neonatal sepsis.**
- **Galactose** is elevated in **plasma**, and **galactose-1-phosphate** is elevated in **red blood cells.**
- Newborn screening programs screen for galactosemia either by measuring **GALT enzyme** activity or **galactose levels.**
- Substituting a **soy-based formula** for breastfeeding, later, a **galactose-restricted diet**.

Also Note

- **IEMs presenting with hypoglycemia:**
  - Organic acidurias.
  - Defects of fatty acid oxidation.
  - Defects of gluconeogenesis (glycogen storage disease type I or fructose-1, 6-bisphosphatase deficiency).

- **Nonketotic hypoglycemia** is the hallmark of **defects in fatty acid oxidation** while **hypoglycemia** associated with **metabolic acidosis** and **ketones** suggests an **organic acidemia** or defect of **gluconeogenesis**.

Defect	Clinical features	Lab features	Treatment
Fatty acid oxidation defect	• Hypoketotic hypoglycemia • Lactic acidosis • Cardiomyopathy • Hepatopathy	Abnormal acylcarnitine profile	Glucose infusion, carnitine (50-100 mg/kg/day), and avoid fasting
Glycogen storage disease	• Typically presents at ***3 to 6 months*** of age • Poor growth • Hypoglycemia • Hepatomegaly	Lactic acidosis, hypertriglyceridemia and hyperuricemia	Avoidance of fasting Frequent or continuous feeding

Ans: (b) Galactosemia

Ref: Nelson, Textbook of Pediatrics, 20th edition, page 726/Manual of Neonatal Care, Cloherty

18. Regarding FeNa, which of the following is true?

(a) FeNa is lower in neonates when compared to children
(b) FeNa is higher in intrinsic renal failure than pre renal failure
(c) Measurement of FeNa is affected by use of diuretic
(d) FeNa is similar in both pre term and term neonate

Explanation:

Fractional Excretion of Sodium (FeNa):

- Test used to assess the **tubular integrity.**
- Used to differentiate **pre renal and intrinsic renal failure.**
- The handling of sodium is often expressed as a **fractional excretion rate**.
- The fractional excretion of sodium (FeNa) is calculated as:

$$\textbf{FeNa (expressed in percentage)} = \frac{UNa/PNa \times 100}{UCr/PCr}$$

(UNa – Concentration of sodium in the urine , PNa – Concentration of sodium in the plasma, UCr – Concentration of creatinine in the urine, PCr – Concentration of creatinine in the plasma)

Parameter	Pre renal failure	Intrinsic renal failure
Specific gravity	>1.020	<1.010
Urine osmolality (UOsm)	> 500 mOsm/kg	< 350 mOsm/kg
Urine sodium (UNa)	< 20 mEq/L	> 40 mEq/L
FeNa	<1% (<2.5% in neonates)	>2% (>10% in neonates)

- Meaurement of FeNa within **6 hours** of **diuretic** may obscure the result.
- FeNa has limited value in **pre-term** neonates due to developmental tubular immaturity
- FeNa in normal individuals ranges from **0.3 to 1.6%,** depending on salt intake.
- In patients with **prerenal azotemia**, FeNa is less than **1%**, whereas it is above **3%** in **acute tubular necrosis** (as tubular integrity is lost).

Ans: (c) Measurement of FeNa is affected by use of diuretic

Ref: Nelson, Textbook of Pediatrics, 20th edition, page 2541

19. All statements regarding plasmodium knowlesi are false *except*:

(a) Occurs only in Africa
(b) Commonly affects children
(c) Causes relapsing malaria
(d) Not transmitted by anopheles mosquito

Explanation:

Plasmodium Knowlesi Infection

- **Plasmodium knowlesi** is a new species of malarial parasite diagnosed in **2004.**
- Plasmodium knowlesi is a primate malarial parasite commonly found in **South East Asia**. It causes malaria in long tailed macaques and has been shown also to infect humans, either naturally or artificially and cause human malaria.
- The infection is documented commonly in **Malaysia, Philippines, Indonesia and Singapore.**
- Plasmodium knowlesi is the most **common cause of malaria in childhood** in the **Kudat district of Malaysia.**
- Plasmodium knowlesi is **absent in Africa**. This may be because there are neither long tailed nor pig tailed macaques, which are the reservoir hosts of plasmodium knowlesi in Africa. **Lack of duffy antigen** in West Africans may also be a reason as duffy antigen is needed for the parasite to invade and hence lack of duffy antigen is protective.
- There has been **no report of plasmodium knowlesi infection from India** mainland but it has been reported in **Andaman islands.**
- Transmitted by the **bite of Anopheles mosquito.**
- Has a **replication period of 24 hours** in **human erythrocytes** and hence it causes **quotidian malaria.**
- **Relapses** are **not seen** in **plasmodium knowlesi infection** due to the **absence of hypnozoites in the exoerythrocytic phase.**
- Based on little evidence **chloroquine plus sulfadoxine pyrimethamine** is effective for treating plasmodium knowlesi infection. **Chloroquine** alone is effective in the treatment of **uncomplicated plasmodium knowlesi infection.**

Ans: (b) Commonly affects children

Ref: Nelson, Textbook of Pediatrics, 20th edition, Volume 1, page 1709,1718 and Vadivelan M, Dutta TK, Recent Advances in the Management of Plasmodium Knowlesi Infection, Trop Parasitol 2014; 4: 31-34

DERMATOLOGY

1. **Tuberculids is associated with:**

(a) Lupus vulgaris
(b) Lichen scrofulosorum
(c) Erythema nodosum
(d) Scrofuloderma
(e) Lupus pernio

Explanation:

Tuberculids

- Hypersensitivity reaction to M. tuberculosis or its products in a patient with significant immunity.
- The main features of tuberculids are:
  - Positive tuberculin test.
  - Evidence of manifest or past tuberculosis.
  - Positive response to antituberculous therapy.
- True tuberculids can be grouped as follows:
  - **Micropapular:** Lichen scrofulosorum.
  - **Papular:** Papulonecrotic tuberculid.
  - **Nodular:** Erythema induratum of Bazin; nodular tuberculid.

Lichen scrofulosorum:

- Lichenoid eruption of minute papules.
- Asymptomatic tiny closely grouped perifollicular lichenoid papules which may be skin coloured or yellowish or reddish-brown.
- The common sites of occurrence are the **trunk** and the **proximal limbs**.
- Occurs predominantly in **children** and **adolescents** with tuberculosis.
- Associated with a **strongly positive tuberculin reaction**. It is because of an immune response to haematological spread from an underlying tuberculous focus.

Papulonecrotic tuberculid:

- It is an eruption of **necrotizing papules.**
- Lesions are hard, dusky papules that crust or ulcerate to heal with atrophic scars.
- Affects **extensor aspect** of the **extremities** occurring in **symmetric crops.**
- Predominantly affecting **young adults**.

Erythema induratum of Bazin:

- Recurrent nodular and ulcerative lesions.
- Occurs secondary to tuberculosis elsewhere in the body.
- Lesions are commonly seen in **lower legs**, but can affect other areas.
- It is more common in women than men.
- The ulcers ragged, irregular and shallow with a bluish edge.

Treatment: Treatment of the tuberculids is by treating the underlying tuberculosis with appropriate anti-tubercular therapy.

(Rook's Textbook of Dermatology, 8th edition, page 31.21-31.23)

A Look at the Other Options Given in the Question:

Lupus vulgaris:

- It is a chronic, progressive, post-primary, paucibacillary form of **cutaneous tuberculosis**, occurring in a person with a moderate or high degree of immunity.
- The characteristic lesion is a plaque, composed of soft, reddish-brown papules, which resembles **'apple jelly' on diascopy**.
- **The edges of the lesion gradually extend in some areas** and heal with scarring in others, sometimes causing considerable tissue destruction over many years.

(Rook's Textbook of Dermatology, 8th edition, page 31.16)

Scrofuloderma:

- Form of **cutaneous tuberculosis** which results from the involvement and breakdown of **the skin overlying a contiguous tuberculosis focus.**
- This is usually a **lymph gland, an infected bone or joint, or a lacrimal gland or duct**.
- It presents as **bluish red nodules** over the **lymph node** or **bone** which break-down to form **undermined ulcers with bluish edge**.

(Rook's Textbook of Dermatology, 8th edition, page 31.14)

Erythema nodosum:

- Erythema nodosum is characterized by painful, erythematous and sometimes ecchymotic nodules on the anterior surface of the legs.
- This commonly occurs in **young women**.
- The condition may be idiopathic or could occur secondary to **streptococcal** infections, and **sarcoidosis**, **Hodgkin's and non-Hodgkin's lymphoma**, **leukemia** and **renal cell carcinoma**. Rarely **tuberculosis** could also be a cause of erythema nodosum.

(Rook's Textbook of Dermatology, 8th edition, page 50.82-50.84)

Lupus pernio:

- It is the **nasal form of sarcoidosis.**
- It is more common in **women**.
- Large bluish-red and dusky **violaceous infiltrated nodules and plaques** occur symmetrically on the nose, cheeks, ears, fingers, hands and toes.
- The lesions may feel soft, doughy or indurated.
- Discrete nodules with a **typical appearance on diascopy** may be found at the edge sometimes.
- The surface is often glistening, and the epidermis stretched, with large pilosebaceous follicles.
- It affects the nasal septum causing obstruction.
- They invariably have multisystem disease.

(Rook's Textbook of Dermatology, 8th edition, page 61.9)

Ans: (b) Lichen scrofulosorum

Ref: Rook's Textbook of Dermatology, 8th edition, page 31.21-31.23

2. **Antibiotic of choice for toxic shock syndrome:**

(a) Linezolid
(b) Clindamycin
(c) Vancomycin
(d) Cephalexin

Explanation:

Management of TSS

- TSS is usually managed in the intensive care setting and the main line of management is **supportive management** along with **appropriate antibiotic therapy** to eradicate Staph. aureus which is mostly the causative organism.
- Because of the increasing frequency of methicillin-resistant Staphylococci in the community, **vancomycin** is often recommended*.

- Beta lactamase resistant penicillins are not very effective due to emerging resistance and they may increase TSST-1 production in vitro probably due to cell lysis. Hence, If they are prescribed they are usually coprescribed with clindamycin which inhibits bacterial protein toxin production.
- Other treatment options are a **combination of vancomycin and clindamycin** for suspected serious staphylococcal infections pending culture and sensitivity.
- **Intravenous immunoglobulin** (IVIG; which presumably acts in part via neutralizing antibodies against toxins) has been used and appears to have significant promise. At present, IVIG is used in severe or recalcitrant cases.

Ans: (c) Vancomycin

Ref: Fitzpatrick, Section 29, Bacterial Disease, page 2155-56

3. **A boy presents with erythematous scaly papules with crusting over on antecubital fossa. He was applying petroleum based emollient in the shower. What is the next step in management?**

(a) Decrease the frequency of petroleum
(b) Decrease the frequency of shower
(c) Mupirocin 1% topical application
(d) Triamcinolone cream topical application

Explanation:

- The given history of erythematous scaly papules with crusting over antecubital fossa in a boy is suggestive of a diagnosis of **atopic dermatitis**. The fact that he was advised emollient in shower also suggests the same as dry skin is quite common in patients with atopic dermatitis.
- The treatment of choice for **limited atopic dermatitis** is **topical corticosteroids**. In the given option Triamcinolone cream is the only topical corticosteroid hence that option is right. This will decrease the inflammation and decrease the lesions.
- Atopic dermatitis shows typical distribution according to the age. In the infants it frequently involves the **face and the extensors**. In the **childhood phase** and **adults flexural involvement** is very common.

Ans: (d) Triamcinolone cream topical application

Ref: Rook's Textbook of Dermatology, 8th edition, page 24.20

4. **Majocchi granuloma is due to:**

(a) Microsporum gypsum
(b) Epidermophyton
(c) Trichophyton rubrum
(d) Microsporum

Explanation:

Majocchi's Granuloma

- Superficial and subcutaneous **fungal infection** caused by **dermatophytes**.
- It involves the deeper portions of the **hair follicles** and presents as scaly follicular papules and nodules that coalesce in an annular arrangement.
- It is caused most commonly by **T. rubrum, T. interdigitale** and **M. canis**.
- Majocchi's granuloma is commonly seen on the **legs** in **women** who become inoculated after shaving or who apply **topical corticosteroids** to the involved area, which facilitates infection. It is also observed increasingly among **immunocompromised individuals.**
- Biopsy may be used to aid in the diagnosis of Majocchi's granuloma in which KOH examination of scale on the surface may more often be negative.

Also Note:

Majocchi's disease (Purpura annularis telangiectodes)

- One should not get confused with the **Majocchi's disease** which is a type of **idiopathic pigmented purpuric dermatosis** which presents as an eruption in young adults of either sex.
- The lesions are small plaques 1–3 cm across that are usually **annular** from their onset.
- Lesions consist of **telangiectases** and **haemosiderin** staining of the skin.
- They may be purple, yellow or brown, and may contain **'cayenne pepper' spots**.

- Treatment is usually ineffective.

Ref: Rook's Textbook of Dermatology (Chapter 49: Purpura and Microvascular Occlusion), 49.22

Ans: (c) Trichophyton rubrum

Ref: Fitzpatrick, 8th edition, Section 30, Fungal Diseases, page 2288 & 2284

5. **Shave biopsy is not done in:**

(a) Viral warts
(b) Seborrheic keratoses
(c) Basal cell carcinoma
(d) Melanoma

Explanation:

Shave Biopsy

- Used for lesions that is predominantly epidermal without extension into the dermis.
- Such lesions include warts, papillomas, skin tags, superficial basal or squamous cell carcinomas and seborrheic or actinic keratoses.
- This type of biopsy is not appropriate for suspicious pigmented lesions.
- Superficial shave removes a thin disk of tissue, typically by scalpel, Dermablade, a double-edged razor blade or scissors.
- This procedure yields a flat, thin specimen of combined epidermis and upper dermis (less than 1 mm).

Indications: Elevated (Exophytic) Neoplasms

- Viral warts.
- Skin tag.
- Non-pigmented benign nevus.
- Keratocanthoma.
- Dermatofibroma.
- Seborrheic keratosis.
- Actinic keratosis.
- Cutaneous horn.
- Possible small localized low-risk cancer.
  - Basal cell cancer.
  - Squamous cell cancer.

Contraindications

- Pigmented lesions.
- Melanomas.
- Subcutaneous lesions.

Ans: (d) Melanoma

Ref: Rook, Histopathology of the Skin: General Principles and Lever's Histopathology, 9th edition, page 7

ANESTHESIOLOGY

1. **Anaphylaxis occurring at the end of anaesthesia is due to:**

(a) Inhalational agents
(b) Opioids
(c) NSAIDs
(d) Latex allergy

Explanation:

*"Anaphylaxis caused by **latex** is more likely to be delayed or to occur later during the procedure compared with muscle relaxants or induction agents." Ref: Mali S. Anesth Essays Res 2012 Jul-Dec; 6(2): 124–133*

*"If the signs appear later, during the maintenance of anesthesia, they suggest an allergy to **latex, volume expanders or dyes."** Ref: Mertes PM et al., Epidemiology of Perioperative Anaphylaxis. Presse Med 2016 Sep;45(9):758-67*

Anaphylaxis During Anesthesia

- Anaphylaxis can be caused by the **opioid** due to release of **histamine**. It is very rare.
- Muscle relaxants – Most common cause of anaphylaxis during anesthesia.
- Inhalation agents: Never causes anaphylaxis.
- NSAIDs: Few cases have been reported of arrhythmia with intravenous diclofenac but not anaphylaxis.
- Latex allergy: 2nd most common cause of anaphylaxis during anesthesia. Mostly noted late during the **perioperative** and never early. Allergic reactions to latex occur late intraoperatively as time is needed to absorb the allergen through the mucosa or peritoneum.
- Anaesthetic drugs which can cause anaphylaxis are:
  - Succinylcholine.
  - Atracurium.
  - Morphine.
  - Propofol (Egg allergy).
  - Thiopenthol sodium (sulfa drug allergy).

Causes of Anaphylaxis During Anesthesia

- Muscle relaxants–Most common cause.
- Latex allergy–2nd Most common cause.
- Drug induced:
  - Antibiotics (Most common drug induced cause)–Beta-lactam antibiotics and vancomycin (Most common antibiotic).
  - NSAIDs – 2nd most common drug induced cause.
  - Anaesthetic drugs which can cause anaphylaxis are:
    - Succinylcholine.
    - Atracurium.
    - Morphine.
    - Propofol (Egg allergy).
    - Thiopenthol sodium (sulfa drug allergy).

Ans: (d) Latex allergy

Ref: Stoelting Pharmacology, 4th edition, page 87

2. **Patient is treated with dantrolene. All the following are adverse effects *except*:**

(a) Hypokalemia (b) Muscle weakness
(c) Breathlessness (d) Bradycardia

Explanation:

Dantrolene is a calcium channel blocker.

MOA:

- Skeletal muscle relaxation by inhibiting Ca^{++} release from endoplasmic reticulum (intracellular storage site) through ryanodine receptor.
- Stabilization of plasma membrane.

Ph/K:

- Available in oral and IV preparations.
- IV preparation is highly alkaline (pH 9.5) and causes thrombophlebitis.
- Injections are always diluted in **Mannitol** to make it isotonic with plasma.
- Metabolized in liver into an active metabolite 5 hydroxy-dantrolene.

Clinical Uses:

- Management of skeletal muscle spasticity due to upper motor neuron lesions.
- Prevention and treatment of malignant hyperthermia.

Side Effect:

- Skeletal muscle weakness.
- Nausea and diarrhea.
- Blurred vision.
- Hyperkalemia.
- Hepatitis (if received > 60 days).

* Breastfeeding is safe after 48 hours of discontinuation of treatment.

Ans: (a) Hypokalemia

Ref: Stoelting Pharmacology, 4th edition, page 596-597

3. **A cardiovascular parameter helpful in diagnosis of anaphylaxis during anaesthesia:**

(a) Dysrhythmia (b) Bradycardia
(c) Increased peripheral vascular resistance (d) Hypotension

Explanation:

"Anaphylaxis always should be considered if immediate, unexpected hypotension develops, with or without bronchospasm, following parenteral administration of a therapeutic agent or the induction of anesthesia."

Anaphylaxis

- Life-threatening syndrome resulting from the sudden release of mast cell- and basophil-derived mediators into the circulation.
- Foods and medications cause most anaphylaxis for which a cause can be identified, but virtually any agent capable of directly or indirectly activating mast cells or basophils can cause this syndrome.
- Histamine activates H1 and H2 receptors. **Pruritus, rhinorrhea, tachycardia**, and **bronchospasm** are caused by activation of the **H1 receptors**, whereas both **H1 and H2** receptors mediate **headache, flushing and hypotension.**
- Histamine binding to H1 receptors during anaphylaxis also stimulates endothelial cells to convert the amino acid L-arginine into **nitric oxide (NO),** a potent autacoid **vasodilator**. NO activates guanylate cyclase, leading to vasodilation and the production of cyclic guanosine monophosphate. Physiologically, NO helps modulate vascular tone and regional blood pressure. Enhanced NO production decreases venous return, thus contributing to the vasodilation that occurs during anaphylaxis.

Grade of Severity in Anaphylaxis

Grade 1	Generalized cutaneous signs: Erythema, urticaria, with or without angioedema
Grade 2	Moderate multiorgan involvement with cutaneous signs, **hypotension** and tachycardia, bronchial hyperreactivity: Cough, difficulty to inflate
Grade 3	Severe life-threatening s multiorgan involvement: Collapse, tachycardia or bradycardia, arrhythmias, bronchospasm. Cutaneous signs may be present or occur only after the arterial blood pressure recovers
Grade 4	Cardiac and/or respiratory arrest

Management:

- Assessment of airway, breathing, circulation and adequacy of mentation.
- Place patient in **supine position** with **elevation of the lower extremities** and monitor vital signs.
- Administer aqueous **epinephrine** 1:1000 dilution, 0.3-0.5 mL (0.01 mg/kg in children; maximum dose, 0.3 mg), intramuscularly into the arm (deltoid) every 5 minutes.
- Aqueous epinephrine 1:1000, 0.1-0.3 mL in 10 mL of normal saline (1:100,000 to 1:33,000 dilution), administered intravenously over several minutes may be used and repeated as necessary in anaphylaxis not responding to epinephrine injections and volume resuscitation. Continuous hemodynamic monitoring is essential.
- Administer oxygen at 6-8 L/min.
- Administer normal saline intravenously for fluid replacement and venous access. If severe hypotension exists, rapid infusion of volume expanders (colloid-containing solutions) is necessary.
- If cardiac arrest then do CPR as per guidelines.

Ans: (d) Hypotension

Ref: Mali S. Anaphylaxis During the Perioperative Period, Anesth Essays Res 2012 Jul-Dec; 6(2): 124–133

4. **True statement regarding 'prone position' ventilation in a polytrauma patient with ARDS:**

(a) Should be tried for 6 –8 hours
(b) Current evidence shows no improvement in outcome
(c) Suited for patients with high PaO_2/FiO_2 ratio only
(d) Definite improvement in PaO_2 in all patients

Explanation:

Prone Position Ventilation

- It is well established that body position can affect the distribution of ventilation.
- Normally during spontaneous breathing, ventilation is higher in the dependent areas of the lungs because the pleural pressure changes during breathing are greater in the dependent areas compared with the independent areas. This may not be true in diseases like **ALI** and **ARDS** because edema and injury occur primarily in the dependent (dorsal) lung region of the supine patient.
- Placing the patient with ARDS in a prone position may:
  - **Improve oxygenation** (increases in PaO_2 can range from 10 to 50 mm Hg or ≥20%); and
  - **Decrease the degree of shunt** present in the lungs (range in one study from 25% to 12%).
- Improvement in PaO_2 may not be seen in all patients (non-responders).
- The mechanisms believed to improve oxygenation with prone positioning are as follows:
  - Blood is redistributed to areas that are better ventilated.
  - Blood redistribution may also improve alveolar recruitment in previously closed areas of lung.
  - Redistribution of fluid and gas results in an improved relation between ventilation and perfusion.
  - Prone positioning changes the position of the heart so it no longer puts weight on underlying lung tissue.
  - Pleural pressure is more uniformly distributed, which could improve alveolar recruitment
  - Prone positioning changes the regional diaphragm motion.

Contraindications of Prone Position Ventilation

- Spinal cord instability.

- Hemodynamic instability.
- Cardiac rhythm disturbance.
- Thoracic and abdominal surgery.
- There is no consensus about the length of time a patient can be placed in the prone position. Recommendations range from 2 to 24 **hours**, although it may require more than **6 hours** of positioning daily, to improve oxygenation status.
- Prone positioning may improve survival in patients with **severe ARDS.**
- Prone positioning is indicated early in the management of all patients with ARDS.
- Patients in prone position are ventilated with a restrict lung protective ventilation protocol characterized by small tidal volumes.

Ans: (a) Should be tried for 6–8 hours

Ref: Pilbeam's Mechanical Ventilation–Physiological and Clinical Applications, 5th edition, page 244-247 and World J Crit Care Med 2016 May 4; 5(2): 121–136

5. A one year child, preterm, low birth weight with delayed milestones is posted for elective hernia repair. Which of the following statement is true?

(a) Wait for complete neurological evaluation
(b) Avoidance of inhalational agent
(c) Avoidance of regional anesthesia
(d) Avoidance of combination of inhalational and muscle relaxation

Explanation:

*"A complete history and physical examination is **essential** before anaesthetizing these children."*

*"In the absence of a **precise diagnosis**, children presenting with an undiagnosed neuromuscular disease **should not have elective surgery or anaesthesia** other than as part of the diagnostic process."*

Ref: Vindra, et al., Anaesthesia for Children with Neuromuscular Disease, Continuing Education in Anaesthesia Critical Care and Pain, Volume 10, Issue 5, 1 October 2010, pages 143–147

- **Inguinal hernia repair** is the most common general surgical procedure performed by pediatric surgeons.
- Males are more frequently affected than females, and the incidence of inguinal hernia is highest in the first year of life.
- Right-sided hernias (60%) occur more frequently than left-sided (30%) and bilateral (10%) hernias.
- Risk factors associated with inguinal hernias are prematurity, chronic respiratory illness, and excessive intraperitoneal fluid (ventriculoperitoneal shunts, ascites, peritoneal dialysis).
- Anesthesia can be induced by mask inhalation of volatile agents or by IV or rectal technique.
- Endotracheal intubation is usually unnecessary for herniorrhaphy, except in infants younger than 1 year, in whom it may be difficult to maintain an adequate airway with bag and mask ventilation without distending the stomach.
- **Premature** infants have a particularly high incidence of **inguinal hernias**. In these infants, for whom an inhalation anesthetic may have increased risks, spinal anesthesia and caudal epidural anesthesia have been used successfully to avoid general anesthesia and endotracheal intubation.
- The history is compatible with **cerebral palsy** or **congenital myopathies**. Since this is an elective surgical repair, complete neurological workup and diagnosis is necessary before anesthetic risk can be assessed.
- These children are ideal for assessment by a **multidisciplinary team** which include anaesthesiologists and pediatrician. **A complete history and physical examination is essential before anaesthetizing these children**, including a discussion of postoperative pain management with the parents. Cognitive and communication problems may make preoperative assessment more difficult. Parents and caretakers are best to be involved during this period not only to gain information but also allay the fears of the child.

Anesthetic Concern in Cerebral Palsy

- Intraoperative hypothermia and slow emergence.
- Suxamethonium does not cause hyperkalaemia in these patients, and a rapid sequence induction may be indicated.

Anesthetic Concern in Neuromuscular Diseases

- The incidence of anaesthesia-induced rhabdomyolysis is significant.
- Succinylcholine and volatile agents should be avoided in at-risk children.

Ans: (a) Wait for complete neurological evaluation

Ref: Smith's Pediatric Anaesthesia, page 749 and Indian J Anaesth 2008;52, page 397

6. **A child during anesthesia with Halothane and succincyl coA develops severe stiffness of masseters. What is the most probable diagnosis?**

(a) Neuroleptic malignant syndrome
(b) Malignant hyperthermia
(c) Anaphylaxis
(d) Halothane hepatitis

Explanation:

Malignant Hyperthermia

- Rare genetic disease (1:15,000 in pediatric patients and 1:40,000 adult patients) characterized by an acute hypermetabolic state within muscle tissue following induction of general anesthesia.
- It is a clinical syndrome observed during GA associated with rapidly increasing temperature of >1degree/ 5 min.

Etiology

- It is due to the abnormality of **Ryanodine receptor**, which is a calcium releasing channel of sarcoplasmic reticulum.
- The abnormality leads to excessive accumulation of calcium which causes sustained contraction of the muscle.

Causative Agents

- ***Muscle Relaxants:*** **Succinyl choline – Most common drug*.**

Inhalational agents	***Local Anesthetic:*** **Lignocaine**
• Halothane – Most common agent • Isoflurane • Desflurane • Enflurane • Sevoflurane • Methoxyflurane	***Other drugs:*** • Tricyclic antidepressants • MAO inhibitors • Phenothiazines

Risk Factors

- **Drugs:**
  - Halogenated general anesthetics (Ether, cyclopropane, halothane, isoflurane, sevoflurane, desflurane, enflurane, methoxyflurane).
  - Nondepolarizing muscle relaxants–Succinylcholine.
- **Family history of malignant hyperthermia.**
- **Myopathy**
  - Duchenne muscular dystrophy.
  - Arthrogryposis multiplex congenita.
  - Osteogenesis imperfecta.
  - Congenital strabismus.
  - Central core diseases.
  - History of neuroleptic malignant syndrome.
- **Pathology**
  - Due to abnormal **ryanodine Ryr1 receptor**. This calcium channel receptor is responsible for calcium release from the sarcoplasmic reticulum and plays a critical role in muscle depolarization.
  - Recent studies have revealed that many MH patients have a normal ryanodine receptor and those abnormalities in **secondary messengers and modulators of calcium release**, such as **fatty acids and phosphatidylinositol**, may be present.
  - An abnormal **sodium channel in skeletal muscle** may also play a role in some patients.

Clinical Features

• Hyperthermia • Hypoxia • Cyanosis • Hyperkalemia	• Muscle rigidity • Tachycardia • Hypertension • Cardiac Arrhythmias	• Renal failure • DIC • Pulmonary edema • Cerebral edema

Sign and Symptoms

Hypermetabolism	Increased sympathetic activity	Muscle damage	Hyperthermia
↑CO_2 production ↑O_2 consumption ↓Mixed venous O_2 tension Cyanosis Mottling	Tachycardia Hypertension Arrhythmia	Masseter spasm Generalized rigidity ↑Serum creatinine kinase ↑K, ↑Na and ↑PO_4 Myoglobinuria	Fever Shivering

Investigations

- Severe metabolic acidosis (pH < 7).
- Increased end tidal CO_2.
- Increased CPK levels.
- Increased myoglobin.

Treatment: Malignant Hyperthermia Protocol

- Stop all anesthetics immediately.
- Hyperventilation with 100% O_2.
- Correct electrolyte imbalance – Hyperkalemia.
- Maintain urine output.
- **Discontinue volatile anesthetic** and succinylcholine.
- Hyperventilate with 100% O_2 at high flows.
- Correct acidosis: Administer **sodium bicarbonate**, 1–2 mEq/kg intravenously.
- **Drug of choice: DANTROLENE SODIUM*** with sterile distilled water and administer 2.5 mg/kg intravenously as soon as possible. 2 mg/kg every 5 minutes to a maximum of 10 mg/kg.
- Institute **cooling measures** (lavage, cooling blanket, cold intravenous solutions).
- Administer **inotropes** and **antiarrhythmic agents** as necessary.
- Change anesthetic tubing and soda lime.
- Monitor urinary output, K+, Ca2+, blood gases, end-tidal carbon dioxide; perform clotting studies.
- Treat severe hyperkalemia with dextrose, 25–50 g intravenously, and regular insulin, 10–20 U intravenously (adult dose).
- Consider invasive monitoring of arterial blood pressure and central venous pressure.

Ans: (b) Malignant hyperthermia

Ref: Ajay Yadav, Short Textbook of Anaesthesia, 5th edition

RADIOLOGY

1. **Which of the following is true?**

(a) I-125 half life is 60 days

(b) I-131 half life is 12 days

(c) I-125 is used for treating thyroid metastasis

(d) I-131 is used in functional thyroid scan

Explanation:

Iodine-125

- Iodine-125, half life–**60 days.**
  - Commonly used in **brachytherapy** in the treatment of cancer especially in **prostate cancer,** enclosed in an implanted titanium capsule.
  - It is also widely used in **Radioimmunoassay** to show presence of hormones in tiny quantities.

Iodine-123

- Half-life–13 hours
- Has **no beta activity only gamma activity** and is more suitable as nuclear imaging tracer to evaluate the **anatomic and physiologic function** of the **thyroid** (thyroid scintigraphy/functional scan/radioactive iodine uptake/RAIU).
- Abnormal results may be caused by disorders such as **Graves' disease or Hashimoto's thyroiditis**.
- **Tc99m pertechnetate** is also used for functional imaging of **thyroid** (used in India due to nonavailability **of I-123).**

Iodine-131

- Half life–8 days.
- Preferred for Radiotherapy, widely used for localizing and treating **thyroid cancer** and **thyroid metastasis** and in **imaging the thyroid.**
- I-131 has **both a beta and gamma decay.**
- Destruction of thyroid tissue by Iodine-131 is due to emission of **Beta Rays.**
- Iodine-131 is also used in tissue targeting radiopharmaceutical agents such as **MIBG.**
- The high energy beta radiation from I-131 causes it to be the most carcinogenic of the iodine isotopes.

Iodine-124

- Iodine-124 is a proton-rich isotope of iodine with a half-life of 4.18 days.
- Its modes of decay are: 74.4% electron capture, 25.6% positron emission.
- Iodine-124 can be made by numerous nuclear reactions via a cyclotron.
- Iodine-124 as the iodide salt can be used to directly image the thyroid using positron emission tomography (PET).

Ans: (a) I-125 half life is 60 days

Ref: Walters and Millers, Textbook of Radiotherapy, 5th edition

2. **Mark the correct statement:**

(a) I-131 is used for radioactive ablation
(b) I-125 is used for thyroid scanning
(c) I-131 is used for thyroid scanning
(d) I-123 is used in radioactive ablation

Explanation:

Radioactive Iodine:

- It is used both as a diagnostic as well as a therapeutic agent. The commonly used radio iodine are I-131 and I-123.
- **Both I-123 and I-131** are tapped by active follicular cells and organified and hence used in the evaluation of thyroid cancers and also in evaluating suspected lingual thyroids and substernal goitres.
- **I-131** is used for radioactive iodine therapy in cancers, as it emits higher levels of beta radiation and is the screening modality of choice in evaluation of metastasis in thyroid cancers and has longer half-life of 8 days.
- **I-123** is used for diagnostic studies as it has low dose radiation and short half-life 12 to 13 hours.
- For diagnostic purpose **I-123** is given orally in empty stomach on previous day (dose—5 micro curie) and patient should not take L-thyroxine for 6 weeks prior to radioisotope study.
- Using Geiger Muller's gamma ray counter, scanning of thyroid gland is done to visualize the gland.
- Hot area suggests more uptake, warm area suggests normal uptake, cold area suggests no uptake.
- Incidence of malignancy is 20% in cold nodules and 5% in warm or hot nodules.

Ans: (a) I-131 is used for radioactive ablation

Ref: Sabiston, Textbook of Surgery, 20th edition, page 897

3. **Radioimmunoassay for thyroid hormones:**

(a) I-131 (b) I-125 (c) I-123 (d) I-127

Explanation:

Refer previous question.

Ans: (b) I-125

Ref: Walters and Millers, Textbook of Radiotherapy, 5th edition

4. **Half-life of which pair is correct?**

(a) I-131- 80 days
(b) I-123-13 hours
(c) I-132- 12 days
(d) I-125- 60 days

Explanation

- Half-life of I-123 is 12 to 13 hours
- Half-life of I-131 is 8 days
- Half-life of Tc 99m is 6 hours

Isotope	Half life
Americium-241	433 years
Antimony-124	60.2 days
Californium-252	2.63 years
Cesium-137	30.1 years
Cobalt-57	271 days
Cobalt-58	71.3 days
Cobalt-60	5.272 years
Iodine-124	4.17 days
Iodine-130	12.4 hours
Iodine-131	8.041 days

Contd.

Iron-52	8.3 hours
Iron-55	2.7 years
Iron-59	44.6 days
Manganese-52	5.63 days
Manganese-54	312.5 days
Molybdenum-99	66.02 hours
Osmium-191	15.3 days
Technetium-99 m	6.02 hours

Ans: (b) I-123-13 hours

Ref: Sabiston, Textbook of Surgery, 20th edition, page 987

5. Which of the following is a radioactive substance?

(a) Bromide (b) P^{32} (c) C^{13} (d) I^{127}

Explanation:

ISOTOPES Used in Medicine

Reactor Radioisotopes (half-life indicated in brackets):

- **Molybdenum-99** (66 h): Used as the 'parent' in a generator to produce technetium-99m.
- **Technetium-99m** (6 h): Used in to image the skeleton and heart muscle in particular, but also for brain, thyroid, lungs (perfusion and ventilation), liver, spleen, kidney (structure and filtration rate), gall bladder, bone marrow, salivary and lacrimal glands, heart blood pool, infection and numerous specialized medical studies.
- Uses of Technetium 99 tegged RBC's.
- Commonly indicated in acute lower gastrointestinal bleeding.
- Relatively sensitive and very specific imaging method for noninvasive diagnosis of liver hemangioma.
- Measurement of left ventricular ejection fraction. Assessment of regional wall motion (left and right ventricles).
- Used of technetium 99 tagged WBC's.
- Detecting infection in bone, joints and soft tissues as well inflammation due to other causes, such as inflammatory bowel disease (ulcerative colitis and Crohn's disease).
- **Chromium-51 (28 d):** Used to label RBC's and quantify gastrointestinal protein loss.
- **Cobalt-60 (10.5 months):** Formerly used for external beam radiotherapy.
- **Copper-64 (13 h):** To study genetic diseases affecting copper metabolism. E.g.: Wilson's and Menke's diseases.
- **Dysprosium-165 (2 h):** Used as an aggregated hydroxide for synovectomy treatment of arthritis.
- **Erbium-169 (9.4 d):** Use for relieving arthritis pain in synovial joints.
- **Holmium-166 (26 h):** Being developed for diagnosis and treatment of liver tumours.
- **Iodine-125 (60 d):** Used in brachytherapy (prostate and brain), to evaluate the filtration rate of kidneys and to diagnose DVT in the leg. It is also used in radioimmunoassays to show the presence of hormones in tiny quantities.
- **Iodine-131 (8 d):** Used in treating thyroid cancer, imaging the thyroid; in diagnosis of abnormal liver function, renal (kidney) blood flow and urinary tract obstruction. A strong gamma emitter, but used for beta therapy.
- **Iridium-192 (74 d):** Supplied in wire form for use as an internal radiotherapy source for cancer treatment.
- **Iron-59 (46 d):** Used in studies of iron metabolism in the spleen.
- **Lutetium-177 (6.7 d):** Emits just enough gammas for imaging while the beta radiation does the therapy on small (e.g., endocrine) tumours. Its half-life is long enough to allow sophisticated preparation for use.
- **Palladium-103 (17 d):** Used to make brachytherapy permanent implant seeds for early stage prostate cancer.

- **Phosphorus-32 (14 d):** Used in the treatment of polycythemia vera (excess red blood cells). Beta emitter.
- **Potassium-42 (12 h):** Used for the determination of exchangeable potassium in coronary blood flow.
- **Rhenium-188 (3.8 d):** Used for pain relief in bone cancer. Beta emitter with weak gamma for imaging.
- **Rhenium-188 (17 h):** Used to beta irradiate coronary arteries from an angioplasty balloon.
- **Samarium-153 (47 h):** Sm-153 is very effective in relieving the pain of secondary cancers lodged in the bone, sold oa Quadramet. Also very effective for prostate and breast cancer. Beta emitter.
- **Selenium-75 (120 d):** Used as seleno-methionine to study the production of digestive enzymes.
- **Sodium-24 (15 h):** For studies of electrolytes within the body.
- **Strontium-89 (50 d):** Very effective in reducing the pain of prostate and bone cancer. Beta emitter.
- **Xenon-133 (5 d):** Used for pulmonary (lung) ventilation studies.
- **Ytterbium-169 (32 d):** Used for cerebrospinal fluid studies in the brain.
- **Ytterbium-177 (1.9 h):** Progenitor of Lu-177.
- **Yttrium-90 (64 h):** For brachytherapy and as silicate colloid for relieving pain of arthritis. Pure beta emitter.
- Radioisotopes of caesium, gold and ruthenium are also used in brachytherapy.

Cyclotron Radioisotopes:

- **Carbon-11, Nitrogen-13, Oxygen-15, Fluorine-18:** Position emitters used in PET.
- F-18 in FDG in detection of cancers and the monitoring of progress in their treatment, using PET.
- **Cobalt-57 (272 d):** Used as a marker to estimate organ size and for in-vitro diagnostic kits.
- **Gallium-67 (78 h):** For tumour imaging and localization of inflammatory lesions (infections).
- **Indium-111 (2.8 d):** Used for specialist diagnostic studies, e.g., brain studies, infection and colon transit studies.
- **Iodine-123 (13 h):** Used for diagnosis of thyroid function, a gamma emitter without the beta radiation of I-131.
- Krypton-81 m (13 sec) from Rubidium-81 (4.6 h): Kr-81m gas can yield functional images of pulmonary ventilation, e.g., in asthmatic patients, and for the early diagnosis of lung diseases and function.
- **Rubidium-82 (65 h):** Convenient PET agent in myocardial perfusion imaging.
- **Strontium-92 (25 d):** Used as the 'parent' in a generator to produce Rb-82.
- **Thallium-201 (73 h):** For diagnosis of coronary artery disease, other heart conditions such as heart muscle death and for location of low-grade lymphomas.

Ans: (b) P 32

Ref: Walters and Millers, Textbook of Radiotherapy, 5th edition

6. **Two nuclides having same number of neutrons but differ in protons number:**

(a) Isotopes (b) Isobars (c) Isotones (d) Isomers

Explanation:

Isotope	• Each of two or more forms of the same element that contain **equal numbers of protons** but different numbers of **neutrons** in their nuclei, and hence differ in relative atomic mass but not in chemical properties; in particular, a radioactive form of an element.
Isobar	• Isobars are atoms (nuclides) of different chemical elements that have the **same number of nucleons.** • They have same **mass number** (Sum of protons plus neutrons).
Isotone	• Two nuclides are isotones if they have the very **same neutron number**, but **different proton number.**
Isomers	• Each of two or more compounds with the **same formula** but a **different arrangement of atoms** in the molecule and different properties

Ans: (c) Isotones

Ref: Walters and Millers, Textbook of Radiotherapy, 5th edition

7. **Time period between occurrence of osteosarcoma following radiation therapy:**

(a) 1 year (b) 3 years (c) 5 years (d) 10 years

Explanation:

Post-radiation Osteosarcoma

- Latent period from radiation is long: Median 11 years.
- Rarely as little as 2 years.
- Latency inversely related to radiation dose.

Osteosarcoma

- The X-ray appearances are variable.
- Hazy **osteolytic areas** may alternate with unusually dense **osteoblastic areas**.
- The **endosteal margin** is **poorly defined**.
- Often the cortex is breached and the tumour extends into the adjacent tissues; when this happens, streaks of new bone appear, radiating outwards from the cortex – the so-called '**sunburst**' effect.
- Where the tumour emerges from the cortex, reactive new bone forms at the angles of periosteal elevation (**Codman's triangle**).
- While both the **sunburst appearance** and **Codman's triangle** are typical of osteosarcoma, they may occasionally be seen in other rapidly growing tumours.

Risk Factors for Osteosarcoma

(a) **Familial cases** where the deletion of chromosome '13q14' inactivates the retinoblastoma gene is associated with a high risk of osteosarcoma development.
(b) **Bone dysplasias,** including Paget's disease, fibrous dysplasia, enchondromatosis, and hereditary multiple exostoses, increase the risk of osteosarcoma.
(c) **Li-Fraumeni syndrome** (germline TP53 mutation) is a predisposing factor for osteosarcoma development.
(d) **Rothmund-Thomson syndrome** (i.e., autosomal recessive association of congenital bone defects, hair and skin dysplasias, hypogonadism and cataracts) is associated with increased risk of this disease.
(e) **Bone irradiation.**

Note:

Characteristic histologic finding of osteosarcoma:

- **Bone forming tumor** (osteo = bone).
- Presence of **osteoid.**

Characteristic radiologic features:

- **Codman's** triangle.

Sunburst appearance.

Ans: (d) 10 years

Ref: Diagnostic Pathology: Bone, By G. Petur Nielsen, Andrew E Rosenberg, 2nd edition, page 77

8. **A patient is worked up for loss of weight and appetite. His spine radiograph is shown in the picture:**

What is the most probable diagnosis?

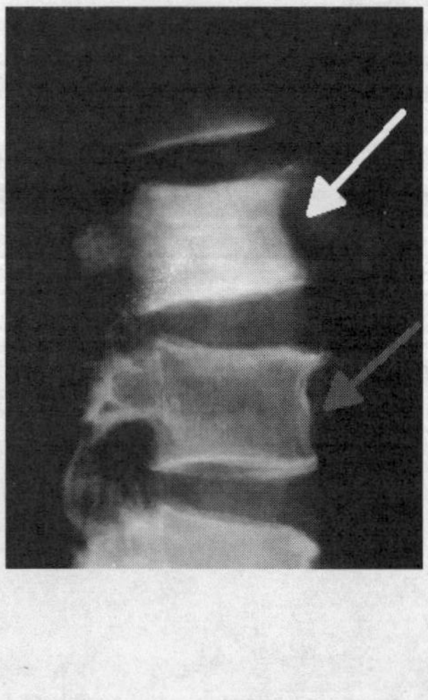

(a) Sarcoma
(b) Hepatocellular carcinoma
(c) Carcinoid
(d) Ca lung with mets

Explanation:

- X-ray shows sclerotic/osteoblastic secondaries in spine. The upper vertebral body is dense (White arrow) and lower vertebral body is normal (red arrow).
- Out of the given options, only carcinoid can cause osteoblastic metastasis in spinal cord.

Vertebral Metastases from Primary Tumours–Sclerotic Vs Lytic

Sclerotic or blastic bone metastases	Lytic bone metastases
• Prostate carcinoma (Most common) • Breast carcinoma (may be mixed) • Transitional cell carcinoma (TCC) • **Carcinoid*** • Medulloblastoma • Neuroblastoma • Mucinous adenocarcinoma of the gastrointestinal tract (e.g., colon carcinoma, gastric carcinoma) • **Lymphoma**	• Thyroid cancer • Renal cell cancer • Adrenal gland carcinoma and pheochromocytoma • Uterine carcinoma • Gastrointestinal carcinomas • Wilms' tumour • Ewing **sarcoma** • Melanoma • Hepatocellular carcinoma • Squamous cell carcinoma of the skin • **Lung cancer** (more commonly lytic, but can be sclerotic, particular if small cell lung carcinoma)

Ans: (c) Carcinoid

Ref: Radiopedia

9. **A 30-year-old male chronic smoker presents with progressive breathlessness for 1 month. Chest X-ray is shown. What is the most probable diagnosis?**

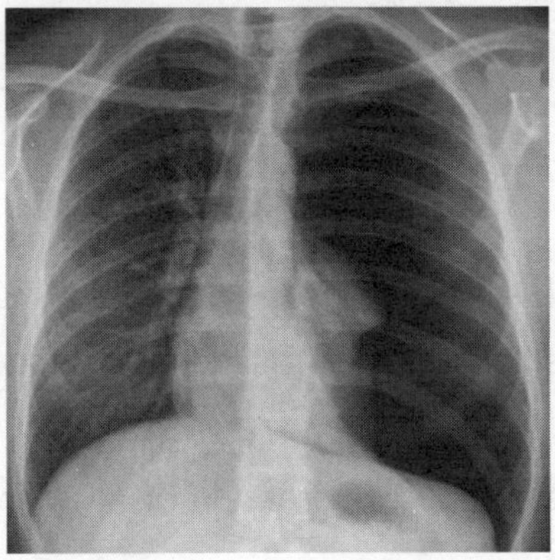

(a) Vanishing lung syndrome
(b) Pneumothorax
(c) Panacinar emphysema
(d) Collapse

Explanation:

Vanishing Lung Syndrome (Idiopathic Giant Bullous Emphysema)

- Characterized by giant emphysematous bullae, which commonly develop in the **upper lobes** and occupy at least **one-third** of a **hemithorax**.
- Progressive condition.
- Associated with several forms of **emphysema**.
- Commonly affects young men 1-2.
- Associated with:
  - o **Cigarette smoking.**

- **Marfan** syndrome.
- **Ehlers-Danlos** syndrome.
- **Alpha-1-antitrypsin deficiency.**

- Affected patients may be asymptomatic or experience hypoxia, severe dyspnea and/or chest pain.
- The bullae commonly involve the **upper lobes** with an **asymmetric** distribution and **paraseptal** location.
- **Plain radiograph**
  - Non-specific features.
  - Bullae occupy more than one-**third** of the affected hemithorax (vary in size 1-20 cm).
  - **Upper lobes** have greater involvement.
  - There is **bilateral** and **asymmetric lung** involvement.
  - May have **compress** effect to adjacent structures (lung parenchyma atelectasis, invert the ipsilateral diaphragm or contralateral displacement of the mediastinum and displacement of junction lines).
- **CT**
  - Bullae predominant in the subpleural location.
  - Size of bullae ranges from 1 to 20 cm in diameter.
  - Usually **asymmetric.**
  - Presence of concomitant foci of **paraseptal and centrilobular emphysema**.
- **Treatment and prognosis**
  - The condition tends to be progressive.
  - Criteria for bullectomy include large bullae with significant symptoms (reduced lung function or infection).
- **Complications**
  - Compression of surrounding lung (atelectasis).
  - Pneumothorax.
  - Bullae infection.
  - Higher risk of lung cancer.

Other Options:

Emphysema: Lungs are large and hyper inflated.

- Signs of hyperinflation are:
  - Low set diaphragm.
  - Flat diaphragm best determined by lateral chest.
  - Hyper lucent lung fields.
  - Increased AP diameter.
  - Increased retro-sternal air.
  - Vertical heart.

Bulla

- Air-filled space in the lung parenchyma due to destruction of alveolar tissue, distal to terminal bronchiole.
- Larger than 2 cm in distended state.
- **Bullae + emphysema** = bullous emphysema (can be congenital or complication of COPD).
- **Giant bulla** = bulla larger than one third of the hemithorax size and compression of adjacent lung parenchyma.

Distinguish Giant Bulla from Pneumothorax

- Important for treatment plan (bulla – no tube thoracostomy; pneumothorax – may need tube thoracostomy if large or symptomatic).
- Differentiation can be difficult on conventional radiography; they can coexist.
- Helpful signs for pneumothorax: **visible visceral pleural line.**
- Expiratory chest radiograph may help delineating a visceral pleural line of pneumothorax.
- **CT scan** is the most accurate mean to differentiate the two diagnoses.
- **"Double wall" sign** described in cases with ruptured bulla causing pneumothorax (air outlining both sides of the bulla wall parallel to the chest wall).

Ans: (a) Vanishing lung syndrome

Ref: Radiopedia

10. **Falsely matched radiological appearance of thorax:**

(a) Batwing appearance in pulmonary edema
(b) Egg-Shell calcification seen in Silicosis
(c) Hampton sign in pulmonary embolism
(d) Pop-corn calcification in tuberculosis

Explanation:

Lungs

- **Ground glass appearance** - Hyaline membrane disease.
- Solitary pulmonary mass lesion > 4 cms – is most commonly due to – **Bronchial adenoma.**
- **Honeycomb appearance:**
  - Sarcoidosis.
  - Histiocytosis X.
  - Interstitial lung disease.
  - Tuberculosis.
  - Collagen disorders.
  - Pneumoconiosis.
  - Drugs–Bleomycin, busulphan, melphalan, cyclophosphamide.
- **Meniscus sign/Crescent sign** (mobile mass in pulmonary cavity) is most commonly seen in –**Aspergilloma** (fungal ball lesion).
- **Egg-Shell calcification**–Silicosis, Sarcoidosis, Coal miner's pneumoconiosis, Lymphoma following radiotherapy.
- **Pop-corn calcification**/Craggy pop-corn calcification–**Pulmonary Hamartoma*.**
- **Pleural calcification**–Most common cause is–Tuberculosis (Asbestosis).
- Diaphragmatic Pleura calcification–is due to–**Asbestosis.**
- Calcification in a pulmonary metastasis–is most commonly due to–**Osteosarcoma.**
- **Coin shadow** in the lung (single), with calcification in the centre–**Epidermoid carcinoma.**
- For radiologically evident pleural effusion–The minimal amount of pleural fluid that should be present is–**250 ml**.
- **Plethoric lung fields–**seen in–L-R shunts (VSD, PDA, ASD).
- **Oligemic lung fields**–Pulmonary atreisa, Stenosis; Ebstein's anomaly.
- **Perihilar fluffy opacities**–seen in–Pulmonary venous hypertension.
- **Batwing appearance** in **pulmonary edema.**
- **Hampton hump sign*** in **pulmonary embolism*.**

Ribs

- **Superior surface notch of ribs**–seen in–Hyperparathyroidism, Neurofibromatosis, Connective tissue disorders.
- **Inferior surface notch of ribs**–seen in–Coarctation of Aorta, SVC obstruction, Chest wall AV fistula, Aortic Thrombosis.
- **Unilateral notching of ribs**–Coarctation of Left subclavian artery, Subclavian artery block, Blalock-Taussig Operation.

Others

- Displacement of tracheal shadow–most common cause is–**Thyroid swelling.**
- **Water Lily sign**–Ruptured hydatid cyst.

Ans: (d) Pop-corn calcification in tuberculosis

Ref: Internet Sources

11. **Hydatid sand is made of:**

(a) Scolex (b) Cyst (c) Protscolex (d) Brood capsule

Explanation:

*"**Ultrasonography** is the most valuable tool for both the diagnosis and treatment of cystic hydatid disease of*

*the liver. The presence of internal membranes or echogenic cyst material (**protoscoleces**, termed **hydatid sand**) can be observed in real time to aid in the diagnosis. Ultrasonography can also be used for **disease staging** used to define **optimal therapy**." – Ref: Nelson*

Hydatid Sand

- It is the granular deposits collected at the bottom of the cyst.
- It consists of:
  - **Scolices***.
  - Detached **brood capsules***.
  - **Hooklets*** liberated from disintegrated scolices.
- It is highly toxic, when absorbed gives rise to anaphylactic symptoms.
- It is an antigenic fluid and used for immunological tests.

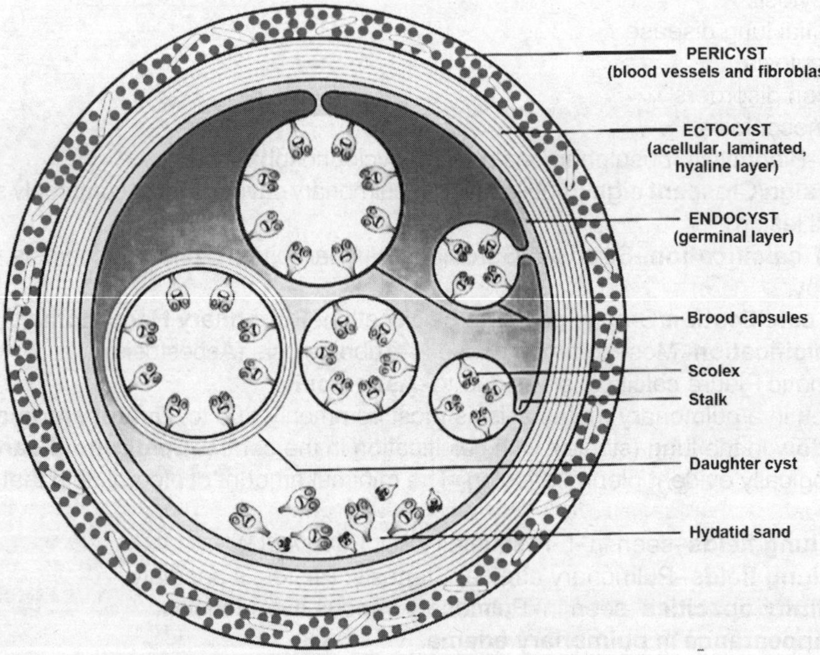

Hydatid Cyst:

- **Hydatid cyst**
  - **Cyst wall**
    - **Laminated layer**
    - **Germinal layer**
  - **contents**
    - **Protoscolex**, **Brood capsules**, **Daughter cysts**, **Granddaughter cysts** — **hydatid sand**
    - **Hydatid fluid**

ECHINOCOCCOSIS (Hydatid Disease or Hydatidosis)

- Widespread, serious human cestode infection.
- Two major Echinococcus groups of species:
  - **Echinococcus granulosus** spp causes **Cystic hydatid disease***.
  - **Echinococcus multilocularis** spp causes **alveolar hydatid disease***.
- The adult parasites are a small (2-7 mm) tapeworm with only **2-6 segments** that inhabit the **intestines** of dogs, wolves, dingoes, jackals, coyotes and foxes. These carnivores pass the eggs in their stool, which

contaminates the soil, pasture and water, as well as their own fur. Domestic animals, such as sheep, goats, cattle, and camels, ingest E. granulosus complex eggs while grazing.

- **Humans** are also infected by **consuming eggs** by **direct contact** with infected **dogs** or from ova in the environment. The larvae hatch, penetrate the **gut**, and are carried by the vascular or lymphatic systems to the liver, lungs, and less commonly bones, brain or heart.

Pathogenesis

- **E. granulosus** complex parasites are often acquired in childhood, but **liver cysts** require **many years** to become large enough to detect or cause symptoms.
- Most common site for cysts:
  - In **children** – **Lung***.
  - In **adults** – **Liver*** (upto 70% cases).
- Other sites for Cysts – Bone, genitourinary system, spleen, subcutaneous tissues and brain.
- The **host** surrounds the **primary cyst** with a **tough, fibrous capsule**.
- Inside this capsule, the parasite produces a **thick lamellar layer** containing **thin germinal layer** of cells responsible for production of **thousands of protoscoleces** that remain attached to the wall or float free or deposit (**Hydatid sand**) in the cyst fluid. Smaller internal daughter cysts may develop within the primary cyst capsule. The fluid in a healthy cyst is clear, colorless and watery.
- Rupture of the cyst, which can occur with trauma or during surgery, can be associated with an **anaphylactic reaction**.
- Protoscoleces released into the tissues can also develop into new cysts.
- **E. multilocularis** almost always involves the **liver***.

Lab Diagnosis

- **USG** – Gold standard screening tool.
- **CT/MRI.**
- **CXR** – Lung cysts.
- **Serologic studies** – Poor sensitivity.
- **Casoni test*** – Immediate hypersensitivity skin test – Seldom used nowadays.

Treatment

• Small cystic lesions **<5 cm** diameter	Albendazole 15 mg/kg/day for 1 – 6 months
• For **large lesions >5 cm**	CT or USG guided '**PAIR**' therapy (**percutaneous aspiration**, **instillation** and **reaspiration**) + Albendazole chemotherapy
• **Complicated cysts** • Cysts communicating with biliary tract • Large pulmonary cysts • Bone/Brain cysts	Surgical removal + Albendazole chemotherapy

Ans: (c) Protoscolex > A and D

Ref: Nelson, Textbook of Pediatrics, 20th edition, page 1755

PSYCHIATRY

1. **A post-natal mother who delivered 2 days back presents with increased tearfulness and sleeplessness. No features of anhedonia, suicidal thoughts or lack of interest present. Most probable diagnosis:**
   (a) Mania (b) Peripartum psychosis
   (c) Postpartum blues (d) Postpartum depression

Explanation:

Psychological disturbances unique for women are:

- Related to **menses**
  - Premenstrual dysphoric disorder.
  - Postmenopausal syndrome.
- Related to **pregnancy**
  - Anxiety.
  - Depression.
- Related to **delivery**
  - Postpartum blues.
  - Postpartum depression.
  - Postpartum psychosis.

The above question deals with postpartum psychological problems.

A. Postpartum blues

- Mild form.
- Characterized by occasional sadness/tearfulness.
- No other significant mood/psychotic/behavioral symptoms present.
- No significant disturbance in sleep, appetite, activities of daily living.
- Treatment is psychotherapy (reassurance and monitoring for symptoms).

B. Postpartum depression

- Moderate form.
- Characterized by:
  - Sadness, loss of interest in previous pleasurable activities (anhedonia).
  - Easy fatigability, feeling of worthless/hopeless/helpless/guilt.
  - Suicidal ideas/attempt, decreased appetite and sleep.
- Depending on the severity, psychotherapy, pharmacotherapy, ECT, may be needed.

C. Postpartum psychosis

- Severe form.
- Characterized by **psychotic symptoms** (hallucination, delusion, and disorganized speech/behaviour).
- This condition needs treatment as inpatient basis with pharmacotherapy ± ECT.
- DDs for postpartum psychosis: **Delirium** (mostly related to events like eclampsia, hemorrhage, thrombosis, especially cortical vein thrombosis and **Sheehan syndrome**–postpartum pituitary gland necrosis).

Ans: (c) Postpartum blues

Ref: Kaplan and Saddock's Synopsis of Psychiatry, 11th edition and Niraj Ahuja's Short Textbook of Psychiatry, 7th edition

2. An example for a bizarre delusion:

(a) Delusion of infidelity (My wife has affair with another person)
(b) Delusion of persecution (My brain is controlled by microchip)
(c) Delusion of grandiosity (I am the greatest person in the world)
(d) Delusion of reference (I am being prosecuted often)

Explanation:

Delusion

- Delusion is a false unshakeable belief.
- It is a disturbance of **thought (content)**.
- Delusion is a psychotic symptom.
- It is seen in:
  - o Organic disturbances (delirium, dementia).
  - o Substance induced psychosis (alcohol – morbid jealousy).
  - o Functional psychosis (affective or non-affective).
- The characteristics of delusion will help in differentiating diagnosis.
  - o Fleeting and fluctuating delusions – **Delirium.**
  - o Delusion of grandeur – **Mania.**
  - o Delusion of guilt – **Depression.**
- Based on the possibility, delusion may be **bizarre or non-bizarre***.
- **Bizarre** means **impossible** from current socio-cultural situation.
- Bizarre delusions are pathognomic of **Schizophrenia** (can be seen in **Mania** also).
- *By definition, **delusional disorder** is characterized by **non-bizarre delusion**.*
- In the above question, all delusions are possible, except being controlled by **microchip**, which is impossible in the current scenario.

COMMON DELUSION THEMES

- **Delusion of Control:**
  - o False belief that another person, group of people, or external force controls one's general thoughts, feelings, impulses, or behavior.
  - o Patient claims that he is able to control phenomena like rotation of earth, rain, flying in air, walking over the sea, curing illnesses, without any logic.
  - o Patient claims that he is being controlled by some external agencies or aliens through some means like black magic, microchips.
- **Cotard delusion:** False belief that one does not exist or has died.
- **Delusional jealousy:** False belief that a spouse or lover is having an affair, with no proof to back up their claim.
- **Delusion of guilt or sin** (or delusion of **self-accusation**): Ungrounded feeling of remorse or guilt of delusional intensity.
- **Delusion of mind being read:** False belief that other people can know one's thoughts.
- **Delusion of thought insertion:** Belief that another thinks through the mind of the person
- **Delusion of reference:** False belief that insignificant remarks, events, or objects in one's environment have personal meaning or significance.
- **Erotomania:** False belief that another person is in love with them.
- **Grandiose religious delusion:** Belief that the affected person is a god or chosen to act as a god.
- **Somatic delusion:** Delusion whose content pertains to bodily functioning, bodily sensations or physical appearance. Usually the false belief is that the body is somehow diseased, abnormal or changed (e.g.: **delusional parasitosis:** Delusion in which one feels infested with parasites).
- **Delusion of poverty:** Person strongly believes they are financially incapacitated.
- **Grandiose delusions** or **delusions of grandeur**

- Subtype of delusional disorder.
- Also seen in schizophrenia and manic episodes of bipolar disorder.
- Characterized by fantastical beliefs that one is famous, omnipotent or otherwise very powerful.

- **Persecutory delusions**
  - Most common type of delusions.
  - Involve the theme of being followed, harassed, cheated, poisoned or drugged, conspired against, spied on, attacked, or otherwise obstructed in the pursuit of goals.
  - Affected person wrongly believes that they are being persecuted. Specifically, they have been defined as containing three central elements. The individual thinks that:
    - Harm is occurring, or is going to occur.
    - The persecutor has the intention to cause harm.
    - They are constantly being prejudged or profiled.

Ans: (b) Delusion of persecution (My brain is controlled by microchip)

Ref: Kaplan and Saddock's Synopsis of Psychiatry, 11th edition and Niraj Ahuja's Short Textbook of Psychiatry, 7th edition

3. Recurrent suicidal tendency, aberrant interpersonal relationship, black and white phenomena are characteristic of:

(a) Borderline personality
(b) Schizotypal personality
(c) Histrionic personality
(d) Narcissistic personality

Explanation:

Personality Disorders

- Personality is defined as a person's persistent and unique way of perceiving, thinking, feeling and behaving.
- Personality disorder is defined when personality is rigid and inflexible and when it causes distress to self/others or dysfunction.
- Personality disorders are grouped as three clusters (DSM), viz.:
  - **Odd, eccentric** (Paranoid, schizoid, schizotypal).
  - **Dramatic** (Narcissistic, histrionic, borderline).
  - **Anxious** (Dependent, avoidant, anankastic).
- **Emotionally unstable** personality disorder has two subtypes:
  - **Borderline.**
  - **Impulsive**.

Borderline Personality Disorder (BPD)

- Seen in almost exclusively **adolescent females**.
- It is characterized by abnormal:
  - **Perception** (self-perception→poor self image, identity crisis).
  - **Thinking** (dichotomous/black and white thinking; micropsychotic episodes).
  - **Feeling** (emotional lability, emotional turmoil).
  - **Behaviour** (easily establishing as well as dissolving relationships, especially with opposite sex; temper tantrums; suicidal behaviour → *wrist slashing*).
- It is the only personality disorder where pharmacotherapy is found useful / indicated.
- Drugs used are: Mood Stabilizers.
- Psychotherapy: DBT (Dialectical Behaviour Therapy).

Ans: (a) Borderline personality

Ref: Kaplan and Saddock's Synopsis of Psychiatry, 11th edition and Niraj Ahuja's Short Textbook of Psychiatry, 7th edition

4. False regarding eating disorder is:

(a) Neurohumoral related
(b) Hereditary 80%
(c) Starvation increases symptom
(d) Penetrance is 50%

Explanation:

- Pathological problems associated with **eating** are many, like **pica, overeating, under-eating**.
- By and large, **eating disorders** denote:
  - o **Anorexia nervosa (AN).**
  - o **Bulimia nervosa (BN); and**
  - o **Binge eating disorder.**
- Etiology-wise, they have more **genetic contribution** (than many psychiatric disorders).
- Studies (especially twin-studies) indicate upto **74%** of phenotypic variation can be accounted by additive genetic factors [option (b) **Heriditary 80%].**
- **Penetrance** is defined as the probability of **expression of an allele**. It can be **complete/incomplete**; highly penetrant/low penetrant. In eating disorders, studies show **higher** degree of **penetrance** (> 50%, some studies state upto 90%) (option (d))
- Like any other psychiatric disorder, eating disorders have **neuro-humoral underpinnings**. Brain regions and chemicals which are involved in appetite are implicated.
- Neurological substrates are mainly hypothalamus, anterior frontal regions.
- Till date, all monoamine neurotransmitter systems were implicated in AN and BN. Among the NTs, dysregulation of 5-HT system appears to have robust data (option (a))
- Starvation and other symptoms of eating disorders are mutually reinforcing each other, may be leading to a vicious cycle as in animal models (p.1119, Biological Psychiatry).

Ans: (d) Penetrance is 50%

Ref: Biological Psychiatry (edited by Hugo A. H. D'haenen, Johan A. Den Boer, Paul Willner) and Yilmaz Z, Hardaway Ja, Bulik Cm. Genetics and Epigenetics of Eating Disorders. Advances in Genomics and Genetics 2015;5, page 131-150

5. **Oneroid state is:**

(a) Twilight state (b) Dream like state (c) Torpor (d) Stupor

Explanation:

- Alteration in consciousness can be **physiological or pathological**.
- **Pathological** alteration in consciousness occurs in several disorders.
- Based on level of awareness (of self and surroundings) and control (over speech and motor movements), they are classified (and specific terms used).

A. Twilight state

- Here one is aware of self but not aware of his current surroundings; behaves oddly even to the extent of violence which might be due to auditory/visual hallucinations occurring in this state.
- *Seen in* – Organic conditions *(concussion, epilepsy, anesthesia)* or functional conditions (hysteria).

B. Dream-like state/Oneroid state

- Here one is neither aware of self nor surroundings, and behave inappropriately– which are not organized as in twilight state.
- [**D**ream–like state **d**isorganized bahavior].
- *Seen in–Prodrome* / acute stage of psychosis, intoxication (*esp. inhalants*).

C. Torpor

- Lowered awareness (self and surroundings) with normal verbal + motor response.
- Seen in Fatigue, hypothyroidism.

D. Stupor is a general term indicating lowered awareness and/or control.

Ans: (b) Dream like state

Ref: Kaplan and Saddock's Synopsis of Psychiatry, 11th edition and Niraj Ahuja's Short Textbook of Psychiatry, 7th edition

6. **Oedipus complex seen in:**

(a) Girls 1 to 3 years (b) Girls 3 to 5 years (c) Boys 1 to 3 years (d) Boys 3 to 5 years

Explanation:

- **Freud** described "stages of life" based on his structural theory (also known as psychosexual stages).
- Psychiatric disorders happens if "arrest" of development occurs in any of these stages.

Sigmund Freud's psychosexual stages

Stage	Years	Disorder / Points
Oral	0 –1½ years	Eating disorder, substance abuse
Anal	1½ – 3 years	OCD
Phallic	3 – 6 years	Oedipus complex (castration anxiety) in males and Electra complex (penis envy) in females
Latent	6 – 12 years	Sexual problems like hypoarousal
Genital	>12 years	Sexual problems like impotence, frigidity

Ans: (d) Boys 3 to 5 years

Ref: Kaplan and Saddock's Synopsis of Psychiatry, 11th edition and Niraj Ahuja's Short Textbook of Psychiatry, 7th edition

7. **Chromosome make up of tall individual with criminal behavior:**

(a) XXY (b) XYY (c) XXXY (d) XXYY

Explanation:

- **XYY** is a condition characterized by **47, XYY** karyotype affecting **males**.
- Around 1 in 1,000 boys are born with a 47, XYY karyotype.
- These boys have **increased growth velocity**. They have **above average height.**
- Some of them might have **learning disabilities**.
- Some of them might have **aggressive behavior**.
- **Criminal behavior** is noted in few studies, though recent evidence disputes the claim.

Ans: (b) XYY

Ref: Kaplan and Saddock's Comprehensive Textbook of Psychiatry and Ahuja–Textbook of Psychiatry

JIPMER–MAY 2017

ANATOMY

1. **Fate of 6th aortic arch:**
   (a) Arch of aorta in between left common carotid artery and left subclavian artery
   (b) Ductus arteriosus
   (c) Right brachiocephalic
   (d) Left subclavian artery

Explanation:

Aortic arch	Develops into
1st Aortic arch	***Maxillary artery****
2nd Aortic arch	***Hyoid artery**** ***Stapedial artery****
3rd Aortic arch	***Common carotid artery**** ***Proximal part of internal carotid and external carotid artery***
4th Aortic arch	**Left side:** ***Arch of aorta*** in between left common carotid artery and left subclavian artery **Right side:** Right ***subclavian artery***
5th Aortic arch	Disappear completely
6th Aortic arch	**Proximal part** – ***Pulmonary artery**** **Distal part disappear** on the **right side** but persist on the ***left side*** as ***ductus arteriosus****

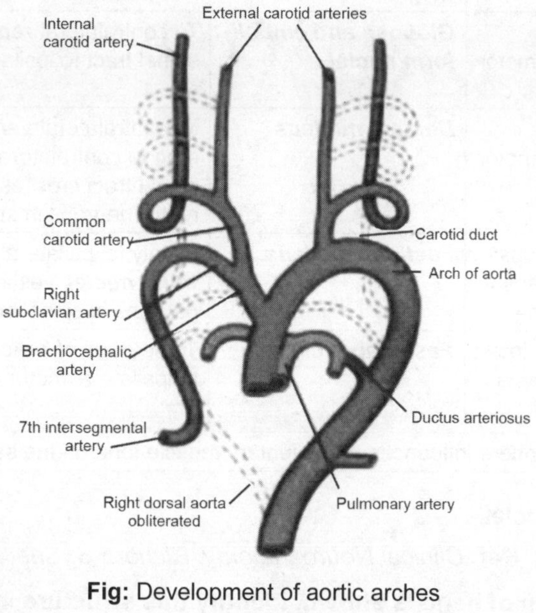

Fig: Development of aortic arches

Ans: (b) Ductus arteriosus

Ref: *Langman's Medical Embryology, 9th Edition, Page 255–259*

2. **Which of the following is the site of cerebellar input?**

(a) Inferior olivary nuclei
(b) Vestibular nuclei
(c) Globose and emboliform nuclei
(d) Dentate nucleus

Explanation:

The Afferent Cerebellar Pathways

Pathway	Function	Origin	Destination
Corticopontocerebellar	Conveys control from cerebral cortex	Frontal, parietal, temporal, and occipital lobes (cerebral ***cortex***)	Via ***pontine nuclei*** and mossy fibers to ***cerebellar*** cortex
Cerebro-olivocerebellar	Conveys control from cerebral cortex	Frontal, parietal, temporal, and occipital lobes (***cerebral*** cortex)	Via ***inferior olivary nuclei*** and climbing fibers to ***cerebellar*** cortex
Cerebroreticulocerebellar	Conveys control from cerebral cortex	Sensorimotor areas (***cerebral*** cortex)	Via ***reticular formation***
Anterior spinocerebellar	Conveys information from muscles and joints	***Muscle spindles, tendon organs, and joint receptors***	Via mossy fibers to ***cerebellar cortex***
Posterior spinocerebellar	Conveys information from muscles and joints	***Muscle spindles, tendon organs, and joint receptors***	Via mossy fibers to ***cerebellar cortex***
Cuneocerebellar	Conveys information from muscles and joints of upper limb	***Muscle spindles, tendon organs, and joint receptors (from upper limb)***	Via mossy fibers to ***cerebellar cortex***
Vestibular nerve	Conveys information of head position and movement	***Utricle, saccule, and semicircular canals***	Via mossy fibers to cortex of ***flocculonodular lobe***
Other afferents	Conveys information from midbrain	Red nucleus, tectum	Cerebellar cortex

The Efferent Cerebellar Pathways

Pathway	Function	Origin	Destination
Globose-emboliform-rubral	Influences ipsilateral motor activity	***Globose and emboliform nuclei***	To contralateral ***red nucleus***, then via crossed rubrospinal tract to ipsilateral motor neurons in spinal cord
Dentothalamic	Influences ipsilateral motor activity	***Dentate nucleus***	To contralateral ***ventrolateral nucleus of thalamus***, then to contralateral motor cerebral cortex; corticospinal tract crosses midline and controls ipsilateral motor neurons in spinal cord
Fastigial vestibular	Influences ipsilateral extensor muscle tone	***Fastigial nucleus***	Mainly to ipsilateral and to contralateral ***lateral vestibular nuclei***; vestibulospinal tract to ipsilateral motor neurons in spinal cord
Fastigial reticular	Influences ipsilateral muscle tone	***Fastigial nucleus***	To neurons of ***reticular formation***; reticulospinal tract to ipsilateral motor neurons to spinal cord
Note: Each cerebellar hemisphere influences the voluntary muscle tone on the same side of the body.			

Ans: (a) Inferior olivary nuclei

Ref: *Clinical Neuroanatomy, Richard S. Snell, 7th Edition, 2010, Page 237–243*

3. **Gross dissected specimen of hand is shown. Identify this structure in Black circle.**

(a) Deep palmar arch
(b) Superficial palmar arch
(c) Radial artery
(d) Ulnar artery

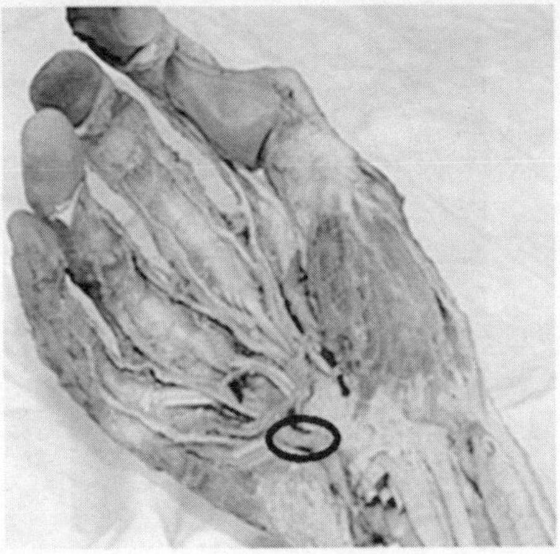

Explanation:

- In this image based question, the circle was marked on the ulnar artery just distal to the flexor retinaculum. So it is **superficial branch of the ulnar artery** not the superficial palmar arch. Superficial ulnar artery not in the option, so **ulnar artery** is the correct answer.

More details about ulnar artery in the hand:

- Ulnar artery enters the palm of hand by passing ***superficial to the flexor retinaculum or passing through Guyon's canal*** [fibers of flexor retinaculum split to form a tunnel for the passage of ulnar nerve and artery] accompanied by ulnar nerve on its medial side.
- In front of the flexor retinaculum and lateral to the pisiform the ulnar artery continues as ***superficial ulnar artery*** after giving deep branch.
- ***Superficial branch*** of ulnar artery ***anastomose with superficial palmar branch of the radial artery or arteria radialis indicis or arteria princeps pollicis*** and forms ***superficial palmar arch.***
- **Branches of superficial palmar arch:**
  - ***Three common palmar digital arteries***–arise from the convexity of the superficial palmar arch.
  - Each common palmar digital artery divides into two ***proper palmar digital arteries*** and supplies the contiguous sides of medial four fingers.
- **Deep branch of the ulnar artery** (accompanies with deep branch of ulnar nerve) joins the **radial artery** to complete the **deep palmar arch.**
- Branches of deep palmar arch:
  - ***Three palmar metacarpal arteries***–which join the common palmar digital arteries from the superficial palmar arch.
  - ***Three perforating branches***–which pass posteriorly between the heads of origin of the dorsal interossei to anastomose with the dorsal metacarpal arteries from the dorsal carpal arch.

EXTRA EDGE:

Look for thumb or little finger in the image.

- Along the side of **thumb:**
  - **Nerve** – Median nerve*.
  - **Artery** – Radial artery* or its branches.
- Along the side of **little finger:**
  - **Nerve** – Ulnar nerve*.
  - **Artery** – Ulnar artery*.

Ans: (d) Ulnar artery

Ref: *Gray's Anatomy, The Anatomical Basis of Clinical Practice, 41st Edition, 2016, Page 889 and 890*

4. Gross dissected specimen of forearm and hand is shown. Identify the structure in Black circle.

(a) Digital branch of radial nerve
(b) Anterior introsseous nerve
(c) Digital branch of ulnar nerve
(d) Median nerve

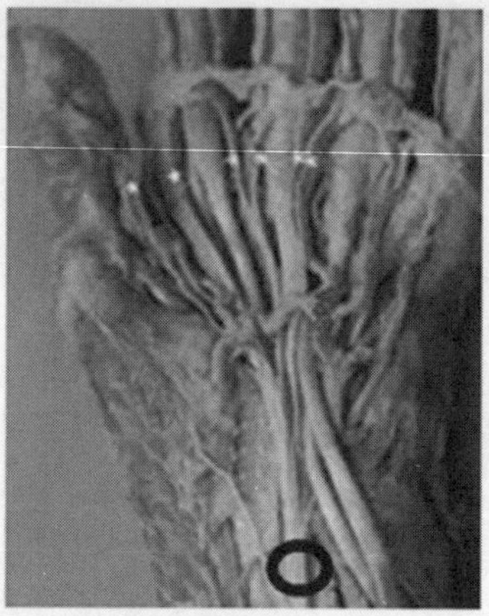

Explanation:

- In this image based question, the circle is marked on the median nerve just distal to the origin of recurrent branch.

More details about median nerve in the hand:

- Median nerve enters the palm of hand by passing ***deep to the flexor retinaculum*** (carpal tunnel).
- ***Branches*** of median nerve in the hand:

Recurrent branch (Motor)	Supply the ***thenar muscles**** • Flexor pollicis brevis • Abductor pollicis brevis • Opponens pollicis
Palmar digital branches (Motor and sensory)	• Supply the ***first and second lumbricals*** • Innervates the skin of ***lateral 3½ fingers*** of palmar aspect of hand

- After giving the recurrent branch the median nerve divides into ***2 proper palmar digital nerves*** and ***2 common palmar digital nerves.*** The 2 proper palmar digital nerves runs along the ulnar side of thumb and radial side of index finger respectively.
- Each common palmar digital nerves divides **into 2 proper palmar digital nerves** which supplies the adjacent sides of index, middle finger and ring finger respectively.
- Palmar digital nerves also gives ***vasomotor*** (blood vessels) and ***sudomotor*** (sweat glands) ***branches*** to lateral 3½ fingers of hand.

Ans: (d) Median nerve

Ref: *Gray's Anatomy, The Anatomical Basis of Clinical Practice, 41st Edition, 2016, Page 891*

5. Sixth pharyngeal arch gives rise to:

(a) Sternohyoid (b) Cricothyroid
(c) Cricoarytenoid (d) Stylopharyngeus

Explanation:

Mesodermal derivatives of the pharyngeal arches and their innervation

Pharyngeal Arch	Nerve	Artery	Muscles	Skeleton
1 arch [Mandibular] (maxillary and mandibular processes)	**V. Trigeminal:** (maxillary and mandibular divisions)	Maxillary	**Mastication** (temporal, Masseter, medial and lateral pterygoids), **mylohyoid, anterior belly of digastric, tensor veli palatinii and tensor tympani**	Premaxilla, maxilla, zygomatic bone, part of temporal bone, **Meckel's cartilage,** Mandible, **malleus, incus**, anterior ligament of malleus and sphenomandibular ligament

Contd.

Contd.

2 arch [Hyoid]	**VII. Facial**	Hyoid and stapedial	**Facial expression** (buccinators, Auricularis, Frontalis, Platysma, orbicularis oris, orbicularis oculi), **posterior belly of digastric, stylohyoid and stapedius**	**Stapes, styloid process,** stylohyoid ligament, lesser horn and upper portion of body of hyoid bone.
3 arch	**IX. Glossopharyngeal**	Common carotid artery, proximal (1st part) of internal carotid artery amd External carotid artery	***Stylopharyngeus***	Greater horn and lower portion of body of ***hyoid bone***
4 arch	**X. Vagus** Superior laryngeal branch	Left side: Arch of aorta Right side: Right subclavian artery	***Cricothyroid, levator veli palatinii and constrictors muscles of pharynx***	***Thyroid cartilage, epiglottis and cuneiform cartilage***
5 arch	Disappears			
6 arch	**X. Vagus** Recurrent laryngeal branch	Right and left pulmonary artery Left side: Distal part persist as ductus arteriosus	***All intrinsic muscles of larynx*** except cricothyroid	***Cricoid, arytenoid, corniculate, and tracheal cartilages***

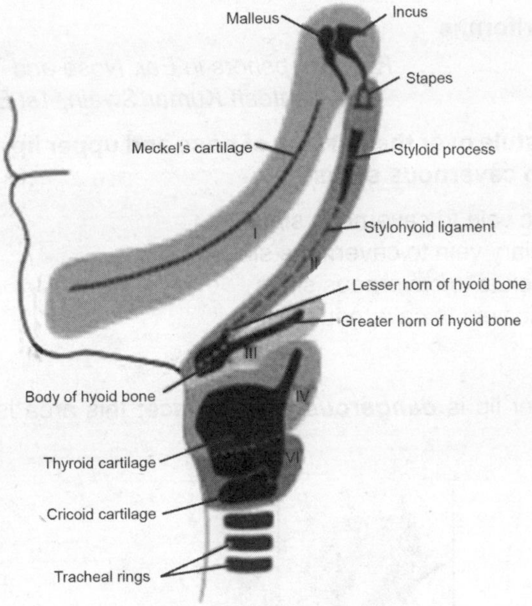

Fig: Mesodermal derivatives of the pharyngeal arches

Ans: (c) Cricoarytenoid

Ref: *Langman's Medical Embryology, 9th Edition, Page 366-372*

6. **During surgery, which of the following anatomical landmark is closely associated with geniculate ganglion?**

(a) Pyramid
(b) Short process of incus
(c) Processes cochleariformis
(d) Oval window

Explanation:

- The complex course of facial nerve through the middle ear is due to its development from ***facioacoustic primordium*** which gives rise to **VII and VIII nerves***.

- To reach the ***second pharyngeal arch mesoderm*** the main trunk of facial nerve courses through the middle ear.

Surgical landmark of facial nerve during middle ear and mastoid surgery

Processes cochleariformis	It demarcates the ***geniculate ganglion***
Cog	It is a bony spur, projecting from the tegmen anterior to the ***head of malleus.*** It is the ***landmark for geniculate ganglion***
Oval window	Facial nerve lies ***above*** the oval window niche
Lateral semicircular canal	Facial nerve lies ***below*** the lateral semicircular canal
Short process of incus	Facial nerve lies ***medial*** to the short process of incus at the level of aditus
Pyramid	Facial nerve runs ***behind*** the pyramid and post tympanic sulcus
Tympanomastoid suture	Vertical or the mastoid segment facial nerve runs ***behind*** this suture
Digastric ridge	Facial nerve leaves the mastoid at the ***anterior end*** of this ridge
Stylomastoid foramen	Facial nerve ***exits*** through this foramen

Surgical landmark of facial nerve during parotid surgery

Tragal point	Facial nerve located ***1 cm deep and inferior*** to this point
Tympanomastoid suture	Facial nerve lies ***6-8 mm deep*** to this suture
Styloid process	Facial nerve crosses ***lateral to styloid*** process
Posterior belly of digastric muscle	Facial nerve is situated ***between digastric groove and styloid*** process
Retromandibular vein	Facial nerve passes ***superficial*** to it

Ans: (c) Processes cochleariformis

Ref: *Snapshots in Ear, Nose and Throat, Head and Neck Surgery, Santosh Kumar Swain, 1st Edition, 2016, Page 195 and 196*

7. A patient presented with pustule over the dorsum of nose and upper lip. Which is the most direct route of spread of this infection to cavernous sinus?

(a) Angular vein to ophthalmic vein to cavernous sinus
(b) Dorsal nasal vein to maxillary vein to cavernous sinus
(c) Facial vein to pterygoid plexus to cavernous sinus
(d) Palatine vein to ophthalmic vein to cavernous sinus

Explanation:

- Dorsum of nose and upper lip is ***dangerous area of face*; this area is drained by facial vein and its tributaries.**

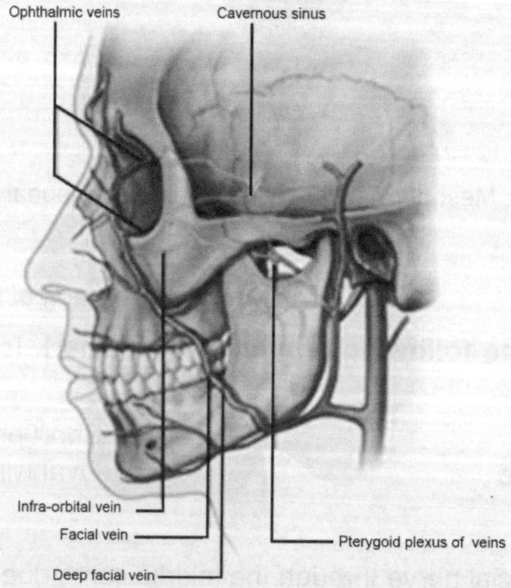

Fig: Communications of facial vein with the cavernous sinus

- Facial vein is ***devoid of valves.***
- Facial vein communicates with the cavernous sinus ***through 2 routes:***
  - ***Directly: Angular vein* and superior ophthalmic vein*.***
  - ***Indirectly: Deep facial vein* and pterygoid venous plexus**** [an emissary vein passing through the foramen ovale connecting the pterygoid venous plexus with cavernous sinus].

Other communications of cavernous sinus:

With ***transverse sinus***	via ***superior petrosal sinus***
With ***IJV***	via ***inferior petrosal sinus*** and plexus of ***veins around ICA***
With ***pterygoid venous plexus***	through ***emissary veins*** passing through foramen ovale, spinosum, lacerum and vesali
With ***opposite cavernous sinus***	via anterior and posterior ***intercavernous sinuses***
With ***superior sagittal sinus***	through ***superficial middle cerebral vein and superior anastomotic vein***

Ans: (a) Angular vein to ophthalmic vein to cavernous sinus

Ref: *Essentials of Human Anatomy, A.K. Datta, 3rd Edition, 2003, Volume-II, Page 82 and 222*

8. **Vein of Labbe is:**

(a) Superior anastomotic vein
(b) Inferior anastomotic vein
(c) Superior cerebral vein
(d) Superficial middle cerebral vein

Explanation:

- French surgeon **Charles Labbé** who described inferior anastomotic vein in his 3rd year of medical school.
- ***Inferior anastomotic vein*** is part of the ***superficial venous system*** of the brain.
- The vein of Labbé is the largest channel that ***crosses*** the temporal lobe ***between the Sylvian fissure and the transverse sinus.***
- It ***connects the superficial middle cerebral vein and the transverse sinus.***
- Its ***location*** is highly variable:
  - **Mid-temporal region: 60%***
  - Posterior temporal: 30%
  - Anterior temporal: 10%

Also Note:

- ***Superior anastomotic vein*** is also called ***vein of Trolard*.***
- ***Superficial middle cerebral vein*** also called ***vein of Sylvius*.***

Ans: (b) Inferior anastomotic vein

Ref: *https://radiopaedia.org/articles/vein-of-labbe-2*

9. **Cranial nerve that lies between superior cerebellar artery and posterior cerebral artery is:**

(a) Oculomotor nerve
(b) Optic nerve
(c) Abducens nerve
(d) Trigeminal nerve

Explanation:

- The oculomotor nerve emerges from the ***ventral surface of the midbrain.***
- It passes forward ***between the posterior cerebral and the superior cerebellar arteries****.
- It then continues into the middle cranial fossa in the ***lateral wall of the cavernous sinus****.

Note: The only cranial nerve which emerges from the **dorsal surface** of brain is **trochlear nerve** and it is the most slender nerve among the cranial nerves.

Ans: Oculomotor nerve

Ref: *Clinical Neuroanatomy, Richard S. Snell, 7th Edition, 2010, Page 340*

10. **In right atrium, triangle of Koch is formed by all these structures *except:***

(a) Coronary sinus orifice
(b) Tendon of Todaro
(c) Sulcus terminalis
(d) Anterior-septal leaflet commissure

Explanation:

Triangle of Koch:

Boundaries:

- ***Inferiorly:*** Septal ***cusp*** of the tricuspid valve.
- ***Basally:*** Ostium of the ***coronary sinus.***
- ***Superiorly: Tendon of Todaro.***
- Triangle of Koch is the ***landmark of atrioventricular node.***

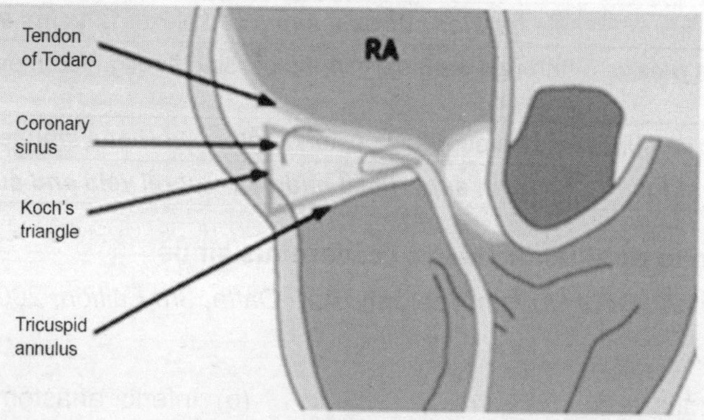

Fig: Triangle of Koch

- ***Location of Sinuatrial node:*** At the junction between **posterior smooth** and **anterior rough** part of **right atrium,** close to the crest of the **right auricle and superior vena cava.**
- ***Sulcus terminalis:*** It is a shallow groove present ***externally*** at the junction between the ***venous part (sinus venarum) and the atrium proper.***
- ***Crista terminalis:*** Sulcus terminalis corresponds ***internally.***

Ans: (c) Sulcus terminalis

Ref: *Gray's Anatomy, The Anatomical Basis of Clinical Practice, 39th Edition, 2005, Page 1000–1012*

11. Two-year-old child presented with retropharyngeal abscess. The retropharyngeal space is a potential space of the head and neck, bounded by:

(a) Between buccopharyngeal and prevertebral fascia
(b) Between pharyngobasilar and prevertebral fascia
(c) Between buccopharyngeal and pharyngobasilar fascia
(d) Buccopharyngeal fascia anteriorly and the alar fascia posteriorly

Explanation:

Retropharyngeal space:

- It lies ***behind the pharynx*** between the ***buccopharyngeal fascia and the alar fascia*** (alar fascia is the anterior layer of prevertebral fascia).
- It extends upwards to the ***base of the skull*** and downwards to the ***retrovisceral space*** in the infrahyoid region.
- It permits the movement of the **pharynx, esophagus, larynx and trachea** during **swallowing.**
- The space is divided into ***two lateral compartments (space of Gillette)*** by a fibrous raphe.
- Each lateral space contains retropharyngeal nodes which usually disappear at 3-4 years of age.
- Parapharyngeal space communicates with the retropharyngeal space.
- Infection of retropharyngeal space can pass down behind the oesophagus into the posterior mediastinum.

Retrovisceral space:

- The retrovisceral space is ***continuous superiorly with the retropharyngeal space.***
- It is situated between the posterior wall of the ***oesophagus and the prevertebral fascia.***
- Inferiorly, the retrovisceral space extends into the superior mediastinum.
- **Prevertebral fascia merge** with the **connective tissue** on the posterior surface of the oesophagus – usually at the level of the **fourth thoracic vertebra** (i.e., bifurcation of trachea).

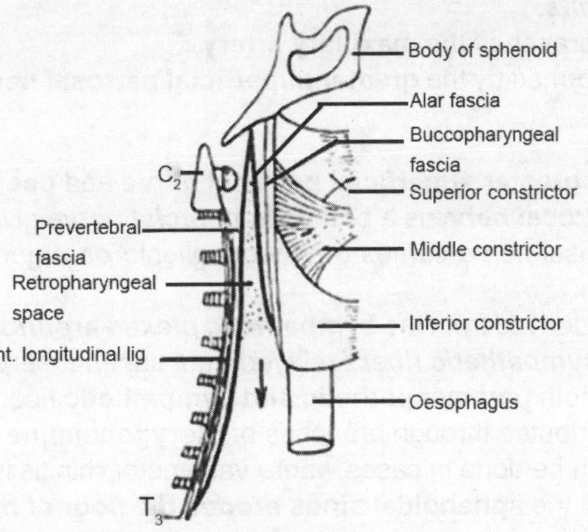

Fig: Schematic diagram showing the retropharyngeal space

More details:

Pharyngobasilar fascia:

- Above the level of ***superior constrictor muscle of pharynx*** the ***fibrous layer*** that supports the pharyngeal mucosa is thickened to form the pharyngobasilar fascia.
- Above it is attached to occipital bone, petrous part of temporal bone, medial pterygoid plate and the pterygomandibular raphe.
- Below it diminishes in thickness but is strengthened posteriorly by a fibrous band (median pharyngeal raphe) attached to the pharyngeal tubercle of the occipital bone.

Buccopharyngeal fascia:

- This fibrous layer is really the ***internal epimysial covering of the muscles*** and their aponeurotic attachment to the base of the skull.
- Which ***covers the superior constrictor*** and passes forwards over the pterygomandibular raphe to cover ***buccinators.***

Prevertebral fascia and Alar fascia:

- The ***prevertebral layer*** of cervical fascia consists of ***dorsal and ventral layers***: ***prevertebral and alar fasciae, respectively.***
- The prevertebral fascia lies closest to the vertebral bodies, covering the anterior surface of longus capitis and longus colli.
- It extends inferiorly from the skull base, descending in front of longus colli into the superior mediastinum, where it blends with the anterior longitudinal ligament.
- The ***prevertebral fascia*** is attached to the ***spinous processes*** of the vertebrae.
- The ***alar fascia*** is a coronally orientated sheet, attached to the ***transverse process*** of the cervical vertebrae.

Ans: (d) Buccopharyngeal fascia anteriorly and the alar fascia posteriorly

Ref: *Gray's Anatomy, The Anatomical Basis of Clinical Practice, 41st Edition, 2016, Page 445, 577 and 578*

12. What structure lies in the floor of sphenoidal air sinus?

(a) Vidian nerve (b) Mandibular nerve
(c) Greater petrosal nerve (d) Maxillary nerve

Explanation:

Vidian canal:

- The vidian canal is located in the ***floor of the sphenoid sinus*** at the junction of the **pterygoid process** and the **sphenoid body** connecting the **pterygopalatine fossa anteriorly** and the **foramen lacerum posteriorly.**

- The vidian canal ***transmits:***
  - o *The **vidian artery*** (branch of the **maxillary artery**).
  - o The ***vidian nerve*** (formed by the **greater superficial petrosal nerve** and the **deep petrosal nerve**).

Vidian nerve:

- Formed by the union of **greater superficial petrosal nerve** and **deep petrosal nerve.**
- ***Greater superficial petrosal nerve*** is a branch from ***facial nerve*** given at the **geniculate ganglion.**
- Greater superficial petrosal nerve carries the preganglionic ***parasympathetic secretomotor fibers*** to pterygopalatine ganglion.
- ***Deep petrosal nerve*** is derived from the ***sympathetic plexus around the internal carotid artery,*** which carries post ganglionic ***sympathetic fibers*** relayed from superior cervical sympathetic ganglia.
- So vidian nerve carries both **parasympathetic and sympathetic** fibers to ***lacrimal, nasal, palatine and pharyngeal glands*** distributed through branches of **pterygopalatine ganglion.**
- ***Vidian neurectomy**** can be done in cases where vasomotor rhinitis is refractory to medical treatment.
- A ***fast-growing tumor*** in the **sphenoidal sinus *erodes the floor of the sinus, endangering the vidian nerve.***

Ans: (a) Vidian nerve

Ref: *Imaging of skull base: Pictorial essay, Abhijit A Raut, Prashant S Naphade, Ashish Chawla, Indian J, Radiol Imaging, 2012, Oct-Dec; 22(4):305–316*

13. Structure passing through Sinus of Morgagni:

(a) Levator veli palatini
(b) Ascending pharyngeal artery
(c) Glossopharyngeal nerve
(d) Tensor tympani

Explanation:

Sinus of Morgagni: [The interval between **base of skull and superior constrictor muscle**].

Structures passing through sinus of Morgagni:

- *Auditory tube.*
- *Levator veli palatini.*
- *Ascending palatine artery.*
- *Palatine branch of ascending pharyngeal artery.*

Structures passing between superior constrictor and middle constrictor:

- *Stylopharyngeus muscle.*
- *Glossopharyngeal* nerve.

Structures passing between middle constrictor and inferior constrictor:

- *Internal laryngeal nerve.*
- *Superior laryngeal vessels.*

Structures passing below the inferior constrictor muscle [in the trachea-oesophageal groove]:

- *Recurrent laryngeal nerve.*
- *Inferior laryngeal vessels.*
- **Killian's dehiscence** – Gap between the thyropharyngeus and cricopharyngeus.
- ***Pharyngeal diverticulum or Zenker's diverticulum*** [mucous membrane of the pharynx bulges] occurs through Killian's dehiscence in neuromuscular incoordination affecting the **thyropharyngeus** and **crico-pharyngeus.**

Ans: (a) Levator veli palatini

Ref: *Essentials of Human Anatomy, A.K. Datta, 3rd Edition, 2003, Volume-II, Page 304 and 305*

14. A child with chronic suppurative otitis media, develops recurrent meningitis. The spread of infection to CNS most probably occurred through:

(a) Hyrtl's fissure
(b) Foramen of Luscha
(c) Fissure of Santorini
(d) Persistent pterosquamous septum

Explanation:

Hyrtl's fissure or tympanomeningeal fissure:

- Hyrtl's fissure is a transient anatomic landmark in the developing fetal petrous temporal bone and is ***usually closed*** by the normal progression of ossification in the ***24th week of gestation.***
- It occasionally ***persists*** into extrauterine life and ***cause recurrent meningitis and spontaneous CSF ottorhoea.***

Fissure of Santorini:

- ***Vertical fissures*** in the anterior portion of the ***external auditory canal*** cartilage in the region of the ***bony-cartilaginous junction.***

Foramen of Luscha:

- ***Lateral apertures in the fourth ventricle of brain.*** Through this opening CSF enters into the subarachnoid space of brain and spinal cord.

Persistent petrosquamous septum [Korner's septum]:

- It is a dense, bony plate found in the mastoid process which represents the ***persistence of the petrosquamous suture line.*** The petrosquamous suture is between the petrous portion and the squamous portion of the temporal bone.

Ans: (a) Hyrtl's fissure

Ref: *Hyrtl's fissure, Rich PM, Graham J, Phelps PD. Otol Neurotol 2002 Jul;23(4):476-82 and Int J Pediatr Otorhinolaryngol 2001, Sep 28; 60(3): 227-37*

15. Which of the following pharyngeal arch give rise to the development of branchial fistula extending from base of tongue to anterior border of sternocleidomastoid?

(a) 1st arch
(b) 2nd arch
(c) 3rd pouch
(d) 4th arch

Explanation:

- ***Branchial fistulas*** occur when the ***second pharyngeal arch fails to grow caudally*** over the **third and fourth arches,** leaving remnants of the **second, third and fourth clefts** in contact with the surface by a narrow canal.
- Such a fistula, found on the lateral aspect of the neck directly ***anterior to the sternocleidomastoid*** muscle, usually provides drainage for a **lateral cervical cyst.**
- **Branchial cysts,** remnants of the cervical sinus, are most often just below the angle of the jaw, although they may be ***found anywhere along the anterior border of the sternocleidomastoid*** muscle.
- ***Internal branchial fistulas*** are rare; they occur when the ***cervical sinus*** is connected to the lumen of the pharynx by a small canal, which usually opens in the ***tonsillar region [base of tongue].***
- Such a fistula results from a ***rupture of the membrane between the second pharyngeal cleft and pouch*** at some time during development.

Ans: (b) 2nd arch

Ref: *Langman's Medical Embryology, T.W. Sadler, 13th Edition, 2016, Page 288 and 289*

PHYSIOLOGY

1. **Deglutitive inhibition:**

(a) Wave of inhibition preceding peristalsis
(b) Inhibition occurs simultaneously with peristalsis
(c) Inhibition occurs after peristalsis
(d) Wave of stimulation preceding peristalsis

Explanation:

Deglutitive inhibition

- **Definition:** A **second swallow,** initiated while an **earlier peristaltic contraction is still progressing** in the striated muscles of esophagus, causing rapid and complete inhibition of the contraction induced by the first swallow.
- It happens secondary to **hyperpolarization** of the circular smooth muscle.
- It is mediated through **nonadrenergic, noncholinergic** neurons in the **myenteric plexus** in GI tract.

Deglutition

- It is the process of swallowing.
- It refers to the passage of food from the oral cavity into the stomach.
- It comprises three stages namely:
  1. Oral phase – voluntary.
  2. Pharyngeal phase – involuntary.
  3. Esophageal phase – involuntary.

Motility events in the esophagus

- During the esophageal phase, food bolus is pushed from esophagus to the stomach by peristalsis.
- Two types of sphincters are seen in esophagus namely:
  - **Upper esophageal sphincter:**
    - Formed by the cricopharyngeal muscle.
    - It is normally contracted tonically and opens only during swallowing.
  - **Upper esophageal sphincter:**
    - Also called as cardiac sphincter.
    - Its main function is to prevent regurgitation of gastric contents into esophagus.

Ans: (b) Inhibition occurs simultaneously with peristalsis

Ref: *Yamada's Textbook of Gastroenterology, 5th Edition, Page 194*

2. **PO_2 (in mm Hg) in skeletal muscle during exercise:**

(a) 3 (b) 10 (c) 20 (d) 30

Explanation:

- PO_2(in mm Hg) in skeletal muscle during exercise can be as low as **1 to 3 mm Hg***.
- This is mainly due to the **compression of blood vessels** supplying the **muscle** during muscle contraction.
- Fortunately, **myoglobin** in the muscle acts as a reservoir for O_2 and enhances its diffusion during exercise.

Skeletal muscle blood flow during exercise:

- At rest, skeletal muscle receives blood flow of **2–4 mL/100 g/min.** But during exercise the value increase by more than **20 times – 80 mL/100 g/min.**
- This increase is mainly because of:
  - Accumulation of **local metabolites** that causes vasodilation.
  - Opening up of **new capillaries** during exercise.

Redistribution of blood flow in the body

- Tremendous increase in skeletal muscle flow is made possible by **redistribution of blood flow.**
- **Sympathetic, nor adrenergic vasoconstriction** occurs in two important vascular beds:
    - **Renal circulation*.**
    - **Splanchnic blood flow*.**
- Vasoconstriction in Renal and Splanchnic system diverts their blood to the exercising muscle.
- **Cutaneous blood** flow **increases** during sustained activities to **dissipate the heat** generated during exercise.
- **Coronary blood flow increases** by more than **four times** than **normal*.**
- **Cerebral blood flow** remains largely **unchanged.**

Ans: (a) 3 mm Hg

***Ref:** West Respiratory Physiology, 9th Edition, Page 91*

3. A man weighing 70 kg has a hematocrit of 45%. What would be his approximate plasma volume?

(a) 2310 ml (b) 2695 ml (c) 2890 ml (d) 3080 ml

Explanation:

- Average blood volume account for **8% of body weight.**
- So, here for 70 Kg man, Blood volume is **5.6 Litres (70 × 8/100).**
- **Blood Volume = Plasma volume/1-Hematocrit.**
- So, **Plasma volume = Blood volume × (1-hematocrit).**
- Here, Plasma volume = 5.6*(1-0.45) = **3080 ml.**

Total Body Water (60% of body weight), 42 liters		
Intracellular fluid	**Extracellular fluid**	
2/3rd of **TBW,** i.e., **40%** body weight (**28 liters**)	**1/3rd** of **TBW,** i.e., **20%** body weight (14 liters)	
	Interstitial Fluid	**Plasma**
	75% or 3/4th of **ECF** or **15%** of body weight (**10.5 liters**)	**25% or 1/4th** of **ECF** Or **5%** of body weight **(3.5 liters)**

Ans: (d) 3080 ml

***Ref:** Ganong Review of Medical Physiology, 21st Edition, Page 2*

4. A patient who underwent extensive bowel resection is on total parenteral nutrition (TPN) for 1 month. Endoscopy done after one month reveals diffuse gastric mucosal atrophy. Which enzyme deficiencies are most likely responsible for gastric mucosal atrophy in this patient?

(a) Gastrin and Ghrelin (b) Secretin and CCK
(c) Gastrin and CCK (d) Gastrin and Secretin

Explanation:

Gastrin

- Produced by **G cells** in the **antral portion** of the gastric mucosa.
- Three forms – **G 34, G 17 and G 14** gastrins.
- **G 17** is the principal form*.
- Acts via **CCK-B receptor*.**
- **Stimuli** that increase gastrin secretion:
    - **Peptides*.**
    - **Amino acids** (Phenylalanine, tryptophan).
    - Gastric distension.
    - **Gastrin releasing peptide*.**
    - Calcium.
    - Epinephrine.
- Stimuli that decrease gastrin secretion:
    - Acid.

- **Somatostatin*.**
- **Secretin*.**
- **GIP.**
- **VIP.**
- **Glucagon.**
- Calcitonin.

- **Actions:**
  - Stimulation of **gastric acid and pepsin secretion.**
  - Stimulation of the growth of the mucosa of GI tract **(Trophic action*).**

Cholecystokinin

- Secreted by **I cells** in the **mucosa** of the **upper small intestine*.**
- Also found in **nerves** in the **distal ileum, colon and brain.**
- Acts via **CCK-A receptor*.**
- **Functions** of CCK:
  - Gut-stimulation of **pancreatic enzyme secretion.**
  - **Contraction** of the **gallbladder*.**
  - **Relaxation** of the **sphincter of Oddi.**
  - Brain-regulation of **food intake.**
  - Production of **anxiety** and **analgesia.**
- **Other actions:**
  - Augments the action of **secretin.**
  - **Inhibits gastric emptying.**
  - Exerts a **trophic** effect on the **pancreas.**
  - Increases the **synthesis** of **enterokinase.**
- Releasing factors that activate CCK secretion:
  - CCK-releasing peptide (intestinal mucosa).
  - Monitor peptide (pancreas).
- **Stimuli that increase CCK secretion:**
  - Peptides and amino acids.
  - Fatty acids (more than 10 carbon atoms).

Ans: (c) Gastrin and CCK

Ref: *Yamada's Textbook of Gastroenterology, 5th Edition, Page 284*

5. Direction of sound is differentiated by:

(a) Auditory cortex
(b) Medial geniculate body
(c) Lateral geniculate body
(d) Inferior colliculus

Explanation:

Central auditory pathway

- Auditory pathway can be easily remembered with the help of a very familiar mnemonic **"E COLI MA".**

Structure	Characteristics
<u>E</u>ighth nerve	• Carries the afferent auditory information
<u>C</u>ochlear nuclei	• 95% of fibers in cochlear nuclei are myelinated fibers that receives input from inner hair cells • Small number (5%) of unmyelinated fibers receives input from outer hair cells
Superior <u>O</u>livary nucleus	• Receives information from both the ears (bilateral) • Helps in localization of sound and the direction from which the sound comes • Also send efferent to outer hair cells in the form of **olivocochlear bundle** modulates the sensitivity of these hair cells and blocks background noise
<u>L</u>ateral lemniscus	• Project auditory information to inferior colliculus
<u>I</u>nferior colliculus	• All auditory pathways ascending through the brainstem converge in inferior colliculi • Helps in localization of sound and the direction from which the sound comes

Contd.

Contd.

Medial geniculate body	• Thalamic nuclei for hearing • Project to auditory cortex
Auditory cortex	• Location – Superior temporal gyrus of the temporal lobe • Also called as **Heschl gyrus** • Tonotopic organization – Low tones are represented anterolaterally and high tones postero-medially • **Planum temporale** – Part of auditory cortex involved in language related auditory processing. It is larger in the left hemisphere

Ans: (d) Inferior colliculus

Ref: *Kandel, Principle of Neural Sciences, 5th Edition, Page 697*

6. A 60-year-old patient, known case of Hypertension for the past 25 years underwent renal artery doppler which showed narrowing and turbulence in right renal artery. If the diameter of lumen is reduced by 50%, how much blood flow will be reduced?

(a) 1/4th (b) 1/8th (c) 1/16th (d) 1/32nd

Explanation:

Blood flow (F)

- Blood flow (F) inside vessel depends on:
  - **Pressure difference** (P_A - P_B) – Directly related*.
  - **Viscosity of the fluid** (η) – Inversely related*.
    - Viscosity is a measure of a fluid's resistance to flow.
    - A fluid with low viscosity flows easily. Such fluids are called **Newtonian fluid.** Example is **water*.**
    - A fluid with high viscosity flows resists motion. Such fluids are called: Non-Newtonian fluid. Example is **blood*.**
    - **Fahraeus-Lindqvist effect** – This effect is seen mainly in **capillaries** where RBCs flow in the center which leaves cell free plasma near the vessel wall. So, the viscosity change per unit change in hematocrit is much less in capillaries.
  - **Radius of the vessel** (r^4) – directly related.
  - **Length of the vessel** (L) – inversely related.
- Inter-relation of these factors are expressed in **Poiseuille-Hagen formula** which is:

$$F = (P_A - P_B) * \pi r^4 / 8 \eta L$$

- According to the above formula, blood flow is directly proportional to the **fourth power of radius*.**
- So, if the radius is **halved,** then blood flow decreases by **2^4 times** which is **16 times*.**

Ans: (c) 1/16th

Ref: *Ganong, 25th Edition, Page 573*

7. PCO_2 at alveoli and expired air is 40 and 30 mm Hg respectively. Calculate dead space to tidal volume ratio.

(a) 0.20 (b) 0.25 (c) 0.30 (d) 0.35

Explanation:

- **Dead space** to **tidal volume** ratio is calculated by **PCO_2 of alveolar air – PCO_2 of expired air/PCO_2** of **alveolar air.** This equation is called **Bohr's equation.**

$$\text{Dead space to tidal volume ratio} = \frac{PCO_2 \text{ of alveolar air} - PCO_2 \text{ of expired air}}{PCO_2 \text{ of alveolar air}}$$

- So, Here it is **40 – 30/40,** that comes around **0.25.**

Dead space ventilation

- Dead space ventilation means the ventilation that is not used for gas exchange.
- It can be of three types:
  1. Anatomic dead space.
  2. Alveolar dead space.
  3. Physiologic or total dead space.

Anatomic dead space

- Is the volume of air present in the conducting zone (first 16 generations) which are not used for gas exchange.
- Volume of anatomic dead space (ml) is approximately equal to the body weight in pounds. For a 70 Kg man (154 pounds) it is 154 ml.

Alveolar dead space

- Is the volume of air present in those alveoli which do not take part in gas exchange.

Physiologic dead space

- Also called as **total dead space.**
- It is obtained by adding anatomic and alveolar dead space.
- Physiologic dead space = anatomic dead space + alveolar dead space.
- In healthy individuals, Physiologic dead space roughly equals anatomic dead space.

Measurement of anatomic dead space

- The technique useful for measuring anatomic dead space is **single-breath Nitrogen method.** This method is also called Fowler's **method.**

Measurement of physiologic (total) dead space

- Physiologic dead space is measured with the help of an equation termed **Bohr's equation.**

Ans: (b) 0.25

Ref: *West Respiratory Physiology, 9th Edition, Page 23*

8. **Alveolar arteriolar O_2 gradient is not increased in:**

(a) Decreased diffusion capacity
(b) Hypoventilation
(c) Shunting of blood
(d) Ventilation perfusion inequality

Explanation:

Alveolar-arterial oxygen difference - (A-a) DO_2

- Also called as **Alveolar–arterial gradient.**
- Normal **alveolar (A) PO_2** is around **104 mm Hg***.
- Normal **arterial (a) PO_2** is around **80 – 100 mm Hg***.
- So the difference **(A-a) DO_2** normally is around **5 to 15 mm Hg***.
- This difference is normally due to some degree of **ventilation perfusion mismatch** normally seen in lung due to shunting of blood.
- Causes of **increased Alveolar–arterial gradient:**
  - Normally with **ageing***.
  - Increased **ventilation-perfusion mismatch***.
  - **Right-to-left** shunt*.
  - **Impaired diffusion***.

Ans: (b) Hypoventilation

Ref: *West Respiratory Physiology, 9th Edition, Page 164*

9. **True regarding Brockenbrough effect:**

(a) Presystolic potentiation
(b) Afterload potentiation
(c) Post extrasystolic potentiation
(d) Post tetanic potentiation

Explanation:

- **Brockenbrough-Braunwald-Morrow effect** is the Paradoxical response to **post extrasystolic potentiation** where there is **decrease in stroke volume** and **pulse pressure** following **post extrasystolic potentiation.**
- Seen in patients with **Hypertrophic cardiomyopathy (HCM).**

Ans: (c) Post extrasystolic potentiation

Ref: *Trevino, Alejandro R. and John Buergler. "The Brockenbrough–Braunwald–Morrow Sign." Methodist DeBakey Cardiovascular Journal* **10.1 (2014): 34-37**

10. What happens when doubling the diffusion capacity of lungs?

(a) Decrease arterial PCO_2 during resting breathing
(b) Increase resting oxygen uptake when the subject breathes 10% oxygen
(c) Increase the uptake of nitrous oxide during anesthesia
(d) Increase maximal oxygen uptake at extreme altitude

Explanation:

- **Oxygen** is normally a **perfusion limited gas*.**
- **Oxygen** transfer becomes **diffusion limited*** only when there is **increase maximal oxygen uptake.**
  - At **extreme altitude*.**
  - **Emphysema*.**
  - **Pulmonary fibrosis*.**

Measurement of Diffusion Capacity

- In clinical practice, **carbon monoxide*** is the **gas of choice** for **measuring diffusion capacity** because it is the **diffusion limited gas*.**
- The procedure is called **diffusion capacity of the lung** for **carbon monoxide** or **DLCO.**

Diffusion capacity of the lung for carbon monoxide (DLCO)

- In this method, subject is made to take a **single breath of gas mixture** containing **dilute concentration (0.01%) of carbon monoxide (CO)** and hold his breath for **10 seconds** followed by **expiration.**
- Carbon monoxide (CO) uptake is calculated from the **difference** between the **inspired air and expired air CO concentration.**
- The **partial pressure of CO (pCO)** is calculated from the **end expiratory sample.**
- Diffusion capacity of the lung for carbon monoxide **(DLCO)** is calculated using the formula:

$$\text{DLCO} = \frac{\text{Carbon monoxide (CO) uptake}}{\text{pCO in alveolar air}}$$

- Normal value of DLCO is **25 mL/min/mm of Hg*.**

Ans: (d) Increase maximal oxygen uptake at extreme altitude

Ref: *West Respiratory Physiology, 9th Edition, Page 34*

11. A patient presents with right to left shunt. Oxygen content in arterial and venous side are 18 and 14 ml/100 ml respectively. Oxygen content at pulmonary capillary is 20. What is the percentage shunting of cardiac output?

(a) 23% (b) 33% (c) 43% (d) 53%

Explanation:

- The shunt as a fraction of cardiac output is given by the formula **(Cc.oxygen-Ca.oxygen)/(Cc.oxygen - Cv. oxygen).**
- **Here in this formula, Cc.oxygen denotes oxygen content in capillaries, Ca.oxygen denotes oxygen content in artery, Cv.oxygen denotes oxygen content in veins.**

- So, here in this question, oxygen content at pulmonary capillary is **20,** oxygen content in arterial and venous side are **18 and 14 ml/100 ml.**
- The answer is **20-18/20-14 = 33%.**

Ventilation – Perfusion ratio (V/Q ratio) – Clinical importance

- Imbalances in ventilation and perfusion commonly leads to ventilation perfusion mismatch that ultimately affects the gas exchange.

Ventilation – Perfusion ratio (V/Q ratio) = Zero (0)

- This means that ventilation (numerator) is zero. So, the ratio becomes zero.
- Physiological cause of non-uniform ventilation is:
  - o Shunt blood perfused regions – Oxygenation of shunt blood doesn't occur because there is no ventilation.
- Pathological causes of non-uniform ventilation are:
  - o Collapse of lung (emphysema).
  - o Foreign body obstruction.
  - o Bronchoconstriction due to asthma.
  - o Compression of airways by tumor.
  - o Pulmonary fibrosis.
  - o Pneumothorax.

Ventilation – Perfusion ratio (V/Q ratio) = ∞ (Infinity)

- This means that the perfusion is nil (denominator). So, the ratio becomes infinity.
- Physiological cause of non-uniform perfusion is:
  - o Dead spaces – No gas exchange happens.
- Pathological causes of non-uniform perfusion are:
  - o Pulmonary embolism.
  - o Compression of pulmonary vessels by high alveolar pressures.
  - o Tumor occluding pulmonary vessels.

Ans: (b) 33%

Ref: *West Respiratory Physiology, 9th Edition, Page 184*

12. If the alveolar PCO is 0.5 mm Hg and the CO uptake is 30 ml·min-1. What is the diffusing capacity of the lung for CO in ml·min-1 mm Hg-1?

(a) 20 (b) 30 (c) 40 (d) 60

Explanation:

- The equation is CO uptake divided by alveolar PCO.
- So, here in this question it is **30/0.5.**
- The answer is **60 ml min-1 mm Hg -1*.**

Factors affecting diffusion of gases across respiratory membrane

According to Fick's law, diffusion is directly proportional to:

- **Membrane surface area**
  - o If membrane surface area decreases, diffusion of gases decreases. This is the case in emphysema where diffusion capacity decreases due to reduction in membrane surface area.
- **Solubility of gases**
  - o The diffusion coefficient of CO_2 is about 20 times that of O_2. So, CO_2 diffuses much faster and easily than O_2.
- **Partial pressure difference.**

According to Fick's law, diffusion is inversely proportional to:

- **Membrane thickness**
  - o If membrane thickness increases, diffusion of gases decreases.
  - o This is the cause for decrease in diffusion capacity in conditions like pulmonary fibrosis where membrane thickness increases.

- **Molecular weight of the gas**

If the molecular weight of a gas is more, rate of diffusion of that gas will be less.

Ans: (d) 60

Ref: *West Respiratory Physiology, 9th Edition, Page 181*

13. If the concentration of inhaled O_2 is doubled, to the resultant effect will be:

(a) Partial pressure of oxygen decreases
(b) Doubles the amount of oxygen in solution
(c) Decrease in amount of oxygen bound with haemoglobin
(d) None of the above

Explanation:

- If the inspired partial pressure of oxygen is doubled, the amount of oxygen in solution doubles but does not double the amount of oxygen in the body because most of oxygen content is bound to haemoglobin.

Transport of oxygen

- Oxygen is transported in blood in two forms. They are:
  - Dissolved form (3%).
  - Combined with hemoglobin (97%).

Oxygen transport in dissolved form

- According to Henry's law, the amount of dissolved gas is proportional to its partial pressure.
- For each mm Hg of PO_2, there is 0.003 ml O_2/100 ml of blood.
- We know that the normal arterial blood have PO_2 of 100 mm Hg. So, the amount of dissolved oxygen is 0.003 ml * 100 = 0.3 ml O_2/100 ml of blood

Oxygen transported in dissolved form = 0.3 ml O_2/100 ml

Oxygen transport combined with hemoglobin

- Once the oxygen enters pulmonary capillaries from alveoli, much of it combines with the oxygen carrier protein in RBCs called hemoglobin.

Ans: (b) Doubles the amount of oxygen in solution

Ref: *Diving and Oxygen, Peter Wilmshurst, BMJ 1998 Oct 10; 317(7164):996–999*

BIOCHEMISTRY

1. A patient's CSF fluid analysis shows a CSF glucose of 30. His CSF/Plasma glucose ratio is 0.4. Which of the following GLUTs transports glucose in brain?

(a) 1 and 2
(b) 3 and 4
(c) 2 and 3
(d) 1 and 3

Explanation:

Glucose transporters mediate the facilitated diffusion of glucose across the membrane. They traverse the membrane 12 times.

Types of GLUT

Type	Organ distribution	Function
GLUT1	**Brain,** RBC, placenta, colon	Basal glucose uptake
GLUT2	**Liver, pancreatic β cells, kidney**	**Glucose sensor*** function
GLUT3	**Brain,** kidney, placenta	Basal glucose uptake
GLUT4	Skeletal and cardiac muscle, adipose tissue	**Insulin dependent** uptake
GLUT5	Small intestine, SPERM	**Fructose transporter***
GLUT6	Product of pseudogene	
GLUT7	Endoplasmic reticulum of hepatocytes	**Glucose-6-phosphate transporter**
GLUT12	Heart, skeletal muscle, brown adipose tissue, and prostate	Basal and Insulin dependent uptake

EXTRA EDGE:

- **Fanconi-Bickel disease** is due to defect in **GLUT2.**

Ans: (d) 1 and 3

Ref: *Harper, 30th Edition, Page 191; Table 19-2*

2. Enzyme catalysing substrate level phosphorylation in TCA cycle:

(a) Fumarase
(b) Succinate dehydrogenase
(c) Succinate thiokinase
(d) Alpha ketoglutarate dehydrogenase

Explanation:

- Main site of production of **ATP** is the **electron transport** chain by **oxidative phosphorylation.**
- Substrate level phosphorylation is phosphorylation of **ADP** without the involvement of **ETC.**
- Only high energy compounds which have free energy of hydrolysis more than that of ATP can participate in substrate level phosphorylation.

$$R\text{-}OPO_3^{2-} \xrightarrow{ADP \rightarrow ATP} R\text{-}OH$$

Glycolysis:

$$\text{1,3 bisphosphoglycerate} \xrightarrow[\textbf{1,3 BPG Kinase}]{ADP \rightarrow ATP} \text{3 bisphosphoglycerate}$$

$$\text{Phosphoenol pyruvate} \xrightarrow[\textbf{Pyruvate Kinase}]{ADP \rightarrow ATP} \text{Pyruvate}$$

TCA Cycle:

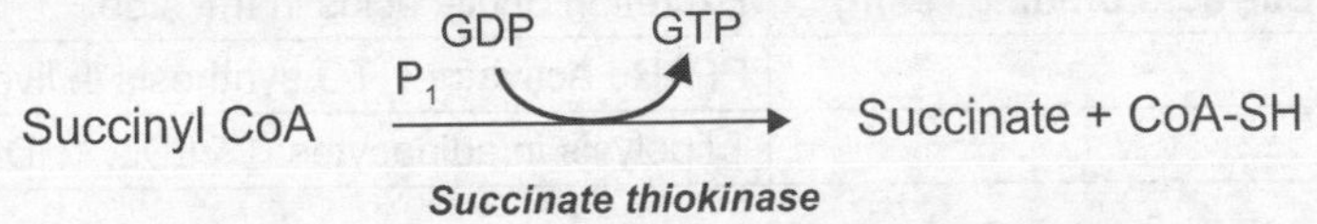

- **Arsenate** is the **uncoupler** of **1,3 BPG kinase** catalysed **substrate level phosphorylation.**

Ans: (c) Succinate thiokinase

Ref: *Harper, 30th Edition, Page 164*

3. The number of high energy bonds required to get 1 molecule of glucose from 2 molecules of lactate in anaerobic metabolism is:

(a) 4 (b) 8 (c) 6 (d) 12

Explanation:

- Energy audit of production of glucose from **2 molecules of lactate**

Reaction	**ATP required**
Pyruvate carboxylase	2 ATPs
Phosphoenol pyruvate carboxykinase	2 GTPs/ATPs
Phosphoglycerate kinase	2 ATPs
Total	6 ATPs

Other ATP requirements to be remembered:

Urea	4 ATP equivalents
Purine–IMP	6 ATP equivalents (5 ATP + 1 GTP)
Gluconeogenesis from 2 lactates	6 ATP equivalents
Gluconeogenesis from malate	4 ATP equivalents
Formation of 1 peptide by ribosome	4 ATP equivalents (Peptidyl transferase reaction needs no ATP).

Ans: (c) 6

Ref: *Harper, 30th Edition, Page 185*

4. Which of the following is the defect in type 2 familial hypercholesterolemia?

(a) Absence of VLDL receptor (b) Absence of hepatic LDL receptor
(c) Defective apoE (d) Over production of VLDL

Explanation:

Disorder	**Defect**
Familial lipoprotein lipase deficiency (type I)	LPL, or apo C-II
Familial hypercholesterolemia (type IIa)	LDL receptors or apoB-100
Familial type III hyperlipoproteinemia	apo E
Familial hypertriacylglycerolemia (type IV)	VLDL over production

EXTA EDGE:

Mechanism of action of hypolipidemic drugs:

Statins	Competitive inhibitor of **HMG CoA reductase**
Ezetimibe	Inhibits intestinal cholesterol absorption **(inhibits Niemann-Pick C1–like 1-NPC1L1)**

Contd.

Contd.

Cholestyramine (Bile acid binding resin)	Excretion of bile acids in the stool
Fibrates	PPARα activator (↓TG synthesis in liver)
Niacin	↓ lipolysis in adipocytes; ↓ VLDL; ↑HDL

5. **A 5-year-old boy presents with mental retardation and self-mutilation behavior. His serum uric acid levels are increased. The most probable enzyme deficient in this boy is:**

(a) Xanthine oxidase
(b) HGPRT transferase
(c) PRPP synthetase
(d) Orotic acid dehydrogenase

Explanation:

Lesch Nyhan Syndrome

- **X-linked recessive** disorder with ***complete*** **absence of HGPRTase** enzyme of purine salvage pathway. Enzymes of *de novo* synthesis of purines are absent in brain. Therefore brain is dependent entirely upon salvage pathway.
- **Reason for hyperuricemia:**
  - HGPRTase enzyme reutilises (salvages) purine bases. When these enzyme is deficient, **guanine, xanthine or hypoxanthine** are not salvaged and therefore degraded to uric acid resulting in hyperuricemia.
- **Clinical Features:**
  - Affected children are usually **male.**
  - Hyperuricemia.
  - Spasticity, Mental retardation.
  - **Self-mutilation*** – Biting tongue, fingers, chewing lips – striking feature of this disease.
- **Treatment:**
  - No curative treatment is available. Removal of deciduous teeth is done to avoid injury. Other managements are symptomatic.
  - Genetic counselling and carrier testing for prevention.

Ans: (b) HGPRT transferase

Ref: *Harper, 30th Edition, Page 354*

6. **Major factor that determines if glucose is oxidized by aerobic or anaerobic glycolysis is:**

(a) NADH
(b) FADH2
(c) Presence of mitochondria
(d) Presence of low glucose

Explanation:

- RBC lacks mitochondria and utilise glucose through anaerobic glycolysis.
- Let's see why pyruvates needs to be converted lactate.
- **Glyceraldehyde 3 phosphate dehydrogenase reaction of glycolysis require NAD⁺ as a cofactor.**

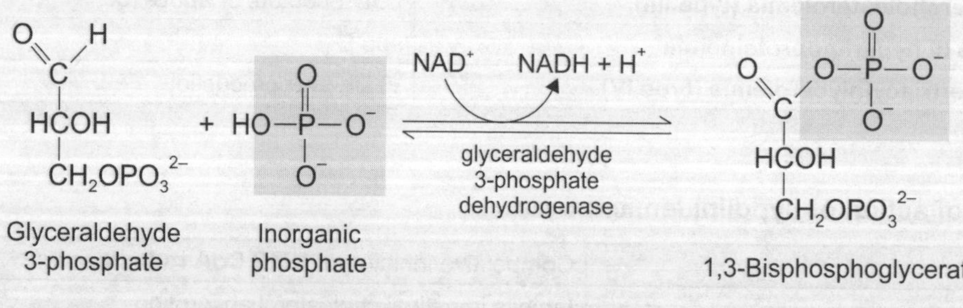

- NADH can be converted to NAD⁺ after donating the electrons to electron transport chain. If there is no mitochondria or there is no oxygen available, there is other way of regenerating the NAD⁺.

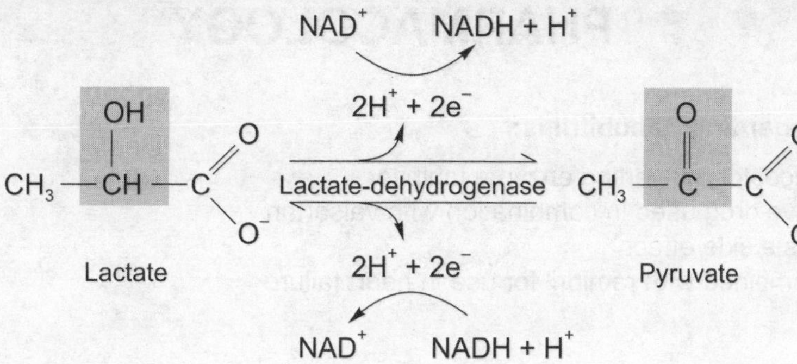

- If there is no mitochondria, to regenerate the NAD^+, pyruvate needs to be converted to lactate (anaerobic glycolysis).

Ans: (c) Presence of mitochondria

PHARMACOLOGY

1. **True statement regarding Sacubitril is:**

(a) Angiotensin receptor converting enzyme inhibitor
(b) Antihypertensive drug used in combination with valsartan
(c) Hypokalemia is a side effect
(d) Sacubitril is combined with ramipril for use in heart failure

Explanation:

Sacubitril

- **Neprilysin** degrades **natriuretic peptides, angiotensin II, bradykinin** and **substance P.**
- **Neprilysin** is inhibited by **Sacubitril** increasing the levels of **natriuretic peptides** and **angiotensin II.**
- To overcome excess of angiotensin II, an Angiotension receptor blocker (ARB) is added along with Sacubitril.
- Sacubitril is a Neprilysin inhibitor and valsartan angiotensin receptor blocker and the combination described as an **"angiotensin receptor-neprilysin inhibitor" (ARNi).**
- Sacubitril is approved for treatment of **heart failure** with along the **valsartan.**
- Combination specifically indicated to **reduce the risk of cardiovascular death** and **hospitalization** for **heart failure** in patients with **chronic heart failure (NYHA Class II-IV)** and **reduced ejection fraction.**

Other options:

- Angiotensin receptor converting enzyme inhibitor: It is not ACE inhibitor.
- Hypokalemia is **NOT** a side effect of sacubitril.
- Sacubitril and valsartan combination has following side effects:
  - ***Hypotension***
  - ***Hyperkalemia****
  - ***Cough***
  - ***Dizziness***
  - ***Renal failure***
- Sacubitril is combined with **valsartan,** not Ramipril for use in heart failure.

Ans: (a) Antihypertensive drug used in combination with valsartan

Ref: *https://www.pharma.us.novartis.com/sites/www.pharma.us.novartis.com/files/entresto.pdf*

2. **Anti-cancer drug causing non-cardiac pulmonary edema:**

(a) Asparginase
(b) Cytosine arabinoside
(c) Gemcitabine
(d) Oxaliplatin

Explanation:

Cytosine arabinoside

- Antimetabolite used in **AML.**
- Most effective agent for **induction of remission** in **AML.**
- An analog **of 2′-deoxycytidine** and interferes with **base pairing.**
- Enters cells via a **nucleoside transporter** and is converted to its active form, the **5′-monophosphate ribonucleotide,** by **deoxycytidine kinase.**
- **Adverse effects:**
  - **Leukopenia, Thrombocytopenia and Anemia.**
  - GI disturbances, stomatitis, conjunctivitis.
  - **Reversible hepatic enzyme elevations.**
  - **Non-cardiogenic pulmonary edema*.**
  - Dermatitis.

Ans: (b) Cytosine arabinoside

Ref: *Goodman and Gillman's, The Pharmacological Basis of Therapeutics, 12th Edition, Page 1700*

3. **All are true regarding amantidine *except*:**

(a) It is an antiviral drug
(b) Indicated in parkinsonism
(c) Acts by increasing adenosine
(d) Causes livedo reticularis

Explanation:

Amantidine:

- Mechanism of Action: Unclear; Proposed mechanisms
  - Block presynaptic DA reuptake.
  - Facilitation of DA release.
  - Postsynaptic DA agonism.
  - Anticholinergic properties.
  - Blocks NMDA glutamate receptors.
- **Uses:**
  - Initial therapy of **mild Parkinson's disease.**
  - As an adjunct in patients on **levodopa** with dose-related **fluctuations** and **dyskinesias.**

Other uses:

- As antiviral against **influenza A.**
- Mechanisms of action
  - Inhibit an early step in **viral replication** (viral uncoating) strains.
  - At late step it **alters hemagglutinin processing.**
- Main action is on **M2 protein,** an integral membrane protein that functions as an ion channel. By interfering with this function of the M2 protein, the drug inhibit the acid-mediate dissociation of the ribonucleoprotein complex early in replication and potentiate acidic pH-induced conformational changes in the hemagglutinin during its intracellular transport later in replication.
- **Rimantadine** is 4-10 times more active than **amantadine.**

Other options:

- **Livedo reticularis** is a known adverse effect of **amantadine.**
- Amantadine doesn't increase adenosine levels.

Ans: (c) Acts by increasing adenosine

Ref: *Goodman and Gillman's, The Pharmacological Basis of Therapeutics,12th Edition, Page 438*

4. **Anti-mycobacterial drug causing anterior uveitis when used along with clarithromycin:**

(a) Rifabutin
(b) Ethambutol
(c) Rifampicin
(d) Isoniazid

Explanation:

- **Uveitis** and **arthralgias** are seen in patients taking **rifabutin** doses >450 mg daily in combination with **clarithromycin.**
- Rifabutin causes an **orange-tan discoloration** of **skin, urine, feces, saliva, tears and contact lenses,** like **rifampin.**
- **Other side effects of Rifabutin:**
  - **Thrombocytopenia**
  - Flu-like syndrome
  - Hemolysis
  - Myositis
  - Chest pain
  - Hepatitis
- Unique side effects include **polymyalgia, pseudojaundice and anterior uveitis*.**

Note:

- **Uveitis** and **arthralgias** are seen in patients taking rifabutin doses >450 mg daily in combination with **fluconazole** also.

Ans: (a) Rifabutin

Ref: *Goodman and Gillman's, The Pharmacological Basis of Therapeutics, 12th Edition, Page 1553*

5. **Beta blocker with nitric oxide releasing property:**

(a) Nebuvilol (b) Sotalol (c) Betaxolol (d) Atenolol

Explanation:

Nebuvilol

- Third-generation cardioselective beta blocker.
- Has **endothelial nitric oxide**-mediated **vasodilation.**
- Has **antioxidant** properties.
- Neutral to favorable effects on both **carbohydrate and lipid metabolism.**
- May increase **insulin sensitivity.**
- Most of the benefits are seen in patients with **metabolic syndrome and hypertension.**

Other points:

Beta blockers releasing nitric oxide (NO)

- ***Nebuvilol***
- ***Celiprolol***
- ***Nipradilol***
- ***Bopindolol***
- ***Carteolol***

Ans: (a) Nebuvilol

Ref: *Goodman and Gillman's, The Pharmacological Basis of Therapeutics, 12th Edition, Page 315*

6. **Ibrutinib drug is used in all the following conditions *except*:**

(a) Mantle cell lymphoma (b) Chronic lymphocytic leukemia
(c) Waldenström's macroglobulinemia (d) AML

Explanation:

Ibrutinib

- Kinase inhibitor indicated for the treatment of patients with:
  - ***Mantle Cell Lymphoma.***
  - ***Chronic Lymphocytic Leukemia.***
  - ***Chronic Lymphocytic Leukemia with 17p deletion.***
  - ***Waldenström's Macroglobulinemia.***

Mechanism of action:

- Small-molecule **inhibitor** of **BTK (Bruton's tyrosine kinase).**
- Forms a covalent bond with a cysteine residue in the BTK active site, leading to inhibition of BTK enzymatic activity.
- BTK is a signalling molecule of the B-cell antigen receptor (BCR) and cytokine receptor pathways.
- BTK's role in signalling through the B-cell surface receptors results in activation of pathways necessary for B-cell trafficking, chemotaxis and adhesion.

Ans: (d) AML

Ref: *https://www.accessdata.fda.gov/drugsatfda_docs/label/2015/205552s002lbl.pdf*

7. **Famciclovir is prodrug of:**

(a) Acylovir (b) Gancilovir
(c) Peniciclovir (d) Valcyclovir

Explanation:

Famciclovir

- Prodrug of **penciclovir***.
- **Nucleoside analogue and inhibitor of DNA polymerase.**

MOA:

- Viral thymidine kinase phosphorylates penciclovir to a monophosphate form that, in turn, is converted by cellular kinases to the active form penciclovir triphosphate.
- Penciclovir triphosphate inhibits **HSV-2 DNA polymerase** competitively with **deoxyguanosine triphosphate.**
- Herpes viral DNA synthesis and replication are selectively inhibited.

Uses:

- ***Herpes labialis.***
- ***Genital herpes.***
- ***Herpes zoster.***
- Treatment of ***recurrent episodes of orolabial or genital herpes*** in **HIV**-Infected Adult Patients.

Adverse Effects:

- Headache, diarrhea and nausea.
- Urticaria and rash.
- Hallucinations or confusional states.

Ans: (c) Peniciclovir

Ref: *Goodman and Gillman's, The Pharmacological Basis of Therapeutics,12th Edition, Page 1601*

8. **Mechanism of action of Bortezomib:**

(a) mTOR inhibitor
(b) Proteosome inhibitor
(c) Histone deacetylase inhibitors
(d) Protein tyrosine kinase inhibitor

Explanation:

Bortezomib

- Reversible inhibitor of the **chymotrypsin-like activity** of the **26S proteasome** in mammalian cells.
- 26S proteasome is a large protein complex that **degrades ubiquitinated proteins.**
- Ubiquitin proteasome pathway plays an essential role in regulating the intracellular concentration of specific proteins, thereby maintaining homeostasis within cells.
- Inhibition of the 26S proteasome prevents this targeted proteolysis, which can affect multiple signalling cascades within the cell.
- This disruption of normal homeostatic mechanisms can lead to **cell death.**
- Bortezomib causes a **delay in tumor growth** in vivo in nonclinical tumor models, including multiple myeloma.

Uses:

- FDA approved as initial therapy for **multiple myeloma (MM).**
- Therapy for **MM after relapse** from other drugs.
- Relapsed or **refractory mantle cell lymphoma.**

Adverse effects

- Thrombocytopenia.
- Fatigue, or weakness.
- Limb pain, Peripheral neuropathy.
- Anemia, Neutropenia.
- Nausea, Vomiting, Diarrhea, Dehydration.

Other options:

- **m TOR inhibitor:** Temsirolimus, Everolimus.
- **Histone deacetylase inhibitors:** Vorinostat, Romidepsin.
- **Protein tyrosine kinase inhibitor:** Imatinib, Dastinib, Sorafenib.

Ans: (b) Proteosome inhibitor

Ref: *Goodman and Gillman's, The Pharmacological Basis of Therapeutics, 12th Edition, Page 1742*

9. **Drug that does not bind to alpha 1 acid glycoprotein:**

(a) Quinidine (b) Lidocaine
(c) Disopyramide (d) Propranolol

Explanation:

- The correct option is **disopyramide.**
- All the drugs given in options bind to **alpha 1 acid glycoprotein**, the least is **disopyramide.**

Drugs highly bound to plasma protein	
To ablumin	**To α_1-acid glycoprotein**
Barbiturates	β-blockers
Benzodiazepines	Bupivacaine
NSAIDs	Lidocaine
Valproic acid	Disopyramide
Phenytoin	Imipramine
Penicillins	Methadone
Sulfonamides	Prazosin
Tetracyclines	Quinidine
Tolbutamide	Verapamil
Warfarin	

Ans: (c) Disopyramide

Ref: *Goodman and Gillman's, The Pharmacological Basis of Therapeutics, 12th Edition, Page 835, Table 29-5*

10. **Olcegepant is:**

(a) CGRP receptor antagonist (b) Serotonin 1F agonist
(c) Bradykinin receptor agonist (d) Kallikrein antagonist

Explanation:

Olcegepant:

- First potent and **selective, non-peptide antagonist** of the **calcitonin gene-related peptide 1 (CGRP1) receptor,** a key modulator in **neurogenic inflammatory pain.**
- An intravenous formulation for treatment of **acute attacks of migraine.**
- **Calcitonin gene-related peptide (CGRP)** is a neuropeptide that acts in the trigeminovascular system and is believed to play an important role in **migraine.**
- CGRP activates two receptors that are both present in the **trigeminovascular system:**
  - The CGRP receptor and
  - The **amylin receptor**
- **CGRP receptor antagonists,** including **olcegepant** and **telcagepant** can treat migraine.
- CGRP is produced in both **peripheral and central neurons.**
- CGRP is a **potent vasodilator** and its levels increased following migraine attack.
- Venous administration of **calcitonin gene-related peptide** to patients prone to migraine can induce **migraine-like headache.**

Other options:

Serotonin 1F agonist	*Lasmiditan (used in migraine)*
Bradykinin receptor antagonist	*Icatibant*
Kallikrein antagonist	*Aprotinin (used in coronary bypass surgery)*

Ans: (a) CGRP receptor antagonist

Ref: *Gang Yao et al.,Therapeutic Effects and Safety of Olcegepant and Telcagepant for Migraine: A Meta-analysis, Neural Regen Res. 2013 Apr 5; 8(10): 938–947*

11. Which of the following drug is not used in the treatment of Tourette syndrome?

(a) Oxcarbazepine (b) Verapamil
(c) Clonidine (d) Haloperidol

Explanation:

- Tourette's syndrome is a developmental neuropsychiatric disorder characterized by:
  - Multiple, brief, recurrent, nonrhythmic movements and one or more vocalizations called tics.
  - The tics may vary in frequency, but persist for more than one year.
- Neurobiological and pharmacological data have implicated **central monoaminergic** and **neuropeptidergic systems.**
- Evidence supports a critical role for **dopamine (DA),** the involvement of **norepinephrine (NE)** and **corticotropin-releasing factor (CRF)** has also been suggested because patients frequently report that tics are more severe during periods of stress.
- Recent interest has been focused on the role of two closely related **neurosecretory nonapeptides, arginine vasopressin and oxytocin.**

Now the main treatments for tics are:

Neuroleptic drugs	*Haloperidol, pimozide*
Atypical antipsychotics risperidone	*Aripiprazole*
Substitute benzamides	*Sulpiride, tiapride*
Presynaptic dopamine depletors	*Tetrabenazine*

Drugs used in treatment of Tourette's syndrome:

Risperidone	Haloperidol	Botulinum toxin
Clonidine	Tetrabenazine	Thioridazine
Aripiprazole	Ziprasidone	Guanfacine
Pimozide	Quetiapine	Oxcarbazepine
Sulpiride	Tetrahydrocannabinol	Atomoxetine
Tiapride	Desipramine	

Ans: (b) Verapamil

Ref: *CMDT 2017, 56th Edition, Page 1018*

12. Example of Bi-specific T-cell engagers (BiTEs):

(a) Alemtuzumab (b) Blinatumomab
(c) Ibritumomab (d) Muromonab

Explanation:

Types of Monoclonal antibodies in cancer therapy:

- Naked monoclonal antibodies.
- Conjugated monoclonal antibodies:
  - Radiolabeled antibodies.
  - Chemolabeled antibodies.
- Bispecific monoclonal antibodies.

Naked monoclonal antibodies:

- Most common type used to treat cancer.
- No drug or radioactive material attached to them.
- Bind to antigens on cancer cells, non-cancerous cells, or target proteins.
- **Example:**
  - **Alemtuzumab** (CD 52 antigen) – Used in Chronic lymphocytic leukemia.
  - **Trastuzumab** (HER2 protein) – Used in Breast cancer.

Conjugated monoclonal antibodies:

- Joined to a **chemotherapy drug or to a radioactive particle.**
- Helpful in delivering the drug to target cells without affecting normal cells.
- Also called as tagged, labelled, or loaded antibodies.

Radiolabeled antibodies:

- Radiolabeled antibodies have small radioactive particles attached to them.
- Example: **Ibritumomab tiuxetan (CD20 antigen).**
- Delivers radioactivity directly to cancerous B.
- This is also as **radioimmunotherapy (RIT).**

Chemolabeled antibodies:

- Chemotherapy drugs are attached.
- Also known as antibody-drug conjugates.
- Example: **Brentuximab vedotin (CD30 antigen):** Used in **Hodgkin lymphoma** and **anaplastic large cell lymphoma.**
- **Denileukin diftitox:** Used in Cutaneous T-cell lymphoma.

Bispecific monoclonal antibodies (BiTE)

- Made up of parts of 2 different mAbs.
- They can attach to 2 different proteins at the same time.
- Example: **Blinatumomab** is a first-in-class bispecific antibody with high affinity toward both **CD19** (expressed primarily on **surface B cells**) and **CD3** (found on **T lymphocytes**) receptors.
- Part of blinatumomab attaches to the **CD19 protein** and another part attaches to **CD3.** By binding to both of these proteins, this drug brings the cancer cells and immune cells together, which is thought to cause the immune system to attack the cancer cells.
- Received accelerated approval for treatment of **Philadelphia chromosome-negative (Ph–) B-cell acute lymphoblastic leukemia (B-ALL) in December 2014.**

Ans: (b) Blinatumomab

Ref: *Maria Ribera J, et al., Profile of Blinatumomab and Its Potential in the Treatment of Relapsed/refractory acute lymphoblastic leukemia, Onco Targets Ther 2015; 8: 1567–1574*

13. Levodopa and carbidopa combination doesn't reduce which of the following side effect?

(a) Psychosis (b) Severe vomiting
(c) Arrhythmia (d) Postural hypotension

Explanation:

Advantages of the Levodopa and carbidopa combination are:

- **Dose** of levodopa **reduced** and its **half-life prolonged.**
- Nausea and vomiting decrease due to less dopamine in circulation.
- Therapeutic doses of levodopa can be attained quickly.
- **Cardiac complications** like arrhythmias are lessened.
- Levodopa effect decreased by pyridoxine does not occur.
- **'On-off' phenomenon** is reduced.
- **Efficacy** of the drug increase.

Disadvantages of the Levodopa and carbidopa combination are:

- **Involuntary movements.**
- Behavioural abnormalities like **psychosis** (Excessive DA action in the limbic system is probably responsible).
- **Excessive day time sleepiness** in some patients.
- **Postural hypotension** (It is more common in patients receiving antihypertensives. Tolerance develops with continued treatment and BP normalizes).
- So from the above points we may conclude that combination of levodopa and carbidopa can reduce side effects such as severe **vomiting and cardiac arrhythmia.**

- But out of other two options postural hypotension and pyschosis.
- Postural hypotension will become normal after few days of treatment but pyschosis persists because of presence of dopamine in brain.
- So psychosis will not reduce even with the combination of levodopa and carbidopa.

Ans: (a) Psychosis

Ref: *Goodman and Gillman's, The Pharmacological Basis of Therapeutics, 12th Edition, Page 615*

14. Mechanism of action of centrally acting muscle relaxant:

(a) Decreases voluntary power and does not paralyse
(b) Increases voluntary power and does not paralyse
(c) Decrease muscle tone without reducing voluntary power
(d) Decreases voluntary power and cause muscle paralysis

Explanation:

Centrally acting muscle relaxants

- **Reduce skeletal muscle tone* without altering consciousness** and **voluntary power of muscle.**
- **Depress spinal and supraspinal polysynaptic reflexes** involved in the regulation of muscle tone.
- They also **depress Polysynaptic pathways** in the ascending reticular formation leading to **mild sedation.**
- No effect is seen on neuromuscular transmission or on muscle fibres.
- They reduce muscle spasticity in chronic spastic conditions, acute muscle spasms, tetanus.
- **Examples:**
  - ***Mephenesin***
  - ***Carisoprodol***
  - ***Chlorzoxazone***
  - ***Chlormezanone***
  - ***Baclofen***
  - ***Thiocolchicoside***
  - ***Tizanidine***
- So among the options the correct one is centally acting muscle relaxants decrease muscle tone without reducing voluntary power.
- But peripherally acting muscle relaxants cause muscle paralysis and loss of voluntary movements, that's why they are used in anesthetic procedures. They primarily block neurotransmission at neuromuscular junction and produce least sedation.

Ans: (c) Decrease muscle tone without reducing voluntary power

Ref: *KD Tripathi - Essentials of Medical Pharmacology, 7th Edition, Page 357*

15. Cardioselective beta blocker with antioxidant property:

(a) Nebuvilol
(b) Sotalol
(c) Metoprolol
(d) Esmolol

Explanation:

Nebuvilol

- Third-generation **cardioselective beta blocker.**
- Has endothelial **NO-mediated vasodilation.**
- Has **antioxidant properties.**
- Neutral to favourable effects on both carbohydrate and lipid metabolism.
- May increase insulin sensitivity.
- Most of the benefits are seen in patients with metabolic syndrome and hypertension.

Ans: (a) Nebuvilol

Ref: *Goodman and Gillman's, The Pharmacological Basis of Therapeutics, 12th Edition, Page 330*

16. True regarding properties of Buspirone is:

(a) Anxiolytic + Muscle relaxant
(b) Anxiolytic alone
(c) Used as sedative hypnotic
(d) Used as Muscle relaxant

Explanation:

Buspirone

- Selective **partial agonist at 5-HT1A receptors.**
- Other drugs include **gepirone** and **ipsapirone.**
- An effective in the treatment of **anxiety.**
- Mimics the anti-anxiety properties of benzodiazepines.
- **Does not interact with GABA A receptors** and or display the sedative and anticonvulsant properties of benzodiazepines.
- So it ***doesn't have sedative*, anti-convulsant** or **muscle relaxant** property.
- It also has **antagonistic effects at dopamine D2 receptors.**
- It **does not impair psychomotor performance** or result in dependence.
- Used in **generalized anxiety disorder.**
- In **panic disorder** patients it increases **anxiety** (buspirone causes increased firing rates of the locus coeruleus) so it is avoided.

Ans: (b) Anxiolytic alone

__Ref:__ Goodman and Gillman's, The Pharmacological Basis of Therapeutics, 12th Edition, Page 349

17. Which of the following is true about steroidal inhibitor of Aromatase?

(a) Exemestane is reversible inhibitor of Aromatase
(b) Exemestane is irreversible inhibitor of Aromatase
(c) Anastrozole is reversible inhibitor of Aromatase
(d) Anastrozole is irreversible inhibitor of Aromatase

Explanation:

- In women **after menopause** more than **90% of the total body oestrogens** are synthesised by **aromatisation of testosterone** and **androstenedione** into **oestrone.**
- The enzyme for this reaction is **aromatase.**
- **Aromatase inhibitors** (AIs) **block** the **synthesis of oestrogen.**
- First–generation: **Aminoglutethimide.**
- Second-generation: **Fadrazole.**
- Third-generation: **Letrozole, anastrozole** and **exemestane.**
- AIs may be subdivided into two classes:
    - **Non-steroidal** AI (NSAI): **Letrozole** and **anastrozole.**
    - **Steroidal** AI (SAI): **Exemestane.**
- NSAIs inhibit the aromatase in a **reversible** manner.
- SAIs bind covalently to aromatase **irreversibly** inactivating the enzyme.
- AIs are used in **Estrogen receptor positive breast cancer** in **postmenopausal women.**
- **Not used in premenopausal women.**

The question specifically asks steroidal drug, so it is exemestane and it is irreversible inhibitor, so the answer is **Exemestane is irreversible inhibitor.**

Ans: Exemestane is irreversible inhibitor

__Ref:__ KD Tripathi - Essentials of Medical Pharmacology, 7th Edition, Page 315

18. Child ingested multiple tablets of metoprolol. Presented with profound hypotension and bradycardia. What is the specific antidote used in this situation?

(a) Atropine (b) Glucagon (c) Adrenaline (d) Isoprenaline

Explanation:

From the above case history it's a clear case of **Beta blocker (metoprolol) poisoning.**

- Poisoning features with this depends on the pharmacological properties of the ingested drug like:
  - β1 selectivity.
  - **Intrinsic sympathomimetic activity.**
  - **Membrane-stabilizing properties.**
- Clinical features seen are:
  - **Hypotension.**
  - **Bradycardia.**
  - **Prolonged AV conduction times.**
  - **Widened QRS complexes.**
  - **Seizures and depression** may be seen.

Treatment:

- If there is **severe bradycardia** treat with **atropine** and may **require pacemaker.**
- Large doses of **isoproterenol** or **an α receptor agonist** may be necessary to treat **hypotension.**
- **Glucagon** acts through its own GPCR and independent of the β adrenergic receptor:
  - Positive chronotropic and inotropic effects on the heart.
- In beta blocker poisoning, **glucagon** is physiological antidote, may use a different cellular mechanism to overcome the effects of a poison:
  - It stimulate an alternative to the blocked β adrenergic receptor and increase cellular cyclic AMP in beta blocker overdose.

So, among the options **Glucagon** is a specific antidote used in this condition.

Ans: (b) Glucagon

Ref: *Goodman and Gillman's, The Pharmacological Basis of Therapeutics, 12th Edition, Page 317*

19. **Which is not a radiosensitizer?**

(a) Amifostine (b) Hydroxyurea
(c) 5FU (d) Bromodeoxyuridine

Explanation:

Radiosensitizers: Compounds that sensitize the tumor cells to radiation during radiotherapy without significant corresponding increase in normal tissue cell death.

• Hyperbaric oxygen	• Fludarabine
• Nicotinamide	• Motexafin gadolinium
• Metronidazole and analogues	• Hypoxic cell toxic agents
• Nicotinamide	• Mitomycin C
• 5-fluorouracil and fluorodeoxyuridine	• Hyperthermia
• Bromodeoxyuridine and iododeoxyuridine	• Novel radiosensitizers
• Hydroxyurea	o **Taxanes**
• Gemcitabine	o **Irnotectan**

Radioprotectors: Compounds that protect the non-tumor (normal) cells from radiation during radiotherapy.

• Amifostine (only clinically approved drug)	• Lipoic acid
• Antioxidants	• Cysteine and cysteamine
• Superoxide dismutase	• Melatonin
• Vitamin A, C, E	• Tetracyclins
• Glutathione	• Fluoroquinolones

Ans: (a) Amifostine

Ref: *Raviraj J, Bokkasam VK, Kumar VS, Reddy US, Suman V. Radiosensitizers, Radioprotectors and Radiation Mitigators. Indian J Dent Res 2014;25:83-89*

20. The risk of carbamazepine induced Stevens-Johnson syndrome is increased in the presence of which of the following genes?

(a) HLA-B 1507
(b) HLA-B 1502
(c) HLA-B 57
(d) HLA-B

Explanation:

Carbamazepine

- Used in treatment of:
  - ***Partial seizures.***
  - ***Bipolar disorder.***
  - ***Trigeminal neuralgia.***
  - ***Chronic pain.***
- Associated with hypersensitivity reactions.
- The reactions may be simple **urticaria** to life-threatening cutaneous disorders, including **Stevens-Johnson syndrome (SJS) and toxic epidermal necrolysis (TEN).**
- These hypersensitivity reactions are associated with **HLA-B*1502** status of the individual.
- There is correlation between **HLA-B*1502** and **carbamazepine-SJS/TEN** in Han Chinese.
- So current guidelines is do genotyping Asian patients before starting the therapy.
- Important to suggest **HLA-B*1502 carriers** to avoid not only **carbamazepine** but also other structurally related anticonvulsants, such as **phenytoin, oxcarbazepine, and possibly Lamotrigine.**

Ans: (b) HLA-B 1502

Ref: *Carbamazepine, HLA-B*1502 and Risk of Stevens-Johnson Syndrome and Toxic Epidermal Necrolysis: US FDA recommendations*

21. Which anti-diarrhoeal acts thru 5HT inhibition?

(a) Alosetron
(b) Clozapine
(c) Tegaserod
(d) Mosapride

Explanation:

Alosetron

- Approved for the treatment of **diarrhea** predominant **IBS** in women.
- **More potent antagonist** of the **5-HT3 receptor** than ondansetron.
- Shows significant **improvements in abdominal pain** as well as **stool frequency, consistency** and **urgency** in IBS patients.
- Also **diminish visceral sensitivity and slow colonic transit.**
- **Pharmacokinetics:**
  - Rapidly absorbed from the GI tract.
  - Duration of action ~ **10 hours.**
  - Metabolized by **hepatic CYPs.**
- It should be started at 1 mg per day for the first 4 weeks and advanced to a maximum of 1 mg twice daily if an adequate response is not achieved.
- Side effects: High incidence of **ischemic colitis***.

Ans: (a) Alosetron

Ref: *Goodman and Gillman's, The Pharmacological Basis of Therapeutics, 12th Edition, Page 1340*

22. Blood therapeutic levels of anti-convulsants are matched correctly in all the following *except*:

(a) Phenytoin 10-20 mg/L
(b) Phenobarbitone 5-10 mg/L
(c) Carbamazepine 6-12 mg/L
(d) Valproate 40 mg/L

Explanation:

Valproate: 50-100 mg/L*

- Monitoring of serum/blood levels of antiepileptic drugs is important in ensuring proper dosing of antiepileptic drug to the patient.

- It is an invaluable surrogate marker for individualizing and optimizing the drug management of patients with epilepsy.
- Therapeutic drug monitoring plays a pivotal role in monitoring adequate blood levels of certain drugs.
- The following is table giving therapeutic range of anti-epileptic drugs.

	Drug	TDM
1	*Phenytoin*	10 – 20 mg/L
2	*Phenobarbitone*	10 – 40 mg/L
3	*Carbamazepine*	4 – 12 mg/L
4	*Leviteracitam*	15 – 45 mg/L
5	*Ethosuximide*	40 – 100 mg/L
6	*Lamotrigine*	2.5 – 15 mg/L
7	*Valproic acid*	50 – 100 mg/L

Ans: (d) Valproate 40 mg/L

Ref: *https://pdfs.semanticscholar.org/b462/b69de9099a9dc35fd76be4caf4265d535fb0.pdf*

23. All are true *except*:

(a) Terlipressin is better than desmopressin for esophageal variceal bleeding
(b) Desmopressin not much effective against nephrogenic diabetes insipidus
(c) Amiloride used for lithium induced diabetes insipidus
(d) Desmopressin used for both pituitary and renal diabetes insipidus

Explanation:

Desmopressin

- Diabetes insipidus of pituitary origin (neurogenic) is the most important indication for **vasopressin.**
- It is **ineffective in renal (nephrogenic) DI,** since **kidney is unresponsive to ADH.**
- **Desmopression** is drug of choice for **central diabetes insipidus** and not much effective against **nephrogenic diabetes insipidus.**
- It can be used **intranasal route and oral route.**
- **Clinical Indications:**
  - **Central diabetes insipidus.**
  - **Nocturnal enuresis** in **children.**
  - **Hemophilia.**
  - **von Willebrand's Disease.**

In case of esophageal variceal bleeding:

- **Terlipressin** is a synthetic analogue of vasopressin with **longer activity** and **fewer side effects.**
- It reduces portal pressure and its effects are still significant 4 hours after administration. So used in **esophageal variceal bleeding.**
- **Desmopressin** has shown no clinical benefits in the setting of **variceal bleeding.**

In case of lithium induced diabetes insipidus:

- **Amiloride** is the drug of choice.
- It blocks entry of **Li+ through Na+ channels** in **the CD cells** and mitigates **diabetes insipidus** induced by **lithium.**
- So among the options, **Desmopressin** used for both **pituitary and renal diabetes insipidus** is a false statement, so it is the option you need to choose.

Ans: (d) Desmopressin can be used for both pituitary and renal diabetes insipidus

Ref: *KD Tripathi - Essentials of Medical Pharmacology, 7th Edition, Page 596*

24. Patient on anti-diabetic medication develops recurrent UTI. Most probable drug:

(a) Sitaglipitin
(b) Dapagliflozin
(c) Linagliptin
(d) Pramlinitide

Explanation

Dapagliflozin:

- **Sodium-glucose cotransporter 2 (SGLT2) inhibitor** indicated as an adjunct to diet and exercise to improve glycemic control in adults with type 2 diabetes mellitus.
- **Mechanism of Action:**
  - Sodium-glucose cotransporter 2 (SGLT2), expressed in the **proximal renal tubules,** is responsible for the majority of the **reabsorption of filtered glucose** from the **tubular lumen.**
  - **Dapagliflozin** is an **inhibitor** of **SGLT2.** By inhibiting SGLT2, dapagliflozin reduces reabsorption of filtered glucose and lowers the renal threshold for glucose, and thereby increases urinary glucose excretion.
- It is **NOT** recommended for patients with **type 1 diabetes mellitus** or for the treatment of diabetic keto-acidosis.
- Should **NOT** be initiated in patients with an **eGFR less than 60 mL/min/1.73 m^2.**
- **Adverse Effects:**
  - Increases the risk of **genital mycotic infections.**
  - **Urinary tract infections.**
  - **Hypotension.**
  - Impairment in **Renal Function.**
  - **Hypoglycemia** with Concomitant Use with **Insulin** and **Insulin Secretagogues.**
  - Increases **in Low-Density Lipoprotein Cholesterol (LDL-C).**
  - **Risk of Bladder Cancer.**

Other options:

- **DPP IV inhibitors:** Sitaglipitin, Linagliptin causes nasopharyngitis, stomatitis and upper respiratory infections.
- **Pramnlinitide:** Nausea, vomiting, anorexia, headache are common ADRs seen. Erythema, edema, or pruritus at the site of injection.
- So among the options dapagliflozin causes recurrent UTIs.

Ans: (b) Dapagliflozin

Ref: *https://www.accessdata.fda.gov/drugsatfda_docs/label/2014/202293s000lbl.pdf*

PATHOLOGY

1. **Mutated gene associated with Wiskott Aldrich syndrome is seen in:**

(a) Y chromosome
(b) Chr-11p22
(c) Chr22q11
(d) X chromosome

Explanation:

Wiskott-Aldrich Syndrome

- **X-linked disease*.**
- **Characterized by:**
  - **Thrombocytopenia.**
  - **Eczema.**
  - **Recurrent infection.**
- Mutations in the gene encoding Wiskott-Aldrich syndrome protein **(WASP),** which is located at **Xp11.23.**
- The WASP protein may be involved in **cytoskeleton-dependent** responses, including:
  - **Cell migration.**
  - **Signal transduction.**
- Thymus is normal, but there is **progressive loss of T cells** from the functional areas of lymph node and spleen.
- Patients do not make **antibodies** to **polysaccharide antigens.**
- **IgM** levels are **low*** (Remember **M** is mirror image of **W - Wiskott**).
- IgG is normal.
- **IgA and IgE levels** are elevated*.

Ans: (d) X chromosome

Ref: *Robbins 9th Edition, Page 171*

2. **Marker associated with systemic mastocytosis is:**

(a) CD 117
(b) CD 25
(c) CD 56
(d) CD 86

Explanation:

WHO 2016 update*

- **Mastocytosis** is now considered as a **separate entity*.**
- In previous **WHO 2008,** it was considered under **Chronic Myeloproliferative neoplasms.**

Systemic Mastocytosis (SM):

One major criterion, and at least one minor criterion is required to make a diagnosis.

- **Major criteria:**
  - Multifocal, dense, compact (≥ 15 mast cells constitute an aggregate), in bone marrow or other organs.
- **Minor criteria:**
  - **< 25%** of Mast cells in bone marrow sections have **spindle shape/atypical morphology,** or **> 25%** of Mast cells in BM smear are **atypical or immature.**
  - **KIT activating point mutation** at codon **D816,** in bone marrow or other extracutaneous organs.
  - **CD25 or CD2 expression** in addition to MCs usual antigens.
  - Persistently elevated **serum tryptase level.**

CD117 vs CD25

- **CD117** – Positive in **normal** as well as **neoplastic Mast cells.**
- **CD25** – Positive only in **neoplastic mast cells** (So it's superior and included in the criteria for diagnosis).

Ans: (b) CD 25

Ref: *WHO Hematological Neoplasms, 4th Edition*

3. **What is CRISPR?**

(a) Bacteria acts against virus
(b) Human defense against bacteriophage
(c) Bacterial defense against bacteriophage
(d) Humans against viruses

Explanation:

CRISPR:

- This was a new update from 10th edition of Robbin's Basic Pathology.
- **CRISPR**-Cas9 is a **genome editing tool***.
- CRISPR Cas9 system is essential in **adaptive immunity** in select bacteria – built-in, gene editing system to the CRISPR-Cas9 system that they use to respond to invading like viruses much like an immune system.
- There are three types of CRISPR mechanisms identified. Of which **type II** is the most commonly explored.
- CRISPRs are transcribed and processed into an RNA sequence that binds and directs the nuclease Cas9 to a sequences (e.g., a phage), leading to its **cleavage** and the **destruction** of the **phage.**
- Gene editing repurposes this process by using **artificial guide RNAs (gRNAs)** that bind **Cas9** and are **complementary** to a **DNA sequence** of interest. Once directed to the target sequence by the gRNA, Cas9 induces double-strand DNA breaks.

CRISPR in medical practice

- Though it's a long way to go in using CRISPR for medical practice. The following are the two methods by which it can be used.
- Repair is done by:
  - **Non-Homologous end joining* (for mutations).**
  - **Homologous recombination*** (to **introduce new sequence**).

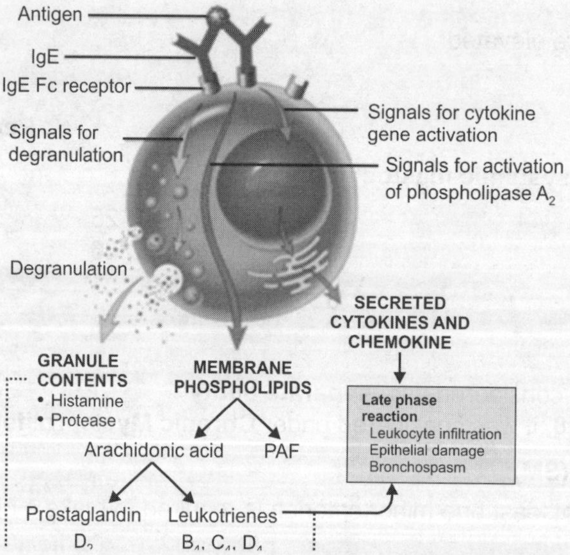

Figure: CRISPR

Ans: (a) Bacteria acts against viruses

***Ref:** Robbins Basic Pathology, 10th Edition, Page 5-6*

4. **FLI 1 gene translocation is associated with:**

(a) Wilm's tumor
(b) Ewing sarcoma
(c) Neurofibroma
(d) Schwannoma

Explanation:

Ewings Sarcoma Family of Tumors (ESFT)

- Account for approximately 6% to 10% of primary malignant **bone tumors** and follow **osteosarcoma** as the second most common group of **bone sarcomas** in children.
- ESFT contain a **(11;22) (q24;q12) translocation** generating in-frame fusion of the **EWS gene** on chromosome **22** to the **FLI1 gene.**

Subtypes	Chromosomal translocations	Fusion transcripts
Lipoblastoma	t(7:8)(q31:q13): t(8:8)(q24:q13)	PLAG1-COL1A2:PLAG1-HAS2
Myxoid liposarcoma	t(12:16)(q13:p11): t(12:22)(q13:q12)	CHOP-TLS; CHOP-EWS
Inflammatory myofibroblastic tumor	t(1:2)(q25:p23): t(2:19)(p23:q13): t(2:17)(p23:q23)	TPM3-ALK: ALK-TPM4; ALK-CLTC
Infantile fibrosarcoma	t(12:15)(p13:q25)	ETV6-NTRK3
Dermatofibrosarcoma protuberans/ Giant cell fibroblastoma	t(17:22)(q22:q13)	COL1A1-PDGF8
Alveolar rhabdomyosarcoma	t(2:13)(q35:q14): t(1:13)(p36:q14)	PAX3-FKHR; PAX7-FKHR
Angiomatoid fibrous histiocytoma	t(12:22)(q13:q12): t(12:16)(q13:p11)	
Synovial sarcoma	t(X:18)(p11.2:q11.2)	SYT-SSX1/2/4
Alveolar soft part sarcoma	t(X:17)(p11:q25)	TFE3-ASPL
Clear cell sarcoma	t(12:22)(q13:q12)	EWS-ATF1
Extraskeletal myxoid chrondrosarcoma	t(9:22)(q22:q12): t(9:15)(q22:q21)	EWS-TEC: CHN-TFC12
Desmoplastic small round cell tumor	t(11:22)(p13:q12) t(11:22)(q24:q12): t(21:22)(q22:q12): t(17:22)(q12:q12): t(7:22)(p22:q12)	EWS-WT1 FLI1-EWS: ERG-EWS E1AF-EWS: ETV1-EWS

Ans: (b) Ewing's sarcoma

***Ref:** Robbins Pathology, 9th Edition, Page 1203*

5. **Myd88 L265p mutation is seen in:**

(a) Multiple Myeloma
(b) Waldenstrom's macroglobulinemia
(c) ALL
(d) Chronic Myeloid leukemia

Explanation:

Waldenstrom Macroglobulinemia

- Indolent neoplasm.
- Also known as **Lymphoplasmacytic lymphoma.**
- Involves **bone marrow** (100%), **liver, spleen, lymph nodes** (15-20%).
- Rare sites of involvement **lung and testis** (PGIMER exam options).
- **IgM secretion.**
- **MYD88 mutation** – virtually in all cases.
- Associated with **cold agglutin AIHA** and **Hyperviscosity syndrome** in 15%.

Ans: (b) Waldenstrom's macroglobulinemia

***Ref:** Robbins, 9th Edition, Page 538*

6. **Which of the following is involved in apoptosis pathway?**

(a) myc
(b) p53 and caspase
(c) APC
(d) VHL

Explanation:

DNA damage:

- Any cell with **DNA damage** will result in **increase in p53 levels.**
- So the p53 **halts** the **cell cycle temporarily** and has two functions:
  - **Repairs** the **damaged DNA.**
  - If the change is **irreparable** results in destruction by **apoptosis.**

P53 protein

- **Guardian of the genome*.**
- DNA damage is sensed by complexes containing kinases of the ATM/ATR family; these kinases phosphorylate p53, liberating it from inhibitors such as **MDM2.**

- Active p53 then upregulates the expression of proteins such as the **cyclin dependent kinase inhibitor p21,** thereby causing **cell-cycle arrest** at the **G1-S checkpoint.** This pause allows cells to repair DNA damage.
- If DNA damage cannot be repaired, p53 induces additional events that lead to cellular senescence or **apoptosis.**
- Rare patients with **Li-Fraumeni syndrome** inherit one defective copy of **TP53** and have a very high incidence of a wide variety of cancers.

Ans: (b) p53 and caspase

***Ref:** Robbins Pathology, 9th Edition, Page 50*

7. **A child is diagnosed with Hypoplasia of thymus. This condition is associated with microdeletion of:**

(a) 22q11.1 (b) 22q11.2 (c) 11q22.1 (d) 11q21.2

Explanation:

DiGeorge syndrome

- Caused by a deletion in the long (or "q") arm of chromosome 22(22q11.2 deletion syndrome).
- **Hypoplasia of 2nd and 3rd pharyngeal pouch derivatives.**
- Symptoms and signs:
  - o **Hypoplasia** of the **hyoid.**
  - o **Thymic hypoplasia** (Immunodeficiency due to a **lack of T-cells**).
  - o **Hypoparathyroidism** (Missing or **hypoplastic inferior parathyroid glands**).
  - o **Outflow tract defects** (Neural crest in this area also contributes to conotruncal cushions of the outflow tract).
- Hypoplasia of the 2nd and 3rd arches can also disrupt the **1st arch,** leading to the following additional findings: (PGIMER)
  - o **Micrognathia (reduced jaw).**
  - o **Cleft palate.**
  - o **Hearing loss.**

Ans: (b) 22q11.2

***Ref:** Robbins Pathology, 9th Edition, Page 163*

8. **Not a property of oncogene:**

(a) Amplification (b) Translocation (c) Point mutation (d) Deletion

Explanation:

Oncogenes and Oncoproteins

- Genes that promote autonomous cell growth in cancer cells are called oncogenes, and their unmutated cellular counter by **mutations in proto-oncogenes and encode proteins called oncoproteins that have the ability to promote cell growth in the absence of normal growth-promoting signals.**
- **Oncoproteins** resemble the normal products of **proto-oncogenes** but bear mutations that are often inactivate internal regulatory elements; consequently, their activity in cells does not depend on external signals.
- Cells expressing **oncoproteins** are thus freed from the normal checkpoints and controls that limit growth, and as a result proliferate excessively.

Now let's come to the question with above information:

- **Normal cell** – **Proto-oncogene*.**
- **Cancer cell (increased** growth) – **Oncogene*.**
- So a cancer cell should have an alteration which activates the proto-oncogene to enable division of the cells without control (neoplasia).
- If the proto-oncogene is deleted, there is no chance of new growth happening. So the answer to above answer is deletion.

Oncogene can undergo following variations (in general gain of function mutations):

- Overexpression.

- Amplification.
- Point mutation.

Ans: (d) Deletion

Ref: *Robbins Pathology, 9th Edition, Page 284*

9. **Factor helping tumor cell to invade tissue is:**

(a) FGF
(b) IL 6
(c) IL 2
(d) Plasminogen activator

Explanation:

Steps of metastasis:

- "Loosening up" of tumor cell–tumor cell interactions.
- Degradation of ECM.
- Attachment to novel ECM components.
- Migration and invasion of tumor cells.

Degradation of the basement membrane and interstitial connective tissue is the second step in invasion.

- Tumor cells may accomplish this by either secreting **proteolytic enzymes** themselves or by inducing stromal cells (e.g., **fibroblasts and inflammatory cells**) to elaborate proteases.
- Many different families of proteases have been implicated in tumor cell invasion
  - **Matrix metalloproteinases (MMPs).**
  - **Cathepsin D.**
  - **Urokinase plasminogen activator.**

Our question also talks about the same process of tissue invasion. The answer is pretty easy now, plasminogen activator.

Ans: (d) Plasminogen activator

Ref: *Robbins Pathology, 9th Edition, Page 307*

10. **vWD is associated with which of the following tumour?**

(a) Ependymoma
(b) Angiosarcoma
(c) Melanoma
(d) Lung carcinoma

Explanation:

This question is about Acquired vWD.

Acquired vWD

- Rare disorders seen in many tumuors.
- In contrast to the vWD, there is no defect in the production of vWD.

Etiology:

- A wide range of disorders (neoplastic, autoimmune, endocrine and drugs) have been implicated as the cause for AvWD.
- Enlisting a few neoplasm which are implicated in the pathogenesis of the same.

Neoplastic Disorders

- Wilms tumor.
- Adrenocortical carcinoma.
- Lung cancer.
- Peripheral neuroectodermal tumor.
- Gastric carcinoma.
- Acute myeloid leukemia.
- Acute lymphoblastic leukemia.

Pathogenesis of Acquired vWD

- Specific inhibitory antibodies to vWF function.
- Non-neutralizing autoantibodies to vWF (immune complexes).

- Adsorption of vWF by malignant cells.
- Increased vWF proteolytic degradation.
- Decreased vWF synthesis.

Diagnosis:
- The laboratory features are same those of vWD.
- One test which can differentiate the congenital vWD from acquired vWD is **measurement of vWF propeptide.**

Treatment:
- Treating the primary disease.

Ans: (d) Lung carcinoma

Ref: *Nathan and Oski's Hematology, Page 1512*

11. A patient presents with anemia and cholelithiasis. Peripheral smear is shown. Most probable diagnosis:

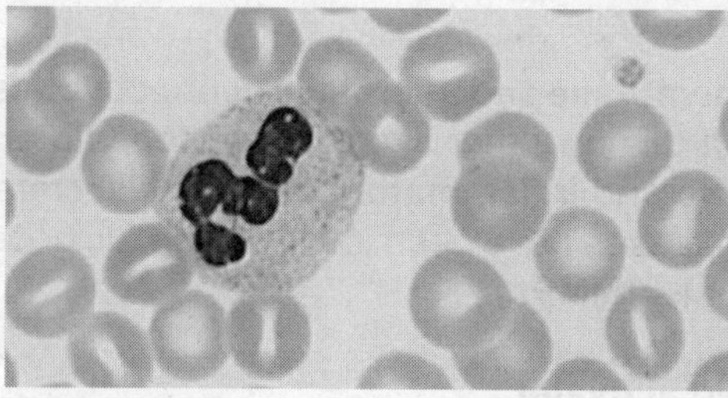

(a) Spherocytes (b) Ovalocytes (c) Stomatocytes (d) Elliptocytosis

Explanation:

Stomatocytosis
- Stomatocytes are erythrocytes with a central slit or mouth-shaped (stoma) area of central pallor when examined on dried smears.
- Stomatocytes are associated with rare hereditary disorders of red cell cation permeability known as the hereditary stomatocytosis syndromes, aberrant Rh blood group antigen expression, sitosterolemia, and familial deficiency of high-density lipoproteins.
- Acquired stomatocytosis has been associated with acute alcoholism and hepatobiliary disease, vinca alkaloid administration, neoplasms and cardiovascular disease.

Spherocyte – Smaller than normal RBC's with no central pallor.

Causes of spherocytes:
- ***Autoimmune hemolytic anaemia*** **– Most common*.**
- *Hereditary spherocytosis*.*
- ***G6PD deficiency*.***
- *Fragmentation syndrome.*

Ans: (c) Stomatocytes

Ref: *Wintrobe, 13th Edition, Page 1666*

12. Dallas Myocarditis criteria is based on:

(a) Lymphocytes and necrosis
(b) Presence of bacterial organism
(c) IHC markers
(d) Imaging studies

Explanation:

Dallas criteria:
- It's a histologic criteria for reporting **viral myocarditis*.**
- It's classified based on the **HPE findings*.**

- Classified into following types:
  - **Active.**
  - **Borderline.**
  - **No evidence of myocarditis.**

Active myocarditis

- Presence of inflammatory infiltrates and damage to adjacent myocytes.
- Frank necrosis with vacuolization with disruption of cellular outlines with lymphocytes closely applied to cell surface.
- Uninvolved adjacent myocardium is normal histologically.

World Health Organization Marburg Classification (most widely used now. Use of IHC and less inter-observer variability).

First biopsy:

- **Acute (active) myocarditis:** A clear-cut infiltrate (diffuse, focal or confluent) of >14 leukocytes/mm^2 (preferably activated T cells). The amount of the infiltrate should be quantified by immunohistochemistry. Necrosis or degeneration is compulsory; fibrosis may be absent or present and should be graded.
- **Chronic myocarditis:** An infiltrate of >14 leukocytes/mm^2 (diffuse, focal or confluent, preferably activated T cells). Quantification should be made by immunohistochemistry. Necrosis or degeneration is usually not evident; fibrosis may be absent or present and should be graded.
- **No myocarditis:** No infiltrating cells or <14 leukocytes/mm^2.

Subsequent biopsies:

- Ongoing (persistent) myocarditis. Criteria as in acute or chronic myocarditis.
- Resolving (healing) myocarditis. Criteria as in acute or chronic myocarditis, but the immunological process is sparser than in the first biopsy.
- Resolved (healed) myocarditis. Corresponds to the Dallas classification.

The amount and distribution of fibrosis should be described similarly as no (grade 0), mild (grade 1), moderate (grade 2) or severe (grade 3). Localisation or formation of fibrosis should be outlined as endocardial, replacement or interstitial.

Ans: (a) Lymphocyte and necrosis

Ref: *Sternberg Diagnostic Pathology, Chapter 29*

13. **CADASIL is associated with:**

(a) NOTCH 1 mutation (b) NOTCH 2 mutation
(c) NOTCH 3 mutation (d) NOTCH 4 mutation

Explanation:

Cerebral autosomal dominant arteriopathy with subcortical infarcts and leukoencephalopathy (CADASIL)

- **Autosomal dominant** disorder.
- Mutations in the **NOTCH 3 gene** that lead to **misfolding** of the extracellular domain of the **NOTCH 3 receptor.**
- NOTCH 3 is preferentially expressed in **vascular smooth muscle.**
- The disease is characterized clinically by:
  - **Recurrent strokes*** (usually infarcts, less often hemorrhages).
  - **Dementia*.**
- **Radiology:** Changes are in **white matter**, usually by around the age of **35 years,** whereas infarcts typically occur 10-15 years later.
- **HPE**: Arteries in the CNS and in other tissues such as skin show concentric thickening of the media and adventitia, loss of smooth muscle cells, and the presence of basophilic, PAS positive deposits.
- The characteristic **deposits** contain the **misfolded NOTCH 3 protein.**
- The diagnosis is made through the identification of these deposits in the walls of vessels in biopsies of other tissues, such as skin or muscle, or by sequencing of **NOTCH 3.**

Ans: (c) NOTCH 3 mutation

Ref: *Robbins Pathology, 9th Edition, Page 1269*

14. Good prognostic factor of Neuroblastoma is:

(a) n-myc
(b) Trk A expression
(c) Near ploidy
(d) Bilateral neuroblastoma

Explanation:

This is one of my favourite topics. The below is a mnemonic in the form of a poem to remember it.

Easy way to remember neuroblastoma prognostic features:

"A young kid with a mature thought
Stands in the corner holding his pot (belly)
Looks at the tiny little beautiful blues on his skin
Wonders if it was the same making his blood thin
Hardly there are less than 200 division in the world
United we stand we can make the enemies go curled
I am hyper and I have A TRicK to express
Rest all are absent so there is nothing to depress"

Deciphering the poem… The good prognostic features are:

"A young kid (<18 months) with a mature thought (schwannian and ganglionic maturation)
Stands in the corner holding his pot (belly) (liver mets and the tumor)
Looks at the tiny little beautiful blues on his skin (skin mets)
Wonders if it was the same making his blood thin (bone marrow – All the above three makes stage 4S)
Hardly there are less than 200 division in the world (<200/5000 mitotic index)
United we stand we can make the enemies go curled (enemy – neuroblastoma)
I am hyper (hyperdiploidy) and I have A TRiCK to express (TRKA expression)

Rest all are absent (all other mutation and chabrrations) so there is nothing to depress." (all are favourable prognostic markers)

- **Prognostic Factors in Neuroblastoma**

Good Prognostic Factors	Bad Prognostic Factors
• Age < 1 year • Stages I and II • **Hyperdiploidy or Triploidy** • Expression of **Trk A gene** • Evidence of **Schwanjian stroma** and **gangliocytic differentiation** • Mitosis-Karryorrhexis index **< 200/5000 cells**	• Age > 1 year • Stage III and IV • **Near diploid tumor** • **TRKB expression** • Deletion of chromosome **1 and 11** • Amplification of **N-MYC** • Telomerase expression • Mitosis-Karyorrhexis Index **> 200/5000 cells**

Ans: (b) Trk A expression

***Ref:** Robbins Patholgy, 9th Edition, Page 475*

15. Cyfra 21-1 is a marker of:

(a) Small cell carcinoma of lung
(b) Non-small cell lung cancer
(c) Melanoma
(d) Adenoid cystic carcinoma

Explanation:

- The trend in exams is changing. Rather from a textbook point of view moving towards practical utility based tests Example **FLI1, Cyfra 21, AML prognostic factors.**
- All these are used in day-to-day for diagnosing and more important in management of a patient. Though the questions seem tough, this change is inevitable and a good move.

CYFRA - 21

- Cytokeratins are structural proteins forming the subunits of epithelial intermediary filaments. Fragments of cytokeratin-19 (CYFRA 21-1) are frequently released into the blood of cancer patients.

- The main indication for CYFRA 21-1 is monitoring the **course of Non-small cell Lung Cancer (NSCLC)** and **detection of recurrent disease after primary therapy.** Successful therapy is accompanied by a rapid fall in the serum level into the normal range.
- An unclear focus in the lung together with values > 30 ng/mL indicate the existence of primary bronchial carcinoma with high probability.
- CYFRA 21-1 has a clear prognostic value in both early and late stages of NSCLC and high serum levels indicate an advanced tumor stage and a poor prognosis.
- CYFRA 21-1 is a valuable marker in the prediction of the response to cytotoxic therapies (such as selective internal radiation therapy (SIRT) or transarterial chemoembolization (TACE)) in diverse cancers such as hepatic cancer or hepatic metastases from other cancers.
- CYFRA 21-1 is also elevated in sera of patients with urological, gastrointestinal and gynaecological cancers (PGIMER).

Ans: (b) Non-small cell carcinoma lung

Ref: *Advances in Tumor Biomarkers, Page 201*

16. MOC 31 in immunohistochemistry is used to differentiate:

(a) Adenocarcinoma vs malignant mesothelioma
(b) Adenocarcinoma from SCC
(c) SCC from malignant melanoma
(d) Small cell carcinoma vs adenocarcinoma

Explanation:

- This is a very practical question. To differentiate between adenocarcinoma of lung and mesothelioma is a nightmare for pathologists. End of the day with all available methods it is tough to differentiate both. Providing you the list of methods which aids is arriving at a correct diagnosis.

Special stain	**Mesothelioma**	**Adenocarcinoma**
Alcian blue with hyaluronidase	Negative	Positive
PAS with diastase	Negative	Positive
Alcian Blue	Positive	Positive

IHC stain	**Mesothelioma**	**Adenocarcinoma**
Cytokeratin 5/6	Positive	Negative
Calretinin	Positive	Negative
D2-40 (podoplanin)	Positive	Negative
WT1	Positive	Negative
B72.3	Negative	Positive
MOC-31	Negative	Positive
TTF-1	Negative	Positive
Claudin-4	Negative	Positive

EM features	**Mesothelioma**	**Adenocarcinoma**
Apical microvilli	Long and thin, no glycocalyx	Shorter and have microvilli
Perinuclear to no filament bundles	Present	Absent
Basal lamina	Present	Absent
Long desmosomes	Present	Absent

High yield – Protocol

- **IMIG** (International Mesothelioma Interest Group) recommends 2 mesothelial markers and 2 carcinoma markers be included in the panel.
- Best positive **mesothelioma markers: Calretinin, CK5 or CK5/6, WT1, D2-40*.**
- Best positive **carcinoma markers: MOC-31, Ber-EP4, CEA and BG8 (Lewis antigen blood group).**
- Best positive **lung adenocarcinoma markers: TTF1 and Napsin*.**

Ans: (a) Adenocarcinoma vs malignant mesothelioma

Ref: *Advances in Tumor Biomarkers*

17. ABCD 1 mutation is seen in:

(a) Adrenoleucodystrophy
(b) Wilson's disease
(c) Adrenal insufficiency in males
(d) Menkes disease

Explanation:

X-linked adrenoleukodystrophy

- Damages the **adrenal gland** (casing **adrenal insufficiency**) and affects the **white matter in brain.**
- Seen in **Males.**
- There are three distinct types of:
  - A childhood cerebral form.
  - Adrenomyeloneuropathy type.
  - Form called Addison disease only.
- Mutations in the **ABCD1 gene** cause X-linked adrenoleukodystrophy.
- The ABCD1 gene provides instructions for producing the **adrenoleukodystrophy protein (ALDP),** which is involved in transporting certain fat molecules called **very long-chain fatty acids (VLCFAs)** into **peroxisomes.**
- Sequence of events appears to be related to an abnormal accumulation of saturated very-long-chain fatty acids **(VLCFA)** in the serum and tissues of the central nervous system, which sets off an abnormal immune response that leads to demyelination.
- Females having the disease - usually develop after age 35, and primarily include progressive stiffness, weakness, or paralysis of the lower limbs, numbness, pain in the joints, and urinary problems.

Ans: (a) Adrenoleucodystrophy

Ref: *Genetic Home Reference*

18. DAX 1 mutation is seen in:

(a) Addison disease
(b) Hashimoto thyroiditis
(c) Cushing syndrome
(d) Graves' disease

Explanation:

- **Mutations** in the **DAX-1** gene give rise to both X-linked adrenal hypoplasia congenita and hypogonadotropic hypogonadism. The closest option is Addison disease.

Below is a list of gene which we use for diagnosis on a day-to-day basis in endocrine

Disorders	**Gene**
DiGeorge syndrome	*TBX1*
Hyperparathyroidism 1, familial isolated primary	*CDC73 (HRPT2)*
Hyperparathyroidism 2 (Hyperparathyroidism-jaw tumor syndrome)	*CDC73 (HRPT2)*
Hyperparathyroidism, neonatal severe	*CASR*
Hypophosphatasia	*ALPL*
Idiopathic infantile hypercalcemia	*CYP24A1*
Pseudohypoparathyroidism Type IA (Albright hereditary osteodystrophy)	*GNAS (maternal)*
Pseudohypoparathyroidism, Type IB	*STX16*
Pseudohypoparathyroidism, Type IC	*GNAS*
Achalasia-Addisonianism-Alacrima syndrome; AAAS (Allgrove syndrome; Triple A)	*AAAS*
ACTH deficiency	*POMC, TBX19*
Adrenal hypoplasia congenita	*NR0B1 (DAX1)*
Adrenoleukodystrophy	*ABCD1*
Pseudohypoaldosteronism	*NR3C2*
Apparent mineralocorticoid excess	*HSD11B2*

Contd.

Contd.

Glucocorticoid-remediable aldosteronism	*CYP11B1*
Glucocorticoid resistance	*NR3C1*
Androgen insensitivity May be minimally affected (MAIS), partial (PAIS) or complete (CAIS)	*AR*
Aromatase deficiency	*CYP19A1*
Aromatase excess syndrome	*CYP19A1*
Estrogen resistance	*ESR1*
17β-Hydroxysteroid Dehydrogenase Deficiency	*HSD17B3*
Leydig cell hypoplasia (M) Luteinizing hormone resistance (F)	*LHCGR*
McCune-Albright syndrome	*GNAS1*
Testotoxicosis, familial	*LHCGR*
Testotoxicosis with pseudohypoparathyroidism type 1a	*GNAS*
Growth hormone insensitivity with immunodeficiency	*STAT5B*
Growth hormone insensitivity syndrome (Laron syndrome)	*GHR*
Kowarski syndrome	*GH1*
Panhypopituitarism, X-Linked	*SOX3*
Hypogonadotropic hypogonadism with or without anosmia(Kallmann syndrome)	*KAL1*
Precocious puberty, central	*KISS1R, MKRN3*
ACTH deficiency	*POMC TBX19*
Diabetes insipidus	*AVP*
Hyperthyroidism, non-autoimmune	*TSHR*
Hypothyroidism, a thyroidal with spiky hair and cleft palate (Bamforth-Lazarus syndrome)	*FOXE1 (TTF-2), POU1F1 (PIT1), PROP1*
Hypothyroidism, congenital with neonatal diabetes mellitus	*GLIS3 103*
Thyroid hormone resistance, generalized (Refetoff Syndrome, GRTH)	*THRB*
T3 Resistance (Allan-Herndon-Dudley syndrome, AHDS)	*SLC16A2*
Autoimmune polyendocrinopathy syndrome (APS1)	*AIRE*
Carney complex	*PRKAR1A*
CHARGE syndrome	*CHD7, SEMA3E*
Culler-Jones syndrome	*GLI2*
Denys-Drash syndrome	*WT1*
IPEX	*FOXP3*
Kenney-Caffey syndrome	*TBCE*
Multiple endocrine neoplasia type 1 (MEN1)	*MEN1*
Multiple endocrine neoplasia type 2A (MEN2A)	*RET*
Multiple endocrine neoplasia type 2B (MEN2B)	*RET*
MEN4	*CDKN1B*

Ans: (a) Addison disease

Ref: *Genetic Home Reference*

19. Favourable prognosis in AML:

(a) FLT3 +ve (b) MLL (c) PML/RARA (d) CEBPA

Explanation:

Risk Category	**Cytogenetic and Molecular classification**
Good	• t(8;21) without KIT mutation • inv(16) without KIT mutation • t(15;17) (PML/RARA) • Intermediate-risk cytogenetics without FLT3-ITD and with either NPM1 or biallelic CEBPA mutation

Contd.

Contd.

Intermediate	• t(8;21) or inv(16) with KIT mutation • t(9;11) • Other cytogenetics, including normal karyotype
Poor	• inv(3), 11q23 abnormalities other than t(9;11) • t(9;22), t(6,9) • 5, del(5q) • 7, del(7q) • 17, 17p abnormalities • Complex cytogenetics (.3 abnormalities)

Ans: (c) PML/RARA

Ref: *WHO Hematological Neoplasms, 4th Edition*

20. Mast cell degranulation is suggested by rise in__________ serum levels.

(a) Histamine (b) Heparin (c) Tryptase (d) Chymase

Explanation:

- The question on mast cell markers in systemic mastocytosis, if you look at it, one of the criteria will be serum tryptase levels.

Mast cell tryptase:

- **Beta-Tryptase** is a neutral **serine protease** and is the most abundant mediator stored in **mast cell granules.**
- The release of beta-tryptase from the secretory granules is a characteristic feature of **mast cell degranulation.**
- Beta-Tryptase activates the **protease activated receptor type 2.**
- It is involved in **airway homeostasis, vascular relaxation and contraction, gastrointestinal smooth muscle activity and intestinal transport and coagulation.**
- Serum mast cell **beta-tryptase concentration** is **increased** in **anaphylaxis** and in other allergic conditions.
- It is increased in **systemic mastocytosis** and other **haematological conditions.**

Mast cell degranulation:

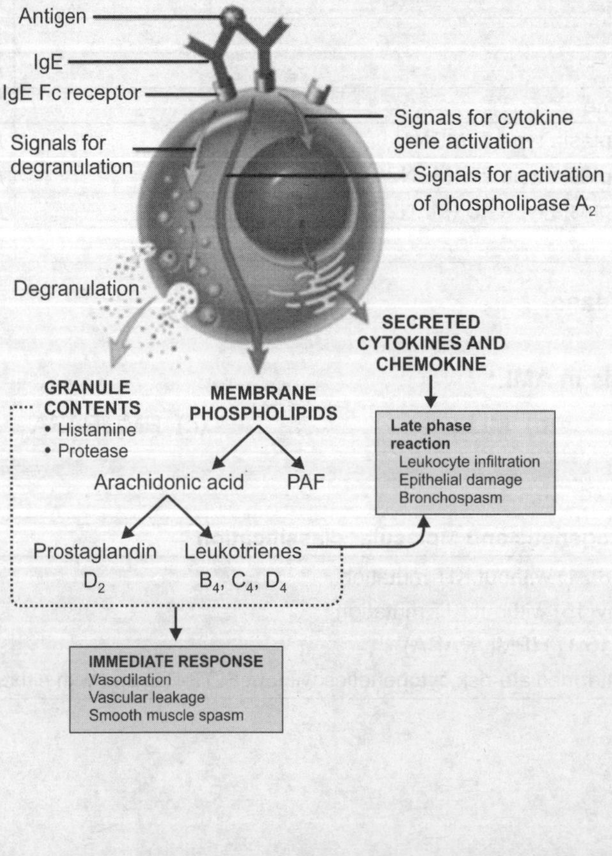

Ans: (c) Tryptase

***Ref:** Hoffman's Hematology, Page 1104*

21. Characteristic CD marker of basophil cells:

(a) CD 34
(b) CD 35
(c) CD 56
(d) CD 13

Explanation:

Below is the list of all consolidated IHC markers asked in exams.

CD1a, S-100, CD-207 (Langherin)	• Langerhan cell histiocytosis
CD 2 3 4 5 7 8	• T-cell markers • CD3 is pan T cell marker
CD10 (aka CALLA antigen)	• Early pre B marker • Immature B cell marker
CD 13, 33, 117, MPO	• Myeloid series marker-AML
CD 14, 64	• Monocyte marker (AML-M4 M5)
CD 15	• RS cell • Neutrophils
CD 13, 14, 203c	• Basophil
CD 15, 30	• RS Cell
CD 16, 56	• NK Cell
CD 19, 20, 21, 22	• B Cell markers • CD 19 is pan B cell marker
CD 23+, CD 5+	• CLL/SLL
CD 23-, CD 5+	• Mantle cell lymphoma
CD 31	• Endothelial cell marker (positive in angiosarcomas)
CD 34	• Stem cell (also positive in angiosarcomas)
CD 41, 61	• Megakaryocyte • Platelet marker • Positive in AML-M7
CD 45 RO	• Memory cell
CD 95/FAS ligand	• Apoptosis marker (extrinsic pathway)
CD 99/MIC-2	• Ewings sarcoma (FLI 1 is most sensitive and specific than CD99)
CD 117	• GIST • Mastocytosis • AML (DOG1 is more useful than CD117 in GIST)

Ans: (d) CD13

***Ref:** Robbins Basic Pathology, 10th Edition*

22. Sialated lewis glycoprotein is:

(a) CEA
(b) CA -125
(c) CA 19-9
(d) PSA

Explanation:

Other name for Ca 19-9 is **sialylated Lewis (a) antigen**

Tumour markers

- Biochemical substances that indicate presence of tumour.
- Tumor markers are not diagnostic, it's mostly used for prognostication of the disease.

Below is the table of tumor marker.

Tumor Markers	Tumor Types
Hormones	
• Human chorionic gonadotropin	• Trophoblastic tumors • Nonseminomatous testicular tumors
• Calcitonin	• Medullary carcinoma of thyroid
• Catecholamine and metabolites	• Pheochromocytoma and related tumors
Oncofetal Antigens	
• α-Fetoprotein	• Liver cell cancer • Nonseminomatous germ cell tumors of testis
• Carcinoembryonic antigen	• Carcinomas of the colon, pancreas, lung, stomach and heart
Isoenzymes	
• Prostatic acid phosphatase	• Prostate cancer
• Neuron-specific enolase	• Small-cell cancer of lung • Neuroblastoma
Specific Proteins	
• Immunoglobulins	• Multiple myeloma
• Prostate-specific antigen and prostate-specific membrane antigen	• Prostate cancer
Mucins and Other Glycoproteins	
• CA-125	• Ovarian cancer
• CA-19-9	• Colon cancer • Pancreatic cancer
• CA-15-3	• Breast cancer

Ans: (c) Ca 19-9

Ref: *Robbins Pathology, 9th Edition, Page 337*

23. A patient's hemogram shows Hb 12, decreased MCV, decreased MCH, RDW is 14. What is the most probable diagnosis?

(a) Iron deficient stores
(b) Sideroblastic anemia
(c) Beta thalassemia trait
(d) Normal lab parameters

Explanation:

This is a pretty straight forward question. Same topic of RDW was asked in the AIIMS exam also.

Data:

- Decreased MCV, MCH, Normal RDW and Hb-12 (without age and gender we will consider Hb-15 to be the ideal) its reduced.
- So it's a microcytic hypochromic anemia with normal RDW.

Red cell distribution width

This is a beautiful concept. We will learn it with the help of a simple fictional example. Examples are always trustworthy. If we arrange RBC's on the basis of their **anisocytosis.** We will get a distribution range–That is RDW.

(1) **Iron Deficiency Anemia** – IDA is an ongoing state. Some days you dates milk shake or a piece of meat – That day your iron requirement will be met with so the RBC produced on the particular day will be looking normal (just for example) and the day preceding and later is going to be iron deficient.
Resultant will be a population of Microcytic and Normal sized RBC's – A bigger range of cells – Wider RDW (holds good for any nutritional def so megaloblastic also has I elevated RDW).

(2) In **thalassemia,** which is a genetic defect. How much ever you are going to eat. All the RBC's from the marrow are going to be small → all are microcytic (gathered over a common point) – the range of RDW will be normal (though it's microcytic). Hope this will clear doubt with RDW.

Normal value:

- RDW-SD 39-46 fL.
- RDW-CV 11.6-14.6% in adult.

Condition with increased RDW:

- Iron deficiency anaemia.
- Folate/vit B_{12} deficiency anaemia.

Now we will see the question again, it's more evident the answer is thalassemia.

Ans: (c) Beta thalassemia trait

Ref: *Robbins Pathology, 9th Edition*

24. Gene defect in Myotonic dystrophy:

(a) CAG repeats (b) CTG repeats (c) Dystophin 1 (d) Dystophin 2

Explanation:

Trinucleotide repeat disorders

- **Expansion of trineuclotide repeats is an important genetic cause of human disease, particularly neurodegenerative disorders.**
- **Some of the disease occurs in coding region and few occurs in non-coding regions.**
- **Friedrich was a myotonic patient with large testis – Remember this for coding region repeat disorders (first three in the table).**

Disease	**Gene**	**Repeat**
Fragile X syndrome	*FMRI (FRAXA)*	CGG
Friedreich ataxia	*FXN*	GAA
Myotonic dystrophy	*DMPK*	CTG
Spinobulbar muscular atrophy (Kennedy disease)	*AR*	CAG
Huntington disease	*HTT*	CAG
Dentatorubral-pallidoluysian atrophy (Haw River syndrome)	*ATNL*	CAG
Spinocerebellar ataxia type 1	*ATXN1*	CAG
Spinocerebellar ataxia type 2	*ATXN2*	CAG
Spinocerebellar ataxia type 3 (Machado-Joseph disease)	*ATXN3*	CAG
Spinocerebellar ataxia type 6	*CACNA2A*	CAG
Spinocerebellar ataxia type 7	*ATXN7*	CAG

Ans: CTG repeats

Ref: *Robbins Pathology, 9th Edition, Page 168*

25. Most common type of lung carcinoma in systemic sclerosis:

(a) Small cell Ca (b) Non-small cell Ca
(c) Carcinoid (d) Synovial sarcoma

Explanation:

Systemic Sclerosis (Scleroderma)

- Abnormal accumulation of **fibrous tissue.**
- The **skin** is most commonly affected, but gastrointestinal tract, kidneys, heart, muscles and lungs also are frequently involved.

Two major categories:

- **Diffuse scleroderma:** Widespread skin involvement at onset and early visceral involvement.
- **Limited scleroderma:** Skin involvement is often confined to fingers forearms and face. Visceral involvement occurs late.

Two ANAs unique to systemic sclerosis:

- **Ab to DNA topoisomerase I (anti-Scl 70)**
  - **Highly specific – Diffuse systemic sclerosis.**

- **Anti centromere antibody:**
  - o **Limited systemic sclerosis.**
  - o Associated with **CREST syndrome** (Calcinosis, Reynaud phenomenon, Esophagealdysmotility, sclerodactyly, telangiectasia).

SLE

- Kidney – Wire loop lesions.
- Skin – Carpet tack sign.
- Joint – Non erosive arthritis.
- CVS – Libmann sacks endocarditis.
- Lungs – Shrinking lungs, carcinoma (NSCLC-Non small cell lung carcinoma).
- Spleen – Onion skin appearance.

Most common cause of death

- 1st 10 years – renal failure.
- Overall – cardiac failure.

Ans: (b) Non-small cell carcinoma

Ref: *Dail and Hammer Pulmonary Pathology, Page 229*

26. Woman is diagnosed with cancer. Karyotyping shows aneupoidy. How will you explain this concept to the patient in layman terms?

(a) Hyperchromatic nuceli
(b) Doubling of DNA base
(c) Amount of DNA less than normal
(d) Number of chromosomes in her defect is not in even numbers

Explanation:

Chromosomal Abnormalities

- Number.
- Structural changes:
  - o Insertions.
  - o Deletion of an arm.
  - o Translocations.
- **Euploidy** – Normal set of chromosomes (46XX or 46XY).
- Aneuploidy – An **aneuploid** is an individual organism whose chromosome number differs from normal individuals, which can be an increase in the number of chromosomes (trisomy – extra chromosome) or decrease (monosomy). So this question is fairly an easy one. Aneuploidy means the number of chromosomes is not in even numbers.

Structural changes:

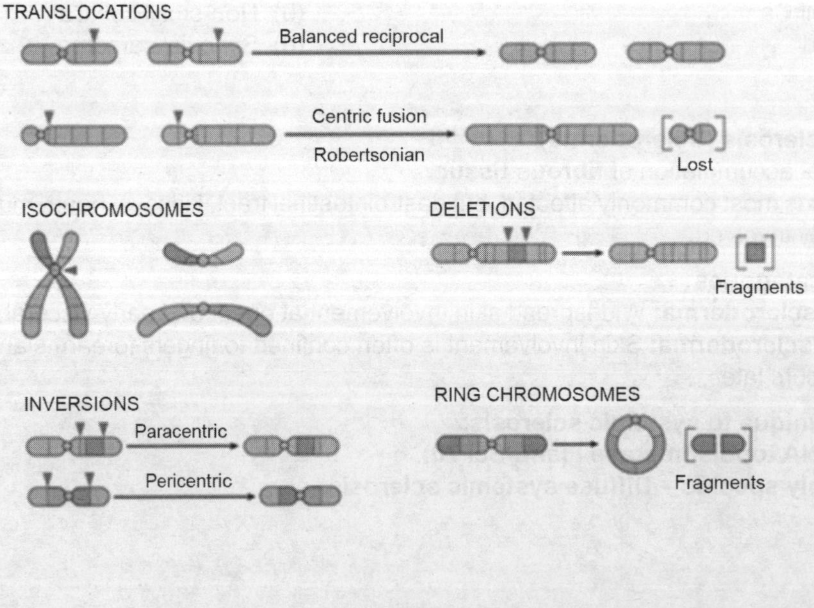

Ans: (d) Number of chromosomes in her defect is not in even numbers

Ref: *Robbins Pathology, 9th Edition, Page 160*

27. Which of the following endogenous molecules plays a significant role in mast cell recruitment?

(a) IL-2 (b) IL-3 (c) IL-4 (d) IL-5

Explanation:

Mast cell

- *Mast cells* are **bone marrow–derived** cells that are widely distributed in the tissues.
- They are abundant near **blood vessels** and nerves and in **subepithelial tissues.**
- Mast cells have cytoplasmic membrane-bound granules that contain a variety of biologically active mediators.
- Mast cells (and their circulating counterpart, basophils) are activated by the cross-linking of high-affinity IgE Fc receptors.
- Cytokines involved in regulation of mast cell growth, recruitment and differentiation:
    - **SCF (stem cell factor)**
    - **IL-3**
    - **IL-9**
- If to choose one option among the three, go for SCF. It's the single most important factor for survival and recruitment of mast cells.

Functions of Mast cell

- Below illustration will be useful in remembering all functions of mast cells.

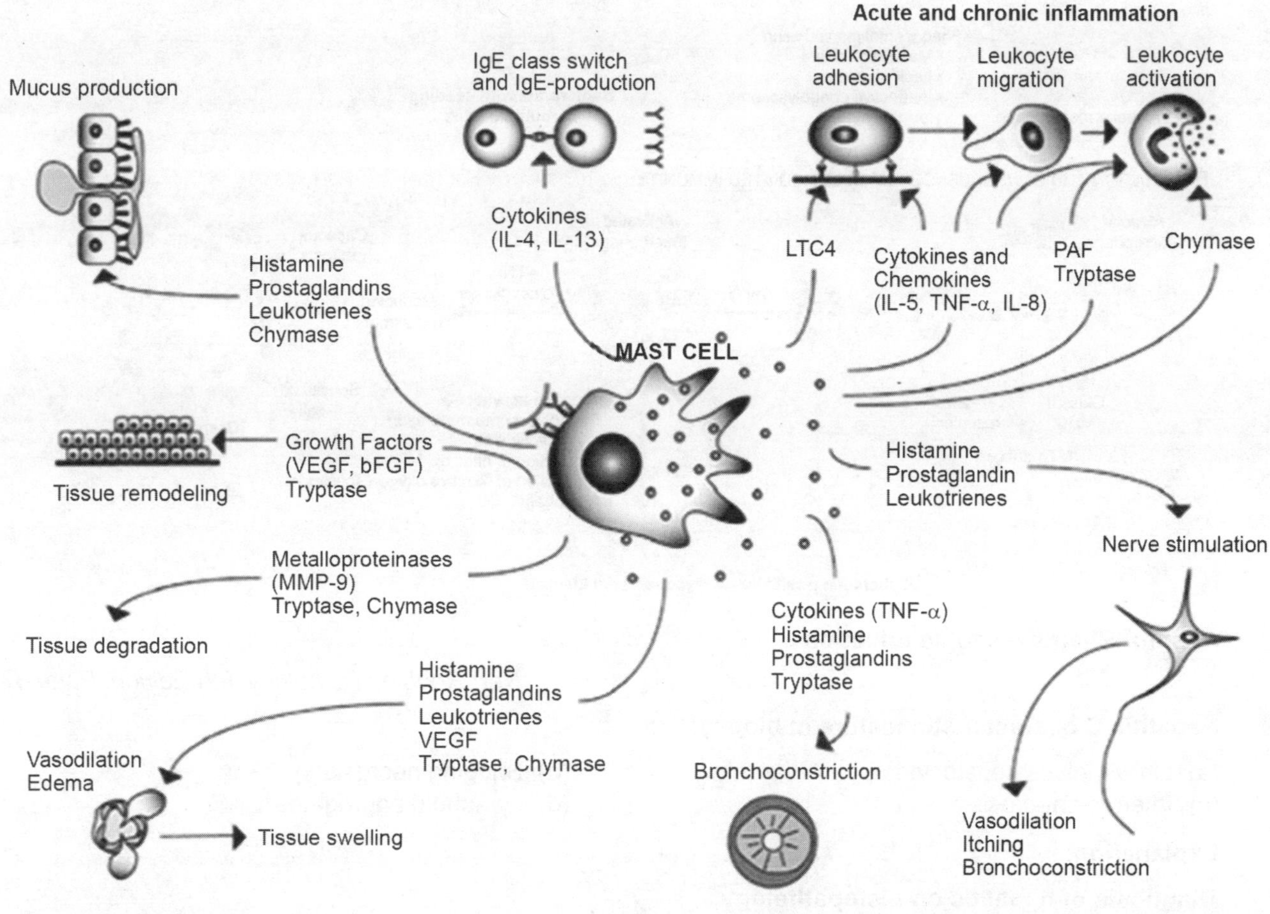

Ans: (b) IL 3

Ref: *Robbins Pathology, 9th Edition, Page 202*

28. Tubercle bacilli are intact even after ingestion of macrophage. This is due to:

(a) Inhibition of complement
(b) Phagolysosome inhibition
(c) Prevents free radical formation
(d) Inhibition of MPO

Explanation:

Infection by *M. tuberculosis* proceeds in steps, from initial infection of macrophages to a subsequent TH1 response that both contains the bacteria and causes tissue damage.

- Early replication in macrophages – Inhibiting phagolysosome formation.
- Th1 response – The alveolar macrophages then secrete IL-12 which converts a T cell predominantly to Th1 response.
- **Macrophage activation** – The IL 12 and the IFN-gamma (secrete predominantly by Th1 cells) causes macrophage activation and kills the tubercle bacilli.
- The end point of the interleukin and cytokines secreted is the granuloma formation – hallmark of tuberculous infection.

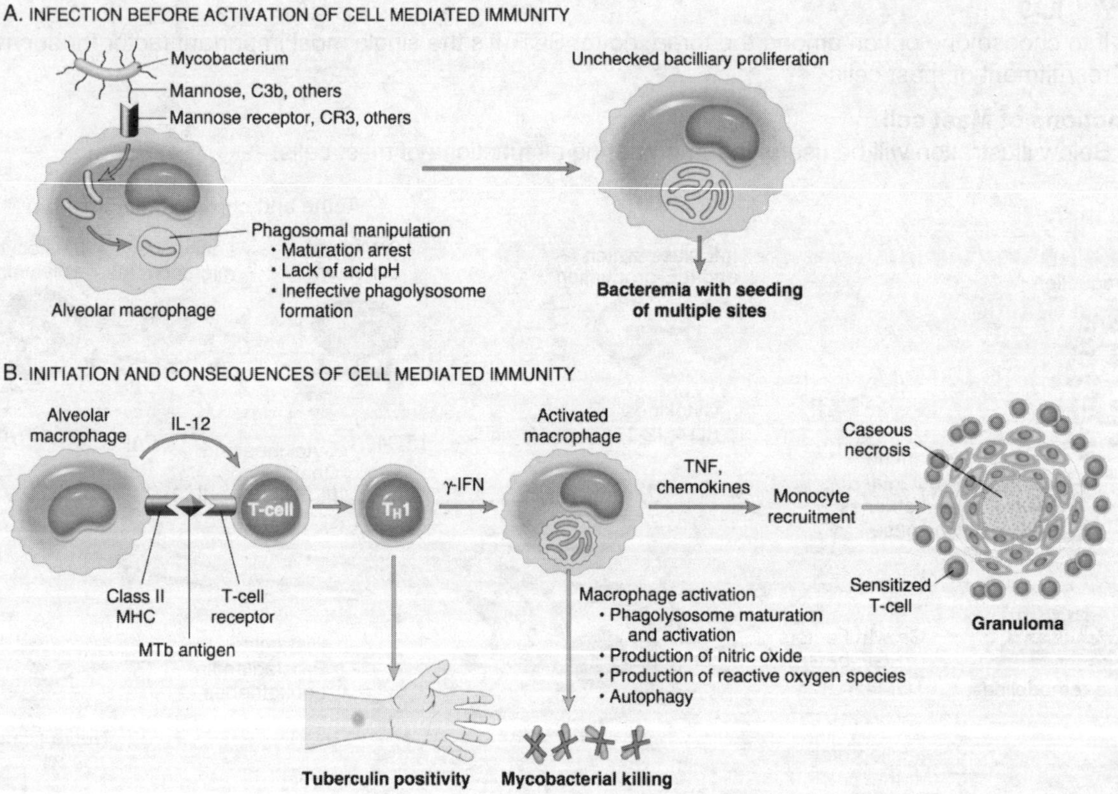

Ans: (b) Phagolysosome inhibtion

Ref: Robbins Pathology, 9th Edition, Page 371

29. Hepatitis C characteristic feature in biopsy:

(a) Groundglass hepatocytes
(b) Bridging necrosis
(c) Interface necrosis
(d) Lymphoid aggregates

Explanation:

Diagnosis of hepatitis on histopathology

- To diagnose hepatitis, liver biopsy is not necessary. Serology is the mainstay.
- The only use of biopsy is to grade the degree of damage and chronicity and to rule out complications.
- Having said that, there are few markers of hepatitis as per etiology on biopsy.

Hepatitis histopathology

- Regardless of etiology, chronic hepatitis is characterized by these features, to variable degrees
- Portal inflammation
- Interface hepatitis
- Parenchymal inflammation and necrosis
- Cirrhosis.

Hepatitis C on HPE

- Predominantly sinusoidal lymphocytic infiltrate, often with lymphoid follicles that surround damaged bile ducts, often involvement of portal tracts.
- Mallory's hyaline, mild and focal macrovesicular steatosis, minimal necrosis.
- Usually no/minimal plasma cells or eosinophils; may have irregular acidophil bodies.
- **Lymphoid aggregates are specific for hepatitis C.**

Hepatitis B on HPE

Acute – Ground glass hepatocytes (finely granular eosinophilic cytoplasm consisting of spherules and tubules of HBsAg) with central ballooning degeneration.

Ans: (d) Lymphoid aggregates

Ref: *Robbins Pathology, 9th Edition, Page 843*

30. Most common antibody seen in anti-phospholipid syndrome:

(a) Anti-cardiolipin antibodies
(b) ANA
(c) Anti-beta2 glycoprotein 1
(d) B2 microglobulin

Explanation:

ANTI-PHOSPHOLIPID ANTIBODY SYNDROME (APLA)

Clinical Criteria

Vascular thrombosis

- One or more clinical episodes of arterial, venous, or small-vessel thrombosis, occurring within any tissue or organ.

Complications of pregnancy

- One or more unexplained deaths of morphologically normal fetuses at or after the 10th week of gestation; or
- One or more premature births of morphologically normal neonates at or before the 34th week of gestation; or

Three or more unexplained consecutive spontaneous abortions before the 10th week of gestation.

Laboratory Criteria

Anticardiolipin antibodies

- Anticardiolipin IgG or IgM antibodies present at moderate or high levels in the blood on two or more occasions at least six weeks apart.

Lupus anticoagulant antibodies (most common)

- Lupus anticoagulant antibodies detected in the blood on two or more occasions at least six weeks apart, according to the guidelines of the International Society on Thrombosis and Hemostasis.

A diagnosis of definite antiphospholipid syndrome requires the presence of at least one of the clinical criteria and at least one of the laboratory criteria. No limits are placed on the interval between the clinical event and the positive laboratory finding.

Ans: (a) Anti-cardiolipin antibodies

Ref: *Thrombotic Complication of Infacny and Childhood, Page 234*

31. Cancers caused by asbestosis includes all *except*:

(a) Mesothelioma
(b) Bladder ca
(c) Ovarian tumours
(d) Laryngeal ca

Explanation:

Asbestosis:

- Localized fibrous plaques or, rarely, diffuse pleural fibrosis.
- Pleural effusions, recurrent.
- Parenchymal interstitial fibrosis *(asbestosis).*
- Lung carcinoma.
- Mesotheliomas.
- Laryngeal, ovarian and perhaps other extrapulmonary neoplasms, including colon carcinomas.
- Increased risk for systemic autoimmune diseases and cardiovascular disease has been proposed.

High Yield Points

- Most common variant of asbestos fibres – **Serpentine*.**
- Most pathogenic variant of asbestos fibres – **Amphibole*.**
- Most common manifestation of asbestos exposure – **Pleural Plaques*.**
- Most common carcinoma following asbestos exposure – **Lung carcinoms*** >> **Mesothelioma*.**
- **Asbestos bodies* (colourless)** and **ferruginous bodies* (brown colour)** findings in **HPE.**

Pleural Plaques

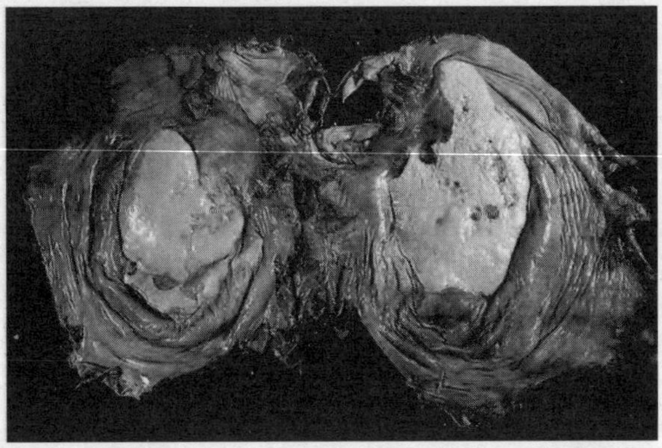

Ans: (b) Bladder cancer

Ref: *Robbins 9th Edition*

MICROBIOLOGY

1. **Post rabies bite leads to hemorrhagic bullous lesion caused by:**

(a) Pseudomonas
(b) *Staphylococcus aureus*
(c) Capnocytophagia
(d) *Vibrio vulnificus*

Explanation:

- **Dog and cat bites** – oral and nasal fluids organism
  - *Pasteurella multocida, S. intermedius, Simonsiella steedae,* ***Capnocytophagia.***
  - Predominant anaerobes – anaerobic gram positive cocci, *Fusobacterium spp, Bacteroides, Porphyromonas and Prevotella spp.*
- **Snake bite** – oral flora (*Pseudomonas, Klebsiella, Proteus and E.coli*).

Ans: (c) Capnocytophagia

Ref: *Harrison's Infectious Disease, 2nd Edition, Page 255-258 and Ananthanarayan and Paniker, 9th Edition, Page 402*

2. **Bacteria that often contaminates disinfectant solution is:**

(a) *Staphylococcus aureus*
(b) Streptococcus
(c) *E.coli*
(d) Enterobacter

Explanation:

- **ESCKAPE group of organisms** important in hospital acquired infections:
  - ***E****nterococcus faecium* and *E. faecalis* (Vancomycin resistant Enterococci).
  - ***S****taphylococcus aureus* (MRSA, VISA, hVISA,VRSA).
  - ***C****itrobacter spp.*
  - ***K****lebsiella pneumoniae* (MDR strains).
  - ***A****cinetobacter baumannii* (MDR strains).
  - ***P****seudomonas aeruginosa* (MDR strains).
  - ***E****nterobacter aerogenes* and other spp.
- ***Pseudomonas aeruginosa***–Bacteria that often contaminates disinfectant solution, especially savlon and Dettol solutions used for placing thermometers.
- Both (a) and (d) are correct, but best answer among the given option is (a).

Ans: (a) Staphylococcus aureus

Ref: *Harrison's Infectious Disease, 2nd Edition, Page 159-168 and Ananthanarayan and Paniker, 9th Edition, Page 644-648*

3. **Bacillary angiomatosis is caused by:**

(a) Borrelia
(b) *Bartonella henselae*
(c) Rickettsia
(d) *Bartonella bacilliformis*

Explanation:

Bartonellosis:

- Short, slightly curved, facultative intracellular pleomorphic gram negative bacillus.
- **Catalase and oxidase negative*.**
- **Twitching motility** seen.
- Species of Bartonella:
  - *B.bacilliformis*: **Carrion's disease/Oraya fever** (Acute form) and **veruga peruana** (chronic form).
  - *B.quintana*: **Trench fever.**
  - *B.henselae, B.elizabethae, B.clarriggeiae, B.vinsonii, B.koehlerae*: **Cat scratch disease.**
  - *B.henselae:* **Bacillary angiomatosis** (opportunistic infection in HIV patients), bacillary peliosis.
- ***Afipiafelis**** another group of organism also responsible for **cat scratch disease.**

- **Vectors:**
  - **Cat fleas:** Cat scratch disease.
  - **Body louse:** Trench fever.
  - **Sand flies** (Lutzomyiaverrucarum): Oraya fever.
- **Diagnosis:**
  - Blood sample, lymph node aspirates and skin biopsies and culture.
  - **Warthin-Starry silver stain**–Bartonella fixed tissues.
  - Antigen detection: ELISA, IFT.
  - PCR assay.
- **Treatment:** Tetracyclines, macrolides, Fluoroquinolones.

Ans: (b) Bartonella henselae

Ref: *Ananthanarayan and Paniker, 9th Edition, Page 412 and 413*

4. **Mechanism by which *Staph aureus* shows methicillin resistance:**

(a) PBP alteration (b) Cell permeability
(c) Antibiotic response (d) Efflux pump

Explanation:

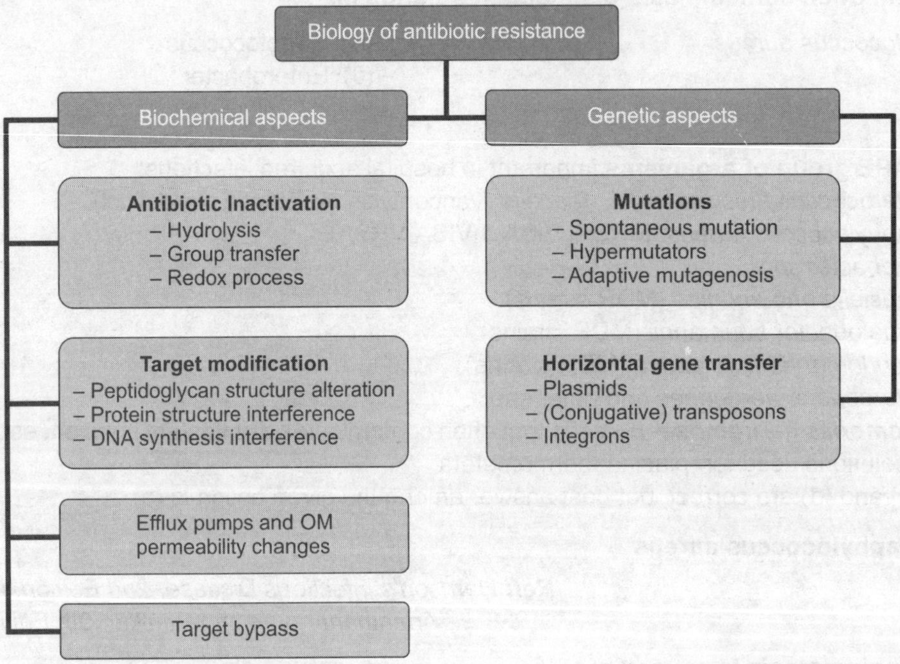

MECHANISM OF RESISTANCE:

(A) Resistance by efflux mechanism:
- Quinolones: NorA in *S. aureus.*
- Chloramphenicol: *cml*A and *flo*-encoded efflux in *E.coli and Salmonella spp*.
- Macrolides: *mef*-encoded efflux in *S. pneumoniae and S.pyogenes.*
- Tetracyclines: *tet* genes encoding efflux proteins in GPB and GNB.

(B) Resistance by Decreased uptake:
- **Aminoglycosides.**
- Changes in outer membrane permeability: *P. aeruginosa.*
- Altered electrical potential (AEP): Bacterial respiration generates AEP (inhibits movements aminoglycosides across cell membrane - anaerobes and facultative anaerobes, e.g., *Enterococci*).

(C) Resistance by Altered target mutation:
- **β-Lactams- Altered PBP(s)**
  - **PBP 2a** (***mec*A** in *S.aureus* and CONS).
  - **PBP 2x, PBP 2b, PBP 1a** (acquired from other Streptococci by transformation *S.pneumoniae*).

- o **PBP 5** (point mutation)– *E.faecium.*
- **Quinolones:**
  - o Mutation leading to reduced binding to active sites (***gyr*A** in enteric GNB and *S.aureus*, ***gyr*A and *par*C** in *S. pneumoniae*).
- **Macrolides:**
  - o Ribosomal active site methylation with reduced binding (*erm*-encoded methylases in *S.aureus, S. pneumoniae and S. pyogenes*).
- **Glycopeptides:**
  - o Altered peptidoglycan cross link target (**D-Ala-D-Ala to D-Ala-D-Lac or D-Ala-D-Ser; VanA gene**–*E.faecalis, E.faecium and S.aureus*, **VanB gene**–*E.faecium and E.faecalis*).
- **Oxazolidinones:**
  - o Mutation leading to reduced binding to active site (G2576U mutation in rRNA in *E.faecium and S.aureus*).
- **Tetracyclines:**
  - o Production of proteins that bind to the ribosome and alter the active site (***tet*(M)** in GPB).
- **Sulfonamides:**
  - o Mutation or recombination of genes encoding **DHPS** (*E.coli, S.aureus and S.pneumoniae*).
  - o Acquisition of new low affinity **DHPS genes (*sul1* and *sul*2** in enteric GNB).
- **Trimethoprim:**
  - o **Mutations in gene encoding DHFR** (***dhfrI* and *dhfrII*** in *E.coli, S.aureus, S.pneumoniae and H.influenzae*).
- **Rifampin:**
  - o Mutation leading to reduced binding to RNA polymerase (**Mutation in *rpo*B** in *S.aureus and M.tuberculosis*).

Ans: (a) PBP alteration

Ref: *Harrison's Infectious Disease, 2nd Edition, Page 406, 430, 500 and Manual of Clinical Microbiology. In Versalovic J, 10th Edition, Washington DC; ASM Press; 2011, Vol 1: 1093*

5. Swollen belly syndrome is caused by:

(a) *Ascaris lumricoides* (b) *Strongyloides fuelleborni*
(c) *Strongyloides stercoralis* (d) *Wucheriria bancrofti*

Explanation:

Synonyms: Swollen stomach sickness, swollen belly, swollen toddler (or stomach) syndrome.

- ***Strongyloides fuelleborni*** is the causative agent of **'swollen toddler (or stomach) syndrome'** in which younger toddlers are most commonly affected.
- Life-threatening GI disease due to *Strongyloides fuelleborni kellyi*; seems in localized areas of **New Guinea.**

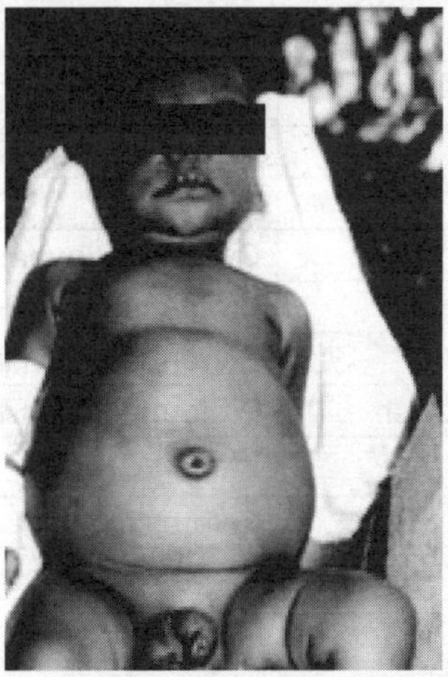

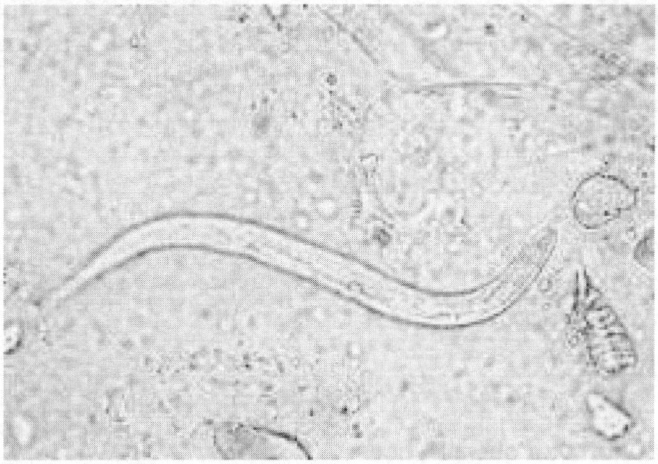

Ans: (b) Strongyloides fuelleborni

Ref: *Jawetz Medical Microbiology, 27th Edition*

6. **Patient presents with watery diarrhea after 24 hours of sea food ingestion. Probable organism is:**

(a) *Vibrio parahemolyticus* (b) *Salmonella typhimurium*
(c) *Shigella flexneri* (d) Campylobacter
(e) Staph food poisoning

Explanation:

Diarrheal diseases:

Mechanism of diarrhea	Pathogens involved	
Noninflammatory (Enterotoxin) Proximal small bowel involved	• *Vibrio cholerae* • ETEC strain of *E.coli* • *Clostridium perfringens* • *Bacillus cereus* • *Staphylococcus aureus* • *Aeromonas hydrophila* • *Plesiomonas shigelloides*	• Rota virus • Norwalk virus • Enteric adeno viruses • *Giardia lamblia* • *Cryptosporidium parvum* • *Cyclospora cayetanensis* • *Microsporidia spp.*
Inflammatory (Invasion or cytotoxin) Colon or distal small bowel involved	• *Shigella spp.* • *Salmonella spp.* • *Campylobacter jejuni* • EHEC and EIEC strain of *E.coli* • *Yersinia enterocolitica*	• *Vibrio parahemolyticus* • *Aeromonas hydrophila* • *Plesiomonas shigelloides* • *Clostridium difficile* • *Entamoeba histolytica*
Penetrating Distal small bowel involved	• *Salmonella typhi* • *Yersinia enterocolitica*	• *Campylobacter fetus*

Bacterial food poisoning:

Time period	Organism involved
1 – 6 hours	*Staphylococcus aureus* (Heat stable toxin) *Bacillus cereus* (Heat stable toxin)
8 – 16 hours	*Clostridium perfringens* (Heat labile toxin) *Bacillus cereus* (Heat labile toxin)
>16 hours	*Vibrio cholerae* ETEC and EHEC strains of *E.coli* *Salmonella spp.* *Shigella spp.* *Campylobacter jejuni* ***Vibrio parahemolyticus***

Organism	Common sources	Pathogenic mechanism
Campylobacter species	Water, poultry, milk	Cytotoxin/invasion
Clostridium perfringens	Meat, poultry	Toxin production in vivo
Clostridium difficile	Antimicrobial therapy	Cytotoxin
Vibrio parahemolyticus	**Seafood**	**Cytotoxin/invasion**
Bacillus cereus	Meat, vegetable, rice	Preformed toxin ingestion
Staphylococcus aureus	Meat, salad, dairy products	Preformed toxin ingestion
Clostridium botulinum	Improperly preserved vegetables, meat, fish	Preformed toxin ingestion
Yersinia enterocolitica	Milk, pork, water	Invasion
Aeromonas sp.	Water	Enterotoxin
Plesiomonas shigelloides	Shellfish	Enterotoxin

Ans: (a) Vibrio parahemolyticus

Ref: *Harrison's Infectious Disease, 2nd Edition, Page 283-289 and Ananthanarayan and Paniker, 9th Edition, Page 311-312*

7. A HIV patient presents with cough for 10 days. Sputum culture by SDA reveals broad budding yeast with thick mucoid wall. Diagnosis:

(a) Histoplasmosis
(b) Coccidiomyocosis
(c) Blastomycosis
(d) Penicillium marneffi

Explanation:

Morphological classification of fungi:

Yeast	**Yeast like fungi**	**Moulds/Filamentous fungi**	**Dimorphic fungi**
Cryptococcus neoformans	Candida Torulopsis Geotrichum	Dermatophytes Aspergillus Zygomycetes Fusarium Cephalosporium Geotrichum Scopulariopsis	*Blastomycosis dermatidis* *Paracoccidioides brasiliensis* *Coccidioides immitis* *Histoplasma capsulatum* *Sporothrix schenckii* *Penicillium marneffi*

Histoplasmosis:

- Intacellular infection of the **reticuloendothelial system.**
- Causative agent: ***Histoplasma capsulatum*** (Dimorphic fungus).
- *H.capsulatum var.capsulatum* **(Darling's disease)** and *H.capsulatum var.duboisii* **(African histoplasmosis).**
- **Lab Diagnosis:**
  - o Blood cultures, sputum and skin biopsies.
  - o Cultured in **glucose-BHI agar and SDA,** incubated **at 37°C and 25°C**–grows as yeast and mycelial forms respectively.
  - o **Mycelial forms** shows spherical spores with tubercles.
  - o **Serology:** Latex agglutination test, CFT and precipitation test.
  - o **Skin tests:** With Histoplasmin antigen (delayed hypersensitivity reaction).

Coccidioidomycosis:

- Causative agent: ***Coccidioides immitis*** (Dimorphic fungus).
- Highly infectious organism; **Agent of bioterrorism.**
- **Not seen in India,** reported in **Central and South America.**
- **Lab diagnosis:**
  - o **Specimens:** Sputum, BAL, urine, pleural, pericardial and peritoneal fluids, skin and lung biopsy.
  - o **Direct examination with KOH mount:** Thick walled **spherules with endoconidia.**
  - o **Culture:** SDA with or without antibiotics at both **room temperature** and **at 37°C (yeast forms) in BHI glucose agar, mold forms** seen both at 25°C and 37°C.
  - o **Fungal stains:** GMS, LCB mount, H and E–**spherules with endoconidia and barrel shaped arthroconidia with alternate cells.**

Blastomycosis:

- Chronic infection of the lungs, also known as **North American Blastomycosis/Gilchrist disease.**
- Disseminated Blastomycosis–**immunosuppressed patients** including AIDS.
- Causative agent: ***Blastomyces dermatitidis*** (Dimorphic fungus).
- **Pathogenesis:** Acquired through inhalation from soil (mycelial fragments and conidia)→ In alveoli they transforms into yeasts→ Causes acute inflammation (neutrophils and macrophages)→ granuloma formation→ grows intracellular and relatively resistant to phagocytosis.
- **Clinical features:**
  - o **Pulmonary blastomycosis:** Asymptomatic or flu like illness sometimes resembles chronic lung disease.
  - o **Cutaneous blastomycosis:** Primary (direct transcutaneous spread) or secondary (hematogenous spread).
  - o Disseminated extrapulmonary blastomycosis.
- **Lab diagnosis:**
  - o **Specimens:** Sputum, BAL, CSF, urine, skin and lung biopsy.

- **Direct examination with KOH mount:** Thick walled **broad based budding yeasts.**
- **Culture:** SDA with or without antibiotics at both **room temperature (mold forms)** and **at 37°C (yeast forms) in BHI glucose agar.**
- **Fungal stains:** GMS, LCB mount, H and E–yeast forms: **Broadbased budding yeast cells (figure of 8 morphology)** and mold forms: **Thick walled terminal chlamydoconidia.**
- **Serology:** CFT, EIA, Immunodiffusion test.
- **PCR:** Labeled DNA/RNA hybrid.

• Treatment: **DOC–amphotericin B.**

Ans: (c) Blastomycosis

Ref: *Ananthanarayan and Paniker, 9th Edition, Page 605-608*

8. **Hepatitis C virus high efficacy testing in blood bank is by:**

(a) NS1 (b) NS2
(c) NS3 (d) Core antigen

Explanation:

Hepatitis C virus (HCV):

- **HCV** is 50-60 nm in size, **linear, ss-RNA genome,** enclosed within a core, surrounded by an envelope carrying glycoprotein.
- Classified under new Genus: **Hepacivirus;** Family: **Flaviviridae.**
- Total **11 genotypes** were identified recently, high mutability present.
- **Clinical features:**
  - **Long incubation period:** 15-160 days.
  - **Acute illness:** Mild and anicteric and **only 5% of population develop jaundice.**
  - It is now the most common cause of **post transfusion hepatitis.**
  - About **50-80%** of the patients **progress to chronic hepatitis** with **remaining develop HCC and cirrhosis.**
  - **Carrier rate:** 1-20%.
  - **1/4th of chronic hepatitis cases** are due to HCV infection.
- **Laboratory diagnosis:**
  - Identification by ELISA for **Anti-HCV antibodies.**
  - **Sensitive:** Anti-HCV antibodies and Radioimmunoblot assay (RIBA) for HCV.
  - **Sensitive and specific test:** Detection of **HCV RNA level.**
  - **Molecular assay:** Reverse transcriptase PCR.

Laboratory diagnosis of Hepatitis:

HAV	HBV	HCV	HDV	HEV
IgM HAV **HAV RNA**	**HBsAg**–Acute, chronic, carrier **HBeAg**–Active infection **Anti HBc**– **IgM**–Acute, window period **IgG**–Chronic infection **Only Anti HBs**–Vaccination **HBV DNA**–Active infection, viral load (monitoring infection) **Anti HBe**–Epidemiological marker	Antibody by 3rd generation **ELISA using:** **C3, C100** **NS 3, 4, 5 Antigen** **HCV RNA** **Genotyping-** 11 sub types	**HBsAg** **Anti HBc** **IgM**–Coinfection **IgG**–Superinfection **HDV Ag** **HDV RNA** **Anti HD IgM**	**Anti HBe Ab** **EM** of stool **HEV RNA**

• **Treatment:** Peg-Interferon α + Ribavirin.

Ans: (d) Core antigen

Ref: *Harrison's Infectious Disease, 2nd Edition, Page 962-963 and Ananthanarayan and Paniker, 9th Edition, Page 548-549*

9. Which of the following transmits resistance in bacteria?

(a) Transposon (b) Plasmid (c) Mitochondria (d) Cell wall

Explanation:

- In addition to chromosomal DNA, most bacteria possess **extrachromosomal genetic elements.**
- These are **not essential for the normal life** and functioning of host bacterium.
- But may **responsible for the drug resistance and toxigenicity,** leading to survival under inappropriate condition.
- Plasmids are **circular double stranded DNA molecules** present in the cytoplasm of the bacteria.
- **Autonomous/independent/self-replicating capability**–Independent replicons.
- They have **ability to transfer genes** from one cell to another.
- Methods of gene transfer–**Conjugation, transformation** (natural and artificial), **transduction.**
- Plasmids have important vectors in **genetic engineering.**
- Plasmid DNA+ Chromosomal DNA = **Episomes.**

Ans: (b) Plasmid

Ref: *Ananthanarayan and Paniker, 9th Edition, Page 55*

FORENSIC MEDICINE

1. True regarding Kevorkian sign are all *except*:

(a) Appears within minutes of death
(b) Persists even 3 years after death
(c) Visualized using ophthalmoscope
(d) These are the breaks seen in blood column in retinal vessels

Explanation:

Kevorkian sign an early postmortem change seen in the eyes.
First described by the Dr. Jack Kevorkian in 1961.

Features:

- It is characterized by fragmentation or segmentation (trucking or shunting) of the blood columns in retinal vessels which are visualized using Ophthalmoscope.
- These appear within minutes after death and persists for about an hour (NOT 3 YEARS).

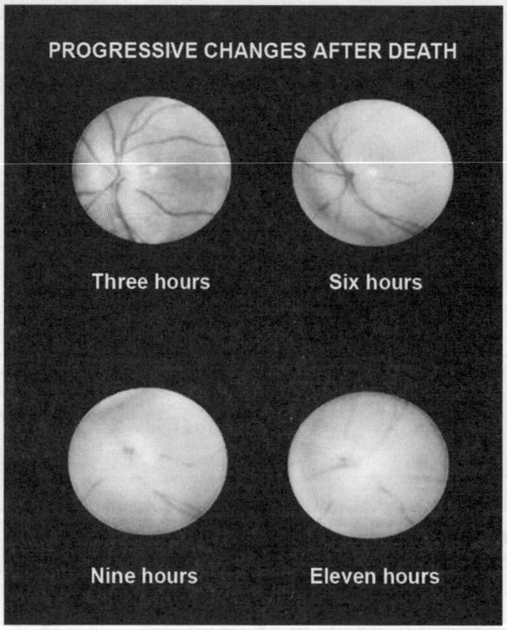

Ocular Changes after Death

- Loss of corneal reflex (not a reliable sign of death).
- Opacity of cornea:
  - Due to drying or dessication.
  - Seen before death in **Cholera**[Q] and Wasting disease.

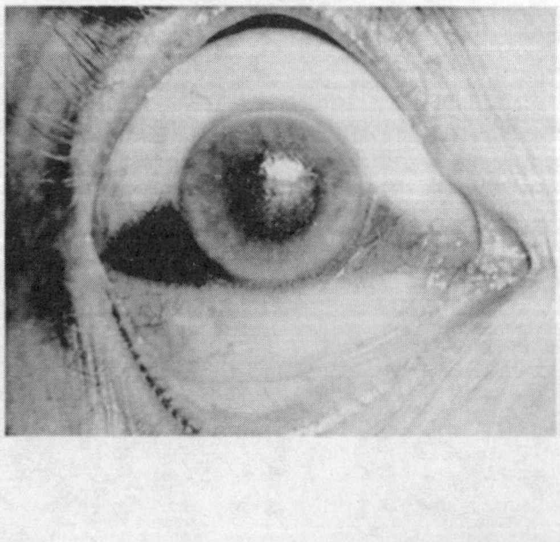

- o **Taches Noire Scleroitiques**[Q] – 2 yellow triangles on the sclera at each side of the iris with apex towards canthus, which later become brown and then black; due deposition of a film of cell debris and mucus if eyelids are open for few hours after death; seen within 3-4 hours.

- **Flaccidity of eyeball** – Due to ↓ IOT
  - o During life – 14 to 25 gm.
  - o Soon after death – <12 gm.
  - o **½ hour after death – < 3 gm.**
  - o 2 hours – nil.
- **Pupils**
  - o Dilated after death (except in phase of rigor mortis where they are constricted).
  - o Reacts to atropine and eserine for about an hour after death but not to strong light.
- **Retina**
  - o **Kevorkian sign**[Q]–Fragmentation or segmentation (trucking) of the blood columns in Retinal vessels.
  - o Pale in first 2 hours.
  - o Hazy disc outline in 6 hours.
  - o Disc outline blurred in 7-10 hours.
- **Chemical changes**
  - o Rise in K+ in vitreous humour[Q] (upto 100 hours).
  - o Fall in Na+, Cl-.

Note: Eyeball being a soft tissue putrefies along with other soft tissues and doesn't persists till 3 years. So this General knowledge also helps pinpoint the answer here.

Ans: (b) Persists even 3 years after death

Ref: *KSN Reddy; The Essentials of Forensic Medicine and Toxicology, 34th Edition, Page 145*

2. Litchenberg flower seen in:

(a) Electrocution (b) Lightening (c) Thermal burn (d) Chemical burn

Explanation:

Lichtenberg's flower (AKA Filigree or Arborescent burns)

- Pathognomonic of lightening injury.
- Superficial, thin, irregular and tortuous marking over skin mainly over shoulders and flanks.
- Resembles branches of a tree (Fern like pattern) of erythema.
- Not associated with burning.
- May be caused by slight staining of tissue by hemoglobin from lysed RBCs along path of current.
- Indicates the path taken by current but *does not correspond to vascular channels.*
- Disappears in 1 or 2 days if survives.

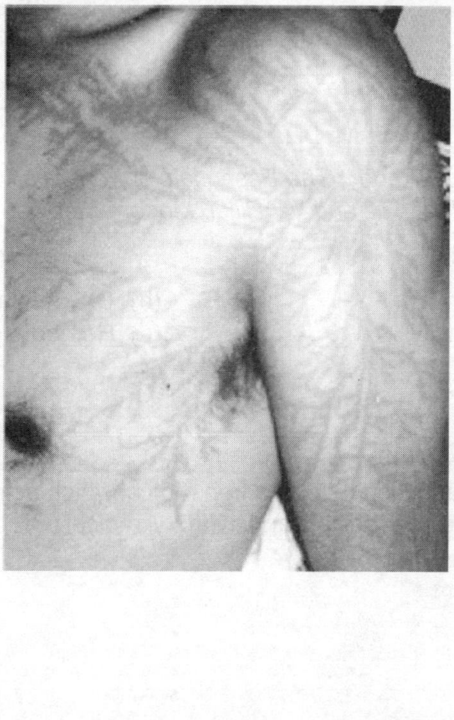

Mechanism of injury in a lightening flash[Q] (According to **Spencer**)

A. Direct effect of high voltage current.
B. Surface flash burn by super heated air.
C. Mechanical effect due to displacement of air around the flash (Expansion and repulsion of air).
D. **Sledge Hammer Effect:** Blow dealt by compressed air pushed before the current produced by lightning may produce bruising is usually at the back of head.

Ans: (b) Lightening

***Ref:** KSN Reddy; The Essentials of Forensic Medicine and Toxicology, 34th Edition, Page 312*

3. **Brick red postmortem lividity seen in:**

(a) Phosphorus
(b) Carbon monoxide
(c) Hydrogen sulfide
(d) Hydrogen cyanide

Explanation:

Postmortem lividity or Hypostasis

- Discolouration under the skin in most superficial layers of dermis (rete mucosum) of dependent parts of body after death due to capillovenos distention.

Colour of PM lividity	Poison
Cherry red[Q] (due to COHb)	Carbon monoxide
Bright (brick) red[Q]/Pink	Hydrocyanic acid (also seen in hypothermia/refrigerated bodies)
Chocolate[Q]/Coffee brown (methaemoglobin formation)	Nitrite, aniline, nitrobenzene, acetanilide, bromates and chlorates
Dark brown/yellow	Phosphorus, copper poisoning
Deep blue (due to reduced Hb)	Carbon dioxide, Potassium cyanide
Bluish green[Q]	H_2S
Blue	Copper sulphate
Black	Opium

- **Note:** KSN Reddy on Page 584 (while dealing with cyanides) Quotes "The colour of the cheek and the postmortem staining may be cherry red in about half the cases, because oxygen remains in the cell as oxyhemoglobin and due to formation of cyanmethemoglobin."
- However on the pages mentioned above, he states the PM lividity in **cyanide** poisoning is **Brick red.**
- Thus there is ambiguity in the answer.
- However the best book on Toxicology by an Indian Author, VV Pillai clearly states PM lividity of **Cyanide** is **Brick red** due to increased haemoglobin oxygen saturation in venous blood because of decreased utilisation of oxygen by tissues.
- Hence it is safe to stick to:
  - **Brick red** for **Cyanide;** and
  - **Cherry red** for **Carbon monoxide*.**

Ans: (d) Hydrogen cyanide

***Ref:** KSN Reddy; The Essentials of Forensic Medicine and Toxicology, 34th Edition, Page 151, 472 and VV Pillai, Modern Medical Toxicology, 4th Edition, Page 34, 365*

4. **Paraquat herbicide ingestion:**

(a) Fast heart rate, confusion
(b) Oxygen helps in rapid recovery
(c) Causes ulceration in oral cavity
(d) Hemodialysis is not useful

Explanation:

Paraquat Poisoning

- Paraquat is a **herbicide/weed killer.**
- MOA: NADPH dependent reduction to form a free radical which acts with molecular oxygen to reform the cation to produce superoxide free radicals and hydroxyl radical (OH) which disrupt cellular function leading to cell death.

- Highest conc. post oral absorption is found in kidneys, lungs followed by muscles.

Clinical features:

System	Signs and symptoms
Local	Irritation and inflammation of skin, cornea, conjunctiva and nasal mucosa
GIT	Ulceration and corrosion of mouth and tongue (Paraquat tongue), oropharynx, and esophagus; nausea, vomiting, hematemesis, diarrhea, dysphagia
Pancreas	Pancreatitis
RS	Cough, hemoptysis, dyspnea due to pulmonary edema, aphonia, aspiration
Renal	Oliguria, renal failure
CVS	Hypovolemia, shock, arrhythmias
Hepatic	Cholestasis
CNS	Coma, convulsions, cerebral edema

- Death occurs from multiorgan failure, or progressive pulmonary fibrosis leading to ARDS.

Treatment:

- Gastric lavage with water.
- Clay (fuller's earth or 7% bentonite) to adsorb paraquat followed by mannitol.
- **N-acetylcystine** and Hemodialysis or hemoperfusion.
- **Oxygen contraindicated** as it enhances **lung damage***.

Autopsy findings:

- Pulmonary edema, effusions and hemorrhages.
- Large, rigid and stiff lungs – In delayed death.
- Fatty degeneration and centrilobular necrosis of liver.
- Renal cortical pallor and diffuse tubular damage.
- Mostly accidental and suicidal.

Ans: (c) Causes ulceration in oral cavity

Ref: *KSN Reddy; The Essentials of Forensic Medicine and Toxicology, 34th Edition, Page 489 and VV Pillai, Modern Medical Toxicology, 4th Edition, Page 398*

PSM

1. A study is planned to check stool occult blood positivity using Hemoccult test among a group of participants aged 50–75 years. The test is repeated if result is positive. No repeating if the test is negative. What is the effect of this on sensitivity and specificity?

(a) ↑ specificity ↓ sensitivity
(b) ↓ specificity ↑ sensitivity
(c) ↑ specificity ↑ sensitivity
(d) No effect

Explanation:

- The **sequential/serial testing** – two sequential tests are used and those who **test positive by the first test** are brought in for the second test. When we retest those who tested positive on the first test, there is a **loss in net sensitivity and a gain in net specificity.**
- The **simultaneous testing,** because an individual who tests positive on any one or multiple tests is considered positive, there is a **gain in net sensitivity and net loss in specificity.**

Basic measures used in evaluation of a diagnostic test are:

a. Sensitivity and specificity
b. Predictive values – positive predictive value and negative predictive value

Sensitivity	Ability of the test to identify **true positives** (TP)
Specificity	Ability of the test to identify **true negatives** (TN)
Positive predictive value	Probability that a patient with positive test result truly has the disease
Negative predictive value	Probability that a patient with negative test result truly does not have the disease

Ans: (a) ↑ specificity ↓ sensitivity

Ref: *Leon Gordis, Epidemiology, 5th Edition, Page 99*

2. New Plasmodium falciparum Malaria Vaccine strain:

(a) PPV 23
(b) RTS s
(c) R14-4
(d) Jeryl Lynn

Explanation:

- RTS,S/AS01 (RTS,S) – also known as **Mosquirix** which is an injectable vaccine that provides partial protection against malaria in young children.
- The vaccine acts against ***Plasmodium falciparum.***
- It is being evaluated in **sub-Saharan Africa** as a complementary malaria control tool.

UPDATES IN IMMUNISATION

JE vaccine

- Given in **UP, WB, Karnataka, Assam and Bihar.**
- First dose at **9-12 months.**
- Second dose at **16-24 months.**
- 0.5 ml **SC** Left upper arm.
- Diluent used – **Phosphate buffer.**
- Maximum age – **15 years.**

Rotavirus vaccine

- Given in **Andhra Pradesh, Haryana, Himachal Pradesh and Odisha** (26th March 2016).
- Expanded in phase-wise manner.
- Total of 3 doses – Given at 6, 10 and 14 weeks.
- 5 drops – Oral.
- Maximum age – Till 1 year.

Pentavalent vaccine

- Total of 3 doses – Given at 6, 10 and 14 weeks.

- IM – 0.5 ml at Anterolateral side of mid-thigh (Left).
- Maximum age – Till 1 year.
- Booster 1 – 16-24 months - DPT - IM 0.5 ml at Anterolateral side of mid-thigh (Left).
- Booster 2 – DPT – 0.5 ml IM Left Upper arm.

April 25, 2016*: "National Switch Day"–In routine immunization, **tOPV** replaced by **bOPV.**

Mission Indradhanush

- **Goal:** To ensure **full immunization** with all available vaccines for children up to **two years** and **pregnant women.**
- The Mission has been launched to accelerate the process of immunization and achieve full immunization coverage for all children in the country.
- The Government of India has identified **201 high focus districts across 28 states** in the country that have the highest number of partially immunized and unimmunized children.

Ans: (b) RTS s

Ref: *http://www.who.int/malaria/media/malaria-vaccine-implementation-qa/en/#What is RTS,S/AS01?*

3. Advantage of random allocation of study participants from community:

(a) Eliminating selection bias during allocation
(b) To make sure samples represent general population
(c) Double blinding
(d) To ensure adequate sample size

Explanation:

Randomization

- In random sampling, everyone in the sampling frame has an equal probability of being chosen.
- Randomization **eliminates "bias"** and allows **comparability.**
- Ensures that the investigator has no control over allocation of participants to either study or control group, thus eliminating **"selection bias".**

Ans: (a) Eliminating selection bias during allocation

Ref: *Park's Preventive and Social Medicine, 23rd Edition, Page 82*

4. Range of Correlation coefficient:

(a) 0 to +1 (b) -1 to +1 (c) -1 to 0 (d) 0 to +2

Explanation:

- The term correlation is used to assess **association** between **two quantitative variables.**
- Correlation denotes that one variable increases or decreases for a unit increase or decrease in the other variable.
- Degree of association is measured by correlation coefficient and represented as **'r'.**
- The correlation coefficient always ranges between **-1 to +1.**
    - **Positive correlation** – one unit increase in one variable increases other variable.
    - **Negative correlation** – one unit increase in one variable decreases other variable or vice versa.
- Complete absence of correlation is represented by **zero (0).**
- Two types of correlation:
    - **Pearson's correlation** – When variables are normally distributed.
    - **Spearman rank correlation** – Non normal distribution of variables.

Ans: (b) -1 to +1

Ref: *Park's Preventive and Social Medicine, 23rd Edition, Page 853*

5. True about Single exposure, common vector outbreak:

(a) All cases does not occur within one incubation period
(b) Frequent secondary cases
(c) Explosive
(d) Secondary wave present

Explanation:

Types of epidemics

Three major types of epidemics may be distinguished:

A. **Common - source epidemics**
   (a) Single exposure or "point source" epidemics.
   (b) Continuous or multiple exposure epidemics.

B. **Propagated epidemics**
   (a) Person-to-person
   (b) Arthropod vector
   (c) Animal reservoir

C. **Slow (modern) epidemics.**

Single exposure or "point source" epidemics

- The graph of the time distribution of epidemic cases is called **'epidemic curve'.**
- All cases occur within a **single incubation period** in a **single peak.**
- There are **no secondary cases.**
- The epidemic tends to be **explosive** with maximum number of cases **clustered** around **one point of time.**
- Epidemic will be **explosive.**

The common source epidemics are frequently but not always due to exposure to an infectious agent e.g.:

- **Bhopal gas tragedy** (air pollution).
- **Minamata** disease in Japan (contaminated food chain).
- **Chernobyl** tragedy (radiation pollution).

Ans: (c) Explosive

Ref: *Park's Preventive and Social Medicine, 23rd Edition, Page 64*

6. **Study in which cases act as their own controls:**

(a) Retrospective study
(b) Cohort study
(c) Prospective study
(d) Case crossover study

Explanation:

Case crossover design

- This study design used for studying the **aetiology of acute outcomes.**
- A case is identified acute condition like myocardial infarction and risk factor, such as level of air pollution.
- Each person who is a case serves as his own control, and comparison is done between the period immediately preceding the adverse outcome with a period after the adverse outcome occurred.

Ans: (d) Case crossover study

Ref: *Leon Gordis, Epidemiology, 5th Edition, Page 206*

7. **The extent to which an intervention does what it is intended to do when used in a community is termed as:**

(a) Efficacy
(b) Effectiveness
(c) Efficiency
(d) Effect modification

Explanation:

- **Efficacy** is a measure of the effect of an agent or intervention in controlled conditions such as 'laboratory settings'.
- **Effectiveness** is a measure of the effect of an agent or intervention in a "real-life" situation such testing effectiveness of a vaccine or a test in a community.
- **Efficiency** of an agent/test is said to be effective when it possible to achieve our goals in a cheaper and better way (Cost-benefit) .

Ans: (b) Effectiveness

Ref: *Leon Gordis, Epidemiology, 5th Edition, Page 310*

ENT

1. **Percentage of SCC of larynx that occur due to HPV infection:**

(a) 10% (b) 15%
(c) 20% (d) 25%

Explanation:

- Approximately **25% of laryngeal squamous cell carcinomas** harbor **HPV infections** on meta-analysis, with common involvement of high-risk **HPV types 16 (highest frequency) and 18.**
- In about **70%, HPV 16 DNA is detected.**
- Other HPV types associated with **laryngeal papillomatosis** include low-risk HPV **types 6 and 11.**
- Other sites of squamous cell carcinoma associated with HPV include **oropharynx and oral cavity.**
- Most common types of cancers associated are **squamous cell carcinoma and verrucous carcinoma.**
- **HPV** associated **laryngeal carcinoma** has a **better prognosis** with better response to **chemoradiation** and improved disease free survival.

Remember

- **Laryngeal squamous cell Ca** – HPV types **16** and **18***.
- **Laryngeal papillomatosis** – HPV types **6** and **11***.

Ans: (d) 25%

Ref: *Kreimer AR, Clifford GM, Boyle P, Franceschi S. Human Papillomavirus Types in Head and Neck Squamous Cell Carcinomas Worldwide: A Systematic Review. Cancer Epidemiol Biomarkers Prev. 2005 Feb; 14(2):467-75*

2. **In Cotton Myer classification for subglottic stenosis, grade 2 will indicate an obstruction of:**

(a) 60-70% (b) <30%
(c) >75% (d) 50-70%

Explanation:

- **Subglottic stenosis classification by Cotton Myer** is based on the circumferential narrowing of the region and is as follows:

Classification	From	To
Grade 1	No Obstruction	50% Obstruction
Grade 2	51% Obstruction	70% Obstruction
Grade 3	71% Obstruction	99% Obstruction
Grade 4	No Detectable Lumen	

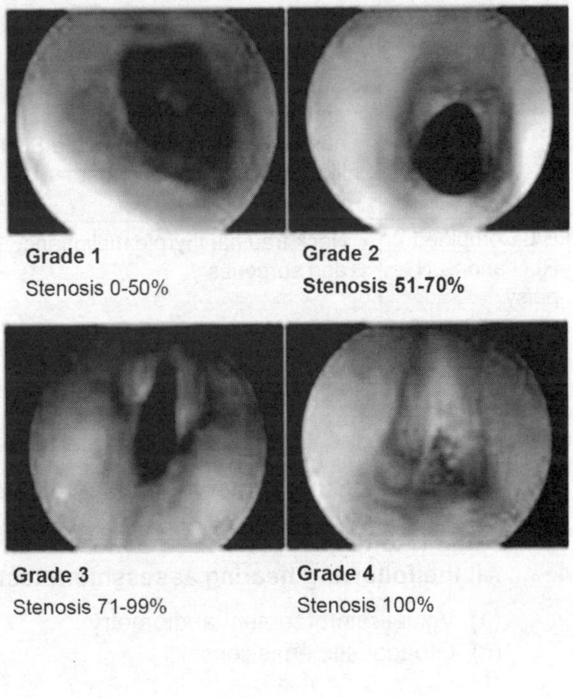

Grade 1 Stenosis 0-50%
Grade 2 **Stenosis 51-70%**
Grade 3 Stenosis 71-99%
Grade 4 Stenosis 100%

- The drawback of the classification is that it does not take into account other factors like the length of the stenosis and involvement of other sites like glottis and trachea; which also have a bearing on the treatment and prognosis of the condition.

Ans: (d) 50-70%

Ref: *A Short Practice of Otorhinolaryngology by Prof KK Ramalingam, 4th Edition, 2014, Page 249*

3. Singer unable to raise the pitch of his voice after thyroid surgery. Most probable nerve affected is:

(a) U/L SLN (b) U/L SLN + RLN
(c) B/L RLN (d) B/L SLN + RLN

Explanation:

Type of Palsy	Etiology	Clinical Features	Treatment
U/L Recurrent laryngeal nerve palsy	• Neck trauma, Thyroid disease/ surgery, carcinoma of cervical esophagus, cervical lymphadenopathy • Bronchogenic carcinoma and mediastinal surgeries [only left RLN palsy]	• Hoarseness of voice	• No treatment as the other vocal cord compensates • Few cases may require Thyroplasty type I [Medial displacement of the vocal cord]
B/L Recurrent laryngeal nerve palsy	• Neck trauma, Thyroid disease/ surgery, carcinoma of cervical esophagus, cervical lymphadenopathy	• Dyspnea and stridor • **The voice will be good**	• Tracheostomy to relieve the stridor • Thyroplasty type II [lateral displacement of the vocal cord] • Laryngeal reinnervation procedures
U/L Superior laryngeal nerve palsy	• Thyroid tumors and surgery, neuritis, diphtheria	• Voice becomes weak and pitch cannot be raised • Mild aspiration because of anesthesia of one side the upper part of larynx	• Speech therapy • No other treatment is required
B/L Superior laryngeal nerve palsy	• Neck trauma, Thyroid disease/ surgery, carcinoma of cervical esophagus, cervical lymphadenopathy	• Voice is weak and husky • Aspiration of saliva and food leading to cough and choking episodes	• Tracheostomy to prevent aspiration • Epiglottoplexy is a reversible procedure to close the laryngeal inlet and prevent aspiration
U/L Combined RLN and SLN palsy	• Thyroid surgery [most common] • Central lesions of the nucleus ambiguous or the part of the vagus nerve before the origin of the SLN like jugular foramen or parapharyngeal space	• Hoarseness of voice • Weak cough • Aspiration	• Speech therapy • Thyroplasty type I
B/L Combined RLN and SLN palsy	• Neck trauma, thyroid malignancy and surgeries	• Aphonia • Aspiration • Weak cough • Bronchopneumonia due to aspiration and inability to cough	• Tracheostomy • Epiglottoplexy • Vocal cord placation to prevent aspiration • Total laryngectomy or laryngotracheal separation for intractable aspiration

Ans: (a) U/L Superior laryngeal nerve palsy

Ref: *Diseases of the Ear, Nose and Throat by PL Dhingra, 6th Edition, 2014, Page 300*

4. All the following hearing assessment tests are used in above 6 months *except*:

(a) Visual reinforcement audiometry (b) Conventional audiometry
(c) Otoacoustic emissions (d) Behavior observation audiometry

Explanation:

Behavior observation audiometry

- Done by presenting an auditory stimulus to the infant and looking for a change in the behavior like stopping of activity or widening of the eyes.
- This is best suited in **infants less than 6 months of age** as most of the reflexes will disappear by then.
- There are certain reflexes which can be looked for:
  - **Moro's reflex** – Sudden movement of head and extension of the limbs in response to sound.
  - **Cessation reflex** – Infant stops activity or may start crying on loud sound.
  - **Cochleopalpebral reflex** – Infant will blink in response to loud sound.

Otoacoustic emissions

- Produced by the **outer hair cells***.
- **Objective test** of hearing.
- Can be done at **any age***.
- MC used for **newborn hearing screening***.

Conventional audiometry

- Subjective test and depends on the patients response to auditory stimulus.
- Can be used only in children **above 5-6 years** of age.

Visual reinforcement audiometry

- Suited for **6 months to 2 years of age.**
- The child is conditioned to respond to auditory stimulus by turning his head.
- This is reinforced by another stimulus like flashing of light or using an animated toy.
- The child will turn his head every time the auditory stimulus is presented and in this way the hearing threshold can be determined.

Ans: (d) Behavior observation audiometry

Ref: *Diseases of the Ear, Nose and Throat by PL Dhingra, 6th Edition, 2014, Page 118*

OPHTHALMOLOGY

1. **Basic pathology Keratomalacia is:**
   (a) Accumulation of desquamated debris
   (b) Absence of mucus
   (c) Breakdown of collagen fibres in corneal stroma
   (d) Infection with cornebacterium xerosis

Explanation:

Keratomalacia
- **Sterile corneal** ulcer secondary to vitamin A deficiency.

Xerophthalmia
- Spectrum of ocular disease ranging from night blindness to corneal melting caused by vitamin A deficiency.
- Nutritional blindness.
- Vitamin A is essential for the synthesis of **retinal photo pigments** and **conjunctival glycoproteins.**
- Vitamin A deficiency is a systemic disease affecting cells and organs throughout the body.

Causes:
- Malnutrition.
- Malabsorption.
- Chronic alcoholics.
- Diseases which precipitate malnutrition like measles, malaria, diarrhoea, acute illness in children.

WHO Classification of Xerophthalmia [in chronological order]

XN	Night blindness
X1A	Conjunctival xerosis
X1B	Bitot's spots
X2	Corneal xerosis
X3A	Keratomalcia < 1/3rd corneal surface
X3B	Keratomalcia > 1/3rd corneal surface
XS	Corneal scar
XF	Xerophthalmic fundus

XN: Night Blindness
- Earliest Symptom; responds rapidly to vitamin A therapy within **24-48 hours.**

X1 A and X1 B: Conjunctival Involvement
- The conjunctival epithelium undergoes **keratanising metaplasia,** i.e., the normal columnar epithelium is transformed into stratified squamous epithelium. **Goblet cells** will be **lost** (mucin secretion is reduced) and **keratinization** occurs.
- **Conjunctival xerosis**–dryness of the conjunctiva starts at the temporal side.
- **Keratin + saprophytic bacilli [Corynebacterium xerosis]** accumulate on the xerotic surface → **Foamy Appearance → Bitot's Spot*.**
- Begin to resolve within **2-5 days** and disappear by **2 weeks** of treatment.
- In chronic cases, the spots will not disappear.

X2: Corneal Xerosis
- Lustreless dry appearance, in the **inferior limbus.**
- Responds within **2-5 days,** disappear within 2 weeks of treatment.

X3A and X3B: Keratomalacia
- **Colliquative Necrosis/Liquefactive Necrosis** → **sterile corneal** melting due to **collagen breakdown without any signs of inflammation*.**

- Round or oval punched out **ulcers** involving the **inferonasal quadrant.**
- Perforation → ***Adherent leucoma, Anterior staphyloma, Phthisis bulbi*.***

XS: Corneal Scarring

- Nebula, macula, leucoma

XF: Xerophthalmic Fundus/Uyemura's Fundus

- Small yellowish white lesions in the peripheral retina.

Treatment:

- Medical emergency especially in malnourished infants.
- **Vitamin A dosage:**
    - 2 lakh I.U. – orally or 1 lakh I.U. – I.M.
    - 3 doses are given = day 1, day 2 and within 1-4 weeks.
    - Children between 6 and 11 months: Half the dose.
    - Chidren < 6 months: Quarter the dose.
- **Ocular lesions:**
    - Lubricants, Broad spectrum antibiotics and cycloplegics.

Ans: (c) Breakdown of collagen fibres in corneal stroma

***Ref:** Kanski Clinical Ophthalmology, 8th Edition, Page 212*

2. A child is diagnosed to have Retinitis pigmentosa. Examination reveals bird shaped head and normal pressure hydrocephalus. What is the most probable diagnosis?

(a) Keane Sayre syndrome
(b) Usher syndrome
(c) Cockayne syndrome
(d) Bassen-Kornzewig syndrome

Explanation:

COCKAYNE SYNDROME (Neill-Dingwall syndrome) • Impaired DNA repair • **Height and Weight below 5th centile*** • **Developmental delay*** • Photosensitivity* and Premature aging • **Sensorineural deafness** • **Retinitis pigmentosa, Cataract** • **Xeroderma pigmentosum** • Dental caries • Premature aging • Bird beak facies • Cardiovascular disease • **Peripheral neuropathy** • **Normal pressure hydrocephalus** • Skeletal dysplasia	**Abetalipoproteinemia, or Bassen-Kornzweig syndrome** • Autosomal recessive inheritance • Mutation in **microsomal triglyceride transfer protein** • Results in deficiencies of apolipoproteins **B-48 and B-100** (used in the synthesis and exportation of **chylomicrons and VLDL**) • Fat malabsorption • Acanthocytosis • **Retinitis pigmentosa** • **Hypocholesterolemia** • Scoliosis • **Developmental delay** • Cognitive impairment
Kearns–Sayre syndrome • Mitochondrial myopathy • **Retinitis pigmentosa – 'Salt and pepper retinopathy'** • Ptosis, **Progressive external Ophthalmoplegia** • AV block • Raised CSF protein • **Cerebellar ataxia**	**Usher syndrome (Hallgren syndrome)** • Autosomal recessive inheritance • **Retinitis pigmentosa** • **Sensorineural nerve deafness** • Cognitive impairment • **Psychosis** • Cataracts

Ans: (c) Cockayne syndrome

***Ref:** Multiple References*

MEDICINE

1. **All are features of Gerstmann syndrome *except*:**

(a) Agraphia
(b) Alexia
(c) Apractagnosia
(d) Finger Agnosia

Explanation:

Gerstmann syndrome:
- **Acalculia** – Impairment of simple arithmetic.
- **Dygraphia** – Impaired writing.
- **Finger anomia** – Inability to name individual fingers such as the thumb and index.
- Alexia.
- Right-left confusion.
- Damage to inferior parietal lobule (especially **angular gyrus**) in the left hemisphere.

Balint's syndrome
- **Spatial disorientation** – Due to bilateral involvement of the network for spatial attention, especially its parietal components.
- **Components:**
  - **Oculomotor apraxia** – deficits in the orderly visuomotor scanning of the environment.
  - **Optic ataxia** – inaccurate manual reaching towards visual targets.
  - **Simultanagnosia** – inability to integrate visual information in the center of gaze with more peripheral information.

Ans: (c) Apractagnosia

***Ref:** Harrison's Principles of Internal Medicine, 19th Edition, Page 179, 2573*

2. **Which of the following is associated with Vitamin B12 deficiency and proteinuria?**

(a) Perinicious anemia
(b) Fanconi anemia
(c) Imerslund Grasbeck syndrome
(d) Tropical sprue

Explanation:

Imerslund Grasbeck Syndrome/Congenital cobalamin malabsorption
- Autosomal Recessive Inheritance.
- Most common cause of **Megaloblastic anemia** due to **cobalamin deficiency** in **Western countries.**
- **Normal Intrinsic factor** and **gastric acid** but are unable to absorb cobalamin.
- 90% of patients have non-specific proteinuria but renal function and renal biopsy are normal.
- **Aminoaciduria** and congenital renal abnormalities, such as **duplication of the renal pelvis** are seen.

Causes of Megaloblastic Anemia
- Cobalamin deficiency or abnormalities of cobalamin metabolism.
- Folate deficiency or abnormalities of folate metabolism.
- Therapy with antifolate drugs (e.g., methotrexate).

Causes of Cobalamin Deficiency Sufficiently Severe to Cause Megaloblastic Anemia
- Nutritional: Vegans.
- Malabsorption: Pernicious anemia.
- **Gastric causes:**
  - Congenital absence of intrinsic factor or functional abnormality.
  - Total or partial gastrectomy.
  - Intestinal causes Intestinal stagnant loop syndrome: Jejunal diverticulosis, ileocolic fistula, anatomic blind loop.
  - Ileal resection and Crohn's disease.
  - Selective malabsorption with proteinuria.
  - Tropical sprue.

- o Transcobalamin II deficiency.
- o Fish tapeworm.

Megaloblastic anemia refractory to cobalamin and folate therapy:

- Some cases of acute myeloid leukemia, myelodysplasia.
- Therapy with drugs interfering with synthesis of DNA (e.g., cytosinearabinoside, hydroxyurea, 6-mercaptopurine, azidothymidine [AZT]).
- **Oroticaciduria** (responds to uridine).
- Thiamine-responsive.

Ans: (c) Imerslund Grasbeck syndrome

Ref: *Harrison's Principles of Internal Medicine, 19th Edition, Page 645*

3. **All are true about Landau-Kleffner syndrome *except*:**

(a) Aphasia
(b) EEG temporal spikes
(c) Present since birth
(d) Behavioural disturbances

Explanation:

LANDAU-KLEFFNER SYNDROME (Acquired epileptic aphasia)

- Characterized by the **abrupt loss of previously acquired language** in young children.
- Most common average age of onset **is 5 to 7 years** and affects **both sexes equally.**
- Language disability is **an acquired cortical auditory deficit (auditory agnosia).**
- Behavioral and neuropsychologic disturbances accompany the progression of LKS.
- EEG is highly **epileptiform** in sleep shows frequent high amplitude spike and sharp waves in the temporal and parietal lobes, the peak area of abnormality in the dominant **perisylvian region** (language areas).
- Diagnosis should be considered for young patients with clear autistic regression, as it is a potentially treatable entity.

EPILEPSY SYNDROMES IN CHILDHOOD

Benign childhood epilepsy with centrotemporal spikes/Benign Rolandic epilepsy

- Most common epilepsy syndrome and usually begins between ages **5 and 10 years.**
- Seizures typically occur only **during sleep or on awakening** usually **focal motor seizures** involving the **face** and **arm.**
- Interictal EEG demonstrates independent **bilateral centro-temporal sharp waves.**
- Seizures usually respond promptly to anticonvulsant therapy.
- Intellectual outcome is normal and the epilepsy resolves after puberty.

Childhood absence epilepsy

- Absence seizures typically begin in the early schoolyears and usually resolve by late childhood or adolescence.
- EEG: **3Hz spike and wave pattern*.**
- **Ethosuximide** is the first-choice therapy.

Juvenile myoclonic epilepsy (of Janz)

- Most common generalized epilepsy among **adolescents and young adults.**
- Onset is typically in **early adolescence** with myoclonic jerks (exacerbated in the morning, often causing the patient to drop objects).
- Seizures resolve promptly with anticonvulsant medication.
- DOC – **Valproic acid.**

Infantile spasms

- Brief contractions of the neck, trunk and arm muscles, followed by a phase of sustained muscle contraction lasting **less than 2 seconds.** Peak age at onset is **3 to 8 months.**
- Spasms occur most frequently when the child is **awakening** from or **going to sleep.**
- Different etiologies have been identified, including:
  - o **Tuberous sclerosis.**
  - o Malformations of cortical development **(lissencephaly).**
  - o Genetic syndromes (trisomy 21).

  - Acquired brain injury (stroke, perinatal hypoxic-ischemic encephalopathy).
  - Metabolic disorders (Phenylketonuria).
- **West syndrome** is the triad of **infantile spasms, developmental regression,** and a dramatically abnormal **EEG pattern (hypsarrhythmia):**
  - **Hypsarrhythmia** consists of chaotic high-voltages low waves, spikes and polyspikes.
- First-line treatment options – **Adrenocorticotropic hormone (ACTH), high-dose oral corticosteroids and vigabatrin.**
- For infants with underlying tuberous sclerosis, **vigabatrin** is the drug of choice*.

Lennox-Gastaut syndrome
- Severe epilepsy syndrome with variable age of onset.
- Most children present **before age 5 years.**
- Frequent, multiple seizure types, including atonic, focal, atypical absence, and generalized tonic, clonic, or tonic-clonic varieties.
- Most patients have significant **intellectual disability.**
- Seizures usually respond poorly to treatment.

Benign neonatal convulsions
- Autosomal dominant genetic disorder linked to abnormal neuronal potassium channels.
- Otherwise well newborns present with focal seizures toward the end of the first week of life, leading to the colloquial term ***fifth day fits*** response to treatment is generally excellent.

Ans: (c) Present since birth

Ref: *Nelsons Essentials of Pediatrics, 7th Edition, Page 621*

4. **Parasite infection causing arthritis includes all *except*:**

(a) Wuchereria bancrofti (b) Trichinella
(c) Dracunculiasis (d) Echinococcus

Explanation:

Protozoal causes of Arthritis

Protozoa	**Musculoskeletal manifestations**
Blastocystis spp	Asymmetric oligoarthritis, Infectious arthritis
Cryptosporidium	Reactive arthritis
Entamoeba histolytica	Reactive arthritis, Infective arthritis, Vasculitis cutaneous, Intestinal
Entamoeba hartmanni	Reactive arthritis
Giardia lamblia	Asymmetrical oligoarthritis, Infectious arthritis Symmetrical polyarthritis, Vasculitis
Isospora belli	Reactive arthritis, Myositis, Vasculitis
Microsporidia	Myositis
Plasmodium spp	Symmetrical polyarthritis, Polymyositis, Vasculitis
Toxoplasma gondii	Arthritis (Still's like), Myositis, Vasculitis
Trypanosoma spp American— *Cruzi* African— *rhododiense, gambiense*	Polymyositis, Vasculitis

Helminthic causes of Arthritis

Helminth	**Musculosketal Manifestations**
Ancylostoma (A duodenale)	Arthritis
Ascaris (A. lumbricoides)	Arthritis, Vasculitis
Dirofilaria (D. immitis, D. tenuis)	Arthritis (reactive), Vasculitis (pulmonary)

Contd.

Contd.

Dracunculus (D. medinensis)	Arthralgia, Myalgia, Arthritis
Echinococcus spp (Hydatid)	Arthralgia, Arthritis, Myalgia, Vasculitis, Bone lesions
Fasciola	Vasculitis
Gnathostoma	Soft tissue mass, Nodular panniculitis
Loa Loa	Arthritis, vasculitis
Onchocerca	Arthritis, Myositis
Paragonimus spp	Myalgia, weakness
Schistosomaspp	Arthralgia, Polyarthritis, Oligoarthritis, Enthesopathy Infectious arthritis, Sacroiliitis, Vasculitis (cerebral)
Strongyloides (S stercoralis)	Arthralgia, Arthritis, Infectious arthritis Reactive arthritis, Sacroiliitis
Taenia saginata	Polyarthritis
Taenia solium (cysticercus)	Bone infection, Myopathy Vasculitis, Localized muscle cysticercosis Generalized muscular pseudohypertrophy
Toxocara (T. canis, T. catis)	Arthalgia/Arthritis, Panniculitis Transient myositis, Eosinophilic arthritis
Trichinella *(Trichinellaspp)*	Myalgia, Myositis, Vasculitis
Trichuris (T. trichuria)	Arthritis
Wuchereria (filiaria)	Arthralgia/Arthritis, Myositis, Vasculitis

Ans: (b) Trichinella

Ref: *Oxford Textbook of Rheumatology, 4th Edition, Page 804*

5. All are features of Allgrove syndrome *except*:

(a) Low aldosterone
(b) Hypoglycemia
(c) Hyperpigmentation
(d) ACTH resistance

Explanation:

Triple A syndrome or Allgrove syndrome

- **Triad** of **adrenal insufficiency** due to **ACTH resistance, Achalasia** and **Alacrima*.**
- Caused by mutations in the ***AAAS* gene,** which encodes **ALADIN,** a **tryptophan/aspartate** WD-repeat–containing protein of the nuclear pore complex.
- Characterized by **isolated glucocorticoid deficiency, hyperpigmentation,** and markedly elevated concentrations of **ACTH.**
- Usually presents during the **first decade of life** with **dysphagia** or severe (occasionally fatal) **hypoglycaemic** or **hypotensive attacks,** related to **adrenocortical insufficiency.**
- Adult patients present with **multisystem neurological disease** with **autonomic disturbances** on presentation.

Causes of Primary Adrenal Insufficiency

Diagnosis	Associated Features
Autoimmune polyglandular syndrome 1(APS1)	Hypoparathyroidism, chronic mucocutaneous candidiasis, other autoimmune disorders, rarely lymphomas
Autoimmune polyglandular syndrome 2(APS2)	Hypothyroidism, hyperthyroidism, premature ovarian failure, vitiligo, type 1 diabetes mellitus, pernicious anemia
Isolated autoimmune adrenalitis	
Congenital adrenalhyperplasia (CAH)	
Triple A syndrome	**Alacrima, achalasia, neurologic impairment**

Contd.

Contd.

Congenital lipoid adrenal hyperplasia (CLAH)	Gonadal failure
Adrenoleukodystrophy (ALD), adreno-myeloneuropathy (AMN)	
Familial glucocorticoid deficiency	Tall stature
Smith-Lemli-Opitz syndrome	Cholesterol synthesis disorder associated with mental retardation, craniofacial malformations, growth failure
Kearns-Sayre syndrome (Mitochondrial disorder)	Progressive external ophthalmoplegia, pigmentary retinal degeneration, cardiac conduction defects, gonadal failure, hypopara-thyroidism, type 1 diabetes
IMAGe syndrome	Intrauterine growth retardation, metaphyseal dysplasia, genital anomalies
Adrenal infections	Tuberculosis, HIV, CMV, Cryptococcosis, Histoplasmosis, coccidioido-mycosis
Adrenal hemorrhage	Meningococcal sepsis (Waterhouse-Friderichsen syndrome), primary antiphospholipid syndrome
Adrenal infiltration	Metastases, lymphomas, sarcoidosis, amyloidosis, hemochromatosis
Drug-induced	Mitotane, aminoglutethimide, abiraterone, trilostane, etomidate, ketoconazole, suramin
Bilateral adrenalectomy	E.g., in the management of Cushing's or after bilateral nephrectomy

Ans: (a) Low Aldosterone

Ref: *Williams Textbook of Endocrinology, 13th Edition, Page 526, 861 and Harrisons Principles of Internal Medicine, 19th Edition, Page 2324*

6. Fulminant hepatitis requiring transplantation of liver is seen with toxicity of which vitamin?

(a) Pyridoxine (b) Riboflavin (c) Thiamine (d) Niacin

Explanation:

Niacin Toxicity

- **Hepatic toxicity** – most serious toxic reaction caused by sustained-release niacin.
- Presents as **jaundice** with **elevated aspartate aminotransferase (AST)** and **alanine aminotransferase** (ALT) levels.
- Doses of **3–9 g/d** causes **fulminant hepatitis** requiring **liver transplantation.**
- Other toxicities are: **flushing, glucose intolerance, hyperuricemia, macular edema and macular cysts.**
- **Flushing** is mediated by prostaglandins and is alleviated with **laropiprant, a selective prostaglandin D2 receptor 1 antagonist,** or **premedication with aspirin.**

Other vitamin toxicities:

Vitamin B6	• Severe sensory neuropathy, photosensitivity and dermatitis
Vitamin C	• **Acute:** >2 g of vitamin C in a single dose causes abdominal pain, diarrhea and nausea • **Chronic:** High-dose vitamin C causes kidney stones
Vitamin A	• **Acute:** Increased intracranial pressure, vertigo, diplopia, bulging fontanels (in children), seizures and exfoliative dermatitis • **Chronic:** Dry skin, cheilosis, glossitis, vomiting, alopecia, bone demineralization and pain, hyper-calcemia, lymph node enlargement, hyperlipidemia, amenorrhea, and pseudotumor cerebri
Vitamin D	• **Hypercalcemia**
Vitamin E	• High doses of vitamin E (>800 mg/d) **reduces platelet aggregation** and interfere with **vitamin K metabolism** and are therefore contraindicated in patients taking **warfarin and antiplatelet agents** (such as aspirin or clopidogrel)

Ans: (d) Niacin

Ref: Harrison's Principles of Internal Medicine, 19th Edition, Chapter 96 e4

7. **A patient is resuscitated and revived following cardiac arrest. Which of the following is a poor prognostic factor in this patient?**

(a) Altered sensorium
(b) Myoclonic seizures
(c) Persistence of dolls eye
(d) No response to painful stimuli

Explanation:

Better neurological outcomes after cardiac arrest:
- Intact brainstem functions.
- Normal pupillary light response.
- Intact oculocephalic and oculovestibular and corneal reflexes.

Poor neurological outcomes after cardiac arrest:
- Absence pupillary reflexes, absent corneal responses.
- Extensor plantar response, no withdrawal to pain.
- Absence motor response to painful stimuli on Day 3.
- Electrophysiologically: Bilateral absence of N20 component of SSEP in the early days.
- Biochemically: Increased serum neuron specific enolase (>33 microg/L).

Ans: (d) No response to painful stimuli

Ref: *Harrison's Principles of Internal Medicine, 19th Edition, Page 1781; Adams and Victor's Principles of Neurology, Edition 10, Chapter 40*

8. **Which organ is spared in familial Mediterranean fever?**

(a) Lung and pancreas
(b) Brain and kidneys
(c) Liver and pancreas
(d) Skin and bone

Explanation:

Hereditary Recurrent Fever Syndromes

	FMF	TRAPS	HIDS	MWS	FCAS	NOMID
Attack length	1-3 days	Often > 7 days	3-7 days	1-2 days	Minutes-3 days	Continuous, with flares
Serosa	Pleurisy, peritonitis; asymptomatic pericardial effusions	Pleurisy, peritonitis pericarditis	Abdominal pain, but seldom peritonitis; pleurisy, pericarditis uncommon	Abdominal pain; pleurisy, pericarditis rare	Rare	Rare
Skin	Erysipeloid erythema	Centrifugally migrating erythema	Diffuse maculopapular rash; oral ulcers	Diffuse urticaria-like rash	Cold-induced urticaria-like rash	Diffuse urticaria-like rash
Joints	Acute monoarthritis; chronic hip arthritis (rare)	Acute monoarthritis, arthralgia	Arthralgia, oligoarthritis	Arthralgia, large joint oligoarthritis	Polyarthralgia	Epiphyseal, patellar overgrowth, clubbing
Muscle	Exercise-induced myalgia common; protracted febrile myalgia rare	Migratory myalga	Uncommon	Myalgia common	Sometimes myalgia	Sometimes myalgia
Eyes, ears	Uncommon	Periorbital edema, conjunctivitis, rarely uveitis	Uncommon	Conjunctivitis, episcleritis, optic disc edema; sensorineural hearing loss	Conjunctivitis	Conjunctivitis, uveitis, optic disc edema, blindness, sensorineural hearing loss
CNS	Aseptic meningitis rare	Headache	Headache	Headache	Headache	Aseptic meningitis, seizures

Contd.

Contd.

Amyloidosis	Most common in M694V homozygotes	~15% of cases, most often cysteine mutations, T50M	Uncommon	~25% of cases	Uncommon	Late complication
Treatment	Oral colchicine prophylaxis, IL-1 inhibitors for refractory case	Glucocorticoids etanercept, IL-1 inhibitors	NSAIDs for fever; IL-1 and TNF inhibitors	Anakinra rilonacept, canakinumab	Anakinra, rilonacept, canakinumab	Anakinra

Ans: (c) Liver and pancreas

***Ref:** Harrison's Principles of Internal Medicine, 19th Edition, Page 2213*

9. Which pollutant released by combustion of fossil fuels causes exacerbation of asthma?

(a) Triethyl lead
(b) Carbon monoxide
(c) Sulphur dioxide
(d) Nitrous oxide

Explanation:

- **Sulphur dioxide** is produced by burning of **fossil fuels, refrigerator, food processing, wood pulp industry** and **bleaching.**
- Air pollution due to increased ambient levels of **sulphur dioxide, ozone and nitrogen oxide** triggers **asthma.**

Asthma triggers:

- **Allergens:** Most common cause Dermatophagoides species.
- **Virus Infection:** Rhinovirus, Respiratory syncytial virus, Corona virus.
- **Pharmacological agents:** All Beta blockers, Aspirin, ACE inhibitors.
- **Exercise.**
- **Physical factors:** Cold and hyperventilation.
- **Food and diet:** Metabisulphite a food preservative, Tartarizine a food colouring agent can trigger asthma.
- **Hormonal:** Premenstrual phase, Hyperthyroidism and Hypothyroidism.
- **GERD.**
- **Stress.**

Ans: (c) Sulphur dioxide

***Ref:** Harrison's Principles of Internal Medicine, 19th Edition, Page 1671*

10. Pickering syndrome:

(a) Flash pulmonary edema of MVP
(b) Flash pulmonary edema of renal artery stenosis
(c) Obesity paradox
(d) Metabolic syndrome

Explanation:

- Flash pulmonary edema is characterized by sudden and recurrent episodes of dyspnea at rest resulting from acute pulmonary venous congestion **in the presence of normal or well-preserved LV systolic function.**
- Described by Pickering *et al.* in 1988 seen with **either bilateral renal artery stenosis or in case of single functional kidney with ipsilateral renal artery stenosis.**
- Most episodes of flash pulmonary edema occur at night.
- Renin angiotensin aldosterone system (RAS) has been implicated in the genesis of flash pulmonary edema with renal artery stenosis.

Renal Artery Stenosis:

- **Most common cause in elderly – Atherosclerosis.**
- **Most common cause in young females – Fibromuscular dysplasia.**

- Common cause in Afro Asian population and Japan in Age <40 years – Takayasu arteritis or Non specific aortoarteritis.
- **Investigations:**
  - Doppler ultrasound – identifies hemodynamically significant lesions (>60% stenosis).
  - Captopril enhanced renography has a strong predictive value when entirely normal.
  - **Renal Angiography – gold standard for diagnosis.**
  - Fibromuscular dysplasis characteristic beads on appearance on angiography.

When to suspect Renal artery stenosis?

- Onset of hypertension before 30 years or after 50 years of age.
- Abrupt onset of hypertension/Severe or resistant hypertension.
- Symptoms of atherosclerotic disease elsewhere.
- Negative family history of hypertension.
- Smoker.
- Worsening renal function after renin-angiotensin inhibition.
- Recurrent "flash" pulmonary edema.
- Abdominal bruit.
- Unilateral small (atrophic)/asymmetric kidney size by ultrasound examination.

Ans: (a) Flash pulmonary edema of renal artery stenosis

Ref: *Harrison's Principles of Internal Medicine, 19th Edition, Page 1627*

11. Lewy body dementia is due to accumulation of:

(a) NF tangles
(b) Amyloid
(c) Alpha synuclein
(d) Tau protein

Explanation:

Protein aggregate in Dementias

Tau protein	**Alpha synuclein protein**	**Amyloid beta protein**
• Picks disease • Progressive supranuclear palsy • Cortico basal degeneration • Familial frontotemporal dementia and parkinsonism	• Sporadic parkinson's disease (Lewy bodies) • Diffuse Lewy body disease (Lewy bodies) • Multiple System Atrophy o Shy Drager syndrome o Striato-nigral degeneration o Olivopontocerebellar atrophy	• Sporadic Alzheimer's disease • Cerebral amyloid angiopathy

Ans: (c) Alpha synuclein

Ref: *Harrison's Principles of Internal Medicine, 19th Edition, Page 2606*

12. Patient with Crohn's disease was given steroids but still clinical features persisted. Next step in management is:

(a) Azathioprine
(b) Sulfasalazine
(c) Cyclosporine
(d) Infliximab

Explanation:

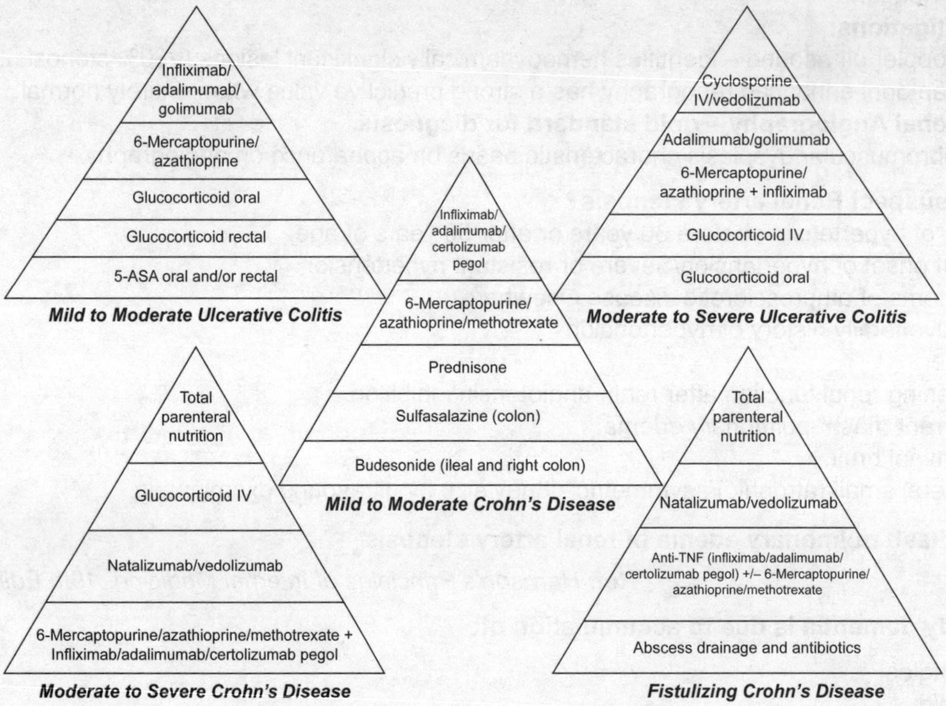

Ans: (a) Azathioprine

Ref: *Harrison's Principles of Internal Medicine, 19th Edition, Page 1963*

13. Elderly lady presents with asymmetric bradykinesia, cogwheel rigidity and dystonia. Probable diagnosis:

(a) Corticobasal degeneration
(b) Progressive supranuclear palsy
(c) Lewy body dementia
(d) Multisystem atrophy

Explanation:

Atypical Parkinsonism

- Group of neurodegenerative condition associated with widespread neurodegeneration than is found in Parkinsons disease.
- Present with rigidity, bradykinesia similar to parkinsonism but characterised by:
  - Early speech and gait impairment.
  - Absence of resting tremor.
  - No motor asymmetry.
  - Poor or no response to levodopa.
  - Aggressive clinical course.

Multisystem Atrophy:

- Combination of **parkinsonism, cerebellar and autonomic features.**
- **Types:** MSA – P and MSA – C.
- Suspected when patient with parkinsonism presents with cerebellar signs and early and prominent autonomic dysfunction usually orthostatic hypotension.
- MRI shows:
  - MSA – P High signal change in the region of external surface of putamen.
  - MSA – C **Hot cross buns sign** due to cerebellar and brainstem atrophies.

Progressive supranuclear palsy

- Early gait disturbances.
- Slow ocular saccades.
- Eyelid apraxia.

- Restricted eye movement with impairment of downward gaze.
- MRI reveals **Humming bird sign** – Atrophy of midbrain with relative preservation of pons.

Corticobasal degeneration:

- Asymmetric onset of rigidity and dystonia.
- **Alien limb phenomenon:** Limb assumes a position in space without the patient being aware of it.
- MRI reveals Atrophy in perirolandic cortex and basal ganglia.

Ans: (a) Corticobasal degeneration

***Ref:** Harrison's Principles of Internal Medicine, 19th Edition, Page 2605, 2609*

14. Brain natriuretic peptide is decreased in:

(a) Pregnancy
(b) Obesity
(c) Restrictive Cardiomyopathy
(d) Postpartum cardiomyopathy

Explanation:

- Natriuretic peptides are useful biomarkers for HF **diagnosis and estimation of HF severity and prognosis and for management.**
- Released from **cardiomyocytes** in response to **stretch.**
- Most commonly measured natriuretic peptides are B-type (i.e., brain) natriuretic peptide (BNP) and its amino-terminal cleavage pro-peptide equivalent, N-terminal pro-B type natriuretic peptide (NT-probnp).

Increased in:

- Valvular heart disease.
- Pulmonary hypertension.
- Ischemic heart disease.
- Atrial arrhythmias.
- Constrictive pericarditis.
- Right ventricular dysfunction.
- Age.
- Renal failure.
- Hyperdynamic state like sepsis.

Reduced in:

- Obesity.

Biomarkers Used in Assessing Patients with Heart Failure (HF)

Inflammation	Oxidative Stress	Myocyte Injury	Myocyte Stress	New Biomarkers
• C-reactive protein • Tumor necrosis factor • Fas (APO-1) • Interleukins 1, 6,18	• Oxidized low-density lipoproteins • Myeloperoxidase • Urinary biopyrrins • Urinary and plasma isoprostanes • Plasma malondialdehyde	• Cardiac-specific troponins I and T • Myosin light-chain kinase I • Heart-type fatty acid protein • Creatine kinase MB	• B-type natriuretic peptide/N-terminal pro-B-type natriuretic peptide • Mid regional proadrenomedullin • ST2	• Chromogranin • Galectin 3 • Osteoprotegerin • Adiponectin • Growth differentiation factor-15

Ans: (b) Obesity

***Ref:** Braunwald's Heart Disease: A Textbook of Cardiovascular Medicine, 10th Edition, Page 478*

15. Organism causing myocarditis with erythema chronicum migrans:

(a) Trichinella
(b) Strongyloides
(c) Borrelia
(d) Ancyclostoma

Explanation:

LYME DISEASE

- Caused by Borreliaburgdoferi. Transmitted by Ixodid ticks.
- **Early Infection Stage 1 (localized):** Erythema chronicummigrans.

- **Early Infection Stage 2 (localized):** Severe headache, mild stiffness of the neck, fever, chills, migratory musculoskeletal pain, arthralgias, and profound malaise and fatigue, meningitis.
- **Meningo-polyneuritis or *Bannwarth's syndrome*:** Characterized by radicular pain, followed by the development of CSF pleocytosis.
- Cardiac Involvement: Fluctuating degree of atrioventricular block (first-degree, Wenckebach, or complete heart block) acute myopericarditis, left ventricular dysfunction.
- **Late Infection Stage 3 (Persistent Infection):** Intermittent attacks of oligoarthritis in large joints (knees), Chronic neurological manifestations like encephalopathy and polyneuropathy.
- **Acrodermatitis chronic atrophicans,** the late skin manifestation of Lyme borreliosis.

Remember:

- **Cutaneous larva migrans** – Ancylostoma braziliense, Ancylostoma caninum.
- **Ground itch** – Ancylostoma duodenale, Necator americanus.
- **Larva currens** – Strongyloides stercoralis.

Ans: (c) Borrelia

Ref: *Harrison's Principles of Internal Medicine, 19th Edition, Page 1151*

16. Interpret the following ABG - pH 7.22, HCO_3 19, pCO_2 62:

(a) Mixed respiratory and metabolic alkalosis
(b) Respiratory acidosis with metabolic compensation
(c) Metabolic acidosis with renal compensation
(d) Mixed respiratory and metabolic acidosis

Explanation:

Pretty straight forward question:

- pH – 7.22 (Acidosis).
- HCO_3 – 19 ↓.
- pCO_2 – 62 ↑.
- Since the arrows are moving in the opposite direction (which is not possible unless a mixed disorder is present) – The answer is Mixed disorder.
- HCO_3 levels are s/o acidosis and pCO_2 levels are suggestive if acidosis as well. Hence the answer is Mixed metabolic and respiratory acidosis.

Ans: (d) Mixed respiratory and metabolic acidosis

Ref: *Harrison's 19th Edition*

17. A young female with bilateral ptosis and weakness of proximal muscles. Which is the most sensitive test to diagnose myasthenia gravis?

(a) Single nerve fibre electromyography test
(b) EMG
(c) Tensilon test
(d) Antibodies against N_m receptor

Explanation:

- **SF-EMG** is the most sensitive investigation for the diagnosis of Myasthenia gravis (with a reported sensitivity of > 95%). What we are planning to look at it is the characteristic "JITTER" that would indicate slowed NM junction transmission. It is not specific though as it can be present in many other diseases.
- Most specific investigation would be Ach R Ab's. Ach R Ab's would be present in approximately 70% of patients with MG and it is not quite sensitive like SFEMG.

Ans: (a) Single nerve fibre electromyography test

Ref: *Harrison's 19th Edition*

18. Complication of DC cardioversion are all *except*:

(a) Ventricular fibrillation
(b) Bradycardia
(c) Myocardial necrosis
(d) Myocardial septal perforation

Explanation:

- DC Cardioversion is extremely safe and effective.
- Complication rates are very low.
- Some complications that can happen include:
  - o **ST segment and T wave changes:** Usually transient.
  - o **Arrhythmias and conduction abnormalities** (Both tachy and brady can occur).
  - o **Myocardial necrosis:** Usually limited to epicardium and NOT associated with elevated troponins. Perforation of Septum or any other structure after cardioversion has not been reported.
  - o **Cutaneous burns.**
  - o **Thromboembolism** – especially after cardioversion of AF.

Ans: (d) Myocardial septal perforation

Ref: *Harrison's 19th Edition*

19. In Wernicke's encephalopathy, the earliest clinical feature to recover is:

(a) Ataxia
(b) Ophthalmoparesis
(c) Confusion
(d) Memory loss

Explanation:

Ophthalmoplegia is the first feature to recover in Wernicke's Encephalopathy.

Wernicke's Encephalopathy – "COAT".

- **Confusion.**
- **Ophthalmoplegia.**
- **Ataxia.**
- **Thiamine** is the treatment.
- Most common cause is **Alcohol** (Secondary to vitamin B1 deficiency) Thiamine treatment results in rapid resolution of ophthalmoplegia in these patients (within hours). Ataxia recovers a bit late followed by confusion/cognitive function which are last to recover.
- More importantly Thiamine treatment may uncover **Korsakoff psychosis.**

Ans: (b) Ophthalmoparesis

Ref: *Harrison's 19th Edition*

20. Paraneoplastic syndrome characterized by antibodies to amphiphysin is:

(a) Cerebellar Degeneration
(b) Stiff Person syndrome
(c) Optic Neuritis
(d) Retinopathy

Explanation:

- Anti Amiphysin Antibodies are characteristically associated with Stiff Person Syndrome.

Important Paraneoplastic Syndromes of CNS and associated Antibodies

Antibody	Associated Cancer	Associated PNS
Anti Hu	SCLC	Encephalitis, Neuropathy, Cerebellar Degeneration, Opsoclonus
Anti Ri	Lung/Breast	Cerebellar Degeneration, Opsoclonus
Anti amiphysin	Lung/Breast	Stiff Person Syndrome
Anti Yo	Breast/Ovary	Cerebellar Degeneration
Anti Tr	Hodgkin	Cerebellar Degeneration
Anti recoverin	SCLC	Retinopathy
Anti VGCC (Presynaptic)	SCLC	Lambert Eaton Myasthenic Syndrome

Ans: (b) Stiff Person syndrome

Ref: *Harrison's 19th Edition*

21. Lambert Eaton myasthenia syndrome clinical picture – Antibodies are directed against:

(a) Pre synaptic anti-voltage gated calcium channel
(b) Post synaptic voltage gated calcium channels
(c) Sodium channel
(d) Potassium Channel

Explanation:

Straightforward question:

- **LEMS** is associated with antibodies against **Presynaptic Voltage Gated Calcium channels.**

Refer to the table of the previous question.

Ans: (a) Pre synaptic anti-voltage gated calcium channel

Ref: *Harrison's 19th Edition*

22. Patient presents with history of recurrent falls. Examination revealed vertical gaze palsy. Most probable diagnosis:

(a) Idiopathic parkinson disease
(b) Multiple system atrophy
(c) Progressive supranuclear palsy
(d) Shy Drager syndrome

Explanation:

Straightforward question again.

History of falls + Vertical gaze palsy in an elderly patient suggests **Steel Richardson syndrome (Progressive Supranuclear Palsy).**

Progressive Supranuclear Palsy

- Elderly.
- Early postural instability – Presents as frequent falls.
- Vertical gaze palsy – Down > Up.
- Apraxia of Eye opening.
- Square wave jerks.
- Surprised look.
- Disease carries a poor prognosis and response to L-Dopa is poor.
- Idiopathic Parkinson's disease does not present with early postural instability and also does not have Vertical gaze palsy.
- Also Shy Drager syndrome would have predominant autonomic features which is a distinguishing feature which this patient does not possess.

Ans: (c) Progressive supranuclear palsy

Ref: *Harrison's 19th Edition*

23. 24 years old female presents with ascending motor weakness with bilateral facial palsy. Which nerve is spared in this condition?

(a) Hypoglossal nerve
(b) Trigeminal nerve
(c) Vestibulocochlear nerve
(d) Oculomotor nerve

Explanation:

Guillain-Barr□ Syndrome: Diagnostic Criteria

I. Required for Diagnosis
1. Progressive weakness of variable degree from mild paresis to complete paralysis.
2. Generalized hypo or areflexia.
II. Supportive of Diagnosis
1. Clinical Features:
a. Symptom progression: Motor weakness rapidly progresses initially but ceases by 4 weeks. Nadir attained by 2 weeks in 50%, 3 weeks 80% and 90% by 4 weeks.
b. Demonstration of relative limb symmetry regarding paresis.

Contd.

Contd.

c. Mild to moderate sensory signs. d. Frequent cranial nerve involvement: **Facial (cranial nerve VII) 50% and typically bilateral but asymmetric; occasional involvement of cranial nerves XII, X and occasionally III, IV and VI as well as XI.** e. Recovery typically begins 2–4 weeks following plateau phase. f. Autonomic dysfunction can include tachycardia, other arrhythmias, postural hypotension, hypertension, other vasomotor symptoms. g. A preceding gastrointestinal illness (e.g., diarrhea) or upper respiratory tract infection is common. **2. Cerebrospinal Fluid Features Supporting Diagnosis** a. Elevated or serial elevation of CSF protein. b. CSF cell counts are <10 mononuclear cell/mm³. **3. Electrodiagnostic Medicine Findings Supportive of Diagnosis** a. 80% of patients have evidence of NCV slowing/conduction block at some time during disease process. b. Patchy reduction in NCV attaining values less than 60% of normal. c. Distal motor latency increase may reach 3 times normal values. d. F-waves indicate proximal NCV slowing. e. About 15–20% of patients have normal NCV findings. f. No abnormalities on nerve conduction studies may be seen for several weeks.
III. Findings Reducing Possibility of Diagnosis 1. Asymmetric weakness. 2. Failure of bowel/bladder symptoms to resolve. 3. Severe bowel/bladder dysfunction at initiation of disease. 4. Greater than 50 mononuclear cells/mm³ in CSF. 5. Well-demarcated sensory level.
IV. Exclusionary Criteria 1. Diagnosis of other causes of acute neuromuscular weakness (e.g., myasthenia gravis, botulism, poliomyelitis, toxic neuropathy). 2. Abnormal CSF cytology suggesting carcinomatous invasion of the nerve roots.

Ans: (b) Trigeminal nerve

***Ref:** Harrison's Principles of Internal Medicine, 18th Edition, Page 3476*

24. Which drug is not used in Lennox-Gastaut syndrome?

(a) Rufinamide (b) Clonazepam (c) Clobazam (d) Lamotrigine

Explanation:

Drug	Principal uses
Carbamazepine	Tonic-clonic Focal-onset
Clobazam	**Lennox-Gastaut syndrome**
Clonazepam	Absence Atypical Absence Myoclonic
Ethosuximide	Absence
Ezogabine	Focal-onset
Felbamate	Focal-onset **Lennox-Gastaut syndrome** Tonic-clonic
Gabapentin	Focal-onset
Lacosamide	Focal-onset
Lamotrigine	Focal-onset Tonic-clonic

Contd.

Contd.

	Atypical absence Myoclonic **Lennox-Gastaut syndrome**
Levetiracetam	Focal-onset
Oxcarbazepine *C*	Focal-onset Tonic-clonic

Drug	**Principal uses**
Phenobarbital	Tonic-clonic Focal-onset
Phenytoin	Tonic-clonic Focal-onset
Primidone	Tonic-clonic Focal-onset
Rufinamide	**Lennox-Gastaut syndrome**
Tiagabine	Focal-onset
Topiramate	Focal-onset Tonic-clonic **Lennox-Gastaut syndrome**
Valproic acid	Tonic-clonic Absence Atypical absence Myoclonic Focal-onset Atonic
Zonisamide	Focal-onset Tonic-clonic

Ans: (b) Clonazepam

***Ref:** Harrison's Principles of Internal Medicine, 19th Edition, Page 2553*

25. Patient with tumorlysis syndrome has hypocalcemia, hyperuricemia, hyperphosphatemia. What should not be done?

(a) Hemodialysis
(b) Rapid alkalinization of urine
(c) Allopurinol prophylaxis
(d) Aggressive hydration

Explanation:

Tumor Lysis Syndrome:

- Characterized by **hyperuricemia, hyperkalemia, hyperphosphatemia and hypocalcemia.**
- Caused by the destruction of a large number of rapidly proliferating neoplastic cells.
- Associated with the treatment of **Burkitt's lymphoma, acute lymphoblastic leukemia, and other rapidly proliferating lymphomas, chronic leukemias and, rarely, with solid tumors.**
- **Hyperuricemia** – treatment kills malignant cells – increased serumuric acid levels from the turnover of nucleic acids precipitates in the tubules, medulla and collecting ducts of the kidney-renal failure.
- **Hyperphosphatemia** – by the release of intracellular phosphate pools by tumor lysis-produces a reciprocal depression in serum calcium – Hypocalcemia/Deposition of calcium phosphate in the kidney and hyperphosphatemia-renal failure.
- **Hyperkalemia** – Due to massive destruction of malignant cells may lead to ventricular arrhythmias and sudden death.
- Standard preventive approach:
  - **Allopurinol.**
  - **Urinary alkalinization.**

- o **Aggressive hydration.**
- **Urinary alkalization** with sodium bicarbonate is controversial. It **increases uric acid solubility,** but **decreases calcium phosphate solubility.** If it is used, it should be discontinued when **hyperphosphatemia** develops.

Ans: (b) Rapid alkalinization of urine

***Ref:** Harrison's Principles of Internal Medicine, 19th Edition, Page 1795*

Prevention and Treatment of Tumor Lysis Syndrome

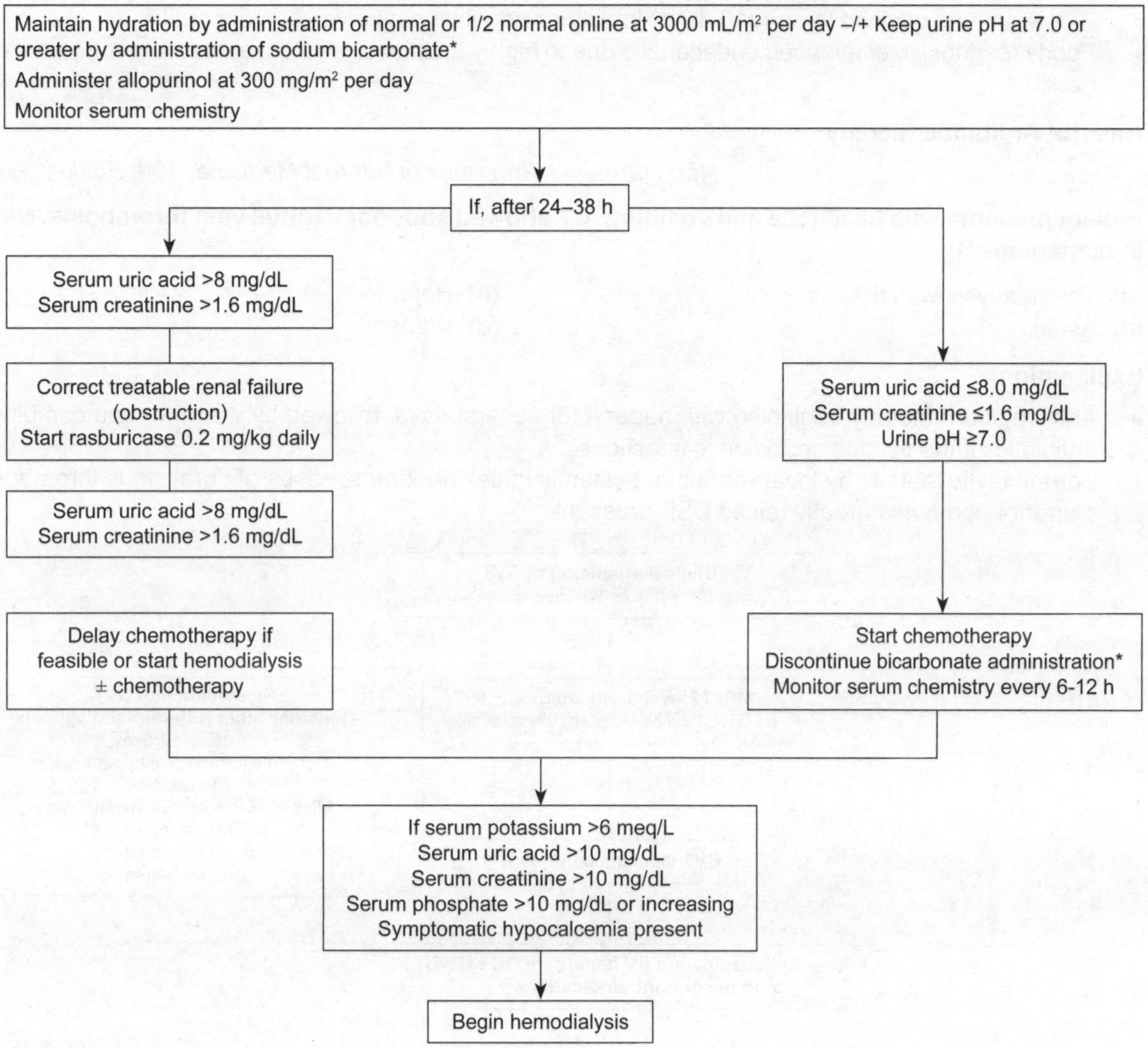

Management of patients at high risk for the tumor lysis sydrome.

26. A pregnant lady is diagnosed to have a heart valve vegetation of 8 mm. Ideal management in this scenario is:

(a) Antibiotic therapy followed by sugery
(b) Antibiotic therapy
(c) Surgery
(d) Surgery followed by Antibiotic therapy

Explanation:

Indications for Cardiac Surgical Intervention in Patients with Endocarditis

Surgery Required for Optimal Outcome

- Moderate to severe congestive heart failure due to valve dysfunction.
- Partially dehisced unstable prosthetic valve.
- Persistent bacteremia despite optimal antimicrobial therapy.

- Lack of effective microbicidal therapy (e.g., fungal or *Brucella* endocarditis).
- *S. aureus* prosthetic valve endocarditis with an intracardiac complication.
- Relapse of prosthetic valve endocarditis after optimal antimicrobial therapy.

Surgery to Be Strongly Considered for Improved Outcome

- Perivalvular extension of infection.
- Poorly responsive *S. aureus* endocarditis involving the aortic or mitral valve.
- **Large (>10 mm in diameter)** hypermobile vegetations with increased risk of embolism, particularly with prior embolic event or with significant valve dysfunction.
- Persistent unexplained fever (≥10 days) in culture-negative native valve endocarditis.
- Poorly responsive or relapsed endocarditis due to highly antibiotic-resistant enterococci or gram-negative bacilli.

Ans: (b) Antibiotic therapy

Ref: *Harrison's Principles of Internal Medicine, 19th Edition, Page 824*

27. **Patient presents with headache and vomiting. CT showed superior sagittal vein thrombosis. Next step in management:**

(a) Thrombolysis with tPA (b) Heparin
(c) Aspirin (d) Warfarin

Explanation:

- Anticoagulant therapy beginning with heparin for several days, followed by warfarin, and combined with antibiotics if the venous occlusion is infectious.
- Thrombolytic therapy by local venous or systemic infusion-extreme cases of dural sinus thrombosis with stupor or coma and greatly raised CSF pressure.

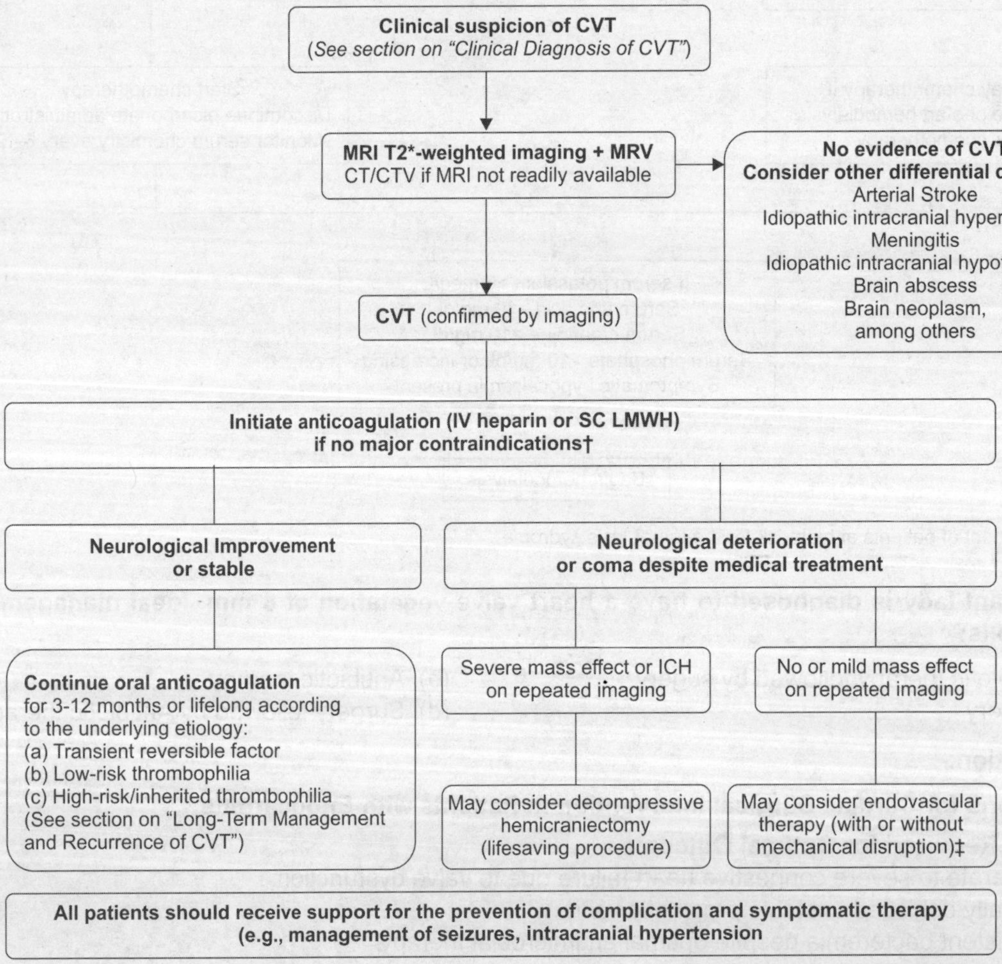

Ans: (b) Heparin

Ref: *Harrison's Principles of Internal Medicine, 19th Edition, Page 2572*

28. Which of the following is true regarding tremors?

(a) Diazepam is helpful in reducing dystonic tremors
(b) Beta blockers effective in Parkinsonian tremor
(c) Valproate induced tremors are cured after withdrawal
(d) Essential tremor is resting tremor

Explanation:

- Tremor consists of alternating contractions of agonist and antagonist muscles in an oscillating, rhythmic manner.
- It can be:
  - **Rest tremor – Parkinsonism.**
  - **Postural tremor – Essential tremor.**
  - **Kinetic tremor – Cerebellar tremor.**
- **Enhanced physiologic tremor (EPT)** in association with anxiety, fatigue, a metabolic disturbance (e.g., hyperthyroidism, electrolyte abnormalities), drugs (e.g., valproate, lithium), or toxins (e.g., alcohol).
- Treatment – Control of any underlying disorder.

Treatment of Essential Tremor:

- Beta blockers (Propanolol) and Primidone – standard drug therapies for ET.
- Gabapentin and topiramate in selected cases.
- Botulinum toxin injections helpful for limb or voice tremor.
- Surgical therapies targeting the VIM nucleus of the thalamus for severe and drug-resistant cases.

Ans: (c) Valproate induced tremors are cured after withdrawal

Ref: *Harrison's Principles of Internal Medicine, 19th Edition, Page 2618*

29. Which drug is not helpful in AML with FLT3 mutation?

(a) Sorafenib (b) Sunitinib (c) Tipifarnib (d) Tandutinib

Ans: (c) Tipifarnib

Ref: *Wintrobe's Clinical Hematology, 13th Edition, Page 3645*

Explanation:

- **FLT3 signaling is an adverse prognostic factor in AML.**

Newer agents in the treatment of Acute Myeloid Leukemia

AC 220	Flt 3 kinase inhibitor
Sorafenib	Flt 3 kinase inhibitor, RET tyrosine kinase inhibitor EGF receptor kinase inhibitor, PDF receptor Kinase inhibitor, angiogenesis inhibitor
Sunitinib	Flt 3 kinase inhibitor, RET tyrosine kinase inhibitor EGF receptor kinase inhibitor, PDF receptor Kinase inhibitor, C kit inhibitor
Tandutinib	Flt 3 kinase inhibitor, RET tyrosine kinase inhibitor, PDF receptor Kinase inhibitor, C kit inhibitor
Midostaurin	Flt 3 kinase inhibitor, Protein kinase C inhibitor, cell cycle inhibitor
Lestaurtinib	Flt 3 kinase inhibitor
Belinostat	Histone deacetylase inhibitor
Entinostat	Histone deacetylase inhibitor
Vorinostat	Histone deacetylase inhibitor

Contd.

Contd.

Mocetinostat	Histone deacetylase inhibitor
Everolimus	mTOR inhibitor, angiogenesis inhibitor
Temsirolimus	mTOR kinase inhibitor
Sirolimus	mTOR inhibitor, angiogenesis inhibitor
Flavopiridol	Cyclin dependent kinase inhibitor
Lenalidomide	TNF alpha antagonist, Immunomodulator
Lintuzumab	Monoclonal antibody CD33
Bortezomib	Proteasome inhibitor
Sapacitabine	Antimetabolite, DNA synthesis inhibitor
Obatoclaxmesylate	Mcl 1 antagonist, Bcl 2 antagonist
Decitabine	DNA methyl transferase inhibitor
Azacitidine	DNA methyl transferase inhibitor
AZD 1152	Aurora kinase inhibitor
Tipifarnib	Farnesyl transferase inhibitor
Voreloxin	DNA topoisomerase ii inhibitor

30. Desert rheumatism is:

(a) Paracoccidiomycosis
(b) Coccidioidomycosis
(c) Blastomycosis
(d) Histoplasmosis

Explanation:

Coccidioidomycosis (Valley fever, Desert rheumatism)

- Acquired by inhalation of arthrospores (arthroconidia).
- Triad of **fever, *erythema nodosum,* and arthralgias** (especially of the knees and ankles) termed "desert rheumatism".
- Pulmonary nodules – Single, frequently in the upper lobes.
- Pulmonary cavities.
- Peripheral blood eosinophilia.
- Hilar/mediastinal adenopathy in chest radiography.

Ans: (b) Coccidioidomycosis

Ref: *Harrison's Principles of Internal Medicine, 19th Edition, Page 1335*

31. 75-year-old man presenting with easy fatiguability and weakness for past 6 months. No H/O fever/ weight loss. Investigations revealed dimorphic anemia with pancytopenia and a cellular bone marrow. What is the diagnosis?

(a) Tuberculosis
(b) CLL
(c) Aplastic anemia
(d) MDS

Explanation:

Differential Diagnosis of Pancytopenia

Pancytopenia with Hypocellular Bone Marrow
Acquired aplastic anemia
Constitutional aplastic anemia (Fanconi anemia, dyskeratosis congenita)
Some myelodysplasia
Rare aleukemic leukemia
Some acute lymphoid leukemia
Some lymphomas of bone marrow

Contd.

Contd.

Pancytopenia with Cellular Bone Marrow	
Primary bone marrow diseases	**Secondary to systemic diseases**
Myelodysplasia	Systemic lupus erythematosus
Myelofibrosis	Overwhelming infection
Myelophthisis	Alcohol
Paroxysmal nocturnal Hemoglobinuria	Hypersplenism
Bone marrow lymphoma	B12, folate deficiency
Some aleukemic leukemia	Brucellosis
Hairy cell leukemia	Sarcoidosis
	Tuberculosis
	Leishmaniasis
Hypocellular Bone Marrow +/- Cytopenia	
Q fever	
Legionnaires' disease	
Anorexia nervosa, starvation	
Mycobacterium	

Ans: (d) MDS

Ref: Harrison's Principles of Internal Medicine, 19th Edition, Page 663

32. A chronic alcoholic and hypertensive presents with high grade fever, chest pain and cough with expectoration. CXR is shown. Probable diagnosis:

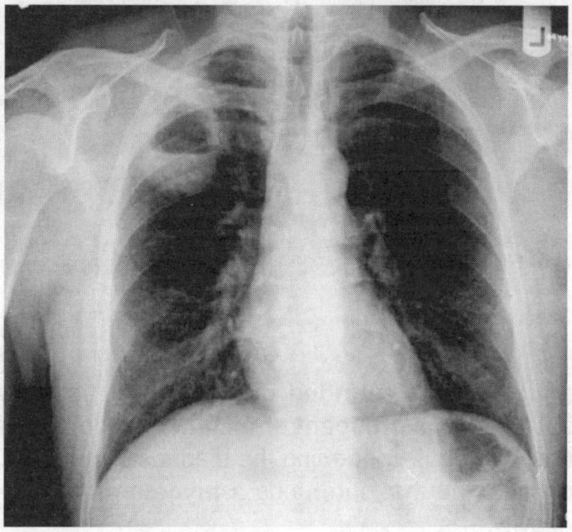

(a) Lung hamartoma (b) Abscess lung (c) Consolidation (d) Bronchiectasis

Explanation

- The clinical picture is clearly suggestive of a **Lung abscess.**
- CXR showing a **thick walled cavity** with clear cut **air fluid level** with characteristic location in the **Right side** which is suggestive of **aspiration.** The diagnosis of lung abscess is also supported by the history – History of **alcoholism** (Patients lie down for longer durations diminishes pharyngeal/laryngeal reflexes making them prone for aspiration of oral contents into the lung) and the history of fever with productive cough +/- changing with posture.
- The classical appearance of a pulmonary abscess is a cavity containing an air-fluid level. In general abscesses are round in shape, and appear similar in both frontal and lateral projections.
- CT is the most sensitive and specific imaging modality to diagnose a lung abscess.
- As aspiration is the most common cause of pulmonary abscesses, the superior segment of the right lower lobe is the most common site.

- For those with lung abscess the primary treatment is **IV clindamycin 600 mg tds.**
- Other options include – **Beta lactam + Beta lactamase inhibitor or Moxifloxacin.**
- Surgical/percutaneous interventions are indicated if **medical therapy fails.**
- Note that metronidazole alone is NOT effective in treating lung abscess.
- Malignancy can present as lung abscess/thick walled cavity due to bronchial obstruction.
- Air fluid levels should NOT be used to differentiate malignant and non-malignant etiologies.
- Further this patient has no risk factors for lung cancer in the history (Age > 45 with History of smoking, loss of weight, Hemoptysis).

Answer: (b) Abscess lung

Ref: *Harrison's 19th Edition*

33. A diabetic presents with chronic cough for more than 2 months. Examine the X-ray carefully. What is the most probable diagnosis?

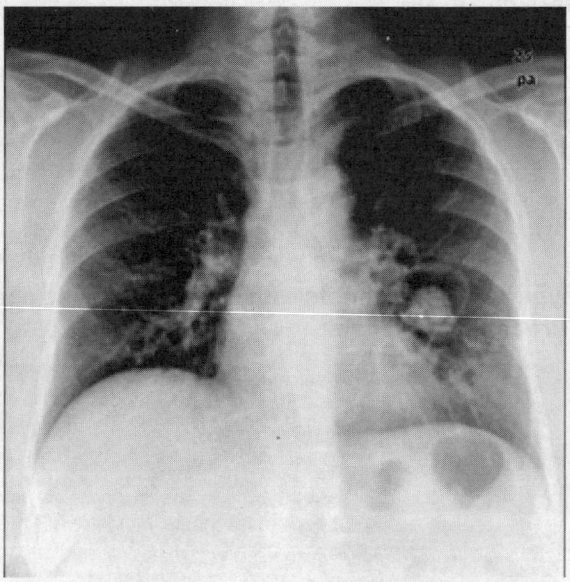

(a) Bronchiectasis (b) Fungal ball (c) Lung abscess (d) Lobar consolidation

Explanation:

The above X-ray shows cystic lesion with:

- **Aspergillomas,** typically appear as **rounded or ovoid soft tissue** attenuating masses located in a surrounding cavity and outlined by a **crescent of air.** Altering the position of the patient usually demonstrates that the **mass is mobile,** thus confirming the diagnosis.
- **Monod sign** simply describes air that surrounds a **mycetoma** (most commonly an aspergilloma) in a pre-existing pulmonary cavity.
- **Pulmonary aspergillosis** is a collective term used to refer to a number of conditions caused by infection with a fungus of the **Aspergillus species (usually Aspergillus fumigatus).**
- There are a number of recognised pulmonary forms–Each form has specific clinical and radiological features.
- **Aspergilloma** (saprophytic/noninvasive aspergillosis): The most common form seen radiographically shows **monod sign.**
- **Allergic bronchopulmonary aspergillosis (ABPA)** shows characteristic **finger in glove opacities*** and **central bronchiectasis*.**
- **Invasive Aspergillosis**-presents with **ground glass attenuation** surrounding the lesion called as **Halo sign.**

Bronchiectasis: CT Chest–HRCT Chest imaging modality of choice

- Airway dilation (detected as parallel **"tram tracks"** or as the **"signet-ring sign"**—a cross-sectional area of the airway with a diameter at least 1.5 times that of the adjacent vessel).

- Lack of bronchial tapering.
- Bronchial wall thickening in dilated airways.
- Inspissated secretions (e.g., the **"tree-in-bud" pattern**).
- **Bilateral predominantly upper lobe bronchiectasis** – CF and allergic bronchopulmonary aspergillosis.
- **Unilateral upper lobe predominance** – tuberculosis.
- **Lower lobe predominance** – childhood viral infections.

Ans: (b) Fungal ball

***Ref:** Harrison's Principles of Internal Medicine, 19th Edition, Page 1695*

34. A patient presented with cough for 2 days and shortness of breath. CXR is given. What is the diagnosis?

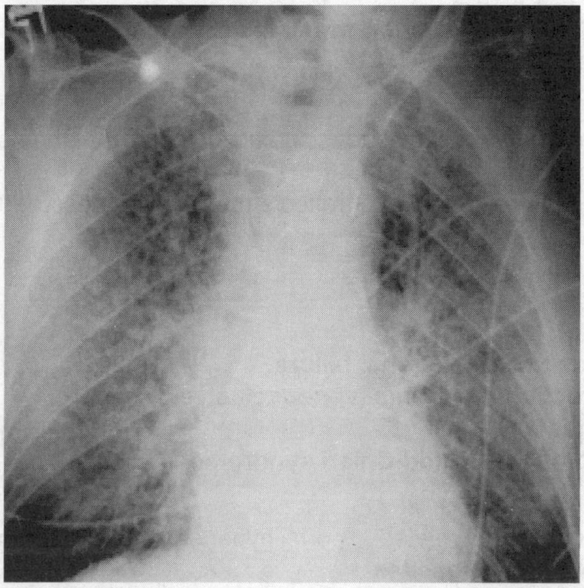

(a) Pulmonary edema (b) Bronchiectasis
(c) COPD (d) ARDS

Explanation:

Features of pulmonary oedema on a plain chest radiograph:

- Bilateral perihilar confluent opacities in a **bat wing distribution.**
- Upper lobe pulmonary venous diversion/pulmonary venous engorgement/**stag's antler sign.**
- Increased cardiothoracic ratio/cardiac silhouette size: Due to an underlying cardiogenic cause.
- Features of **pulmonary interstitial oedema:**
  - o Peri-bronchial cuffing and perihilar haze.
  - o Septal lines/Kerley lines.
  - o Thickening of interlobar fissures.
  - o May have air bronchograms.
- Pleural effusions and fluid in interlobar fissures (including **'vanishing' pulmonary pseudotumour**).
- There is a progression of signs on a plain radiograph that occurs as the pulmonary capillary wedge pressure (PCWP) increases.

Correlation between the pulmonary vascular pattern and pulmonary capillary wedge pressure (PCWP)

CXR Findings	PCWP
Normal	< 8 mm Hg
Cephalization	10-12 mm Hg
Kerley B lines (thickening of interlobular septa)	12-18 mm Hg
Pulmonary Interstitial edema	18-20 mm Hg
Pulmonary Alveolar edema (batwing appearance)	>20 mm Hg

Ans: (a) Pulmonary edema

Ref: *Braunwald's Heart Disease: A Textbook of Cardiovascular Medicine, 10th Edition, Page 266*

35. High SAAG *(serum-ascites albumin gradient)* ascites is seen in all *except*:

(a) Cirrhosis of liver
(b) Congestive heart failure
(c) Chronic renal failure
(d) Nephrotic syndrome

Explanation:

- The **SAAG** is useful for distinguishing **ascites** caused by **portal hypertension** from **non-portal hypertensive ascites.**
- The SAAG reflects the **pressure within the hepatic sinusoids** and correlates with the **hepatic venous pressure gradient.**
- The SAAG is calculated by **subtracting the ascitic albumin** from the **serum albumin** and does **not change with diuresis.**

SAAG ≥ 1.1 g/dL

- This reflects the presence of portal hypertension and indicates that the ascites is from an increased pressure in the hepatic sinusoids.
- According to Starling's law, a high SAAG reflects the oncotic pressure that counterbalances the portal pressure.
- Possible causes include:
  - **Cirrhosis.**
  - **Cardiac ascites.**
  - **Fluid overload** due to **chronic renal failure.**
  - **Sinusoidal obstruction syndrome** (**venoocclusive** disease).
  - Massive **liver metastasis**.
  - **Hepatic vein thrombosis (Budd-Chiari syndrome).**

SAAG <1.1 g/dL

- It indicates that the ascites is not related to portal hypertension as in **tuberculous peritonitis, peritoneal carcinomatosis,** or **pancreatic ascites.**
- In nephrotic syndrome, due to reduced oncotic pressure (serum albumin), SAAG is < 1.1 g/dL.

Ans: (d) Nephrotic syndrome

Ref: *Harrison's 19th Edition*

36. A 22-year-old female presented with fever, cough for 6 months, chest X-ray shows mediastinal widening and blood tests revealed increased ACE levels. That is the most probable diagnosis:

(a) Sarcoidosis
(b) Tuberculosis
(c) Churg Strauss syndrome
(d) Lymphoma

Explanation:

- Raised ACE levels points towards Sarcoidosis. The given history is also compatible with pulmonary tuberculosis, but serum ACE levels will be normal.

SARCOIDOSIS

- It is a multisystem granulomatous disease and lesions may occur anywhere in the body.
- The clinical manifestations depend on the extent and degree of granulomatous inflammation and are extremely variable.
- **Children** may present with **non-specific symptoms,** such as **fever, weight loss,** and general **malaise.**
- In adults and older children, **pulmonary involvement** is most frequent, with **infiltration** of the **thoracic lymph nodes** and **lung parenchyma.**
- **Isolated bilateral hilar adenopathy** on chest radiograph is the most common finding, but **parenchymal infiltrates** and **miliary nodules** may also be seen.
- Patients with lung involvement are commonly found to have **restrictive changes** on pulmonary function testing.
- **Extrathoracic lymphadenopathy** and **infiltration** of the **liver, spleen** and **bone marrow** leading on to isolated **hepatomegaly** and **splenomegaly.**

- **Cutaneous disease,** such as **plaques, nodules, erythema nodosum** in acute disease, or lupus **pernio** in chronic sarcoidosis.
- **Red-brown to purple maculopapular lesions** <1 cm on the **face, neck, upper back,** and **extremities** are the most common skin finding.
- **Ocular involvement** is frequent, **anterior** or **posterior uveitis, conjunctival granulomas, eyelid inflammation,** and **orbital** or **lacrimal gland infiltration.**
- The **arthritis** in sarcoidosis can be confused with JRA.
- **Central nervous system (CNS) involvement** is rare in childhood but may manifest as seizures, **cranial nerve involvement, intracranial mass lesions,** and **hypothalamic dysfunction.**
- **Kidney disease** also occurs infrequently in children but typically manifests as renal insufficiency, proteinuria, transient pyuria, or microscopic hematuria as a result of either early monocellular infiltration or granuloma formation in kidney tissue.
- Only a small fraction of children have **hypercalcemia or hypercalciuria,** which is therefore an infrequent cause of kidney disease.
- **Sarcoid granulomas** can also infiltrate the **heart** and lead to **cardiac arrhythmias** and **sudden death.**
- In contrast to the variable clinical presentation of sarcoidosis in older children, early-onset sarcoidosis classically manifests as the triad uveitis, arthritis and rash.
- Pulmonary disease and lymphadenopathy are less common.
- The **arthritis** is **polyarticular** and **symmetric,** with large **boggy effusions.**
- The **rash** is **diffuse, erythematous, papular.**
- **Noncaseating granulomas** are demonstrated with biopsy of the skin or joint synovium.

Laboratory Findings

- There is no single laboratory test diagnostic of sarcoidosis.
- **Anemia, leukopenia** and **eosinophilia** may be seen.
- **Hypergammaglobulinemia** and elevations in **acute-phase reactants (ESR and CRP).**
- **Hypercalcemia** and/or **hypercalciuria.**
- **Angiotensin-converting enzyme (ACE)** is produced by the epithelioid cells of the granuloma, and its serum value may be **elevated,** but this finding **lacks diagnostic sensitivity and specificity.**
- Fluorodeoxyglucose F18 positron emission tomography **(18FDG PET)** can help identify **nonpulmonary sites** for a diagnostic biopsy.
- A **positive gallium scan** can support the diagnosis if increased activity is noted in the **parotids** and **lacrimal** glands **(panda sign)** or in the right **paratracheal and left hilar area (lambda sign).**

Ans: (a) Sarcoidosis

Ref: *Harrison's Principles of Internal Medicine, 19th Edition*

37. All except are features plummer vinson syndrome:

(a) Hypertrophy of oral mucosa
(b) Dysphagia
(c) Glossitis
(d) Iron deficiency anemia

Explanation:

Plummer–Vinson syndrome (PVS)

- Also called **Paterson–Brown–Kelly syndrome** or **sideropenic dysphagia.**
- **It is Premalignant.**
- Presents as a triad of:
  - Dysphagia.
  - Esophageal webs.
  - Iron deficiency anemia.
- It most usually occurs in postmenopausal women.

Clinical features:

- Burning sensation with the tongue and oral mucosa.
- **Atrophy of lingual papillae** produces a smooth, shiny, red dorsum of the tongue.
- Dysphagia.
- Pain.
- Weakness.

- Odynophagia.
- **Atrophic glossitis.**
- Angular stomatitis.
- The condition is associated with **koilonychia, glossitis, cheilitis** and **splenomegaly.**
- Hemogram – **Microcytic hypochromic** anemia suggestive of iron deficiency.
- Increased risk of **squamous cell carcinoma of Esophagus.**

Ans: (a) Hypertrophy of oral mucosa

Ref: *Harrison's Principles of Internal Medicine, 19th Edition*

SURGERY

1. **A 25-year-old male presented with painless testicular swelling and with history of fever and weight loss. All the following investigations are indicated in this patient *except*:**

(a) USG scrotum
(b) CT abdomen and pelvis
(c) Chest X-ray
(d) Transscrotal biopsy

Explanation:

- Painless testicular swelling in a 25-year-male with history of fever and weight loss amounts to a diagnosis of **Malignant Testicular swelling, i.e., Testicular cancer.**
- The diagnosis of testicular cancer includes **history and physical examination** of the both testes, **abdomen examination** to rule out para aortic nodes.
- The radiological imaging in the form of **ultrasonogram** will have a better accuracy in identifying the tumor in both the testes.
- To confirm the histopathological evidence of testicular cancer, **Orchidectomy** in form of **High inguinal Orchidectomy** to be done after a Maneuver known as CHEVASU Maneuver**
- **Trans scrotal biopsy** is **contraindicated***, as Tunica albuginea will be breached during biopsy. Since Tunica albuginea is a natural barrier to testicular cancer, following biopsy, this will be breached and extend into the **scrotum.**
- Before orchidectomy, **Serum tumor markers** specific for testicular cancers like **AFP, LDH and Beta HCG** to be quantified.
- If tumor markers are elevated, **metastatic work up to be done,** to rule out lung metastases and liver metastases and nodal metastases.
- Chest X-ray PA view can pick up **cannon ball metastases,** if in doubt CT scan of the abdomen and pelvis and Thorax to be done.

Ans: (d) Transscrotal biopsy

Ref: *Bailey and Love, 26th Edition, Page 1385-1388*

2. **Carcinoma breast is diagnosed in second trimester of pregnancy. Which should not be done?**

(a) Breast conservation surgery/BCS
(b) Chemotherapy
(c) Modified radical mastectomy
(d) 3D focal radiotherapy to local area

Explanation:

- Pregnant women with breast cancer often present at a later stage of disease because breast tissue changes that occur in the hormone-rich environment of pregnancy obscure early cancers. However, they have a prognosis, stage by stage, that is similar to that of nonpregnant women with breast cancer.
- Ultrasonography and needle biopsy specimens are used in the diagnosis of these nodules. Mammography is rarely indicated because of its decreased sensitivity during pregnancy and lactation; however, the fetus can be shielded if mammography is needed.
- Breast surgery can be safely performed in all trimesters of pregnancy; however, patients and surgeons may choose to wait until after the 12th week of gestation when the risk of spontaneous abortion may be lower. A modified radical mastectomy can be performed during the first and second trimesters of pregnancy.
- During the third trimester, lumpectomy with axillary node dissection can be considered if adjuvant radiation therapy is deferred until after delivery. Lactation is suppressed.
- Chemotherapy administered during the first trimester carries a risk of spontaneous abortion and a 12% risk of birth defects. There is no evidence of teratogenicity resulting from administration of chemotherapeutic agents in the second and third trimesters.
- For this reason, many clinicians now consider the optimal strategy to be delivery of chemotherapy in the second and third trimesters as a neoadjuvant approach, which allows local therapy decisions to be made after the delivery of the baby.

- If the patient meets criteria for post mastectomy radiation therapy or they have had breast-conserving surgery, radiation therapy should be administered and this is recommended only after delivery of the fetus. Radiation exposure during pregnancy may result in fetal death, malformations, growth and/or mental impairment, and induction of cancers or hereditary defects.

Ans: (d) 3D focal radiotherapy to local area

Ref: *Diseases of The Breast, 5th Edition, Page 850-860; Schwartz Principles of Surgery, 10th Edition, Page 554*

3. A 55-year-old male patient with gastritis symptoms diagnosed to have gastric ulcer for which he had undergone partial gastrectomy three years back and currently on high dose omeprazole. Follow up endoscopy reveals two ulcerative lesions in gastric mucosa. What is the next step in management?

(a) H pylori serology
(b) Insulin tolerance
(c) Gastrin level
(d) CT scan

Explanation:

- The clinical scenario makes us think that the patient **underwent partial gastrectomy** for an **intractable gastric ulcer** 3 years ago and during follow up he was found to have **two gastric mucosal lesions** despite high dose omeprazole.
- High dose omeprazole is generally given in patients with **Gastrinoma or Zollinger-Ellison syndrome** to **control acid secretion.**
- **Gastrinoma** is a condition, which is associated with **acid hypersecretion** secondary to the increased **production of gastrin.**
- **Diagnosis of gastrinoma** should be considered in cases of:
  - Intractable peptic ulcers.
  - Multiple ulcers.
  - Ulcers at uncommon sites.
  - Recurrent ulcers.
- Hence, patient with recurrent ulcer following surgery, should be evaluated with **Serum gastrin** to rule out **ZES.**
- Patients with **serum gastrin >1000 pg/ml** is diagnosed to have **ZES.**

Ans: (c) Gastrin level

Ref: *Sabiston Textbook of Surgery, 20th Edition, Page 1210-11; Schwartz Principles of Surgery, 10th Edition, Page 1071-73*

4. A patient presents with upper abdominal pain and vomiting. His pulse is 110/min and BP is 70/40 mm of Hg. A diagnosis of pancreatitis is made. What is the next appropriate management?

(a) Immediate IV fluids
(b) Removal of necrosed pancreatic tissues
(c) Start enteral nutrition first
(d) IV antibiotics

Explanation:

- Regardless of the cause or the severity of the disease, the cornerstone of the treatment of AP is **aggressive fluid resuscitation** with **isotonic crystalloid solution.**
- The rate of administration should be individualized and adjusted on the basis of age, comorbidities, vital signs, mental status, skin turgor and urine output.
- In addition to fluid resuscitation, patients with AP require **continuous pulse oximetry** because one of the most common systemic complications of AP is **hypoxemia** caused by the **acute lung injury** associated with this disease.
- Patients should receive **supplementary oxygen** to maintain arterial saturation **above 95%.**
- It is also essential to provide effective **analgesia. Narcotics** are usually preferred, especially **morphine.**
- There is no proven benefit in treating AP with antiproteases (e.g., gabexatemesilate, aprotinin), platelet-activating factor inhibitors (e.g., lexipafant), or pancreatic secretion inhibitors.
- Nutritional support is vital in the treatment of AP. Oral feeding may be impossible because of **persistent ileus, pain, or intubation.**

- The main options to provide this nutritional support are **enteral feeding** and **total parenteral nutrition (TPN).** Although there is no difference in the mortality rate between both types of nutrition, enteral nutrition is associated with fewer infectious complications and reduces the need for pancreatic surgery.
- Although TPN provides most nutritional requirements, it is associated with mucosal atrophy, decreased intestinal blood flow, increased risk of bacterial overgrowth in the small bowel, antegrade colonization with colonic bacteria, and increased bacterial translocation.
- Recent meta-analyses and systematic reviews that have evaluated multiple randomized controlled trials have proved that **prophylactic antibiotics do not decrease** the **frequency of surgical intervention, infected necrosis, or mortality in patients with severe pancreatitis.**

Ans: (a) Immediate IV fluids

Ref: *Sabiston Textbook of Surgery, 20th Edition, Page 1525-1530*

5. **A 3 days old neonate presents with respiratory distress, vomiting and cyanosis after every feeding. Examination reveals froth from nose. Most likely diagnosis:**

(a) Tracheoesophageal fistula with esophageal atresia
(b) Cleft palate causing recurrent aspiration
(c) Bilateral choanal atresia
(d) Cleft palate

Explanation:

- **Esophageal atresia and TEF** can occur alone or in combination.
- The incidence of this anomaly **is 1 in 1500 to 3000 live births,** with a slight **male predominance.**
- In 10% of patients, there is a non-random, non-hereditary association of anomalies referred to by the acronym **VATER (vertebral, anorectal, tracheal, esophageal, renal or radial limb);** an alternative acronym is **VACTERL** (vertebral, anorectal, cardiac, tracheal, esophageal, renal and limb).
- Five anatomic variants of esophageal atresia are there. In the **most common type (C lesion) of proximal esophageal atresia with distal TEF, the proximal blind pouch ends approximately the distance of one or two vertebral bodies from the distal TEF.** The distal TEF is typically located approximately 1 cm above the carina in the membranous portion of the trachea.
- The anatomic variant of infants with EA-TEF predicts the clinical presentation. When the esophagus ends either as a blind pouch or as a fistula into the trachea (as in types A, B, C or D), infants present with excessive drooling, followed by chocking or coughing immediately after feeding is initiated as a result of aspiration through the fistula tract.
- As the neonate coughs and cries, air is transmitted through the fistula into the stomach, resulting in abdominal distention. As the abdomen distends, it becomes increasingly more difficult for the infant to breathe. This leads to further atelectasis and respiratory compromise.
- In patients with type C and D varieties, the regurgitated gastric juice passes through the fistula where it collects in the trachea and lungs and leads to a chemical pneumonitis, which further exacerbates the pulmonary difficulties.
- The diagnosis of EA is confirmed by the **inability to pass an orogastric tube into the stomach.** The dilated upper pouch may be occasionally seen on a plain chest radiograph. If a soft feeding tube is used, the **tube will coil in the upper pouch,** which provides further diagnostic certainty.

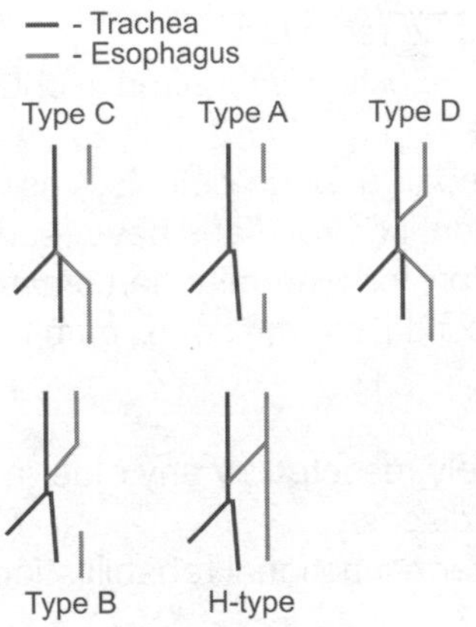

Ans: (a) Tracheoesophageal fistula with esophageal atresia

Ref: Schwartz Principles of Surgery, 10th Edition

6. **A patient is on total parental nutrition for more than a month via Central Venous Catheter. All are done *except*:**

(a) Change Central Venous Catheter tube every two weeks routinely
(b) LFT, BUN must be done weekly once
(c) Electrolytes must be checked every 2-3 days once
(d) Sudden glucose intolerance is an early sign of sepsis

Explanation:

Patients on long term TPN via central venous catheter:

- Central venous catheter must be managed very carefully with **full sterile precautions.**
- Inspect daily the catheter site for **infection.**
- Early sign of catheter related sepsis is **Sudden Glucose intolerance.**
- Suspected catheter sepsis – **Remove the catheter** and send for **Culture and sensitivity.**
- Catheter is changed only in suspected infections – Not changed routinely.
- Increased risk of catheter related infections is seen in **Multi lumen catheter.**
- Risk is highest with **Femoral Vein** catheter > **IJV** > **Subclavian** vein catheter.
- Monitor **LFT** and **RFT** every **week once.**
- Monitor **Electrolytes** level every **2-3 days.**
- **Elevation of Liver enzymes** is associated with **Steatosis** due to **Overfeeding.**

Ans: (a) Change Central Venous Catheter tube every two weeks routinely

Ref: Schwartz, 10th Edition, Page 56

7. **A patient is diagnosed with Liposarcoma of 8×6×4 cm involving the posterior part of thigh. Treatment of choice in this patient is:**

(a) Above thigh amputation
(b) Extra compartmental excision
(c) Chemotherapy
(d) Wide local excision

Explanation:

- Among soft tissue sarcoma, the most common site is **Extremity sarcoma***, among **extremities,** the most common site being **Thigh*.**
- The most common histological variant of STS is **Liposarcoma*** (previously MFH, i.e., Malignant fibrous Histiocytoma which has been reclassified as High grade undifferentiated pleomorphic sarcoma).
- Nowadays, the treatment goal is to do **function sparing resection** of the tumors and not amputation.

Principles of Surgery:

1. **Wide Local Excision** is to remove the tumor with approximately **1 to 2 cm of surrounding normal soft tissue** outside the **Pseudocapsule** (Zone of compressed reactive tissue that surrounds the soft tissue sarcoma).
2. Tumor adjacent to or displacing major neurovascular structures, these need not be resected, but the adventitia or perineurium should be removed.
3. In cases of Bony invasion, Bone resection is required to obtain an adequate surgical margin and to achieve adequate local control.
4. For locally advanced tumors, repair of bone defects, vascular reconstruction, tendon transfers and soft tissue reconstruction using regional or free flaps have resulted in good functional outcomes.
5. All patients undergoing resection for extremity sarcomas should undergo physical therapy beginning immediately after surgery and continuing until maximum function is achieved.

Amputation: (In 5% of tumors)

1. Tumors that cannot be completely resected by any other means.
2. Without evidence of metastatic disease.
3. Have propensity for good long term functional rehabilitation.

Ans: (d) Wide local excision

Ref: *Sabiston Textbook of Surgery, 20th Edition, Page 762-764*

8. **Saw tooth appearance in abdominal barium enema X-ray:**

(a) Multiple polyposis
(b) Prediverticulosis
(c) Ischemic colitis
(d) Ulcerative colitis

Explanation:

- **Diverticula** are **abnormal outpouchings** or sacs of the colon wall that occur most commonly because of:
  - o **Interactions of high intraluminal pressures.**
  - o **Disordered motility.**
  - o **Alterations in colonic structure.**
  - o **Diets low** in fiber.
- Diverticula are formed on the **mesenteric side** of the **antimesenteric taeniae coli** in areas of relative weakness in the bowel where small arterioles (vasa recta) penetrate the muscular layers as they traverse the colon wall.
- This results in the **protrusion of the mucosa** and **submucosa** through the layers of muscle, termed a **pseudodiverticulum** or **false diverticulum.**
- The sigmoid and descending colon are the most commonly affected areas and in this disease process are characterized by hypertrophy of the muscular layers and associated decreased luminal diameter.
- The resulting disordered motility in these segments and increase in luminal pressure facilitate the herniation of diverticula through the muscular coat.
- The diagnosis of diverticulitis can often be made by eliciting these findings on a thorough history and physical examination.
- Barium enema studies were primarily used before the advent of computed tomography (CT) scans and have largely been abandoned as a primary tool as they provide information only about the luminal surface of the colon and cannot be performed if perforation is suspected.
- The findings include:
  - o ***Saw-tooth*** **appearance** to the colon, usually **sigmoid,** with **shortening of bowel, crowding of haustra** and **picket-fencing of folds** is seen in **prediverticular disease.**

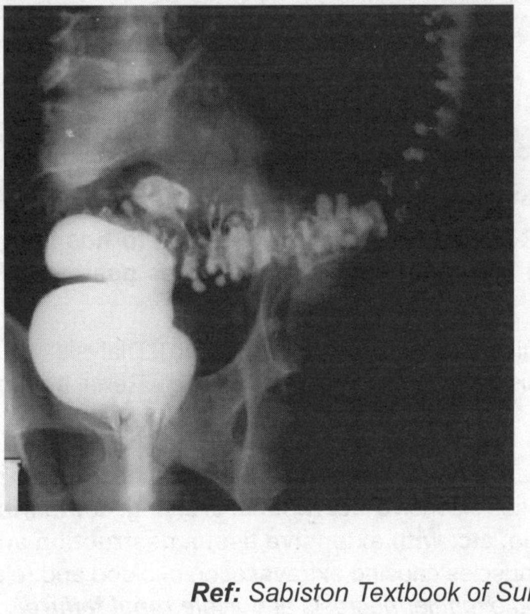

Ans: (b) Prediverticulosis

Ref: *Sabiston Textbook of Surgery, 20th Edition, Page 1330-32*

9. **A coin foreign body is stuck in esophagus at 25 cm from incisors. This located is approximately situated at which of the following levels?**

(a) Left mainstem bronchus
(b) Arch of aorta
(c) Cricopharyngeal constriction
(d) Gastroesophageal junction

Explanation:

It is rather a straightforward clinically oriented anatomy question.

- The esophageal silhouette resembles an **hourglass.**
- There are **three distinct areas of narrowing** that contribute to its shape:
  - Measuring **14 mm** in diameter, the **cricopharyngeus** muscle is the **narrowest point** of the gastrointestinal tract and marks the superior most portion of the hourglass-shaped esophagus.
  - Located just below the carina, where the left mainstem bronchus and aorta abut the esophagus, the **bronchoaortic constriction** at the level of the **fourth thoracic vertebra** creates the center narrowing and measures **15 to 17 mm.**
  - Finally, the **diaphragmatic constriction,** measuring **16 to 19 mm,** marks the inferior portion of the **hourglass** and is located where the esophagus passes through the diaphragm.
- Between these three distinct areas of anatomic constriction are two areas of dilation known as the superior and inferior dilations. Within these areas, the esophagus resumes the normal diameter for an adult and measures approximately 2.5 cm

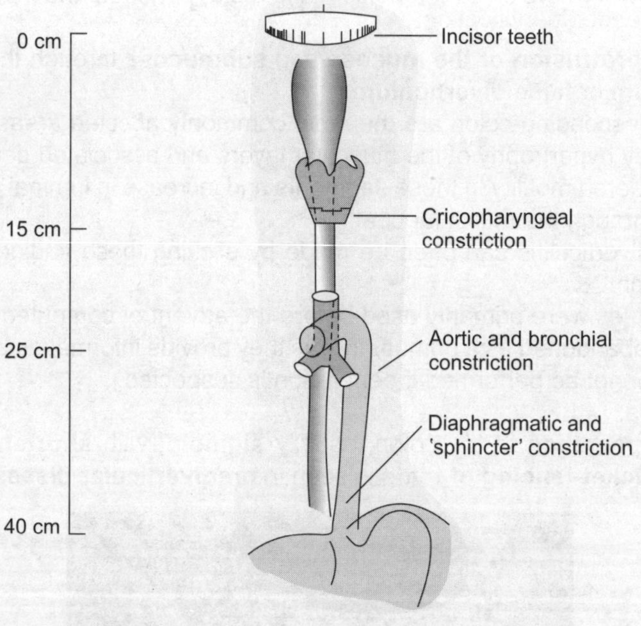

Ans: (a) Left mainstem bronchus

Ref: *Sabiston Textbook of Surgery, 19th Edition, Page 1015-1016; Bailey and Love, 26th Edition, Page 987*

10. A 20-year-old male with RTA and crush injury presents to hospital. On day 1 of admission, he has reduced urine output and his urine myoglobin becomes positive. What should not be done for this patient?

(a) Crystalloids should be given
(b) Dialysis
(c) Mannitol alkaline diuresis
(d) Renal transplant

Explanation:

- **Crush injury** is one where a part of the body is being **squeezed/compressed** between two high force or pressure systems. It causes extensive **lacerations, bruising, compartment syndrome, crush syndrome, fractures, haemorrhage, etc. with extensive tissue destruction and devitalisation.**
- It is due to crushing of muscles causing extravasation of blood and release of **myohaemoglobin** into the circulation leading to *acute tubular necrosis* and *acute* ***renal failure.***
- Initially **tension increases** in the **muscle compartment** commonly in the limb, which itself impedes the circulation and increases the *ischaemic damage.*
- Patient will be associated with **Renal failure, Toxaemia, Septicaemia, Disability** with extensive tissue loss and **Gas gangrene.**

- Treatment includes **Fasciotomy** to relieve compartment pressure.
- **Low molecular weight dextran, or mannitol** is given to improve the urine output by improving the renal function.
- **Alkalisation of urine** is done by giving **sodium citrate** or **sodium bicarbonate.** It increases the **solubility of acid haematin** in the urine and so promotes its **excretion.**
- **Haemodialysis** is done sometimes as a life-saving procedure.
- Other measures include **Catheterization, Oxygen therapy, Antibiotics, Blood transfusion and Correction of severe hyperkalaemia.**

Ans: (d) Renal transplant

Ref: *Bailey and Love, 26th Edition, Page 26-28*

11. A 48 years male patient, victim of RTA presents to emergency room. Primary survey of this trauma patient includes all the following *except*:

(a) Measuring BP
(b) Exposing body to rule out injuries
(c) CT abdomen for bleeder identification
(d) Checking airway

Explanation:

Primary Survey

- Airway with cervical spine protection.
- Breathing and ventilation.
- Circulation and hemorrhage control.
- Disability: Neurologic status.
- Exposure/Environment control: Completely undress the patient; control hypothermia.

ABCDE's	Assessment	Management
Airway with C spine	Verbal response Suctioning and inspection of foreign bodies, facial, mandibular/laryngeal fractures Assessment of GCS Gentle care in holding the neck	Jaw Thrust Chin Lift Maneuver C spine Collar GCS < 8, airway equipment needed like Oropharyngeal airway
Breathing and ventilation	JVP, Tracheal position and Chest wall excursion Inspection, Palpation and Auscultation of the chest	Tension, open pneumothorax, massive hemothorax and flail chest with pulmonary contusion require immediate intervention
Circulation with hemorrhage control	Skin colour and temperature Pulse, blood pressure Heart sounds Look for any active external bleed Level of consciousness	Massive Hemothorax, Cardiac tamponade, Major internal bleed like abdominal and pelvic bleed should be managed Minimum of 2 large IV catheters needed
Disability	Neurological evaluation by GCS Alcoholics, Narcotics or any drugs	
Exposure	Completely undressed Get rid of toxins in dress (e.g., OPC poisoning)	Covered by warm blankets or external warming device, warm IV fluids

Resuscitation:

- Proper airway maintenance with airway equipments.
- Ventilation assistance given if needed.
- Circulation control established with control of bleeds, tourniquet application and insertion of two large bore IV cannulas with 1 to 2 L bolus of isotonic warm solutions to achieve response.
- Control of hypothermia with warm blankets, warm fluids and warming devices.

Adjuncts to Primary Survey:

- ECG, Pulse Oximetry, ABGs.

- Urinary and Gastric catheters.
- Chest and Pelvic X-rays.
- FAST and DPL.

Secondary Survey:

- This does not begin until the primary survey is completed, resuscitative efforts are underway and normalization of vital functions has been demonstrated.
- Complete head to toe evaluation, with complete history and reexamination of vital signs and detailed examination of each part of the body.

History:

- From the prehospital personnel, mode of injury, mechanism of impact, blunt or penetrating, any associated thermal injuries and detailed mechanism of injury recorded.
- AMPLE history – Allergies, Medications currently used, Past illness/Pregnant, Last meal intake, Events/ Environment related to injury.

Physical Examination:

- **HEAD** – Look for scalp (lacerations/avulsions), Eyes, Pupils, visual acuity, any penetrating injury or globe ruptures etc.
- **MAXILLOFACIAL** – Palpate all the facial bones, intra oral examination and assessment of any facial fractures.
- **CERVICAL SPINE AND NECK** – Inspect, palpate spine for tenderness, tracheal position, laryngeal apparatus palpation for any crepitus and carotids for bruits. Penetrating injuries should not be explored in the ER itself.
- **CHEST and ABDOMEN** examination as usual.
- **VAGINA, PERINEUM and RECTUM** examination are necessary if suspect pelvic injuries, and done prior to urinary catheterization.
- **MUSCULOSKELETAL SYSTEM** – Palpation of all the bones and muscles and spine to elicit tenderness, abnormal mobility and movement restriction.
- **NEUROLOGICAL SYSTEM** – Start again with GCS, Sensory and motor system examination.

Adjuncts to Secondary Survey:

- Complete CT screening of spine.
- CT abdomen and pelvis.
- CT chest.
- CT brain.
- All these may be needed for further evaluation of injuries, which helps in the definitive care.

Ans: (c) CT Abdomen for bleeder identification

Ref: *Schwartz Principles of Surgery, 10th Edition, Page 161-165; Bailey and Love, 26th Edition, Page 303-305*

12. **Scalloping of edge of sigmoid colon seen in:**

(a) Diverticulitis (b) Crohn's disease
(c) Ulcerative colitis (d) Sigmoid volvulus

Explanation:

Double-contrast barium enema (DCBE) is the radiological examination of choice to show disease extent and severity.

- **Crypt abscesses:** May erode through the muscularis mucosae and spread laterally within the submucosa:
  - ***En face appearance*:** Linear, transverse, serpiginous or rounded.
  - ***Tangential appearance*:** Undercutting of the mucosal edge can give a 'T' or 'collar stud' shape.
- **Ruptured crypt abscesses** lead to superficial erosions which fill with barium to produce a typical granular mucosal pattern (producing continuous ulceration on a background of diffusely abnormal mucosa – discrete ulceration with normal intervening mucosa is not seen).
- **Reflux ileitis:** There is a patulous ileocaecal valve and a granular distal ileum.
- **Postinflammatory polyps:** When an acute attack remits, the granulation tissue forming at the ulcer base undermines the residual oedematous mucosal flap at the ulcer edge – this is therefore prevented from sealing down, resulting in sessile, filiform, frond-like polyps (less commonly found in Crohn's disease).

- **Chronic colitis:** A tubular, shortened, featureless ('lead-pipe') colon.
- **Strictures:** Chronic hypertrophy of the muscularis mucosa (and submucosal thickening with fat) can cause generalized colonic shortening as well as localized left-sided colonic strictures (10–20%):
  - The strictures are smooth, tapering and symmetrical (cf. asymmetrical strictures in Crohn's disease).

US

- Wall thickening (– 4 mm)
  - A stratified appearance with differentiation between the submucosa and muscularis propria.
  - Ulceration (with focal disruption of the bowel wall layers which may be outlined by intracolonic gas).
  - Inflammatory echogenic pericolic fat.

CT

- ***Acute disease:*** Wall thickening (– 4 mm) tending to be less marked than with Crohn's disease:
  - **Absence of formed faecal residue** within any affected segments.
  - **Normal pericolonic tissues** (unless perforation has occurred).
- *Chronic disease:* A widened presacral space due to fibrofatty proliferation.
- ***'Target' sign:*** Due to chronic muscularis mucosae thickening and fatty submucosal infiltration (visible even with NECT).

Ans: (c) Ulcerative colitis

Ref: *Grainger Allison Radiology, Page 294-295*

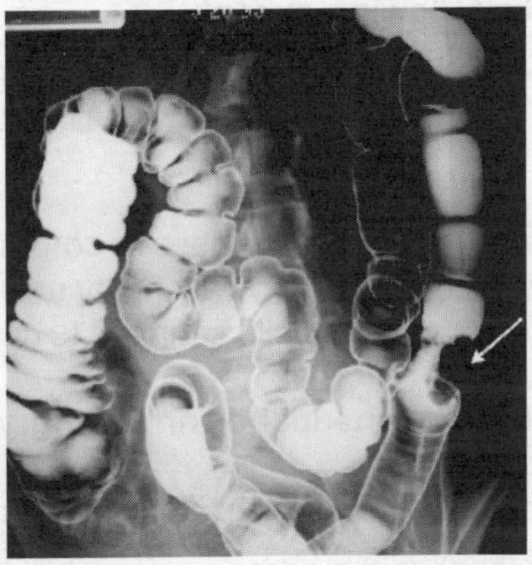

Figure: Figure showing series of indentations or erosions on a normally smooth margin of a structure

13. Following esophagus perforations, non-operative treatment methods are preferred in all *except*:

(a) Mediastinum involvement
(b) Cervical perforation
(c) Boerhaave syndrome
(d) Perforation caused by fiberoptic endoscopy

Explanation:

- **Perforation of the oesophagus** usually leads to **mediastinitis.** The aim of treatment is to limit mediastinal contamination and prevent or deal with infection.
- The decision between operative and non-operative management rests on four factors. These are:
  - The **site** of the perforation (cervical versus thoracoabdominal oesophagus).
  - The **event** causing the perforation (spontaneous versus instrumental).
  - Underlying **pathology** (benign or malignant).
  - The **status of the oesophagus before** the perforation (fasted and empty versus obstructed with a stagnant residue).
- It follows that most perforations that can be managed non-operatively occur in the context of small instrumental perforations of a clean oesophagus without obstruction, where leakage is likely to be confined to the nearby mediastinum at worst.
- Instrumental perforations in the cervical oesophagus are usually small and can nearly always be managed conservatively.

- General guidelines for non-operative management include:
  - Pain that is readily controlled with opiates; absence of crepitus, diffuse mediastinal gas, hydropneumothorax or pneumoperitoneum; mediastinal containment of the perforation with no evidence of widespread extravasation of contrast material; no evidence of ongoing luminal obstruction or a retained foreign body.
- Surgical management is required whenever patients: are unstable with sepsis or shock; have evidence of a heavily contaminated mediastinum, pleural space or peritoneum; have widespread intrapleural or intraperitoneal extravasation of contrast material.

Factors that favour non-operative management	Factors that favour operative repair
Small septic load	Large septic load
Minimal cardiovascular upset	Septic shock
Perforation confined to mediastinum	Pleura breached
Perforation by flexible endoscope	Boerhaave's syndrome
Perforation of cervical oesophagus	Perforation of abdominal oesophagus

Ans: (c) Boerhaave syndrome

Ref: *Bailey and Love, 26th Edition, Page 992-994*

14. High fiber diet reduces risk of the following *except*:

(a) IBD (b) Ca colon
(c) Sigmoid volvulus (d) Diverticulitis

Explanation:

- **Sigmoid volvulus** accounts for two thirds of all cases of **colonic volvulus.** The condition is permitted by an elongated segment of bowel accompanied by a lengthy mesentery with a narrow parietal attachment, a situation that allows the two ends of the mobile segment to come close together and to twist around the narrow mesenteric base.
- **Associated factors** include **chronic constipation and aging,** with the average age at presentation being in the seventh to eighth decade of life.
- There is an increased incidence of the condition in institutionalized patients afflicted with neuropsychiatric conditions and treated with psychotropic drugs.
- The increased incidence of volvulus in the so-called volvulus belt countries has been attributed to a diet high in fiber and vegetables.
- Diverticula are abnormal outpouchings or sacs of the colon wall that occur most commonly because of interactions of high intraluminal pressures, disordered motility, alterations in colonic structure, and diets low in fiber. Treatment is mainly focused on High fiber diet.
- Worldwide, the prevalence of colorectal cancer is closely associated with intake of red meat. The protective effect of dietary fiber is also suggested by epidemiological studies. The hypothesis is that increased roughage is associated with reduced transit times, and this inturn reduces the exposure of the mucosa to dietary carcinogens.
- Although the cause of ulcerative colitis is unknown, its prevalence in industrialized countries and the increased incidence in individuals who migrate from low-risk to high-risk areas suggest an environmental influence. Speculation on the influence of dietary factors has included inadequate fiber intake, chemical food additives, refined sugars, and cow's milk.

Ans: (c) Sigmoid volvulus

Ref: *Sabiston Textbook of Surgery, 20th Edition 1330, 1334 and 1339; Bailey and Love, 26th Edition, Page 1163*

15. A patient presents with head injury. Non-contrast CT scan of head is indicated in all the following situations *except*:

(a) Age < 65 (b) Loss of consciousness
(c) Vomiting (d) Seizures

Explanation:

National Institute for Health and Clinical Excellence **(NICE) guidelines** for computed tomography (CT) in head injury.

- **GCS <13** at any point.
- **GCS 13 or 14 at 2 hours.**
- **Focal neurological deficit.**
- Suspected **open, depressed** or **basal skull fracture.**
- More than one episode of **vomiting.**
- Any patient with a **mild head injury over the age of 65 years** or with a **coagulopathy,** for instance warfarin use, should be scanned urgently.
- Dangerous mechanism or injury or **antegrade amnesia >30 minutes** warrants CT within 8 hours.

Ans: (a) Age < 65

Ref: *Bailey and Love, 26th Edition, Page 314-315*

16. **A 45 years old male having multiple sexual partners presents with lesion in the anus. Biopsy reveals early stage of squamous cell carcinoma of anus. Correct management for this patient is:**

(a) Wide local excision
(b) APR
(c) Chemoradiation nigro regimen
(d) Antiviral therapy

Explanation:

- Historically, treatment consisted of **surgery alone or radiation therapy alone.**
- **Epithelial or subepithelial** tumors were **locally excised,** and more advanced lesions underwent **APR.**
- The introduction of **multimodality therapy** combining **chemotherapy and radiation therapy** promised to **preserve continence,** to **avoid colostomy,** and to offer similar or improved survival.
- Nigro was the first to promote **radiation therapy** with **chemotherapy** as definitive treatment for squamous cell cancers of the anal canal.
- The current protocol includes **infusional 5-FU with mitomycin C** and **external beam radiation to the pelvis with a minimum dose of 45 Gy.** The **inguinal nodes, pelvis, anus, and perineum should be included** in the radiation fields.
- Patients with advanced and residual disease after **45 Gy,** or **node-positive disease** are usually treated with an additional **9 to 14 Gy for a total dose of 54 to 59 Gy.**

Ans: (c) Chemoradiation nigro regimen

Ref: *Sabiston Textbook of Surgery, 20th Edition, Page 1414-15*

17. **Which of the following is not a bariatric surgery?**

(a) Laparoscopic Gastric Banding
(b) Roux en Y Gastric Bypass
(c) Laparoscopic Sleeve Gastrectomy
(d) Pylorus exclusion Gastrojejunostomy

Explanation:

- Bariatric Surgery is the Surgery done in Morbid Obesity patients to attain better weight control. **Morbid obesity is defined as patients with BMI >40 kg/m^2.**
- **Why is it necessary?** Morbid Obesity patients have several complications related to Cardiovascular, pulmonary, Metabolic, Gastrointestinal, Musculoskeletal, Genitourinary, Neurologic, Psychiatric systems and they have been socially abused based on the physical form and has employment issues.
- **Indications for Bariatric Surgery:**

  Patients must meet the following criteria:
  - BMI >40 or BMI >35 with associated medical comorbid condition or worsened by obesity.
  - Failed Dietary therapy.
  - Psychiatrically stable without alcohol dependence or illegal drug use.
  - Knowledgeable about the operation and its sequelae.
  - Motivated individual.
  - Medical problems not precluding probable survival from surgery.

- **Bariatric Multidisciplinary Team:**
  - Surgeon
  - Assisting surgeon
  - Nutritionist
  - Anesthesiologist
  - Operating room nurse
  - Operating room scrub tech or nurse
  - Nurse care coordinator or educator
  - Secretary or administrator
  - Psychiatrist or psychologist
  - Primary care physician
  - Medical specialists for cardiac, pulmonary, gastrointestinal, endocrine, musculoskeletal and neurologic conditions as indicated.
- **Preoperative Evaluation:**
  - Full blood count, urea and electrolytes, liver function tests.
  - Fasting lipid profile, Fasting glucose, HbA1C (if diabetic).
  - Vitamins A, D and E.
  - Parathyroid hormone.
  - Magnesium, calcium and phosphate.
  - Ferritin, vitamin B12, folate and coagulation screen.
  - Zinc, selenium, copper and C-reactive protein.

Surgical Procedures:

Restrictive	Largely Restrictive, Moderately malabsorptive	Largely Malabsorptive, Mild restrictive
Laparoscopic Adjustable Gastric (LAGB) Laparoscopic Sleeve Gastrectomy (LSG)	Roux en Y Gastric Bypass (RYGB)	Biliopancreatic diversion (BPD) Duodenal Switch (DS)

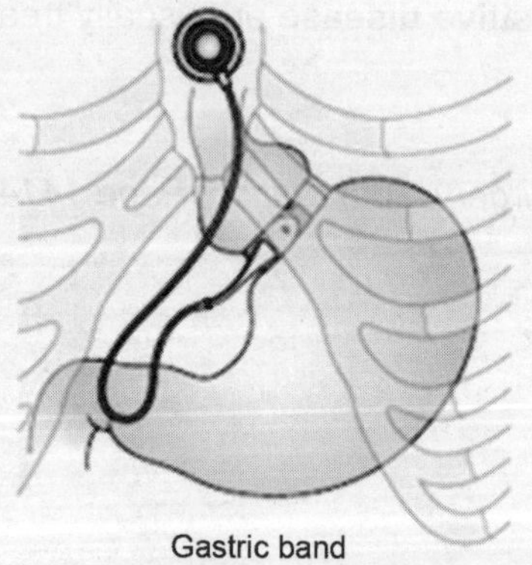

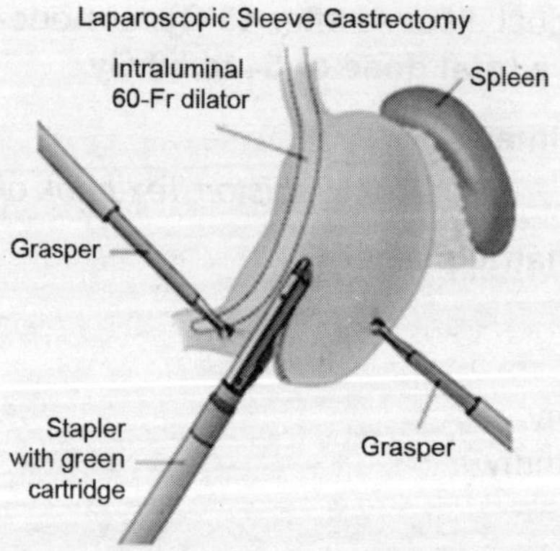

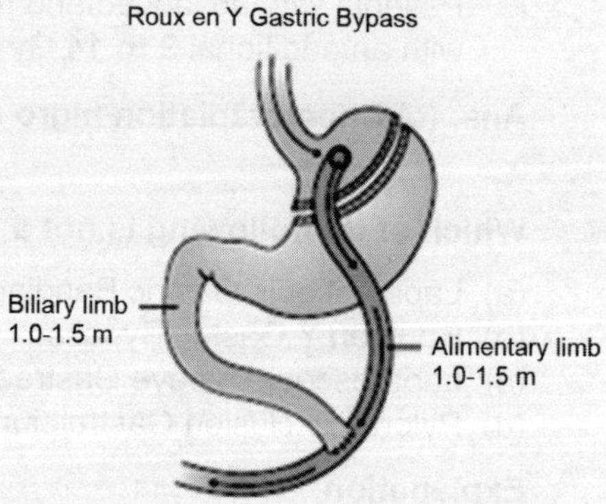

- The above surgical procedures are classified based on the mechanism of action. The restrictive procedures involves restriction of calorie intake by causing early satiety and weight loss occurs with inducing satiety and appetite loss through stretch receptors. All these techniques are done laparoscopically, which is considered standard.

SOME IMPORTANT MECHANISM OF ACTION

Procedure	Mechanism
Laparoscopic adjustable gastric banding (LAGB)	Patient controlled adjustable banding, which constricts the stomach thereby restricting entry and creating early satiety
Laparoscopic Sleeve Gastrectomy (LSG)	Most of the stomach is resected, hence Ghrelin levels will be very low and also the stomach will be tubular leading to activation of stretch receptors even with lesser food intake, leading to early satiety and decrease in appetite

Contd.

Contd.

Roux-en-Y Gastric Bypass (RYGB)	Food contents bypass the stomach, thereby entering into small bowel with stimulation of anti-incretin factors and stimulate the release of insulin
Biliopancreatic diversion with Duodenal switch (BPD/DS)	These are malabsorptive procedures, as the food bypass the stomach as well as absorptive portions of the jejunum thereby creating rapid weight loss.

- Pylorus exclusion procedure is done in advanced carcinoma of the antrum where it is fixed to pancreas, thereby doing Gastrojejunostomy bypass by excluding pylorus (Devine's procedure).

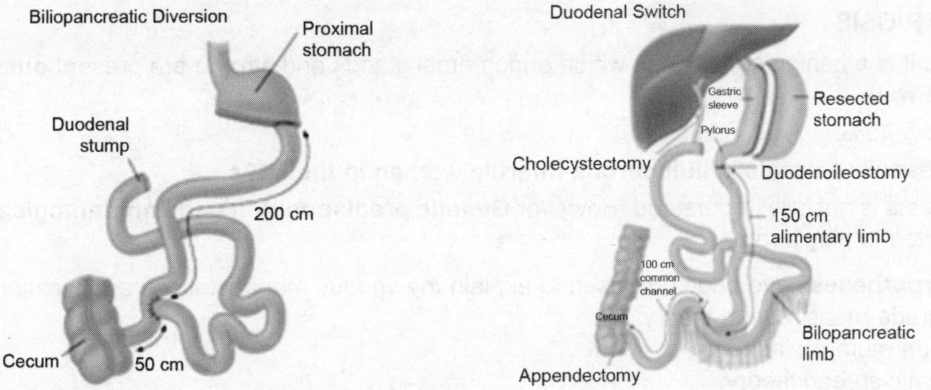

Ans: (d) Pylorus exclusion Gastrojejunostomy

***Ref:** Sabiston's Textbook of Surgery, 20th Edition, Page 1160-1186; Bailey and Love, 26th Edition, Page 1058-1062*

OBSTETRICS AND GYNECOLOGY

1. **Most common site of endometriosis:**

(a) Ovary
(b) Pouch of douglas
(c) Uterosacral ligament
(d) Broad ligament

Explanation:

ENDOMETRIOSIS

Definition: It is a benign condition in which endometrial glands and stroma are present **outside the uterine cavity and wall.**

Incidence: 5-15%.

Age: It classically presents in **nulliparous infertile women in their 30s.**

Pathogenesis is not fully understood. However **Genetic predisposition and Immunological changes** have been reported to play a role.

Several hypotheses have been proposed to explain the various manifestations and location of the disease.
- Retrograde menstruation theory.
- Mullerian metaplasia theory.
- Lymphatic spread theory.
- Hematogenous spread theory.

Sites of occurrence: Most commonly found in the dependent portions of the pelvis.
- **Ovaries*** – **Most common site** (2 out of 3 women with endometriosis).
- Broad ligament.
- Peritoneal surfaces of the cul-de-sac–uterosacral ligaments and Pouch of Douglas.
- Rectovaginal septum.
- Rectosigmoid colon, appendix, and vesicouterine fold of the peritoneum are sometimes involved.
- Endometriosis can develop in **Laparotomy scars** especially after Cesarean section or myomectomy where uterine cavity has been entered.

Endometriosis of ovary:
- Cysts filled with **thick chocolate coloured fluid** – This characteristic fluid **represents aged, haemolysed blood** and desquamated epithelium.
- May have a **black tarry consistency** sometimes.

Risk factors:
- Reproductive age group (usually, late teens to 40s).
- Nulliparity.
- Infertility.
- A first degree relative with endometriosis.
- Frequent menstrual cycle.
- Prolonged menstruation of > 8 days.

Symptoms:
- **Severe dysmenorrhea – 90% (most common symptom).**
- Chronic pelvic pain – 70%.
- Dyspareunia – 75%.
- Infertility – 55%.

On examination, patient may have:
- Pelvic pain.
- Firm, fixed tender adnexal mass.
- **Tender nodularity in cul-de-sac and uterosacral ligament.**

Diagnosis:
- Confirmed by doing a **diagnostic laparoscopy.**
- Advantage of laparoscopy – treatment can be offered in the same sitting.

Characteristic appearance of endometriostic lesions in laparoscopy

- Red, dark brown, or black peritoneal implants.
- **Chocolate cysts of the ovary.**
- White or yellow spots or nodules.
- **Powder burn lesions.**
- Normal appearing peritoneum (microscopic disease).

TREATMENT OF ENDOMETRIOSIS

Medical Management

- **Prostaglandin synthetase inhibitors** (naproxen, ibuprofen) – for dysmenorrhea and menorrhagia.
- **Combined OCP** for 6-9 months – inhibits ovulation and menstruation.
- **Progestogen** – Oral medroxyprogesterone acetate 10-30 mg daily for 6-9 months.
- **Danazol** – Given orally 400-800 mg/day for 6-9 months.
- **GnRHagonist:**
  - **Nafarelin:** Intranasally using a nasal spray, 200 micrograms twice daily.
  - **Goserelin:** 3.6 mg injected SC every 4 weeks.
  - **Triptorelin:** 3.75 mg injected IM every 4 weeks.

Surgical management

Conservative surgery

- Minimal to mild disease – can be removed by **LASER or electrocautery.**
- Pre-sacral neurectomy has been used to treat severe dysmenorrhea.

Definitive surgery – Total hysterectomy and bilateral salpingo-oophorectomy in patients above 40 years or after completion of family.

Ans: (a) Ovary

Ref: *Berek and Novak's Gynecology, 14th Edition, Page 523-524*

2. **AMSTL criteria includes all *except*:**

(a) Controlled cord traction (b) Uterine massage
(c) Oxytocin (d) Methergine

Explanation:

Third stage of labor includes the period from **delivery of the baby to delivery of placenta and membranes.**

Active management of third stage of labor for prevention of postpartum hemorrhage (PPH) includes:

- Intramuscular oxytocin 10 U given at the delivery of anterior shoulder.
- Controlled cord traction to deliver the placenta.
- Uterine massage holding the fundus of uterus after delivery of placenta.

WHO definition of PPH – Blood loss of **500 ml or more following vaginal delivery or blood loss 1000 ml or more following a caesarean section** is defined as PPH.

Clinical definition – Any amount of bleeding from or within the genital tract, following birth of the baby upto the end of puerperium, which adversely affects the general condition of the mother, as evidenced by rise in pulse rate or fall in BP is termed as PPH.

Primary PPH – Defined as hemorrhage that occurs **within 24 hours following birth of the baby.** It can be:

- **Third stage hemorrhage** – Occurs before expulsion of placenta.
- **True PPH** – Occurs after expulsion of the placenta.

Important causes of PPH: (Acronym – remember 'four Ts')

- Tone (atonic uterus).
- Trauma (genital tract).
- Tissue (retained products of conception).
- Thrombin (coagulopathy).

The most common cause of primary PPH is atonic uterus (80%).

Risk factors of PPH

- Grand multipara.

- Uterine overdistension—multiple pregnancy and hydramnios.
- Anemia.
- Antepartum hemorrhage.
- Prolonged labor.
- Morbidly adherent placenta.
- Genital tract trauma.

Management of PPH

- **Call for help** – To alert obstetric and anesthetic seniors.
- Start IV line with two wide bore cannula and start **IV infusion with crystalloids.**
- Send **blood** for blood grouping, cross matching and transfuse blood as soon as available.
- Give **O_2 by mask.**
- Catheterize the bladder to monitor hourly urine output.
- Palpate the uterus:
  - If uterus is relaxed – atonic PPH.
  - If uterus is well contracted – traumatic PPH, explore the genital tract.

Management of Atonic PPH

Bimanual uterine compression – Massage the uterus to stimulate uterine contractions.

Medical management for atonic PPH:

- Start 20 units of **oxytocin** in normal saline IV at the rate of 60 drops/minute.
- **Injection Methergin** 0.2 mg IV.
- **Injection Carboprost** (PGF2 alpha) 250 mcg IM, can be repeated at intervals of > 15 minutes, upto maximum of 8 doses.
- **Intramyometrial Injection carboprost** 250 mcg may be given.
- **Misoprostol (PGE1)** 1000 mg can be placed per rectum.

Surgical measures to control PPH

- **Explore** the uterus and genital tract.
- **Repair** any genital tract injuries in case of traumatic PPH.
- **Uterine tamponade with** Hydrostatic balloon catheters (Sengstaken - Blakemore esophageal catheter) can be used for hemostasis.
- **Hemostatic compression sutures** – Hemostatic suture techniques are effective in controlling severe PPH.
  - **B lynch sutures**
  - **Modified B lynch suture**
  - **Multiple square sutures**
- **Uterine devascularization procedures:**
  - Bilateral **ligation of uterine vessels** and utero-ovarian vessels.
  - Bilateral **Internal iliac artery ligation** is an effective method to control PPH.
  - **Uterine artery embolization** – It requires the equipment and interventional radiologist to perform the procedure.
  - **Hysterectomy** – final step if patient is not responding to the above methods.

PREVENTIVE MEASURES FOR PPH

Antenatal measures:

- Correction of anemia.
- Blood group and Rh typing for all antenatal women.
- Localization of placenta by ultrasound.

Intrapartum measures: Active management of third stage of labor (AMTSL).

Ans: (d) Methergine

Ref: *WHO 2012 Recommendations; FIGO 2006 Recommendations*

3. **A milky white watery discharge with fishy odour from vagina and minimal itching is due to:**

(a) Bacterial vaginosis (b) Gonorrhoea
(c) Trichomonas (d) Candida

Explanation:

GARDNERELLA VAGINOSIS

- Alteration in normal vaginal flora.
- **Decrease in number of lactobacilli in vaginal discharge** – lactobacilli reduce pH and release hydrogen peroxide toxic to other bacteria.
- 100 fold increase in anerobic bacteria.
- **Hemophilus vaginalis, Gardnerella, Mobiluncus and Mycoplasma hominis**–cause.
- Vaginal discharge without discharge.
- White, milky non-viscous discharge, **pH** of discharge more than **4.5.**
- **Whiff Test – Fishy odour** when vaginal discharge is mixed with 10% KOH – due to release of amino metabolites from various organisms.
- Presence of **Clue Cells** – epithelial cells with granular cytoplasm caused by gram negative bacilli adhering on the surface.
- Wet smear, gram stain and culture are investigations.
- **Treatment:**
    - o **Metronidazole** 500 mg bd for 7 days.
    - o Ampicillin 500 mg or cephalosporin 500 mg bd for 7 days.
    - o Tetracycline 500 mg 4 times a day.
    - o Doxycycline 100 mg bd.
    - o Sulphafurazole 1 g 4 times daily for 10-14 days.
    - o Clindamycin 300 mg daily for 7 days.
    - o Clindamycin 2% cream locally.
    - o Ornidazole 500 mg vaginal tablet for 7 days.
    - o **Lacteal** is protein free acidifying lactate gel neutralises vaginal ph 5 ml applied for 7 days.

AMSEL CRITERIA for diagnosing Bacterial Vagninosis

- Thin, white, yellow, homogeneous discharge.
- Clue cells on microscopy.
- pH of vaginal fluid >4.5.
- Release of a fishy odor on adding alkali—10% potassium hydroxide (KOH) solution.
- **At least three of the four criteria** should be present for a confirmed diagnosis.

Ans: (a) Bacterial vaginosis

Ref: *Berek and Novak's Gynecology, 14th Edition, Page 542-544*

4. **All the following are sling operations for uterine prolapse *except*:**

(a) Khanna (b) Shirodkar
(c) Abdominocervicopexy (d) Manchester

Explanation:

Sling operations provide a substitute for the weakened supports of the uterus by using nylon or Dacron tapes as slings to support the uterus.

Indications: 2nd or 3rd degree uterine prolapse in women who are desirous of retaining their child bearing and menstrual functions.

The various sling operations are:

A. **Purandare's sling**
    - The tape is fixed **anteriorly** to the uterine isthmus and lateral edges brought between leaves of broad ligament and **fixed to the rectus sheath** on either side.
    - Plication of round ligament.
    - **Moschowitz's repair** – abdominal correction of enterocele.

B. **Shirodkar's sling operation**
    - Mesilene tape (originally fascia lata) is fixed to posterior aspect of the cervix and to the **anterior longitudinal ligament of the sacral promontory.**
    - Sling taken through the **Psoas loop on the left side** due to the presence of sigmoid colon.

C. **Khanna's sling operation**
- Merseline tape fixed to the isthmus of cervix posteriorly and fixed to **anterior superior iliac spine** on either sides.

D. **Abdominocervicopexy**

MANCHESTER OPERATION

Indications
- Suitable for women less than 40 years, completed their family with the intention of preserving menstrual function.
- II or III degree uterine prolapse with cystocele/rectocele with or without supravaginal elongation of cervix.

Principle steps
- Preliminary D and C.
- Amputation of cervix.
- Shortening of Mackenrodt's and anchoring in front of cervix.
- Anterior colporrhaphy.
- Posterior colpoperineorrhaphy.

Disadvantages is mainly due to cervical amputation
- Cervical Incompetence leading to:
  - Habitual abortions.
  - Preterm deliveries.
- Cervical stenosis leading to:
  - Dystocia during labor.
  - Hematometra.
- **Hence usually preferred in women who have completed family.**

Ans: (d) Manchester

Ref: *Berek and Novak's Gynecology, 14th Edition, Page 994*

5. **Longest fetal diameter:**

(a) Biparietal
(b) Suboccipitobregmatic
(c) Occipitofrontal
(d) Mentovertical

Explanation:

DIAMETERS OF FETAL SKULL

Fetal Skull Diameter	**Borders**	**Length**
Suboccipitobregmatic	From **nape of neck** to **center of bregma**	9.5 cm
Suboccipitofrontal	From **nape of neck** to **anterior fontanelle** or center of sinciput	10 cm
Occipitofrontal	From **occipital eminence** to **root of nose**	11.5 cm
Mentovertical	From **midpoint of chin** to **highest point of sagittal suture**	14 cm
Submentovertical	From **junction of floor of the mouth and neck** to **highest point of sagittal suture**	11.5 cm
Submentobregmatic	From **junction of mouth** and **neck to center of bregma**	9.5 cm
Biparietal	Extends **between two parietal eminences**	9.5 cm
Super sub-parietal	From a point placed **below one parietal eminence** to a point placed above the **other parietal eminence on opposite side**	8.5 cm
Bitemporal	Distance **between two anterior ends of coronal suture**	8 cm
Bimastoid	Distance between **tips of mastoid processes**	7.5 cm

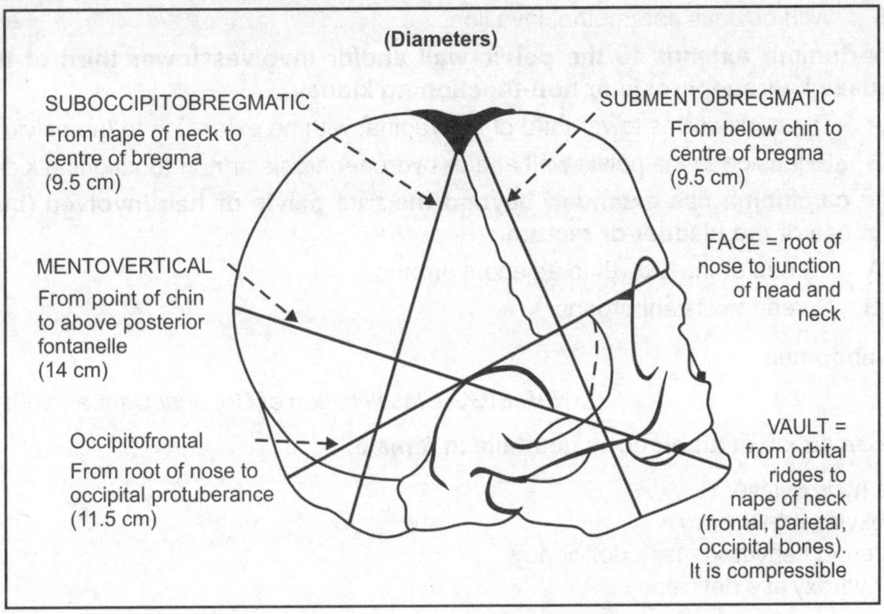

Ans: (d) Mentovertical

***Ref:** DC Dutta Textbook of Obstetrics, 8th Edition, Page 96*

6. **In a woman diagnosed with cervical cancer, all the following investigations are included for FIGO staging *except*:**

(a) IVP (b) CT abdomen
(c) Cystoscopy (d) CXR

Explanation:

FIGO staging system of carcinoma cervix is mainly **based on clinical examination** rather than surgical findings. It allows **only the following diagnostic tests in determining the stage:**

- Palpation
- Inspection
- Colposcopy
- Hysteroscopy
- Endocervical curettage
- IVP (intravenous pyelogram)
- Chest X-ray
- Cervical conization

Carcinoma of the cervix - FIGO 2009

Stage I The carcinoma is strictly confined to the cervix

IA Invasive carcinoma which can be diagnosed only by microscopy, with deepest invasion $\leq$5 mm and the largest extension $\geq$7 mm.

IA1 Measured stromal invasion of $\leq$3.0 mm in depth and extension of $\leq$7.0 mm.

IA2 Measured stromal invasion of >3.0 mm and not >5.0 mm with an extension of not >7.0 mm.

IB Clinically visible lesions limited to the cervix uteri or pre-clinical cancers greater than stage IA.

IB1 Clinically visible lesion $\leq$4.0 cm in greatest dimension.

IB2 Clinically visible lesion >4.0 cm in greatest dimension.

Stage II Cervical carcinoma invades beyond the uterus, but not to the pelvic wall or to the lower third of the vagina

IIA Without parametrial invasion.

IIA1 Clinically visible lesion $\leq$4.0 cm in greatest dimension.

IIA2 Clinically visible lesion >4.0 cm in greatest dimension.

IIB With obvious parametrial invasion.

Stage III The tumour extends to the pelvic wall and/or involves lower third of the vagina and/or causes hydronephrosis or non-functioning kidney

IIIA Tumour involves lower third of the vagina, with no extension to the pelvic wall.

IIIB Extension to the pelvic wall and/or hydronephrosis or non-functioning kidney.

Stage IV The carcinoma has extended beyond the true pelvis or has involved (biopsy proven) the mucosa of the bladder or rectum.

IVA Spread of the growth to adjacent organs.

IVB Spread to distant organs.

Ans: (b) CT abdomen

Ref: *FIGO Classification of Cervical Cancer, 2009 Recommenations*

7. **Least common cause of ambiguous genitalia in female:**

(a) 17 Alpha hydroxylase
(b) 21 Hydroxylase deficiency
(c) 3 Beta steroid dehydrogenase deficiency
(d) 11 Beta hydroxylase deficiency

Explanation:

CONGENITAL ADRENAL HYPERPLASIA:

- It is a familial disorder of adrenal steroid biosynthesis with autosomal recessive inheritance.
- The defect is expressed as adrenal enzyme deficiency.
- **5 major Enzymes deficiency** are clinically important:
  - ***21-Hydroxylase* – most common*.**
  - *11-Beta-Hydroxylase.*
  - *17-Alpha-Hydroxylase.*
  - ***3-Beta-steroid dehydrogenase* – *Least common*.***
  - *20,22 Desmolase deficiency.*

21 hydroxylase deficiency

- **Most common type, accounts for >80% of cases.**
- Incidence is 1:5000 to 1:15000 live birth.
- Gene is located on **the short arm of chromosome 6** in close association with HLA genes.
- Heterozygous carriers can be detected by ACTH stimulation test.
- It is characterized by **reduced production of cortisol and aldosterone and increased production of progesterone, 17-OH-progesterone and sex steroids.**
- The urinary steroid metabolites (17-ketosteroids and pregnanediol) are elevated above normal levels.
- Decreased secretion of aldosterone results in **salt loss with hyponatremia and hyperkalemia; plasma renin activity is therefore elevated.**
- In partial enzyme deficiencies, the aldosterone deficiency is not expressed, and patients remain normonatremic and normokalemic.
- The **excess androgens causes virilization of girls and ambiguous genitalia and dark scrotum in boys.**
- 2 forms, classic early virilization type with or without salt-losing crisis and non-classic type with late-onset virilization.
- Male babies with non salt-losing, non-classic type remains asymptomatic till late childhood when they may show signs of sexual precocity.

11 Beta hydroxylase deficiency

- Accounts for 5-10% of cases of CAH.
- Gene is located on the **long arm of chromosome 8.**
- It is characterized by **low plasma renin activity and elevation of serum 11-Deoxycortisol and 11-deoxycorticosterone.**
- Because of the strong mineralocorticoid activity of deoxycorticosterone, the condition is **characterized by salt retention, hypertension and hypokalemic alkalosis.**

- The elevated plasma androgens may cause **virilization of the female fetus.**

17α-Hydroxylase Deficiency

- Impaired conversion of pregnenolone and progesterone to 17-hydroxypregnenolone and 17-hydroxyprogesterone.
- Impaired cortisol production → ACTH hypersecretion → increased DOC, corticosterone, and 18-hydroxycorticosterone in the adrenals → salt and water retention HTN and hypokalemia.
- Phenotype may dictate gender assignment.

3β-Hydroxysteroid Dehydrogenase Deficiency

- A very rare disorder.
- **Incomplete masculinization with salt-wasting** → impaired aldosterone and cortisol synthesis – a small phallus, hypospadias with labioscrotal fusion, a urogenital sinus, and a blind-ending vaginal pouch. Testes are often scrotal, and wolffian ducts develop normally.
- Diagnosis – increased levels of 3β-hydroxysteroids (pregnenolone, 17-hydroxypregnenolone and DHEA).

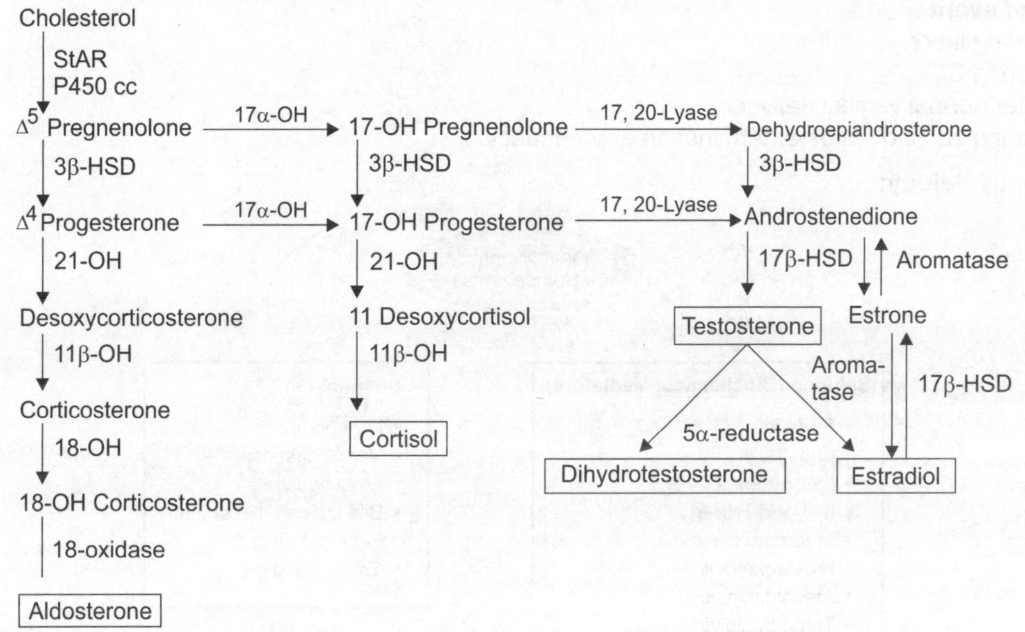

Approach to ambiguous genitalia:

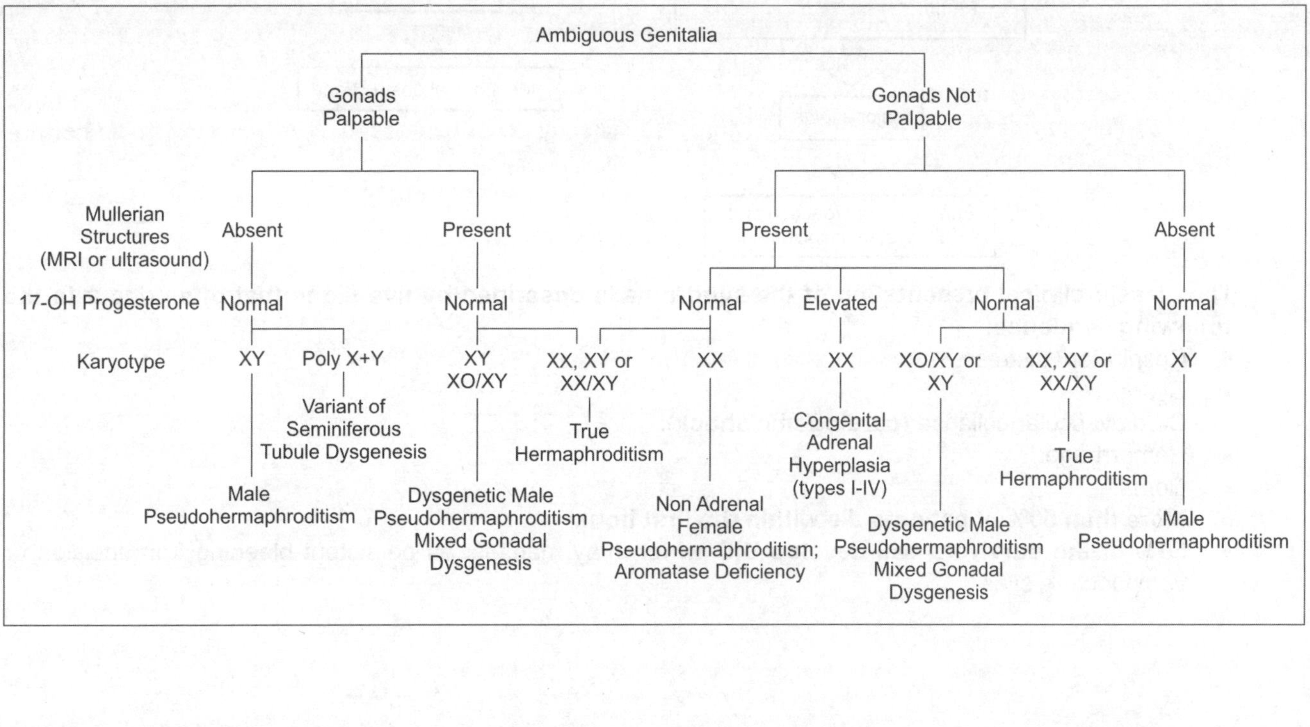

Ans: (c) 3 Beta steroid dehydrogenase deficiency

Ref: *Berek and Novak's Textbook of Gynecology, 14th Edition, Page 443*

8. **A patient who delivered few hours back collapses and dies. During autopsy, alveolar fluid analysis shows presence of hair and squamous epithelial cells. Most likely cause of death:**

(a) Amniotic fluid embolism (b) Fat embolism
(c) DIC (d) Pulmonary embolism

Explanation:

Amniotic Fluid Embolism

- Complex condition characterized by **abrupt onset of pulmonary embolism, shock and DIC which is due to entering of amniotic fluid into the maternal circulation.**

Incidence – 1 in 8,000 to 1 in 80,000 pregnancies.

Time of event

- During labor.
- During C/S.
- After normal vaginal delivery.
- During second trimester termination of pregnancy.

Pathophysiology:

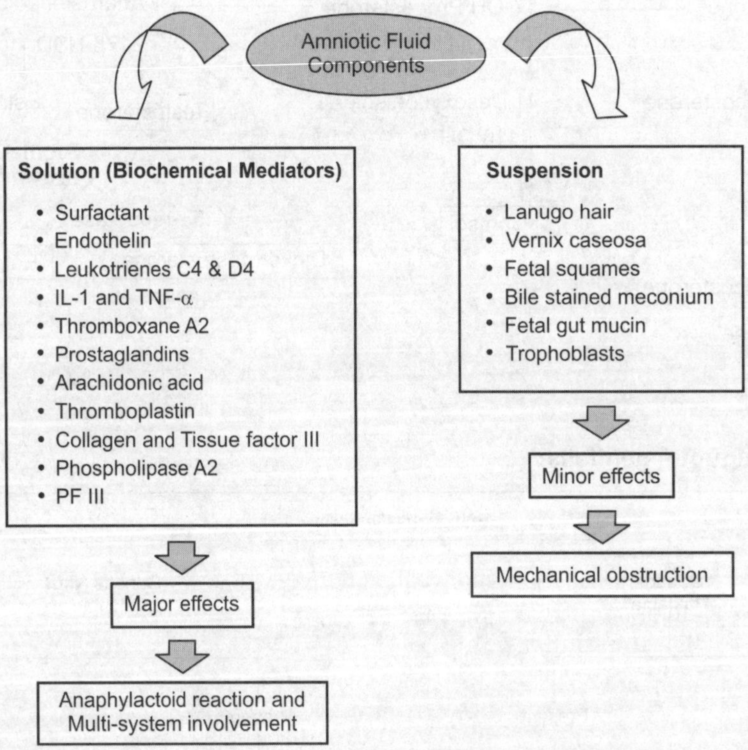

The classic clinical presentation of the syndrome is described by five signs that often occur in the following sequence:

- Respiratory distress.
- Cyanosis.
- Cardiovascular collapse **(cardiogenic shock).**
- Hemorrhage.
- Coma.
- **More than 50% of patients die within the first hour.**
- **50% of the survivors will develop DIC which** may manifest as persistent bleeding from incision or venipuncture sites.

- 10-15% of patients will develop grand mal seizures.
- CXR may be normal or shows effusions, enlarged heart or pulmonary edema.
- ECG may show a right strain pattern with ST-T changes and tachycardia.
- The presence of **squamous cells in the pulmonary vasculature once considered pathognomonic for AFE is neither sensitive nor specific** (only 73% of patients dying from AFE had this finding).
- **The monoclonal antibody TKAH-2** may eventually prove more useful in the rapid diagnosis of AFE.
- Invesigations: CBC, ABG, PT, aPTT, fibrinogen, FDP.

Goals of Management
- **Restoration of cardiovascular and pulmonary equilibrium**
  - Maintain systolic blood pressure >90 mm Hg.
  - Urine output > 25 ml/hr.
  - Arterial pO_2 > 60 mm Hg.
- **Re-establishing uterine tone.**
- **Correct coagulation abnormalities.**
- As intubation and CPR may be required, it is necessary to have easy access to the patient, experienced help, and a resuscitation tray with intubation equipment, DC shock and emergency medications.

IMMEDIATE MEASURES
- Set up IV Infusion, O_2 administration.
- Airway control → endotracheal intubation → maximal ventilation and oxygenation.

Ans: (a) Amniotic fluid embolism

Ref: *DC Dutta Textbook of Obstetrics, 8th Edition, Page 703*

9. **Karyotyping of the patient is 45X0/46XY. What is the diagnosis?**

(a) Mixed gonadal dysgenesis (b) Ovotestis
(c) Testicular feminization syndrome (d) Turner syndrome

Explanation:

Mixed gonadal dysgenesis
- Combined features of **Turner's syndrome and male pseudohermaphroditism.**
- Short stature.
- **Streak gonad on one side with a testis on the other.**
- **Unicornuate uterus and fallopian tube on the side of streak gonad.**
- **Mosaic Karyotype 46XY/45X0.**
- Considerable variation in the sexual phenotype.

True hermaphroditism
- **Gonads:** Ovary one side and testis on the other or bilateral ovotestis.
- **Karyotype: 46, XX most common;** XX/XY(30%) and XY(13%).
- **Internal genitalia:** Both mullerian and wolffian derivatives.
- Phenotype is variable.
- **Gonadal biopsy is required for confirming diagnosis.**

Klinefelter's syndrome
- Syndrome characterized by **enuchoidism, gynecomastia, azoospermia, increased gonadotropin levels and small, firm testes.**
- **47 XXY karyotype.**
- **Nondisjunction during meiosis.**
- **Incidence–1 of 1000 liveborn males.**
- **Gynecomastia can be quite marked at pubertal development.**
- **8 times risk for breast carcinoma compared with normal males.**
- Seminiferous tubules degenerate and are replaced with hyaline.
- **Decreased androgens prevents normal secondary sexual development.**
- **Normal amounts of pubic and axillary hair, but facial hair is sparse.**
- Muscle development, fat distribution is more like female than male.
- **Patients tend to be taller than average, due to disproportionately long legs.**

- Predisposed to **malignant neoplasms of extragonadal germ cell origin.**
- **Management – Androgen supplementation to improve libido and reduction mammoplasty.**
- Surveillance for breast carcinoma.

Turner's syndrome

- 1 in 2500 live births.
- **60% are 45, XO and 40% are mosaics.**
- No oocytes remain in the ovaries, which become streaks.
  - Ovum donation for those with bilateral streaks.
- **Four classic features:**
  - Female phenotype.
  - Short stature.
  - Lack of secondary sexual characteristics.
  - A variety of somatic abnormalities.
- **If Y chromosomal material is present → masculinization and gonadoblastoma (30%).**
- **30-60% have structural or positional abnormalities of the kidney:**
  - Horseshoe kidney – 10%.
  - Duplication or renal agenesis – 20%.
  - Malrotation – 15%.
  - Multiple renal arteries – 90%.

PURE GONADAL DYSGENESIS

- **Features:**
  - Normal female external genitalia.
  - Normal Müllerian ducts with absence of wolffian duct structures.
  - Normal height.
  - Bilateral streak gonads.
  - Sexual infantilism.
  - Normal 46,XX karyotype.
- Streak gonads → elevated serum gonadotropins.
- **Management of 46, XX pure gonadal dysgenesis:**
  - Cyclic hormone replacement with estrogen and progesterone.
  - Growth is basically normal, so GH is not needed.
- Possibly autosomal recessive trait.

Female pseudohermaphroditism:

- 46, XX individuals with ovaries.
- Have a partially masculinized phenotype and ambiguous genitalia.
- **CAH is most common cause.**
- Uncommon etiologies:
  - Maternal ingestion of androgens.
  - Virilizing tumors in the mother.

Congenital adrenal hyperplasia:

- Error in cortisol biosynthesis pathway.
- **The most commonly recognized syndromes result from a deficiency of 21-hydroxylase or 11-hydroxylase. 21-hydroxylase is responsible for 95% of cases of CAH.**
- Formation of hydrocortisone is impaired, causing a compensatory increase in the secretion of **ACTH →** enhances formation of adrenal steroids, proximal to the enzymatic defect and a secondary increase in the formation of testosterone, the active androgen in CAH.
- Incidence is 1 in 5,000 to 1 in 15,000. The highest incidence 1 in 490 is seen in the **Alaskan Eskimo.**

Ans: (a) Mixed gonadal dysgenesis

***Ref:** Berek and Novak's Gynecology, 15th Edition, Page 1044*

10. An obese diabetic and hypertensive patient presented to OPD with post menopausal bleeding and was diagnosed to have endometrial carcinoma with invasion of more than 50 percent of myometrium with extension to vagina, but no involvement of paraaortic or inguinal lymph nodes. What is the staging of endometrial Ca?

(a) Stage 2A
(b) Stage 2B
(c) Stage 3A
(d) Stage 3B

Explanation:

Carcinoma of the Endometrium staging

IA	Tumor confined to the uterus with < ½ myometrial invasion.
IB	Tumor confined to the uterus with > ½ myometrial invasion.
II	Cervical stromal invasion, but not beyond uterus.
IIIA	Tumor invades serosa or adnexa.
IIIB	Vaginal and/or parametrial involvement.
IIIC1	Pelvic node involvement.
IIIC2	Para-aortic involvement.
IVA	Tumor invasion bladder and/or bowel mucosa.
IVB	Distant metastases including abdominal metastases and/or inguinal lymph nodes.

Risk factors for endometrial cancer

- **Early age** at **menarche.**
- **Late age** at **menopause** (>52 years – 2.5 fold increased risk).
- **55–70 age group** – majority of endometrial carcinoma occur in this age group.
- **H/o Obesity, Diabetes, Hypertension (Cancer corpus syndrome).**
- Nulliparity – 2 fold increased risk.
- Chronic anovulation due to any cause.
- Endometrial hyperplasia.
- Long term unopposed use of **estrogen** (HRT increases risk by 4-8 times).
- **Tamoxifen therapy** – 2-3 fold increased risk.
- Family history of endometrial, ovarian, colon cancer.
- **HNPCC** (hereditary non-polyposis colonic cancer) – Women with HNPCC have 40-60% life time risk of endometrial carcinoma.

CAUSES OF POST MENOPAUSAL BLEEDING

Uterine causes

- Endometrial atrophy – 60-80%.
- Endometrial polyps – 2-12%.
- Endometrial carcinoma – 10%.
- Endometrial hyperplasia – 5-10%.
- Hormone replacement therapy – 15-20%.

Non uterine causes

- Carcinoma cervix.
- Atrophic vaginitis.
- Decubitus ulcer.
- Vulval carcinoma.

Non genital causes

- Bleeding P/R.
- Hematuria.
- **Most common** genital malignancy presenting with post menopausal bleeding in India is **cervical carcinoma*.**

Ans: (d) Stage 3B

Ref: *FIGO 2009 Guidelines*

ORTHOPEDICS

1. **Agnes Hunt traction is used in:**

(a) Flexion deformity of hip
(b) Inter-trochanteric fracture
(c) Fracture shaft femur
(d) Low backache

Ans: (a) Flexion deformity of hip

Ref: *Fundamentals of Orthopedics by Mohindra and Jain, 1st Edition, Jaypee Publishers, Page 24*

Explanation:

- **Agnes Hunt traction** has conventionally been used for correction of mild flexion deformity of the hip in patients with poliomyelitis.

List of important traction systems used in Orthopedics

Agnes Hunt traction	Hip flexion deformity
Bryant's traction, Gallows traction, 90-90 traction	Fracture shaft femur
Buck's traction	Skin traction applied in lower limb
Crutchfield tongs, head halter traction, Gardner well tongs, halo-pelvic traction	Cervical spine injury
Dunlop traction, Smith traction	Supracondylar fracture humerus
Halo-pelvic traction	Spinal deformities (scoliosis)
Perkin's traction	Tibial and femoral fractures
Pelvic belt traction	Low back ache (given on OPD basis)
Russel's traction	Trochanteric fracture, femoral shaft fracture
Supracondylar femoral traction	Proximal femoral and shaft fracture
Upper tibial traction	Femoral fracture
Well leg traction	Correction of adduction or abduction deformities of hip joint

2. **Russell's traction is used in:**

(a) Inter-trochanteric #
(b) # Shaft of femur
(c) Low back ache
(d) Flexion deformity of hip

Explanation:

- Since inter-trochanteric fractures are mostly encountered in patients aged > 70 years, many a times fitness for surgery cannot be obtained.
- Conservative management involves use of special traction method called as Russel's traction (Fig. 1).

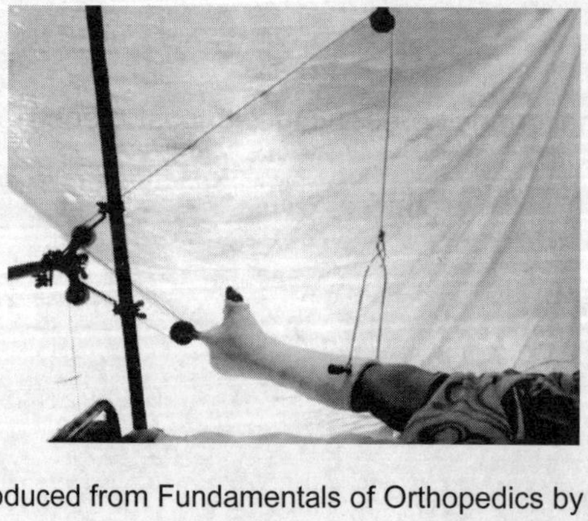

Fig. 1: Russel's traction (Reproduced from Fundamentals of Orthopedics by Mohindra and Jain, 1st Edition)

Ans: (a) Inter-trochanteric #

Ref: *Fundamentals of Orthopedics by Mohindra and Jain, 1st Edition, Jaypee Publishers, Page 110*

3. Intraosseous skeletal tumor is best detected by:

(a) Bone scan with CT
(b) X-ray
(c) Bone scan
(d) MRI

Explanation:

- **Bone scans** have limited ability to determine **intraosseous extent** of bone lesions or to demonstrate extra osseous soft tissue extensions.
- **X-rays**
  - Used in initial evaluation of suspected bone tumor.
  - Guides in determining location, mineralization and margins.
  - Best overall modality for characterizing a primary bone tumor.
  - Limited assessment of soft tissue component.
- **Computer tomography (CT)**
  - Confirms osseous origin when radiographs are ambiguous.
  - Demonstrates lesion features that may be subtle on radiographs, margins, internal matrix, mineralization, cortical destruction and periosteal reaction.
- **MRI**
  - Good for assessing size and location of marrow and soft tissue extension.
  - **Not sensitive** for detection of **calcification** or **periosteal** reaction.
  - Allows assessment of **tumour vascularity** and helps target areas amenable to biopsy.
  - Can be useful in monitoring response to therapy and recurrence.
  - Investigation of choice for **intraosseous tumour** (Osteosarcoma).

Ans: (d) MRI

Ref: *Bone Tumors; A Practical Guide to Imaging by Jim S.Wu and Mary Hochman, Springer Publications, Chapter 3*

4. Most radioresistant tumor:

(a) Osteosarcoma
(b) Malignant fibrous histiocytoma
(c) Ewing's sarcoma
(d) Multiple myeloma

Explanation:

- Osteosarcoma is most **radioresistant** and **chemoresistant** bone tumor and has a **very poor survival rate.**
- It is the **most common tumor** to **metastasize** and metastases commonly involve **lungs.**
- Radiotherapy has role in treatment of both **Multiple myeloma** and **Ewing sarcoma.**
- Treatment of choice in Ewing sarcoma is **chemotherapy.**

Highly radiosensitive tumours are:

- ***Lymphoma****
- ***Wilm's tumour****
- ***Myeloma****
- ***Ewing's sarcoma****
- ***Seminoma****

Moderately radiosensitive tumours are:

- Small cell lung carcinoma
- Carcinoma of breast
- Teratoma
- Ovarian carcinoma
- Basal cell carcinoma
- Medulloblastoma
- Dysgerminoma

- Nasopharyngeal carcinoma
- Relatively Resistant tumours are:
  - Squamous cell carcinoma of lung
  - Hypernephroma (Renal Cell Carcinoma)
  - Rectal carcinoma and carcinoma colon
  - Bladder carcinoma
  - Soft tissue carcinoma such as fibrosarcoma
  - Carcinoma of cervix

Highly Resistant tumours are:

- ***Melanoma****
- ***Osteosarcoma****
- ***Pancreatic carcinoma****
- ***Hepatoma****

Ans: (a) Osteosarcoma

Ref: *Fundamentals of Orthopedics by Mohindra and Jain, 1st Edition, Jaypee Publishers, Page 263-264*

PEDIATRICS

1. **A 10 years boy presented with Cola coloured urine, oliguria for 3 days, facial puffiness, edema and hypertension. Urine albumin is positive and C3 levels are reduced. BP is 130/80. He had skin infection two weeks back. What is the next appropriate management?**

(a) Renal biopsy (b) *Conservative therapy*
(c) Cyclosporine (d) Steroids

Explanation:

- The above clinical scenario is compatible with a diagnosis of **Post Streptococcal Glomerulonephritis (PSGN).** PSGN is quite likely in a child presenting with acute nephritic syndrome, evidence of recent streptococcal infection, and a low C3 level.

POST STREPTOCOCCAL GLOMERULONEPHRITIS (PSGN)

- **Second most common glomerular causes** of **gross hematuria** in children, **after IgA nephropathy*.**
- It follows infection of the **throat (serotype 12)** or **skin (serotype 49)** by certain **"nephritogenic" strains of group A β-hemolytic streptococci.**
- Acute glomerulonephritis may also follow infection with **coagulase-positive and coagulase-negative staphylococci, Streptococcus pneumoniae, and gram-negative bacteria*.**
- **Bacterial endocarditis** may produce a **hypocomplementemic glomerulonephritis** with **renal failure.**
- **Light microscopy findings:**
  - o All glomeruli appear enlarged.
  - o Relatively bloodless.
  - o Diffuse mesangial cell proliferation.
  - o Increase in mesangial matrix.
- **Immunofluorescence microscopy** reveals:
  - o **'Lumpy-bumpy' deposits** of immunoglobulin and complement (GBM) and in the mesangium.
- **Electron microscopy:**
  - o Electron-dense deposits, or **"humps"**, seen on the **epithelial side** of GBM.

Clinical features:

- Most common in children aged **5-12 years.**
- Presents with **acute nephritic syndrome (edema, hypertension and oliguria).**
- **1-2 weeks** after an antecedent **streptococcal pharyngitis** or **3-6 weeks** after a streptococcal **pyoderma.**
- Range from **asymptomatic microscopic hematuria** with normal renal function to **acute renal failure.**
- May develop **encephalopathy** and/or heart failure owing to hypertension or hypervolemia.
- The acute phase generally **resolves – 6-8 weeks.**
- Urinary protein excretion and hypertension usually **normalize – 4-6 weeks** after onset.
- Persistent microscopic hematuria may **persist – 1-2 years.**
- **Supportive Diagnosis:**
  - – Urinalysis shows **hematuria, RBC casts, proteinuria and polymorphonuclear leukocytes.**
  - – Normochromic anemia due to hemodilution and low-grade hemolysis.
  - – **Serum C3 level is reduced.**
  - – Confirmation of the diagnosis-clear evidence of invasive streptococcal infection (ASLO titer/Culture).
  - – The best single antibody titer to document **cutaneous streptococcal infection** is the deoxyribonuclease **(DNase) B antigen*.**
  - – **The Streptozyme test** – detects antibodies to streptolysin O, DNase B, hyaluronidase, streptokinase and nicotinamide-adenine dinucleotidase using a slide agglutination test.

Complications:

- **Hypertension**
- Heart failure
- **Hyperkalemia***
- **Hyperphosphatemia***

- **Hypocalcemia***
- Acidosis
- Seizures
- Uremia

Management:

- Treating the acute effects of renal insufficiency and hypertension (Sodium restriction, diuresis, and pharmacotherapy with calcium channel antagonists, vasodilators, or angiotensin-converting enzyme inhibitors are standard therapies used to treat hypertension).
- Antibiotic therapy **does not affect** the natural history of glomerulonephritis.
- **Prognosis and Outcome:**
  - Complete recovery in >95% of children.
  - Glomerular hyalinization and chronic renal insufficiency.

Option A

Indications for Renal biopsy in PSGN

- Persistent Hematuria and proteinuria.
- Diminished renal function.
- Low C3 level persist more than 2 months after onset.
- Nephrotic syndrome.
- Absence of evidence for streptococcal infection.

Option C and D: Cyclosporine and steroids are **NOT** used in poststreptococcal glomerulonephritis.

Ans: (b) Conservative Management

Ref: *Nelson Textbook of Paediatrics, 20th Edition, Page 2501*

2. **An infant brought to emergency, unresponsive, bradycardia, shallow breathing. Next step of management:**

(a) IV epinephrine
(b) IV atropine
(c) Stabilise the airway and assist breathing
(d) Cardiopulmonary resuscitation

Explanation:

Approach to bradycardia in children: (PALS Algorithm)

(A) Child is stable then:

- Support Basics (ABCs) and give oxygen if indicated.
- 12 Lead ECG – if available.
- Observe and Consider Cardiology consultation – to identify the cause and treat it.

(B) Child is unstable (altered level of consciousness or signs of poor perfusion), then:

- Be sure that the airway is patent and assist breathing.
- Administer oxygen as needed (O_2 saturation less than 94% or the presence of shortness of breath).
- Apply cardiac monitor, take and monitor vital signs including pulse oximetry obtain IV or IO access.

(C) If HR <60/min with poor perfusion despite O_2 and ventilation then:

- Begin CPR.
- Administer Epinephrine 0.01 mg/kg (0.1 ml/kg) of 1:10,000.
- Can be repeated every 3-5 minutes if bradycardia does not resolve.
- If IV/IO assese in not available then epinephrine can be given endoatracheally at dose of 0.1 ml/kg of 1:1000 dilution.

Note: In our case the child is unresponsive and bradycardic (HR not mentioned), hence the next immediate step will be **Stabilise the airway and assist breathing.**

Option A and D: Epinephrine/Cardiopulmonary resuscitation have to be done (though this is not the immediate step) if the HR< 60/min despite of the initial steps of airway stabilisation and assisting breathing.

Option B: Atropine can be given in increased vagal tone or in AV block, but this is not the immediate step.

Ans: (c) Stabilise the airway and assist breathing

Ref: *Pediatrics Advanced Life Support Provider Manual (2015)*

3. **True about Pott shunt:**

(a) Ascending aorta and right pulmonary artery
(b) Left pulmonary artery with descending aorta
(c) Subclavian artery and pulmonary artery
(d) Superior vena cava and right pulmonary artery

Explanation:

Table 1: Important Shunt procedures in Cyanotic heart diseases

Shunt	Between the structure	Indication	Mechanism of action
Pott shunt	**Descending thoracic aorta** and the **left pulmonary artery**	Palliative surgery for **TOF**	Improves pulmonary blood flow and thus the cyanosis
Sano shunt	Extra cardiac conduit between the **right ventricle** and **main pulmonary artery** stump	As a step in **Norwood procedure** for **hypoplastic left heart syndrome**	Reduces coronary steal phenomenon associated with *Blalock-Taussig shunt*
Waterston shunt	Between the **ascending aorta** and the **right pulmonary artery**	Palliative surgery performed in patients with **tetralogy of Fallot**	Improves pulmonary blood flow and thus the cyanosis
Blalock-Taussig shunt	Branch of the **subclavian artery** separated and connected with the **pulmonary artery**	Palliative procedure performed in patients with **tetralogy of Fallot**	To increase pulmonary blood flow for palliation in duct dependent cyanotic heart defects like pulmonary atresia
Glenn shunt	Anastomosis of the **side of** the **SVC** with the **distal end of the divided right pulmonary artery**	**Single ventricle, Hypoplastic Left Heart Syndrome**	The systemic venous return is redirected to the pulmonary circulation, bypassing the right heart

Ans: (b) Descending thoracic aorta and the left pulmonary artery

Ref: *Park's Pediatric Cardiology for Practitioners, 7th Edition; Nelson, 20th Edition, Page 2215*

4. **Urine osmolality in preterm:**

(a) 200 (b) 400 (c) 500 (d) 800

Explanation:

- The physiological range for urine osmolality in neonates varies from a lower limit of 50 mmol/L to an upper limit of **500 mmol/L in preterms and 800 mmol/L in term infants.**

Ans: (c) 500 mmol/L

Ref: *Manual of Neonatal Care, 7th Edition, John P Cloherty*

5. **A 4 months old infant with UTI was treated for 14 days with IV cefotaxime. What is the next step in management?**

(a) USG only
(b) USG + MCU
(c) USG + DMSA
(d) USG + MCU + DMSA

Explanation:

UTI management in children:

- **Diagnosis of UTI:**

Growth of significant organism in single urine sample
• (Significant pyuria is defined as >10 leukocytes per mm^3 in a fresh **uncentrifuged sample,** or >5 leukocytes per high power field in a **centrifuged sample**)/(Significant bacteriuria Colony count of **>10^5/mL** of a single species in a midstream clean catch sample)

Contd.

Contd.

PLUS
Urinary symptoms
• Other causes of leukocyturia: fever, glomerulonephritis, renal stones or presence of foreign body in the urinary tract.

- **Evaluation for first episode of UTI (Fig. 1).**

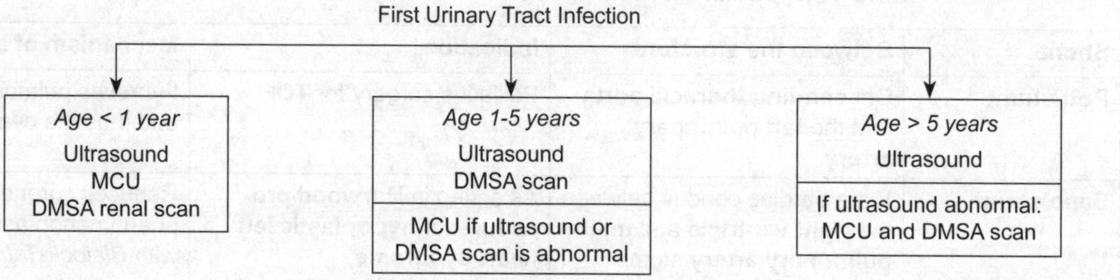

Fig. 1: Approach to first episode of UTI in children

  - **Ultrasonography** should be done soon after the diagnosis of UTI. (Information on kidney size, number and location, presence of hydronephrosis, urinary bladder anomalies and post-void residual urine).
  - **DMSA scintigraphy** is a sensitive technique for detecting renal parenchymal infection and cortical scarring and is carried out 2-3 months after treatment of UTI.
  - **Micturating Cysto Urethrogram** detects VUR and provides anatomical details regarding the bladder and the urethra. The MCU is recommended 2-3 weeks after the treatment of UTI.
- **Antibiotic prophylaxis in UTI:**

Indicated in	**Not indicated in**
• UTI below 1 year of age, while awaiting imaging studies • VUR (Till 1 year for grades I and II reflux; for higher grades prophylaxis till 5 years, or longer in case of bowel bladder dysfunction or breakthrough UTI • Frequent febrile UTI (3 or more episodes in a year) even if the urinary tract is normal	• In patients with urinary tract obstruction (e.g., posterior urethral valves) • Urolithiasis and neurogenic bladder • In patients on clean intermittent catheterization

Table 2: Drugs used for urinary prophylaxis in children

Medication	Dose, mg/kg/day	Remarks
Cotrimoxazole	1-2*	Avoid in infants <3 months, glucose-6-phosphate dehydrogenase deficiency
Nitrofurantoin	1-2	May cause vomiting and nausea; avoid in infants <3 months, G6PD deficiency, renal insufficiency
Cephalexin	10	Drug of choice in first 3-6 months of life
Cefadroxil	5	An alternative agent in early infancy

Ans: (d) USG + MCU + DMSA

Ref: *Principles and Practice of Pediatric Nephrology, 2nd Edition – Vijayakumar M; Nelson, 20th Edition, Page 2560*

6. **Congenital lobar emphysema is commonly seen in which lobe?**

(a) Left lower (b) Right upper (c) Left upper (d) Right lower

Explanation:

Congenital lobar emphysema:

- Caused by localized obstruction due to:
  - ***Congenital deficiency of the bronchial cartilage***

- ***External compression by aberrant vessels***
- ***Bronchial stenosis***
- ***Redundant bronchial mucosal flaps***
- ***Kinking of the bronchus caused by herniation into the mediastinum***

- Diagnosed by **antenatal ultrasonography.**
- CLE affects **the upper and middle lobes,** with the **left upper lobe*** being the **most common** site.
- A radiolucent lobe and a mediastinal shift are often revealed by radiographic examination.
- A CT scan may demonstrate the aberrant anatomy of the lesion.
- MRI/MRA will demonstrate any vascular lesions, which might be causing extraluminal compression.
- **Treatment** by immediate surgery and excision of the lobe may be lifesaving in the presence of cyanosis and severe respiratory distress.
- **Overinflation of all three lobes of the right lung** has been produced by **anomalous location of the left pulmonary artery,** which impinges on the right main stem bronchus.
- Hyperinflation also occurs in patients with the **absent pulmonary valve type of tetralogy of Fallot** and secondary aneurysmal dilatation of the pulmonary artery, which partially compresses the main stem bronchi.

Congenital Cystic Adenomatoid Malformation

• Consists of **hamartomatous or dysplastic lung tissue** mixed with more **normal lung.** • Usually confined to **one lobe** (less frequent in **middle lobe**). • Due to embryologic insult, **before the 35th day of gestation,** with **maldevelopment** of **terminal bronchiolar structures.**
• Three histologic patterns: o **Type 1** (50%) is **macrocystic** (>2 cm in diameter) cysts lined with ciliated **pseudostratified** epithelium. Good prognosis for survival. o **Type 2** (40%) is **microcystic** small cysts with similar histology to that of the type 1 lesion and carries a **poor prognosis.** o **Type 3** (<10%) is solid with **bronchiole-like structures** lined with **cuboidal ciliated epithelium** and separated by areas of **nonciliated cuboidal epithelium.** Usually **fatal.**
• Diagnosed in utero by ultrasonography. • Postnatal CT allows for accurate sizing of the lesion.
• Presents in early infancy with respiratory distress, **recurrent respiratory infection** and **pneumothorax.**
• Often confused with a **diaphragmatic hernia.**
• **Antenatal treatment:** o Excision of the affected lobe for microcystic lesions. o Aspiration of macrocystic lesions. o **Open fetal surgery.** • **Postnatal surgery** is indicated for all symptomatic patients.

Pulmonary Sequestration

• Aberrant formation of segmental lung tissue that has no connection with the bronchial tree or pulmonary arteries. • Intrapulmonary or extrapulmonary, depending on the location within the visceral pleura, they functions as a space-occupying lesion. • **Most common is intrapulmonary*.** • Lung tissue in a sequestration does not connect to a bronchus. • Receives its **arterial** supply from the systemic arteries (commonly off the aorta). • Returns its **venous** blood to the right side of the heart through the inferior vena cava in extralobar or pulmonary veins in intralobar. • **Gastric or pancreatic tissue** may be found within the sequestration. • **CT with contrast** can demonstrate both the extent of the lesion and its vascular supply.
• Surgical removal is recommended. o ***Intrapulmonary sequestration* – seen in lower lobe** and does not have its own pleura. Segmental resection occasionally suffices.

Contd.

Contd.

- *Extrapulmonary sequestration* – **more common in males and almost always involves the left lung** and it is enveloped by a pleural covering and is associated with **diaphragmatic hernia*** and other abnormalities such as **colonic duplication*, vertebral abnormalities***, and **pulmonary hypoplasia***. Surgical resection of the involved area is recommended.

Pulmonary Agenesis

- Complete absence of a lung, Unilateral agenesis.
- Bilateral agenesis is incompatibility with life.
- **Right lung** agenesis has a **higher morbidity** and **mortality** than left lung agenesis.
- Associated with **VACTERL sequence** (**v**ertebral anomalies, **a**nal atresia, **c**ongenital heart disease, **t**racheo **e**sophageal fistula, **r**enal anomalies and **l**imb anomalies.
- **X-ray** shows **unilateral lung or lobar collapse** with a **shift of mediastinal structures** toward the affected side.
- CT of the chest is **diagnostic**.

Pulmonary Hypoplasia

- Secondary to other **intrauterine disorders** that produce an impairment of normal lung development like:
  - ***Deformities of the thoracic spine and rib cage (thoracic dystrophy)***
  - ***Pleural effusions with fetal hydrops***
  - ***Cystic adenomatoid malformation***
  - ***Congenital diaphragmatic hernia***
  - ***Oligohydramnios***
- Involves a **decrease** in both the number of **alveoli** and the number of **airway generations.**
- Inhaled **nitric oxide/ECMO** may provide gas exchange for a critical period of time and permit survival.
- **Rib expanding devices** may improve the survival of patients with thoracic dystrophies.

Congenital Diaphragmatic Hernia

- Common site is the **left hemithorax***, with the defect in the diaphragm being posterior **(foramen of Bochdalek*)** in 70% of infants.
- 1 in 4,000 live births.
- Associated with **trisomies 13 and 18, and 45 XO,** and **Goldenhar, Beckwith-Wiedemann, Pierre Robin** syndromes.
- Present at birth with cyanosis, respiratory distress, a **scaphoid abdomen,** decreased or absent breath sounds on the side of the hernia, and **heart sounds displaced** to the side opposite the hernia.
- Small hernias, right-sided hernias, sac-type hernias, and **substernal hernias of Morgagni** may have a more subtle presentation, manifested as feeding problems and mild respiratory distress.

Diagnosis

- **Prenatal Diagnosis.** Occur after the routine **16-week** prenatal ultrasonography; therefore, many of these cases are not diagnosed until postnatally.
- The development of **polyhydramnios** can prompt a later fetal ultrasonography that will detect DH.
- Presence of **liver in the thorax*** correlates with **increased severity and poorer prognosis.**

- **Lung-to-head ratio** (LHR measured prenatally predict severity of involvement and help guide initial therapy.
  - LHR <1 – No survivors
  - LHR >1.4 has a 100% survival rate
  - LHR between 1 and 1.4 – has a 38% survival rate with a high need for extracorporeal membrane oxygenation (ECMO).

- Severe cases that have been diagnosed before birth may be best managed with delivery by the **EXIT (Ex Utero Intrapartum Treatment Procedure) procedure and ECMO.**

Ans: (c) Left upper lobe

***Ref:** Nelson Textbook of Paediatrics, 20th Edition, Page 2051 and Manual of Neonatal Care, 7th Edition – John P Cloherty*

7. **Lorenzo oil used in treatment of:**

(a) Gaucher disease
(b) Adrenoleucodystrophy
(c) Fabry's disease
(d) Hurles disease

Explanation:

Lorenzo's oil

- Lorenzo's oil (**4 : 1** mixture of **glyceryl trioleate** and **glyceryl trierucate**).
- Only available to patients participating in a clinical trial.
- **Indication:**
  - o **Adrenoleukodystrophy** ALD in children (asymptomatic boys < 8 years old, with normal MRI reduces the risk of developing the childhood cerebral phenotype).
  - o Adrenomyeloneuropathy in adults.
- **Lorenzo's oil dosage:**
  - o Upto **3 mL/day** in children **8 years of age** (average) has been used in a clinical study.
  - o Case studies in Zellweger syndrome report using Lorenzo's oil 2 g/kg daily.
- **Thrombocytopenia** has been reported following treatment with Lorenzo's oil.

CLASSIFICATION OF PEROXISOMAL DISORDERS

(A) Disorders of Peroxisome Import

- *A1: Zellweger syndrome*
- *A2: Neonatal adrenoleukodystrophy*
- *A3: Infantile Refsum disease*

(B) Defects of Single Peroxisomal Enzyme

- *B1: X-linked adrenoleukodystrophy*
- *B5: Classic Refsum disease*
- *B10: Glutaric aciduria type III*

ZELLWEGER SYNDROME

- Typical facial appearance
  - o High forehead
  - o Unslanting palpebral fissures
  - o **Hypoplastic supraorbital ridges***
  - o **Epicanthal folds***
- **CNS:** Severe **weakness**, **hypotonia** and neonatal*.
- **Eye abnormalities** (Cataracts, Glaucoma, **Corneal clouding*, Brushfield spots*, pigmentary retinopathy,*** and nerve dysplasia).
- **DD: Down syndrome** may be suspected due to hypotonia and "mongoloid" appearance.

ADRENOLEUKODYSTROPHY (X-LINKED)

- Accumulation of un-branched saturated VLCFA.
- Progressive dysfunction of:
  - o **Adrenal cortex.**
  - o **Central** nervous system **white matter.**
  - o **Peripheral** nervous system **white matter.**
- Key biochemical defect – Impaired function of **peroxisomal lignoceroyl CoA ligase** leads to excess accumulation of **hexacosanoic acid** (C26:0).
- **Lamellar cytoplasmic inclusions** – Electron microscope in:
  - o Adrenocortical cells (mainly **zona fasciculata***).
  - o **Testicular Leydig cells.**
  - o **Nervous system macrophages.**

Types:

- **Childhood cerebral form** of ALD, sy 4 and 8 years (hyperactivity, which is often mistaken for an attention deficit disorder) **Auditory discrimination** is often impaired. Other initial symptoms are disturbances of vision, ataxia, poor handwriting, seizures and strabismus.

- **Adolescent ALD** 10 and 21 years. Similar to childhood cerebral ALD except slow progression.
- **Adrenomyeloneuropathy** presents in adulthood as a progressive paraparesis.
- **Laboratory finding** – Abnormally high levels of VLCFA in plasma, red blood cells, or cultured skin fibroblasts.
- CT/MRI shows cerebral white matter lesions which are symmetric and involve the periventricular white matter in the posterior parietal and occipital lobes.
- Lorenzo Oil and bone marrow transplant were the treatment available.

Available Enzyme replacement therapy:

Disease	Deficiency	Accumulation of	Enzyme replacement available
Gaucher Disease Lysosomal storage disorder	Enzyme glucocerebrosidase	Glycolipid glucocerebroside	Imiglucerase Velaglucerase alfa
Fabry disease Lysosomal storage disorder	α-galactosidase A	Globotriaosylceramide	Agalsidasealfa and beta
Pompes disease Glycogen storage disease type II	Acid maltase	Glycogen	Alglucosidasealfa
Hurlers disease Mucopolysaccharidoses type 1	Alpha-L-iduronidase	Macromolecular glycosaminoglycans	laronidase
Hunter syndrome Mucopolysaccharidosis II	Iduronate-2-sulfatase,	Glycosaminoglycans	Idursulfase
Maroteaux-Lamy syndrome Mucopolysaccharidosis type VI	Arylsulphatase B	Dermatan sulphate	Galsulfase

Ans: (b) Adrenoleukodystrophy

Ref: *Nelson Textbook of Paediatrics, 20th Edition, Page 691*

8. **A child with tetralogy of Fallot and polydactyly is diagnosed to have vaginal atresia. Likely diagnosis:**

(a) Ellis-van Creveld syndrome
(b) Rubinstein-Taybi syndrome
(c) McKusick-Kaufman syndrome
(d) Edwards syndrome

Explanation:

McKusick-Kaufman syndrome

- Autosomal recessive disease.
- Postaxial polydactyly (PAP).
- Congenital heart disease (CHD).
- In Females: Hydrometrocolpos.
- In Males: Hypospadias or Cryptorchidism.

Polydactyly:

Post-axial	Extra finger or toe present on the **ulnar border** of the hand
Pre-axial	Extra finger or toe present on the **radial border** of the hand

Common Syndromes Associated with Polydactyly

- Carpenter syndrome.
- Ellis-van Creveld syndrome.
- Meckel-Gruber syndrome.
- Trisomy 13.
- Rubinstein-Taybi syndrome.

Option A:

Ellis-van Creveld syndrome
- Short limb dwarfism.
- Polydactyly.
- Abnormal development of fingernails.
- **Single common atrium** is most common cardiac defect.

Option B:

Rubinstein-Taybi syndrome
- Growth delays.
- Intellectual disability.
- Abnormally broad and often angulated **thumbs and great toes (halluces).**
- Feeding difficulties (dysphagia).
- The characteristic facial features:
  - Downward slanted eyes (downslanted palpebral fissures).
  - Long eyelashes.
  - High-arched eyebrows.
  - Low-hanging nasal septum (columella).
  - High palate.
  - Grimacing smile.
  - Extra cusp on the lingual side of a front tooth **(talon cusps).**
- **Patent ductus arteriosus** is the most common cardiac anomaly*.

Option D:

Bardet-Biedl syndrome
- Polydactyly.
- **Cardiomyopathy** is the most common cardiac anomaly*.
- Congenital heart disease.
- Nyctalopia.
- Obesity.
- Anosmia.
- Dental anomalies.
- Renal anomalies.

Ans: (b) McKusick-Kaufman syndrome

Ref: *Nelson Textbook of Paediatrics, 20th Edition, Page 2214*

9. **RBC lifespan in preterm babies:**

(a) 60–75 (b) 35–50 (c) 75–90 (d) 100–120

Explanation:

Life span of RBCs
- In **Adults – 120 days.**
- **Term** neonate – **60 and 90 days.**
- **Preterm** neonates – **35 to 50 days.**

Ans: (b) 35 to 50 days

Ref: *Manual of Neonatal Care, 7th Edition, John P Cloherty*

10. **Osteogenesis imperfecta with normal dentition and sclera:**

(a) Type 1A (b) Type 2 (c) Type 3 (d) Type 4B

Explanation:

Osteogenesis Imperfecta/OI (brittle bone disease):
- Most common genetic cause of **osteoporosis***.
- Autosomal dominant disorder.

- Quantitative defects in **type I collagen** – heterotrimer, composed of two α1(I) chains and one α2(I) chain (primary component of the extracellular matrix of bone and skin).
- The structural defects are 2 types:
  - 80% – point mutations, substitutions of **helical glycine residues.**
  - 20% are single exon **splicing defects.**
- One third of mutations in the **α1** chain are **lethal** while **glycine substitutions** in α2 **(I)** are predominantly nonlethal.
- **OI congenital** – forms detectable at birth.
- **OI tarda** – forms detectable later in childhood.

Triad of Osteogenesis Imperfecta (OI)

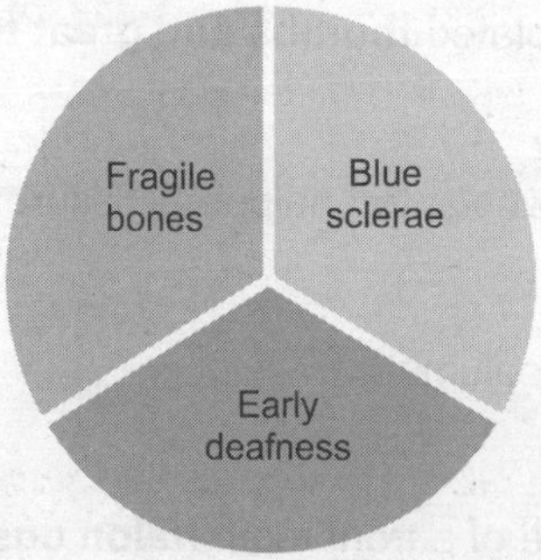

The **Sillence classification** divides OI into 4 types based on **clinical and radiographic** criteria

OI type	Severity	Classical features	Other features
I	Mild	**Blue sclerae,** recurrent fractures in childhood, and presenile hearing loss	Easy bruising, joint laxity, and mild short stature
II	Perinatal/Lethal	Birthweight and length are small for gestational age, multiple intrauterine fractures of long bones, frog-leg position, **dark blue to gray sclera**	Respiratory insufficiency, enlarged anterior and posterior fontanelles
III	Progressive Deforming	Most severe nonlethal form of OI, Fractures usually occur in utero, **"popcorn" appearance** at the **metaphyses, sclera blue or white**	Scoliosis and vertebral compression, extreme short stature
IV	Moderately severe	Moderate bowing even with infrequent fractures, recurrent fractures after ambulation. Fracture rates decrease after puberty, **Sclera blue or white**	Moderate short stature. Scleral hue may be blue or white
Other	Type V (Hyperplastic Callus), Type VI (Mineralization Defect), and Type VII (Autosomal Recessive).		

Both types I and IV are divided – **Absence (A) or Presence (B)** of **dentinogenesis imperfecta.**

Diagnosis:

- Sequencing of **cDNA** using **fibroblasts** cultured from a **skin punch biopsy.**
- Severe OI can be detected **prenatally** by **level II ultrasonography** as early as **16 weeks of gestation.**
- In the neonatal period, the normal to **elevated alkaline phosphatase** levels present in OI distinguish it from **hypophosphatasia.**

Complications:

- Recurrent pneumonias and declining pulmonary function occur in childhood.
- Corpulmonale is seen in adults.
- Basilar invagination.
- Brainstem compression.

- Hydrocephalus.
- Syringohydromyelia.

Management

- There is no cure for OI.
- **Growth hormone** improves bone histology in growth-responsive children (usually types **I and IV**).
- **Bisphosphonates** – beneficial for vertebrae (trabecular bone) than long bones (cortical bone).

Option A: Type IA – Have normal dentition but blue sclera.

Option B: Type 2 – Have blue sclera.

Option D: Type 4B – Normal sclera but presence of dental findings.

Ans: (c) Type 3

Ref: *Nelson Textbook of Paediatrics, 20th Edition, Page 3380*

11. All are the features of Digeorge syndrome *except*:

(a) Recurrent infection
(b) Mandibular hypoplasia
(c) Impaired B cell function
(d) Hypocalcaemia seizures

Explanation:

DiGeorge syndrome

- **Also known as 22q11.2 deletion syndrome and velocardiofacial syndrome.**
- Occurs in **both sexes.**
- **Microdeletions** from chromosome **22q11.2*.**
- Mutation of **T-box transcription family member, *TBX1,*** has been implicated as an etiology.
- Disorder of **T cell production*.**
- **Basic pathology:**
  - **Dysmorphogenesis of 3rd and 4th pharyngeal pouches*.**
  - **Hypoplasia** of the **thymus (Recurrent infection)** and **parathyroid glands (Hypocalcemia).**
- **Associated anomalies:**
  - **Right-sided aortic arch*.**
  - **Esophageal atresia.**
  - **Bifid uvula*.**
  - Congenital heart disease (**conotruncal*,** atrial and ventricular septal defects).
  - Cleft palate/a short philtrum of the upper lip.
  - Hypertelorism, antimongoloid slant, **mandibular hypoplasia,** and low-set, notched ears.
- **Complete DiGeorge syndrome:**
  - Aplasia of the thymus and parathyroid glands resemble **severe combined immunodeficiency (SCID*).**
  - **Associated with CHARGE syndrome** in 1/3rd patients (coloboma, heart defect, choanal atresia, growth or developmental retardation, genital hypoplasia, and ear anomalies including deafness).
- **Partial DiGeorge syndrome:**
  - Variable hypoplasia of the thymus and parathyroid glands.
- Concentrations of serum immunoglobulins are **normal*.**
- **Absolute lymphocyte counts** are **low** for age. The CD3 T-cell counts are variably decreased in number.
- **Lymphocyte** responses to **mitogen** stimulation are **absent/reduced*.**
- **Treatment:**
  - Cultured unrelated thymic tissue transplants.

Ans: (c) Impaired B cell function

Ref: *Nelson Textbook of Paediatrics, 20th Edition, Page 1020*

12. Which of the following is true about Gilles de la Tourette syndrome?

(a) Coprolalia
(b) Echolalia
(c) Methylphenidate may unmask this syndrome
(d) All of the above

Explanation:

Tics in childhood classified into 3 subgroups

- Transient tics of childhood.
- Chronic tics.
- Gilles de la Tourette syndrome (TS).

Gilles de la Tourette syndrome (TS)

- It is a lifelong condition.
- Onset between **2 and 21 years** of age.
- **Autosomal dominant** inheritance.
- **Clinical features:**
  - **Multiple motor tics** in different parts of the body (face, eyelids, neck and shoulders).
  - At least one **vocal tic** beginning before age **18 years.**
  - Waxing and waning over a period of more than a year.
- **Examples of vocal ticks:**
  - Throat clearing, sniffling and barking.
  - **Coprolalia** (Obscene words).
  - **Echolalia** (Repetition of words addressed to the patient).
  - **Palilalia** (Repetition of one's own words).
  - **Echokinesis** (Imitation of movement of others).
- **Treatment:**
  - **Methylphenidate** may unmask TS.
  - **Haloperidol** or **Clonidine** is effective in treating this condition.

DSM-V Criteria for diagnosis of TOURETTE'S DISORDER*

A. Both multiple **motor** and one or more **vocal** tics have been present at some time during the illness, although not necessarily concurrently.

B. The tics may wax and wane in frequency but have persisted for **more than 1 year** since first tic onset.

C. **Onset** is **before age 18 years.**

D. The disturbance is **not attributable** to any **drugs** (e.g., cocaine) or another **disease** (e.g., Huntington's disease, post-viral encephalitis).

Ans: (d) All of the above

Ref: *Nelson Textbook of Paediatrics, 20th Edition, Page 140*

DERMATOLOGY

1. **A 20 years male presents with erythematous papule over penis after taking an over the counter medicine. Most likely causative drug:**

(a) Aceclofenac (b) Doxycycline (c) Ofloxacin (d) Azithromycin

Explanation:

- The clinical condition described here is **Fixed drug eruption** that has occurred only on the genitalia.
- In the case of **isolated male genital fixed drug eruption** (often affecting only the **glans penis**), the drugs most commonly implicated are:
  - o **Co-trimoxazole (trimethoprim–sulfamethoxazole).**
  - o **Tetracycline, Doxycycline and Minocycline.**
  - o **Ampicillin.**

Fixed Drug Eruption (FDE)

- Reddish brown **solitary,** erythematous round oval lesion.
- Rarely can be multiple or in form of plaque, bulla or erosion.
- Natural course: **Erythematous papule → edematous → desquamation → Hyperpigmentation.**
- Site of eruption is fixed, i.e., whenever the individual takes the drug, eruptions occur at the same site.
- Recurs at **same site** within hours of **re-challenge.**
- May become generalised or blistering.
- Healing occurs over **7–10 days.**
- Melanin is increased in epidermis and dermis (melanophages).
- Pathogenesis not well understood.
- Common drugs involved:
  - o Paracetamol, Phenacetin, pheynlbutazone.
  - o Antibiotics: Sulphonamide, tetracycline group.
  - o Barbiturates.

Dermatological adverse effects of other options:

- **Tetracyclines** also can cause **photosensitivity** and **pigmentation.**
- **Ofloxacin** can cause **pustular eruption** and **photo-onycholysis.**
- **Azithromycin** has caused **toxic pustuloderma.**

Ans: (b) Doxycycline

Ref: *Rook's Textbook of Dermatology, 8th Edition, Page 28, 75*

2. **Positive Darier's sign is seen in:**

(a) Smooth muscle hamartoma (b) Urticaria pigmentosa
(c) Darier's disease (d) Lichen planus

Explanation:

Urticaria pigmentosa

- It is the most common type of **cutaneous mastocytosis.**
- Occurs due to the accumulation of **mast cells in the skin.**
- Caused by a **point mutation** at **amino acid 816** of the **proto-oncogene c-kit.**
- The skin lesions are itchy, small, yellow tan to reddish brown macules scattered all over the body.
- Mild **Trauma** such as **scratching** or **rubbing** the lesions may cause **urtication** and **erythema** around macules **(Darier's sign*).**
- Symptoms exacerbated by Temperature, spicy foods, alcohol and drugs.
- **Diagnosis:** HPE shows **mast cell infiltration** of the **dermis.**
- **Treatment:** Avoidance of **precipitating factors** and **anti-histaminics.**
- **Nifedipine,** a calcium channel blocker may reduce mast cell degranulation.
- Another mast cell stabilizer **Gastrocrom,** a form of **cromoglicic acid** has also been used to reduce mast cell degranulation.

EXTRA EDGE

Pseudo-Darier sign

- Firm stroking may provoke temporarily increased induration or piloerection.
- Seen in **Smooth muscle hamartoma.**

Darier's disease

- Multiple, symmetrical, dirty, warty, papular excrescences.
- Commonly involves face, trunk and flexures of the limbs.
- Associated with **acrokeratosis verruciformis** like papules.
- **White cobblestone-like papules** may be seen on the **palate** and **tongue.**
- **Nail changes:**
  - o Longitudinal subungual, red and white streaks with subungual keratosis.
  - o Thinning of the nail plate, fragility and splintering.
  - o Triangular nicking of the free edges.
- HPE: Hyperkeratosis, acanthosis and papillomatosis.
- **Treatment** options **Vitamin A** and its derivatives like etretinate.

Ans: (b) Urticaria pigmentosa

***Ref:** Rook, 8th Edition, Page 14, 22, 31 and 35*

3. **Boggy swelling of scalp in a child is caused by:**

(a) Trichophyton mentagrophytes (b) T. violaceum
(c) Microsporum canum (d) M. furfur

Explanation:

- The history of boggy inflammatory swelling of scalp in a child is suggestive of the diagnosis of inflammatory type of **tinea capitis** called as **Kerion.**
- Among given options, **Trichophyton mentagrophytes** is commonly implicated in Kerion.

TINEA CAPITIS

- Cutaneous fungal infection of scalp.
- Endothrix and Ectothrix.
- Most common – **Trichophyton violaceum.**

Varieties:

(A) Non inflammatory

- Gray patch
- Black dot
- Seborrheic dermatitis

(B) Inflammatory

- Favus
- Kerion, agminate folliculitis

(I) ***Non inflammatory Tinea capitis:***

Black dot/Grey patch

- Breakage of hair gives rise to **'black dots'.**
- Patchy alopecia, often circular, numerous broken-off hairs, dull grey.
- Wood's lamp examination: Green fluorescence (occasional non-fluorescent cases).

(II) ***Inflammatory Tinea capitis***

Tinea capitis: Kerion, agminate folliculitis

- Inflammatory variety.
- Painful, inflammatory boggy swelling with purulent discharge.
- Caused by:
  - o ***Microsporum.***
  - o ***Trichophyton verrucosum.***
  - o ***Trichophyton mentagrophytes.***
- Hairs may be matted, easily pluckable.
- Lymphadenopathy.

- Co-infection with bacteria is common.
- May heal with scarring alopecia.

(III) *Tinea capitis: Favus*
- Inflammatory variety.
- Seen in Kashmir.
- Most common cause – **Trichophyton schoenleinii.**
- Yellowish, cup-shaped crusts develop around a hair with the hair projecting centrally.
- Extensive patchy hair loss with **cicatricial alopecia.**

Ans: (a) Trichophyton mentagrophytes

Ref: *Rook, 8th Edition, Page 20, 27, 36*

4. A 9-month infant presented with yellow crust, greasy scales on scalp and crusting of flexures. Most probable diagnosis:

(a) Atopic dermatitis (b) Infantile Seborrheic dermatitis
(c) Allergic contact dermatitis (d) Irritant dermatitis

Explanation:

- As such there is some confusion if the two diseases **Atopic dermatitis** and **Infantile seborrheic dermatitis** are two different entities or part of same clinic-pathological spectrum.
- This is because many infants diagnosed with **infantile seborrheic dermatitis** go on to develop classical **atopic dermatitis** later in life.
- The question tells that the infant is 9-month-old. Usually infantile **seborrheic dermatitis** is seen during the **first three months** of life, usually between the **third and eighth** week.
- If the question had the age of the child within **three months,** infantile seborrheic dermatitis seems to be the best option among the choices provided because of the greasy nature of the scales which is classical of seborrheic dermatitis.
- Similarly the sites of involvement mentions **scalp and flexures.** Atopic dermatitis in infants usually **extensor** aspects of limbs are involved and **not the flexures. Flexural lichenification** of **Atopic dermatitis** is a feature in **adults** and not infants. Atopic dermatitis is **pruritic** but Infantile seborrheic dermatitis is **not pruritic.**
- Infantile SD involves the **eyebrows, paranasal areas,** and the **flexural areas,** this distribution of lesions is also helpful in distinguishing between Infantile SD and Atopic dermatitis.
- A family history of **Atopy** is helpful to aid in the diagnosis of **Atopic dermatitis.**
- Infantile **seborrheic dermatitis spontaneously resolves** but **atopic dermatitis** can **relapse.**
- The term infantile **'seborrheic' dermatitis** is widely used to describe an allegedly **distinctive eczematous** or **psoriasiform eruption** seen in infants, having a predilection for the scalp and the proximal flexures, and a favourable prognosis compared with atopic dermatitis.

ATOPIC DERMATITIS
- In infancy begins as erythema and scaling of the cheeks.
- The eruption may extend to the scalp, neck, forehead, wrists and extensor extremities.
- The lesions may be popular or exudative.

The major criteria to diagnose Atopic dermatitis are: Must have 3 of the following:

(A) Pruritus

(B) Typical morphology and distribution
- Flexural lichenification in adults.
- Facial and extensor involvement in infancy.

(C) Chronic or chronically relapsing dermatitis.

(D) Peronal or **family** history of **atopic disease** (asthma, allergic rhinitis, atopic dermatitis).

The minor criteria are: Must have 3 of the following:
- Xerosis, Ichthyosis/hyperlinear palms/Keratosis pilaris.
- IgE reactivity, Elevated serum IgE.
- Early age of onset, Dennie-Morgan infraorbital fold, Keratoconus.
- Tendency to cutaneous infections, Tendency to Nonspecific hand/foot dermatitis, nipple eczema, cheilitis.

- Recurrent conjunctivitis, anterior subcapsular cataracts, orbital darkening, facial pallor/facial erythema.
- Pityriasis alba, Itch when sweating, intolerance to wool and lipid solvents, perifollicular accentuation.
- Food hypersensitivity, course influenced by environmental and/or emotional factors and white dermographism or delayed blanch to cholinergic agents.

Allergic Contact Dermatitis:

- It is an acquired sensitivity to various substances that produce inflammatory reactions in those and only those, who have been previously sensitized to the allergen.
- It is a delayed hypersensitivity reaction.
- Some common causes of allergic contact dermatitis are nickel, neomycin, gold, formaldehyde etc.
- Eczematous reaction occurs and itching is the classical symptom.
- It can be diagnosed using patch testing.

Irritant Dermatitis:

- It is an inflammatory reaction in the skin resulting from exposure to a substance in sufficiently high concentration that causes an eruption in most people who come in contact with it.
- **No previous exposure** is needed and the effect is evident within minutes or a few hours at most.
- Common causes of Irritant dermatitis are alkalies such as soaps, detergents etc and acids like HCl, Hydrofluoric acid etc.
- Symptomatically **pain and burning** are more common in irritant dermatitis unlike itch of allergic contact dermatitis.

Ans: (b) Infantile Seborrheic dermatitis

Ref: *IADVL Textbook of Dermatology, 2nd Edition, Page 497-99; Rook, 8th Edition, Page 17, 28, 499; Andrews' Diseases of the Skin, Clinical Dermatology, 10th Edition, Page 69-70, 91*

5. **A 34-year-old female presents with itchy, maculopapular lesion in the inner aspect of wrists, ankles and forearms. Her oral mucosa has a white lace like eruptions in tongue with oral ulcers. What is the most probable diagnosis?**

(a) Lichen planus (b) Eczema (c) Pityriasis rosea (d) Psoriasis

Explanation:

LICHEN PLANUS

- Lichen planus is a **pruritic,** inflammatory **papulosquamous** disorder affecting the **skin, mucous membranes, nails** and **hair follicles.**
- ***Etiology*** **– unknown**
  - o Genetic predisposition: **HLA B8–oral LP; HLA-Bw35-cutaneous LP.**
  - o Exogenous: **Primary biliary cirrhosis, alcoholic cirrhosis, hepatitis B, hepatitis C.**
  - o Drugs cause lichenoid drug eruptions.
  - o Metals like **mercury** (dental amalgams), **palladium, gold** – oral lichenoid eruptions.
- ***Clinical features:***
  - o 30-60 years; children–4% of cases, childhood LP more common in India.
  - o **Skin:**
    - ▪ Intensely pruritic, flat topped, shiny, polygonal, violaceous papules and plaques.
    - ▪ Predominantly flexor distribution – flexor of wrist, forearm, legs, trunk, glans penis (cf–psoriasis another papulosquamous disorder has predominant extensor distribution).
    - ▪ **Wickham's striae** – network of greyish white streaks on papules seen on pressing with glass slide after application of oil – corresponds to wedge shaped hypergranulosis seen on histopathology.
    - ▪ **Koebner/isomorphic phenomenon** common.
    - ▪ Annular LP – glans penis.
    - ▪ Hypertrophic LP – shins.
    - ▪ Actinic LP – sun exposed areas.
  - o **Oral:**
    - ▪ Classical type is **reticulate pattern** – white/**violaceouslacy reticular network** of coalesent papules in buccal mucosa and tongue; usually asymptomatic.
    - ▪ Most common pattern – ulcerative/erosive LP.

- o **Nail:**
  - 5-10% cases.
  - **Thinning of nail plate** (cf psoriasis – thickening of nail plate), **longitudinal ridging,** roughening of nail plate **(trachyonychia)** and nail dystrophy involving all 20 nails called 20 nail dystrophy (also seen in alopecia areata).
  - Classical/characteristic nail finding (but not common finding) – **pterygiumformation** (proximal nail fold fuses with nail bed).
- o **Hair follicles: Lichen planopilaris – scarring alopecia.**

- ***Histopathology:***
  - o Hyperkeratosis.
  - o Wedge shaped hypergranulosis (psoriasis – hypogranulosis).
  - o Irregular acanthosis (psoriasis – regular acanthosis).
  - o **Saw tooth rete ridges** (psoriasis – elephant foot/camel foot like/ club shaped rete ridges).
  - o Basal layer vacuolar degeneration.
  - o Band like dermal lymphocytic infiltrate hugging epidermis.
  - o **Max Joseph spaces** – subepidermal clear zone (subepidermal clear zone in lepromatous leprosy is called Grenz zone).
  - o Melanin incontinence.
- ***Treatment*** – Steroids (topical/intralesional/systemic), retinoids, cyclosporine, PUVA photochemotherapy, dapsone, methotrexate.

Remember:

- **Lichen planus – "8 P's":**
  - o Papulosquamous disorder characterized by:
    - **P**ruritic.
    - **P**lane topped.
    - **P**olygonal/**P**olyangular.
    - **P**urple coloured.
    - **P**apules and **P**laques.
    - Heal with **P**igmentation.
    - Shows characteristic **P**terygium formation in nails.

OTHER OPTIONS

Psoriasis

- Pruritic papulosquamous disorder characterized by well defined erythematous papules and plaques covered by **silvery white micaceous scales** with predominant **extensor** distribution.
- Mucosal lesions are very rare–annular plaques, diffuse erythema, **geographic tongue.**
- **Auspitz sign** will be positive.

Pityriasis rosea

- Papulosquamous disorder with pruritic or asymptomatic lesions with an initial herald or mother patch on trunk followed by daughter patches two weeks later in a **Christmas tree pattern** along lines of cleavage with a **peripheral collarette of scale** producing the hanging curtain sign when stretched.
- No oral lesions.
- Common in adolescents and young adults.

Eczema

- Pruritic papulovesicular dermatitis.
- Oozing, erythema, edema and crusting in **acute phase.**
- Crusting and scaling in **subacute phase.**
- Hyperkeratosis and lichenification in **chronic phase.**

Ans: (a) Lichen planus

Ref: *Andrew's Diseases of the Skin, 11th Edition, Page 213-27*

6. **Poikiloderma vasculare atrophicans is associated with:**

(a) SLE (b) Dermatomyositis (c) Mycosis fungoides (d) Kawasaki disease

Explanation:

- **Poikiloderma vasculare atrophicans is now recognized as a clinical form of patch-stage of mycosis fungoides.**
- In Poikiloderma vasculare atrophicans, **mottled pigmentation, atrophy** and **telangiectasia** of the **involved skin** are observed.
- A mix of **hyper- and hypopigmentation** may remain after regression of the skin lesions following treatment.
- **Poikiloderma** is also a feature of some inflammatory 'connective tissue' diseases, and is particularly characteristic of **dermatomyositis.**
- It is also seen in **lupus erythematosus** and rarely in **systemic sclerosis.**

Ans: (c) Mycosis fungoides

Ref: *Andrews' Diseases of the Skin, 10th Edition, Page 728*

7. **A pregnant woman presents with vulval warts. What is the ideal treatment?**

(a) Cryothearpy (b) Tricholoracetic acid
(c) Excision (d) Observation

Explanation:

*"**Cryotherapy** is a safe treatment of vulval warts in pregnancy."*

– IADVL Textbook of Dermatology, 2nd Ed., Page 1921

Pregnancy and genital warts:

- **Imiquimod, sinecatechins, podophyllin, and podofilox should not be used** during pregnancy.
- Genital warts can proliferate and become **friable** during pregnancy.
- Although removal of warts during pregnancy can be considered, resolution might be **incomplete or poor** until pregnancy is complete.
- Rarely, HPV types **6 and 11** can cause **respiratory papillomatosis** in infants and children, although the route of transmission (i.e., **transplacental, perinatal, or postnatal**) is not completely understood.
- Whether cesarean section prevents respiratory papillomatosis in infants and children also is unclear; therefore, cesarean delivery should not be performed solely to prevent transmission of HPV infection to the newborn.
- **Cesarean delivery** is indicated for women with **genital warts** if the pelvic outlet is obstructed or if vaginal delivery would result in excessive bleeding.
- Pregnant women with genital warts should be counselled concerning the low risk for warts on the **larynx (recurrent respiratory papillomatosis)** in their **infants** or **children. – CDC STD Treatment Guidelines 2010.**

Ans: (a) Cryotherapy

Ref: *IADVL Textbook of Dermatology, 2nd Edition, Page 1921 and CDC STD Treatment Guidelines, 2010*

8. **A 1 year boy with chronic diarrhea present with refractory peri-oral erosion and peri-anal erosions. History of intermittent diaper use is present. Probable diagnosis:**

(a) Irritant contact dermatitis (Diaper dermatitis)
(b) Acrodermatitis enteropathica
(c) Olmsted syndrome
(d) Biotin deficiency

Explanation:

- Presence of peri-oral lesions rules out diaper dermatitis.

Irritant contact dermatitis

- Also known as **Diaper dermatitis** or **Napkin dermatitis** or **Primary irritant napkin dermatitis.**
- Lesions limited to **exposed surfaces** and the **folds are spared,** in contrast to **intertrigo, inverse psoriasis** and **candidiasis,** where the **folds are frequently involved.**
- In severe cases, **superficial erosion** or **even ulceration.**
- **Constant maceration** of the skin is **critical.**

- Not seen in the absence of diaper use.
- **Moist skin** is more easily **abraded by friction** of the diaper as the child moves.
- It is also **more permeable to irritants** and also allows the **growth of bacteria** and **yeast,** which **raise** the **local pH,** increasing the **activity of fecal lipases** and **proteases.**
- **Candidiasis** may be a **secondary phenomenon.**
- Diaper dermatitis as we saw above is **irritant dermatitis** and not **Allergic Contact dermatitis.**

Acrodermatitis enteropathica:

- Inherited **autosomal recessively.**
- **Premature** infants are at risk.
- The dermatitis is typically seen in **acral** and **periorificial distribution.**
- Lesions are patchy, red, dry scaling with exudation and crusting.
- Commonly involves the **face,** in the **groin,** and other **flexors.**
- **Angular cheilitis** and **stomatitis** may be present.
- Chronic lesions may be **psoriasiform.**
- **Diarrhea** is present in most cases.
- Therefore a **chronic diaper rash** with **diarrhea** in an infant should lead to evaluation for **zinc deficiency.**
- In our question there is **no history of diarrhea** that has been mentioned. Hence, this is unlikely.

Olmstead Syndrome:

- Olmsted syndrome is a rare disorder characterized by the combination of **periorificial, keratotic plaques** and **bilateral mutilating palmoplantar keratoderma** associated with **flexion deformities** of the digits, leading to **constriction or spontaneous amputation.**

Biotin deficiency:

- It is rare. The **skin** and **nervous system** are primarily affected.
- A **dermatitis** similar to that found in cases of **zinc deficiency** and **essential fatty acid deficiency** is seen.
- It is **periorificial** and is characterized by **patchy, red, eroded lesions** on the **face** and **groin.**
- **Total alopecia** may occur.
- Conjunctivitis may be present.
- **Neurologic symptoms** include, depression, lethargy, hallucinations and limb paresthesias.

Ans: (b) Acrodermatitis enteropathica

Ref: *IADVL Textbook of Dermatology, 2nd Edition;*
Andrews' Diseases of the Skin, 10th Edition, Page 214, 483

9. A patient with a known autoimmune disease presents with oral mucosal and skin lesions. In this condition, antibodies are most likely to be present against which of the following antigens?

(a) Desmoglein 1 (b) Desmoglein 3 (c) BP230 (d) BP180

Explanation:

- The history of **oral mucosal** and **skin lesions** in a patient with **autoimmune disease** suggests a diagnosis of **Pemphigus vulgaris.**
- It can be differentiated from **Pemphigus foliaceus** in which **oral mucosal** lesions are **NOT** seen.
- Similarly mucosal lesions are **rare** in **bullous pemphigoid.**
- **Desmoglein-3 is found in desmosomes** and possibly elsewhere on the cell membrane of keratinocytes. It is detected early in keratinocyte differentiation, primarily in the lower epidermis and is **expressed more strongly in buccal mucosa and scalp skin** than in skin from the trunk. This contrasts with the pattern of expression of the **pemphigus foliaceus antigen, desmoglein-1,** which is present throughout the epidermis, more intensely in the upper layers, but **only weakly expressed in mucosae.** Since oral mucosal lesions are present in the patient, the patient is likely to have **Pemphigus vulgaris** and hence antibodies against **Desmoglein 3** are likely to be present.
- In **Bullous pemphigoid, IgG antibodies** against **BP 230 and BP 180 antigens,** which are part of **hemi-desmosomes,** are found.

PEMPHIGUS

- Autoimmune blistering disorder characterized by ***auto-antibody formation*** against the intercellular cementing substance called ***desmogleins*.***

- The mechanism of cell separation is called ***acantholysis****–loss of intercellular substance causing separation of the epidermal keratinocytes which become rounded → result in **intraepidermal blister.**
- These large rounded keratinocytes with **large nucleus, perinuclear halo** and **peripheral condensation** of cytoplasm are called the ***acantholytic cells*** – seen in **Tzanck smear.**

Types of pemphigus:
- Pemphigus vulgaris (variant-pemphigus vegetans)–most common type.
- Pemphigus foliaceus (variant-pemphigus erythematosus; endemic pemphigus or fogoselvagem).
- Paraneoplastic pemphigus.
- Drug induced pemphigus.
- IgA pemphigus.
- Neonatal pemphigus.

Clinical features:
- Fluid filled bullae→Rupture→painful erosions with no tendency to spontaneous healing.
- Painful mucosal erosions–oral (**most common;** almost in all cases in pemphigus vulgaris); genital mucosa, pharynx, larynx, conjunctiva, urethra.
- ***Bulla spread sign/Asboe Hansen sign–positive.***
- ***Nikolsky sign*** – Peeling of skin leaving behind erosions when tangential pressure applied over areas of normal looking skin or over bony prominences (other conditions–staphylococcal scalded skin syndrome, toxic epidermal necrolysis).

Diagnosis:
- Tzanck smear-acantholytic cells.
- Histopathology.
- Direct and indirect immunofluoresence.

Treatment:
- ***Systemic steroids*** are mainstay of treatment.
- Adjuvants – cyclophosphamide, azathioprine, methotrexate, mycophenolate mofetil, dapsone.
- Plasmapheresis, IV immunoglobulins.
- Biological agent – **Rituximab (anti CD20).**

Characteristics of Various Pemphigus disorders (High yield table)

Features	**Pemphigus vulgaris**	**Pemphigus foliaceus**	**Bullous pemphigoid**	**Dermatitis herpetiformis**
Antigen	**Desmoglein 3***	**Desmoglein 1***	BP 180, BP 230	Unknown
Level of split	Intraepidermal - suprabasal	Intraepidermal-subcorneal	Subepidermal	Subepidermal
Mechanism of blister	Acantholysis	Acantholysis	Basement membrane zone disruption	Basement membrane zone disruption
Age	40-60 years	40-50 years	>60 years	20-55 years
Symptoms	Pain	Pain (less severe)	Pruritus	Intensely pruritic
Type of blister	**Flaccid bullae** on normal or erythematous skin	Transient blisters	**Tense bullae** on normal or erythematous or urticated skin	Grouped erythematous papules and papulovesicles; vesicles excoriated
Nature of erosion	Painful erosions with no tendency to spontaneous healing	Crusted moist scaly erosions	Erosions heal spontaneously	-
Distribution	Scalp, face, trunk, axilla, groins, pressure sites	Seborrheic distribution	Flexural aspect of limbs, lower abdomen, groin, axilla	Extensor aspect of limbs (elbows, knees), buttock, nasal cleft, shoulder, upper back, face, scalp

Contd.

Contd.

Bulla spread sign	+	Transient vesicles	+/-	Vesicles not seen as excoriated
Nikolsky sign	+	+	-	-
Mucosal involvement	Almost in all patients; may be presenting or the only feature (80-90%)	Uncommon	Rare; never presenting feature; desquamative gingivitis (40%)	Common but asymptomatic
Tzanck smear	Acantholytic cells	Acantholytic cells	Eosinophils	Neutrophils
HPE	Suprabasal cleft with row of tomb stone appearance	Subcorneal split	Subepidermal blister with eosinophils	Neutrophilic microabscess at tips of dermal papillae
DIF	**Intercellular IgG** deposits throughout the *epidermis* in fish net pattern	**Intercellular IgG** deposits in upper *epidermis*	**Linear IgG** and **C3** deposits in *basement membrane zone*	**Granular IgA** deposits in *dermal papilla*
IIF	Antibody titres correlate with disease severity	Antibody titres correlate with disease severity	Antibody titres do not correlate with disease severity	Negative or anti basement membrane zone or dermal autoantibodies. Antithyroid or antigliadin antibodies present
Associations	Thymoma, myasthenia gravis, lymphoma, bronchogenic carcinoma	-	Gastric carcinoma, diabetes, rheumatoid arthritis, psoriasis	Gluten sensitive enteropathy
Mainstay of treatment	Steroids + adjuvants	Steroids + adjuvants	Steroids + adjuvants	Dapsone Gluten free diet

Ans: (b) Desmoglein 3

***Ref:** IADVL Textbook of Dermatology, 2nd Edition; Rook's Textbook of Dermatology, 8th Edition, Page 40.5, 27*

10. Groove sign is present in:

(a) Diffuse fasciitis with eosinophilia
(b) Polymyalgia rheumatica
(c) Syphilis
(d) Granuloma inguinale

Explanation:

Eosinophilic fasciitis

- Uncommon scleroderma-like disorder.
- Characterised by **induration of the skin, peripheral eosinophilia, hypergammaglobulinaemia,** and elevated ESR.
- **Groove sign*** is a characteristic finding of **eosinophilic fasciitis,** consisting of a **depression** along the course of the superficial veins, more marked on elevation of the affected limb.
- Because the **upper dermis and epidermis** are **spared** by the fibrotic process, and the connective tissue around the veins is **relatively immobile,** the superficial layers of skin can bow inward as the peripheral venous pressure falls.

Extra EDGE

- There is also one more **"Groove sign of Greenblatt"** that is seen in **Lymphogranuloma venereum,** where there is a groove formed due to enlarged lymph nodes on either side of the inguinal ligament.

Ans: (a) Diffuse fasciitis with eosinophilia

***Ref:** IADVL Textbook of Dermatology, 2nd Edition, page 1236, 1896; Lancet 2014, Nov 15; 384(9956)*

11. **Telangiectasia macularis eruptive perstans is characteristically seen in:**

(a) Eczema
(b) Cutaneous T cell lymphoma
(c) Cutaneous mastocytosis
(d) Pemphigus vulgaris

Explanation:

Telangiectasia macularis eruptive perstans (TMEP)

- Described by **Parkes Weber in 1930.**
- Rare variant of **mastocytosis.**
- Typical lesions are **telangiectatic macules** with background color ranging from light to dark brown.
- More common in **adults** than **children.**
- **Darier's sign** and **dermatographism** are often present, but there is little whealing and no blistering.
- Extra-dermal manifestations – **Chest and extremities, systemic** involvement may occur.
- Associated with **multiple myeloma** and **polycythemia vera.**
- Histologically, infiltrates consisting of **mast cells around venules** and **dilated capillaries** of the superficial venous plexus of the dermis.
- Symptomatic treatment. No gold standard treatment till date.

Ans: (c) Cutaneous mastocytosis

***Ref:** J Clin Aesthet Dermatol, 2011 Oct; 4(10): 52–54 and IADVL Textbook of Dermatology, Page 1468*

12. **Girl presented with itching and oozing from lesion of ear following wearing gold ear rings. How will you confirm the diagnosis?**

(a) Patch test
(b) History
(c) Clinical examination
(d) RAST

Explanation:

- Itching and oozing are classical signs of acute stage of **dermatitis (eczema).**
- Eczema could be due to **exogenous** causes or **endogenous.**
- In the question given above, the history is suggestive of eczema due to the **allergen** in the **ear rings** which is **gold** in this case.
- **Allergic contact dermatitis** can be diagnosed with the help of **patch testing***.
- **Patch testing:**
  - The test consists of applying specified concentrations of chemicals or the prepared readymade objects in suitable bases, on the normal-looking skin of the individual and covering these areas with occlusive patches for 48 hours.
  - At the end of 48 hours, the patches are removed and the sites examined for evidence of an inflammatory reaction.
  - Dermatitis at the site of a patch test indicates that the individual has **contact hypersensitivity** to the agent applied at the site.

Ans: (a) Patch test

***Ref:** IADVL Textbook of Dermatology, Page 62 and Rook, 8th Edition, Page 26.85s*

ANESTHESIOLOGY

1. Most commonly used anesthetic agent for induction is:

(a) Desflurane (b) Sevoflurane (c) Isoflurane (d) N_2O

Explanation:

Inhalational agents	Property
N_2O	• **Secondary gas effect*** • Mild analgesic effect • **Diffusion Hypoxia** • **Megaloblastic anemia***
Halothane	• Potent inducing and maintenance agent • Causes **halothane hepatitis*** • With **adrenaline** causes **arrhythmia**
Isoflurane	• Potent maintenance agent • Causes **coronary steal phenomena*** • With dry and exhausted sodalime produces **carbon monoxide***
Sevoflurane	• Causes smooth and fast induction – **Most common inducing agent in Children*** • Not a good maintenance agent because it causes **'Emergence Excitation'** reaction • With dry and exhausted sodalime produces **'Compound A'** which is a nephrotoxic agent
Desflurane	• Causes faster induction and faster recovery • Require special vaporizer and very costly – not commonly available
Trilene	• With dry and exhausted sodalime produces **'Phosgene gas'***

Ans: (b) Sevoflurane

Ref: *Stoelting's Pharmacology and Physiology in Anesthetic Practice, 4th Edition*

2. Minimum alveolar concentration of anesthetic is closely correlated with:

(a) Efficacy (b) Effectiveness (c) Potency (d) Half life

Explanation:

- **Potency** is a measure of **drug activity** expressed in terms of the amount required to produce an effect of given intensity.
- Lesser amounts of drug required to produce maximum effect is called as more **potent drug.**
- For inhalational anaesthetic agents potency are measured by **MAC value.**
- Lesser the **MAC** more is the **potency [MAC ∝ 1/Potency].**
- Inhalational agents order from maximum potent to minimum potent.
- ***Methoxyflurane > Trilene > Halothane > Chloroform > Isoflurane > Enflurane > Sevoflurane > Ether > Sevoflurane > Xenon > N_2O*.***

MAC (Minimum alveolar concentration)

- **MAC** is the concentration of inhalational agent in alveoli at 1 atm that prevents skeletal muscle movement in response to a supra-maximal painful stimulus (surgical skin incision) in 50% of patients.
- It is used to measure **potency** of inhalational agents.
- **MAC ∝ 1/Potency**

Inhalational agents	MAC
Methixyflurane	**0.16**
Trilene	**0.2**
Halothane	**0.75**

Contd.

Contd.

Chloroform	**0.8**
Isoflurane	**1.17**
Enflurane	**1.63**
Sevoflurane	**1.8**
Ether	**1.9**
Sevoflurane	**6.6**
Xenon	**71**
N_2O	**104**

- **Factors affecting MAC:**

Increase of MAC	Decrease of MAC	No Change of MAC
• Hyperthermia • Hypernatremia (↑ Na) • Sympathomimetic drugs • Cyclosporine • ↑Pheomelanin production (red hair)	• Hypothermia • Increasing age (6% per decades) • Alpha 2 agonist agents • Acute alcohol ingestion • Pregnancy and Postpartum upto 72 hours • Lithium • Lidocaine • Hyponatremia • Ketanserine • Adrenergic antagonist agents • BP <40 mm Hg • PaO_2 <38 mm Hg	• Chronic alcohol abuse • Gender • Duration of Anaesthesia • $PaCO_2$ 15-95 mm Hg • PaO_2 >38 mm Hg • BP > 40 mm Hg • Hyper or Hypokalemia • Thyroid dysfunction • Anesthetic metabolism

Ans: (c) Potency

Ref: *Stoelting's Pharmacology and Physiology in Anesthetic Practice, 4th Edition*

3. **Mechanism of action of Etomidate:**

(a) Na channel blocker (b) Block t-type ca channels in thalamus
(c) K channel blocker (d) Opening of chloride channel

Explanation:

- All intravenous anaesthetic agent except Ketamine are GABA Agonist.
- GABA decreases the excitability of neurons by its action at the GABA–A receptor complex.
- When GABA occupies the binding site of this complex, *it allows inward flux of chloride ion,* resulting in hyperpolarizing of the cell and subsequent resistance of the neuron to stimulation by excitatory transmitters.

	Anaesthetic agents	Thiopenthol sodium	Propofol	Ketamine	Midazolam	Etomidate
Pharmaco-kinetics	**MOA**	GABA receptor agonist	GABA receptor agonist	NMDA antagonist	GABA receptor agonist	GABA receptor agonist
	Metabolism	Liver by hydroxy-lation	Liver by conjuga-tion	Liver by demethy-lation-active meta-bolite nor ketamine	Liver by hydro-xylation	Liver by ester hydro-lysis
	Excretion	Renal	Renal ans lung	Renal	Renal	Renal
	PPB in %	80	75	70	98	75
	pH	11	4.4	7.5	6.15	6.9
	T1/2 (min)	8-10	10	2 hrs	2 hrs	30
	Onset of action	One arm circula-tion time	1 min	1 min	One arm circula-tion time	One arm circulation time
	Duration of action	12 hrs	24 hrs	3 hrs	4 hrs	6 hrs

Contd.

Contd.

Pharmaco-dynamics	**CNS**	↓ ICT, CMRO2,CBF	↓ ICT, CMRO2,CBF	↑ICT, CMRO2, CBF	↓ ICT, CMRO2,CBF	↓ ICT, CMRO2,CBF
	CVS	↑ HR ↓MAP	No change-HR ↓MAP	↑↑HR, ↑↑ BP	↑ HR ↓MAP	↑ HR ↓MAP
	RS	↓ RR, Bronchoconstriction	↓ RR, Bronchoconstriction	↓ RR, Bronchodilation	↓ RR	↓ RR, Bronchoconstriction
	Renal	↓RBF	↓RBF	↑RBF	↓RBF	↓RBF
	Hepatic	↓HBF	↓HBF	↑HBF	↓HBF	↓HBF
Indication		• Induction of anesthesia • **Status epilepticus**	• Induction of Anesthesia • TIVA • ICU sedation • Agent of choice for **day care surgery**	• Induction of anesthesia in **asthmatic** patients and **shock** • **Neuroleptic anesthesia** • **Refractory bronchospasm**	• Anxiolytic • **TIVA** • Induction of anesthesia • Sedation	• Induction agent of choice in patient with and **shock, trauma and cardiac disease**
Contraindication		1. Acute intermittent porphyria 2. Sulpha drug allergy	1. Hypotension and shock 2. Egg allergy	1. ↑ ICT 2. CAD 3. HTN 4. Acute glaucoma 5. ICSOL 6. Bleeding diathesis	1. Hypotension	Non-specific
Specific adverse effects		• Anaphylatic reaction • Intra arterial injection causes gangrene of finger	• Pain on injection • Thrombophlebitis • Propofol infusion syndrome • Abuse potential	• Emergence delirium • ↑ all pressures • Bleeding by inhibition platelet aggregation	• Respiratory depression and hypotension	• Adrenocortical suppression • Myoclonic movements

Ans: (d) Opening of chloride channel

***Ref:** Stoelting's Pharmacology and Physiology in Anesthetic Practice, 4th Edition*

4. **Regarding Neuraxial Anesthesia, which of the following statement is true?**

(a) Aspirin should be stopped 7 days before surgery
(b) Unfractionated heparin should be stopped 7 days before surgery
(c) Fondaparinux should be stopped 7 days before surgery
(d) Clopidrogrel should be stopped 7 days before surgery

Explanation:

Drug therapy during neuraxial anesthesia

Anticoagulants	**When to stop before neuraxial block**	**When to start after neuraxial block**
IV Heparin	6 hrs (APTT < 40 sec)	2-4 hrs
SC Heparin	12 hrs (APPT < 40 sec)	2-4 hrs
LMWH (Enoxaparine)	24 hrs	12 hrs
Aspirine	No need to stop	No restriction
Clopidogrel	7-10 days	2 hrs
Warfarin	4-5 days (INR < 1.4)	2 hrs
Fondaperinoux	72 hrs	12 hrs
Rivaroxaban	24 hrs	6 hrs (24 hrs if truamatic puncture and major risk of bleeding)
Aoixaban	48 hrs	

Contd.

Contd.

Thrombin inhibitor (desirudin, lepirudin, bivalirudin)	**5 days (wait upto APTT <40 sec)**	**2 hrs**
Fibrinolytics–Streptokinase, Altiplase, Reteplase, Tenecteplase	10 days	10 days
Glycoprotein IIb/IIIa inhibitors–Abciximab, Eptifibatide and Tirofibane	**48 hrs** **8 hrs**	**2 hrs**

Ans: (d) Clopidrogrel should be stopped 7 days before surgery

Ref: *ASRA Guidelines*

5. **A woman who underwent surgery by spinal anesthesia presents after 3 days with history of headache. How will you manage?**

(a) Foot end elevation
(b) Sumatriptan
(c) IV fluids
(d) Autologous blood patch

Explanation:

Post spinal headache (Post lumbar puncture headache)

- **Definition:** Headache which occurs **within 24 hours to 2 weeks** after dural puncture.
- It presents usually after **24 to 48 hours.**
- Usually **Occipital** but can be **frontal** also.
- May be associated with **pain** and **stiffness** in **neck.**
- It is **throbbing** and the typical presentation is that pain **increases on sitting** and **relieved on lying down.**
- External stimuli like **strong light** and **noise aggravates** the pain.
- Incidence: **3–30%.**
- In most cases (90%) it lasts for **7–10 days** and is relieved in almost all cases in 3 weeks.

Risk factors

- Young age.
- Females > Males.
- Pregnancy.
- Large needle.
- Cutting point needle.
- Dural fibers cut transversely.
- Multiple punctures.
- Large bore needle.
- Cutting needle.
- History of migraine.

Etiological factors

- Single most important factor is **needle size:** Incidence with 16 G needle is 75% while with 25 G needle is 1–3%.
- **Type of needle:** Incidence less with dural separating needle.
- **Altitude:** High incidence with high altitude.
- **Type of patient:** Previous **history of headache.**
- **Inadequate dehydration.**
- **Cause:** It is a low pressure headache due to seepage of CSF from dural rent created by spinal needle.
- The loss can be around **10 ml/hr.**
- CSF leakage results in changes in hydrodynamics of brain causing traction on pain sensitive structures like dura, vessels, tentorium producing pain.

Symptoms:

- It is ***bilateral, frontal or retroorbital***, and occipital and extends into the neck.

- It may be throbbing or constant and associated with ***photophobia*** and nausea and aggravate with change in body position.
- The pain is aggravated by sitting or standing and relieved or ***decreased by lying down flat.***

Classification:
- **Mild** – Subsides after rest and lots of fluid, no disturbance in routine activity.
- **Moderate** – Subsides only after medicine and rest, some disturbance in routine activity.
- **Severe** – Not subsided with medicine and severe disturbance in routine activity.

TREATMENT

A. Preventive
- Use of small bore needle.
- Adequate hydration.
- To avoid pillow for next 24 hours.
- Supine position after lumbar puncture.
- If possible, prone position can be tried.
- Avoid spinal if history of headache.
- Avoid sitting in postoperative period.
- Atraumatic needle.

B. Curative
- Bed rest (Supine position).
- Ask patient to lie **supine** in slight **trendelenburg position.**
- **Analgesics – NSAIDs.**
- **Intravenous fluids** (15 ml/kg/hr) or **Oral fluids** 3 litres/day. Adequate hydration to increase CSF production.
- Abdominal binders.
- **Desmopressin:**
  - **Inhalation of 5–6% CO_2 in oxygen.** CO_2 is cerebral vasodilator and will promote CSF production.
  - **Oral or IV caffeine** (500 mg) inhibits vasospasm cycle in cerebral vessels.
- **Epidural blood patch: Autologous blood** given in same epidural space will cause blood to clot and seal the rent.

Other causes of headache after spinal anesthesia
- **Meningeal irritation:** Related to high pressure headache and is not related to postural changes.
- **Queckenstedt's test:**
  - To differentiate between **high pressure and low pressure headache.**
  - Applying **pressure on jugular veins increases** the **headache high pressure** and **relieves headache** in **low pressure** headache.

So, answer would be option C first, followed by option D.

Ans: (c) IV fluids

Ref: *Stoelting's Pharmacology and Physiology in Anesthetic Practice, 4th Edition*

6. **Fluosol DA is:**

(a) Local anesthetic
(b) Artificial whole blood
(c) Intravenous anesthetic agent
(d) Intralipid

Explanation:
- Artificial blood is a product made to act as a substitute for red blood cells, blood substitutes are used to fill fluid volume and/or carry oxygen and other blood gases in the cardiovascular system.
- **Advantages:**
  - Long shelf life.
  - No need for refrigeration and the ability to sterilize.
  - Artificial blood does not need specifically matched type.
- It is also called as blood substitutes.
- The half life of blood is **42 days.**
- High levels of nitric acid packed in it.

PROBLEMS ASSOCIATED WITH ARTIFICIAL BLOOD

- Body immune systems may sometimes react negatively to the foreign blood that is injected into the body.
- Trauma patients are often frequent recipients of blood products or plasma during surgery, it becomes challenging to understand the effect of individual blood product.

Composition of Artificial Blood:

- Perfluoro-octyl bromide – 28%
- Fo-9982 – 28% – 12%
- Yolk lecithin – 2.4%
- DSPE-50H – - 0.12%
- Distilled water – 57.48%

Types of Artificial Blood:

Type	Perflurocarbon (PFC) Emulsions (Fluosol DA and Fluosol 43)	Haemoglobin based oxygen carriers based (HBOCS)
Chemical compound	1. PFC'S are derived from a group of hydrocarbons in which the hydrogen atoms are replaced by fluorine atoms. 2. These are chemically inert due to the strength of the carbon-fluorine bond.	• Haemoglobin is a tetramer with 2-α and 2-β polypeptide chains, each are bound to an iron heme group which successively binds to oxygen molecule. • Haemoglobin's heme bond allows, it to have a higher affinity for oxygen, thus having excellent source of blood substitute.
Example	**Perflurodecalin** **Perflubron**	**Polyheme**
Advantage	1. PFCs do not react with oxygen 2. PFCs allow easy transportation of the oxygen to the body 3. They allow increased solubility of oxygen in plasma.	1. Available in much larger quantities. 2. Can be sterilized via Pasteurization.
Disadvantages	1. Often causes flu like symptoms. 2. It decreases platelets count.	1. Reduced circulation half life. 2. It releases free radicals into the body.

Other Promising Technique:

(1) Stem cells
(2) Dendrimers
(3) Biodegradable micelles
(4) Placental umbilical cord blood

Ans: (b) Artificial whole blood

Ref: *Internet Reference*

RADIOLOGY AND RADIOTHERAPY

1. Twin peak sign in ultrasound is seen in:

(a) Monochorionic diamniotic twins
(b) Dichorionic diamniotic twins
(c) Dichorionic monoamniotic twins
(d) Monochorionic Monoamniotic twins

Explanation:

Dichorionic Diamniotic Twins

- The **twin peak sign** (also known as the **lambda (λ) sign**) is a triangular appearance of the chorion insinuating between the layers of the intertwin membrane and strongly suggests a dichorionic twin pregnancy.
- It is always **dichorionic and diamniotic,** but can be **monozygotic or dizygotic.**
- **T Sign*** is seen in **Monochorionic diamniotic** twin gestation.

Twin peak or lambda sign:

- It is characteristic of **dichorionic** pregnancies and is due to the chorionic tissue between the two layers of the intertwin membrane at the placental origin.
- A potential space exists in the intertwin membrane which is filled by proliferating placental villi, giving rise to a twin peak sign.
- Twin peak appears as a triangle with base at chorionic surface and apex in intertwin membrane.
- In **monochorionic** twins there is no chorionic tissue, and intertwin membrane is composed of 2 amnion only giving rise to the **"T" sign** on ultrasound.
- Monochorionic pregnancies have a dividing membrane that is so thin, it may not be seen until the second trimester.
- The membrane is generally less than 2 mm thick and magnification reveals only 2 layers (of amnion).

Ans: (d) Dichorionic Diamniotic Twins

Ref: *Nyberg DA, Diagnostic Imaging of Fetal Anomalies, Page 780*

2. Contrast induced nephropathy defined as:

(a) Rise in Serum Creatinine by 0.5 mg in 48 hours
(b) Rise in Serum Creatinine by 1 mg in 48 hours
(c) Rise in Serum Creatinine by 1.5 mg in 48 hours
(d) Rise in Serum Creatinine by 2 mg in 48 hours

Explanation:

Contrast-induced nephropathy

- Defined as the impairment of renal function within **48-72 hours** of intravenous contrast administration—measured as either:
  - **25% increase in serum creatinine** from baseline (or)
  - **0.5 mg/dL increase in absolute Serum Creatinine** value.
- For renal insufficiency (RI) to be attributable to contrast administration, it should be **acute,** usually occurring **within 2-3 days;** it should also not be attributable to any other identifiable cause of renal failure.
- Following contrast exposure, **Serum Creatinine levels** peak between **2 and 5 days** and usually return to normal in **14 days.**
- **Hydration*** is cornerstone in **prevention** of contrast induced nephropathy.

Ans: (a) Rise in serum creatinine by 0.5 mg/dl in 48 hours

Ref: *Gore RM, Textbook of Gastrointestinal Radiology E-Book, Page 21*

3. A child is diagnosed to have renal cortical scarring. Best imaging to demonstrate this lesion:

(a) DMSA (b) USG (c) MCU (d) DTPA

Explanation:

- **Tc99m DMSA scan** is a **static** or **anatomical imaging** suitable for imaging **renal morphology*** and **cortical function*.**

- It is the **agent of choice** for evaluation of **scar** in the **kidney** and for differential **renal cortical function/ split renal function.**
- **99m Tc dimercapto succinic acid (99 m Tc-DMSA)** is an agent that is actively taken up by the **proximal** and **distal** renal tubular cells, directly from the **peritubular vessels,** and accumulates in the **renal cortex.**
- This modality is primarily used for imaging functioning cortical mass and individual renal function. It is the most reliable method for assessing **chronic cortical scarring.**
- **DTPA isotope*** scan used for functional image of kidneys.

Ans: (a) DMSA

Ref: *Nelson, 20th Edition*

4. Investigation of choice to detect myocardial viability:

(a) MUGA scan
(b) Thallium 201
(c) TC99m tetrofosmin
(d) PET

Explanation:

The investigation of choice for detection of Myocardial viability is 18FDG PET as it detects the metabolism of the myocardial cells.

Myocardial imaging

Infarct scanning: Tc-99 m Pyrophophate is used for Myocardial infarct imaging and the Infarct appears as Hot spot.

Myocardial Perfusion scanning: Looks at the blood flow through the coronary arteries; and is useful in diagnosis of CAD,Thallium-201 is most commonly used radionuclide for this purpose. Other isotopes used are Technetium-99 tetrofosmin and MIBI.

Multigated equilibrium studies: Assesses the left ventricular function and ejection fraction. MUGA is also known as radionuclide cardiac ventriculography. Tc-99-albumin is also used most commonly.

Ans: (d) PET

Ref: *Multiple sources*

5. Which of the following cardiac imaging modalities is useful in evaluating Hypertension?

(a) 18 FDG PET CT
(b) Colour Doppler
(c) MR angiogram
(d) Radionuclide Angiography

Explanation:

Cardiac Imaging in Hypertension

Imaging modality	Cardiac/vascular applications					
	Ejection fraction	**Left ventricular mass**	**Left ventricular volume**	**Diastolic function**	**Regional wall motion (contraction) abnormalites**	**Great vessel anatomy**
Radionuclide angiography	Yes	No	Yes	Yes	Yes	No
Conventional computed tomography	No	No	No	No	No	Yes
Computed tomography	Yes	Yes	Yes	Yes	Yes	Yes
Magnetic resonance imaging	Yes	Yes	Yes	Yes	Yes	Yes

Ans: (d) Radionuclide Angiography

Ref: *Izzo JL, Hypertension Primerl, 4th Edition*

6. New emerging technology to identify cancer metastasis:

(a) SPECT
(b) FDG glucose PET
(c) Bone scan
(d) MR spectroscopy

Explanation:

- **18 FDG PET** is better than **MRI** and **Bone scan** in determining cancer metastasis.
- Molecular imaging with **positron emission tomography (PET)** using **tumour-seeking radiopharmaceuticals** has gained wide acceptance in oncology with many clinical applications.
- The hybrid imaging modality PET/CT allows assessing **molecular** as well as **morphologic information** at the same time. Therefore, PET/CT represents an efficient tool for whole body staging and restaging within one imaging modality.
- In oncology the **glucose analogue 18F-fluorodeoxyglucose (FDG)** is the most widely used **PET** and **PET/CT** radiopharmaceutical in clinical routine.
- FDG PET and PET/CT have been used for **staging and restaging tumour** patients in numerous studies.
- The most important current clinical applications of **18F-FDG PET/CT** in **breast cancer patients** are for the detection and evaluation of **recurrent or metastatic disease.**

Ans: (b) FDG glucose PET

Ref: *Ann Saudi Med., 2011 Jan-Feb; 31(1): 3–13*

7. **Earliest anomaly to be detected in ultrasound is:**

(a) Anencephaly (b) Spina bifida (c) Meningocele (d) Horseshoe kidney

Explanation:

- **Anencephaly** may be sonographically detectable as early as **10-11 weeks.** Ultrasound can be a non-invasive, cost effective and fast method to detect anencephaly and has an accuracy of approximating 100% at 14 weeks.
- **Findings of anencephaly:**
  - o **No brain parenchymal tissue** is seen above the orbits.
  - o **Calvarium is absent.**
  - o **Acrania** with loosely arranged brain parenchyma.
  - o **"Frog eye"** or **"mickey mouse"** appearance may be seen when seen in the coronal plane due to absent cranial bone/brain and bulging orbits.
  - o May show evidence of **polyhydramnios.**

Remember:

- **Spina bifida/Meningocele** – Large defects can be detected as early as 12 weeks.

Ans: (a) Anencephaly

8. **A 50-year-old patient with ischemic heart disease develops chest pain. ECG shows ST segment elevation and Q waves. Myocardial necrosis in this patient can be best demonstrated by:**

(a) Technetium 99 tetrofosmin (b) Sestambi scan
(c) Technetium 99 Pyrophosphate (d) Thallium 201

Explanation:

- **Myocardial Necrosis** is best demonstrated by **Tc99m Pyrophosphate.**
- Tc 99m pyrophosphate binds to the calcium released at the site of necrosis and gives the area of infarct as **HOT** uptake.
- **Thallium 201, Tc99m Tetrofosmin and Tc99m Pyrophosphate** are used for detecting **myocardial perfusion** and the area of infarct appears **cold** on **Nuclear imaging.**
- **MUGA scan is** used to detect **ventricular function.**

Ans: (c) Technetium 99 pyrophosphate

Ref: *Wackers FJT, Thallium-201 and Technetium-99m-Pyrophosphate Myocardial Imaging, 2012*

9. **Which of the following is true?**

(a) I-125 half life is 60 days
(b) I-131 half life is 12 days
(c) I-125 is used for treating thyroid metastasis
(d) I-131 is used in functional thyroid scan

Explanation:

Iodine-125

- Iodine-125, half life-**60 days.**
- Commonly used in **brachytherapy** in the treatment of cancer especially in **prostate cancer,** enclosed in an implanted titanium capsule.
- It is also widely used in **Radioimmunoassay** to show presence of hormones in tiny quantities.

Iodine-123

- Half-life –13 hours.
- Has **no beta activity only gamma activity** and is more suitable as nuclear imaging tracer to evaluate the **anatomic and physiologic function** of the **thyroid** (thyroid scintigraphy/functional scan/radioactive iodine uptake/RAIU).
- Abnormal results may be caused by disorders such as **Graves' disease or Hashimoto's thyroiditis.**
- **Tc99m pertechnetate** is also used for functional imaging of **thyroid** (used in India due to **nonavailability of I-123**).

Iodine-131

- Half life –8 days.
- Preferred for Radiotherapy, widely used for localizing and treating **thyroid cancer** and **thyroid metastasis** and in **imaging the thyroid.**
- I-131 has **both a beta and gamma decay.**
- Destruction of thyroid tissue by Iodine-131 is due to emission of **Beta Rays.**
- Iodine-131 is also used in tissue targeting radiopharmaceutical agents such as **MIBG.**
- The high energy beta radiation from I-131 causes it to be the most carcinogenic of the iodine isotopes.

Iodine-124

- Iodine-124 is a proton-rich isotope of iodine with a half-life of 4.18 days.
- Its modes of decay are: 74.4% electron capture, 25.6% positron emission.
- Iodine-124 can be made by numereous nuclear reactions via a cyclotron.
- Iodine-124 as the iodide salt can be used to directly image the thyroid using positron emission tomography (PET).

Ans: (a) I-125 half life is 60 days

10. Osteolytic metastasis in lumbar spine with CA breast investigation of choice:

(a) PET scan (b) SPECT
(c) Bone scan (d) X-ray

Explanation:

- NaF PET is found to be more sensitive and specific for detecting **bone metastasis** in patients with skeletal metastasis especially **osteolytic metastasis**, better than **18FDG PET or bone scan.**

Sensitivity and specificity of imaging modalities in bone metastasis

	Sensitivity	**Specificity**
18NaF PET/CT	100	97
MRI	95	90
SPECT	87	91
18 FDG PET	98	56
CT	74	56
Bone scintigraphy	78	48

Ans: (a) PET SCAN

Ref: *World J Radiol 2015 Aug 28; 7(8): 202–211*

11. Following is used in PET scan:

(a) FDG (b) DTPA (c) MAG-3 (d) I^{131}

Explanation:

*"**Fluorine-18 Fluorodeoxyglucose (FDG)** is the most common positron-labeled radiotracer in positron emission tomography **(PET).** In most tissues, including cancer, there is little phosphatase activity. The intracellular metabolite, FDG-6-phosphate cannot undergo further conversions and is therefore trapped inside the cell. FDG is useful in staging and metastasis of Renal cell cancer by PET." (Ref: Wolfgang)*

Positron emission tomography (PET)

- It is a nuclear medicine imaging technique that produces a three-dimensional image or picture of functional processes in the body.
- The system detects **pairs of gamma rays** emitted indirectly by a **positron-emitting radionuclide (tracer),** which is introduced into the body on a biologically active molecule. Three-dimensional images of tracer concentration within the body are then constructed by computer analysis. In modern scanners, three dimensional imaging is often accomplished with the aid of a CT X-ray scan performed on the patient during the same session, in the same machine.
- If the biologically active molecule chosen for PET is **FDG,** an analogue of **glucose,** the concentrations of tracer imaged then give tissue metabolic activity, in terms of regional glucose uptake.
- The electron-positron **decays** result in **two 511 keV gamma photons** being emitted at almost **180 degrees** to each other; hence, it is possible to localize their source along a **straight line of coincidence** (also called the **line of response,** or **LOR**).
- A **collimator** is a device that narrows a beam of particles or waves. Lead collimators are used in X-rays and linear accelerators.

Ans: (a) FDG

Ref: *Radiology by Wolfgang Dahnert, 5th Edition, Page 1113*

12. Rotting fence post appearance of femur is seen in:

(a) Fibrous dysplasia
(b) Hyper parathyroidism
(c) Paget's disease
(d) Fracture neck of femur

Explanation:

Renal Osteodystrophy:

- CRF leading on to Hyperparathyroidism.
- **Signs of chronic renal failure:**
  - o Findings of Osteomalacia.
  - o Hyperparathyroidism.
  - o Bone sclerosis.
- ***Rugger jersey spine*.***
- ***Rotting fence post appearance*:*** Due to Rickets + Hyperparathyroidism.
- In children, **metaphyseal** changes resembling rickets are seen, which together with **cortical** erosions can give rise to the so-called 'rotting fence-post' appearance, particularly at the **femoral neck.**
- ***Looser's zone.***

Ans: (b) Hyperparathyroidism

Ref: *Harrison's Principles of Internal Medicine, 18th Edition*

13. Rat tail tapering of lower esophagus in barium swallow is seen in:

(a) Diffuse esophageal spasm
(b) Achalasia cardia
(c) Ca esophagus
(d) Gastroesophageal reflux

Explanation:

X-RAY FINDINGS – ABDOMEN (CONTRAST)

(A) Barium

- Bird's Beak deformity of lower oesophagus – Achalsia cardia (Barium Swallow).
- Rat tail tapering of lower oesophagus – Carcinoma oesophagus (Barium Swallow).
- Cork screw oesophagus – Diffuse oesophageal spasm (Barium Swallow).
- Most common radiological appearance of gastric carcinoma (in barium meal follow through) is – filling defect in antrum/body of stomach.

- Trifoliate duodenum – Chronic duodenal ulcer with scarring (Barium Meal).
- Hour Glass stomach – Peptic ulcer.
- Cup and Spill/Cascade stomach – Volvulus of stomach.
- Constriction of transverse duodenum – Superior mesenteric artery syndrome.
- Bull's eye lesion (in barium meal) – Leiomyosarcoma.
- Single-bubble appearance – Pyloric stenosis.
- Double-bubble sign – Duodenal atresia, duodenal stenosis, annular pancreas.
- Triple-bubble sign – Jejunal atresia.
- Coffee bean sign – Strangulation of incompletely obstructed loop of small intestine.
- String of Beads – Small bowel obstruction.
- Coiled spring appearance – Intussusception.
- Pincer-shaped ending in barium enema – Intussusception.
- Bird of Prey sign – Sigmoid volvulus.
- Moulage sign (flocculation of barium, with mucosal thickening) – seen in – malabsorption syndrome.
- String sign of Kantor – Crohn's disease.
- Pipe-stem appearance (Loss of Haustrations) – Ulcerative Colitis (Barium Enema).
- Saw-tooth appearance and/or diverticula – Diverticular disease/Diverticulosis (Barium Enema).
- Scalloping of edge of sigmoid colon on barium enema – Ulcerative colitis.
- Napkin ring sign – Annular carcinoma of colon.
- Porcelain gallbladder – Carcinoma of gallbladder.
- Pad sign – Carcinoma pancreas (Barium Meal).

(B) ERCP (Endoscopic retrograde cholangiopancreatography)

- Scrambled-egg appearance – Carcinoma of pancreas.
- Chain of Lakes appearance – Chronic pancreatitis.
- Double duct sign – Carcinoma of pancreas.

(C) PTC (Percutaneous transhepatic cholangiography)

- Meniscus sign – Choledocholithiasis.

Ans: (c) Ca esophagus

Ref: *Multiple sources*

PSYCHIATRY

1. Mood stabilizer not used for mania in pediatric group:

(a) Lithium (b) Valproate (c) CBZ (d) Oxcarbazepine

Explanation:

Bipolar affective disorder in children is different from adults from various perspectives.

- **Symptomatology:**
  - More of irritability, non-goal directed hyperactivity than euphoria and goal-directed hyperactivity.
  - Well formed delusions are uncommon, rather oddities in speech common. The so-called **"mixed"** type is common in this age group.
- **Course:**
  - Typical cyclic course with inter-episode recovery is uncommon.
  - If cyclic course is seen, it would be rapid-cycling (females, hypothyroid patients are other groups).
- **Comorbidity:**
  - **ADHD** is comorbid and may be difficult to differentiate from **BPAD.**

Treatment of BPAD:

- Treatment of manic episode is mainly **pharmacological.**
- **Lithium, anti-epileptics** and **antipsychotics** are mainstay of treatment (Benzodiazepines are adjuvant drugs).
- **In children, commonly used mood stabilizers include:**
  - **Lithium**
  - **Carbamazepine**
  - **Divalproex**
  - **Lamotrigine**
- **Antipsychotics** used in children:
  - **Olanzapine**
  - **Quietapine**
  - **Risperidone**
- Choice of drug depends upon efficacy and side-effect profile.
- In childhood bipolar mania, **Oxcarbazepine** has been demonstrated less efficacious among the options as per studies.
- Regarding side-effects, **lithium** is most dangerous given the **narrow therapeutic window** (need for close monitoring).

Ans: (d) Oxcarbazepine

***Ref:** Washburn JJ, West AE, Heil JA. Treatment of Pediatric Bipolar Disorder: A Review, Minerva Psichiatrica 2011;52(1):21-35*

2. According to DSM 5 criteria, all are true about ADHD *except*:

(a) Adult ADHD symptoms similar to children
(b) Diagnosed before 12 years
(c) Diagnosed before 7 years
(d) Symptoms should be present in more than one setting

Explanation:

- Like any other psychiatric disorder, ADHD also has specific diagnostic criteria.
- DSM has revised its manual and come up with **fifth edition.**

In DSM, ADHD criteria are grouped into two categories viz.:

1. Inattention.
2. Hyperactivity/impulsivity:
   - Each group has 9 symptoms and at least 6 should be present.
   - If only inattention group symptoms present – predominantly **inattentive type.**

- If only hyperactivity/impulsivity group symptoms present – predominantly **hyperactive/impulsive type.**
- If both inattention and hyperactivity/impulsivity group symptoms present – **combined type.**
    A. Symptoms should be present for **at least 6 months.**
    B. Symptoms should be severe enough to cause **academic, occupational, social dysfunction.**
    C. Symptoms should be present in **more than one setting,** i.e., child should be inattentive/hyperactive/impulsive not only in own **home** but also in **school, public place** etc. (These two criterias B and C exclude normal hyperactivity).
    D. Symptoms should start **from childhood,** and **12 years** was kept as cut-off.
- Symptoms can start upto 12 years. Hence, answer is C.

Ans: (c) Diagnosed before 7 years

Ref: *Diagnostic and Statistical Manual of Mental Disorders, 5th Edition, American Psychiatric Association*

3. Suicidal tendency is least with which of the following drugs?

(a) Carbamazepine (b) Lithium (c) Valproate (d) Escitalopram

Explanation:

Suicide has many causes and can be grouped under following headings:

- Psychological
- Physical
- Social
- Financial
- Others

These groups are not water-tight compartments and multiple reasons can be present in a given case and these reasons are interactive in nature.

Psychiatric disorders which increase the risk of suicide are:

- **Depression** (*Bipolar depression carries more risk than unipolar depression*).
- **Schizophrenia** and other non-affective psychotic disorders (secondary to insight, command hallucinations).
- **Adjustment disorder with depressive symptoms** (here comes life events, stress like interpersonal relationship strain, failure in exams or love etc.).
- **OCD** (due to depression secondary to having such a chronic illness).

Drugs and Suicide

- Drugs reducing the risk of suicide are rare and if so, acts by indirect means (for example, anti-psychotic drugs reduce hallucinations → lowering the risk of suicide attempt).
- Only two drugs have been shown to reduce the risk of suicide by studies.
    - ***Lithium****
    - ***Clozapine****
- The exact mechanism of such reduction of risk is not known.
- Lithium has neuroplastic effect also.
- No antidepressant (Escitalopram was given as a distracter) has been shown to reduce the risk of suicide till date. Rather **SSRIs** have **increased risk of suicide** in initial course due to **increased anxiety.** That is why benzodiazepines are given with them in early phase.

Ans: (b) Lithium

Ref: *Stephen and Stahl Psychopharmacology*